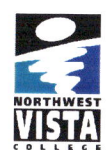

Northwest Vista College
Learning Resource Center
3535 North Ellison Drive
San Antonio, Texas 78251

RA
1242
.T44

NORTHWEST VISTA COLLEGE

Veterans and agent orange.

Veterans and Agent Orange

Update 2000

Committee to Review the Health Effects in
Vietnam Veterans of Exposure to Herbicides
(Third Biennial Update)

Division of Health Promotion and
Disease Prevention

INSTITUTE OF MEDICINE

NATIONAL ACADEMY PRESS
Washington, D.C.

NATIONAL ACADEMY PRESS • 2101 Constitution Avenue, NW • Washington, D.C. 20418

NOTICE: The project that is the subject of this report was approved by the Governing Board of the National Research Council, whose members are drawn from the councils of the National Academy of Sciences, the National Academy of Engineering, and the Institute of Medicine. The members of the committee responsible for the report were chosen for their special competences and with regard for appropriate balance.

Support for this project was provided by the Department of Veterans Affairs. The views presented in this report are those of the Institute of Medicine Committee to Review the Health Effects in Vietnam Veterans of Exposure to Herbicides (Third Biennial Update) and are not necessarily those of the funding agencies.

Library of Congress Cataloging-in-Publication Data

Institute of Medicine (U.S.). Committee to Review the Health Effects in Vietnam Veterans of Exposure to Herbicides

    Veterans and agent orange : update 2000 / Committee to Review the Health Effects in Vietnam Veterans of Exposure to Herbicides, Division of Health Promotion and Disease Prevention, Institute of Medicine.

    p. cm.

Includes index

ISBN 0-309-07552-1

    1. Agent Orange—Health aspects. 2. Agent Orange—Toxicology. 3. Vietnamese Conflict, 1961-1975—Veterans—Health risk assessment—United States. I. Title.

RA1242.T44 I57 2001

363.17'9—dc21   2001026682

Additional copies of this report are available for sale from the National Academy Press, 2101 Constitution Avenue, N.W., Box 285, Washington, D.C. 20055. Call (800) 624-6242 or (202) 334-3313 (in the Washington metropolitan area), or visit the NAP's home page at www.nap.edu. The full text of this report is available at www.nap.edu.

For more information about the Institute of Medicine, visit the IOM home page at: www.iom.edu.

Copyright 2001 by the National Academy of Sciences. All rights reserved.

Printed in the United States of America.

    The serpent has been a symbol of long life, healing, and knowledge among almost all cultures and religions since the beginning of recorded history. The serpent adopted as a logotype by the Institute of Medicine is a relief carving from ancient Greece, now held by the Staatliche Museen in Berlin.

*"Knowing is not enough; we must apply.
Willing is not enough; we must do."*
—Goethe

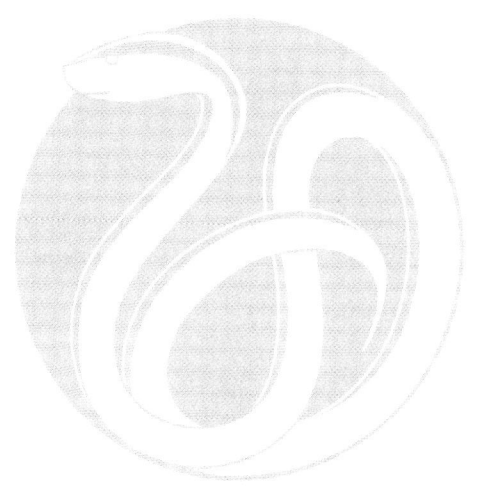

INSTITUTE OF MEDICINE
Shaping the Future for Health

THE NATIONAL ACADEMIES

National Academy of Sciences
National Academy of Engineering
Institute of Medicine
National Research Council

The **National Academy of Sciences** is a private, nonprofit, self-perpetuating society of distinguished scholars engaged in scientific and engineering research, dedicated to the furtherance of science and technology and to their use for the general welfare. Upon the authority of the charter granted to it by the Congress in 1863, the Academy has a mandate that requires it to advise the federal government on scientific and technical matters. Dr. Bruce M. Alberts is president of the National Academy of Sciences.

The **National Academy of Engineering** was established in 1964, under the charter of the National Academy of Sciences, as a parallel organization of outstanding engineers. It is autonomous in its administration and in the selection of its members, sharing with the National Academy of Sciences the responsibility for advising the federal government. The National Academy of Engineering also sponsors engineering programs aimed at meeting national needs, encourages education and research, and recognizes the superior achievements of engineers. Dr. Wm. A. Wulf is president of the National Academy of Engineering.

The **Institute of Medicine** was established in 1970 by the National Academy of Sciences to secure the services of eminent members of appropriate professions in the examination of policy matters pertaining to the health of the public. The Institute acts under the responsibility given to the National Academy of Sciences by its congressional charter to be an adviser to the federal government and, upon its own initiative, to identify issues of medical care, research, and education. Dr. Kenneth I. Shine is president of the Institute of Medicine.

The **National Research Council** was organized by the National Academy of Sciences in 1916 to associate the broad community of science and technology with the Academy's purposes of furthering knowledge and advising the federal government. Functioning in accordance with general policies determined by the Academy, the Council has become the principal operating agency of both the National Academy of Sciences and the National Academy of Engineering in providing services to the government, the public, and the scientific and engineering communities. The Council is administered jointly by both Academies and the Institute of Medicine. Dr. Bruce M. Alberts and Dr. Wm. A. Wulf are chairman and vice chairman, respectively, of the National Research Council.

COMMITTEE TO REVIEW THE HEALTH EFFECTS IN VIETNAM VETERANS OF EXPOSURE TO HERBICIDES (THIRD BIENNIAL UPDATE)

Irva Hertz-Picciotto, Ph.D. (Chair),[1,2] Professor, Department of Epidemiology, University of North Carolina at Chapel Hill
Margit L. Bleecker, M.D., Ph.D., Director, Center for Occupational and Environmental Neurology, Baltimore, Maryland
Thomas A. Gasiewicz, Ph.D., Professor of Environmental Medicine and Deputy Director of the Environmental Health Sciences Center, University of Rochester
Tee L. Guidotti, M.D., M.P.H., Professor and Chair of the Department of Environmental and Occupational Health, The George Washington University School of Public Health and Health Services
Robert Herrick, Ph.D., C.I.H.,[1,2] Lecturer on Industrial Hygiene, Department of Environmental Health, Harvard School of Public Health
David G. Hoel, Ph.D.,[1,2] Distinguished University Professor, Medical University of South Carolina
Loren D. Koller, D.V.M., Ph.D., Professor, Oregon State University, College of Veterinary Medicine
Howard Ozer, M.D., Ph.D.,[1,2] Eason Chair and Chief of the Hematology/Oncology Section, Director of the Cancer Center, and Professor of Medicine, University of Oklahoma
John J. Stegeman, Ph.D., Senior Scientist and Chair of the Biology Department, Woods Hole Oceanographic Institution
David S. Strogatz, Ph.D., M.S.P.H., Associate Professor and Chair of Epidemiology, School of Public Health, State University of New York at Albany

Staff
David A. Butler, Study Director
James Bowers, Research Assistant
Jennifer A. Cohen, Research Assistant
Rose Marie Martinez, Director, Division of Health Promotion and Disease Prevention
Marjan Najafi, Research Associate
Patricia Spaulding, Project Assistant
Anna Staton, Project Assistant
Kathleen Stratton, Acting Director (1997–1999), Division of Health Promotion and Disease Prevention
Donna D. Thompson and **Rita Gaskins,** Division Assistants
Melissa French, Financial Associate

Staff Consultants
Michelle Catlin, Program Officer
Florence Poillon, Contract Editor

---

[1]Member of the committee responsible for *Veterans and Agent Orange: Herbicide/Dioxin Exposure and Type 2 Diabetes.*
[2]Member of the committee responsible for *Veterans and Agent Orange: Update 1998.*

Reviewers

This report has been reviewed in draft form by individuals chosen for their diverse perspectives and technical expertise, in accordance with procedures approved by the NRC's Report Review Committee. The purpose of this independent review is to provide candid and critical comments that will assist the institution in making its published report as sound as possible and to ensure that the report meets institutional standards for objectivity, evidence, and responsiveness to the study charge. The review comments and draft manuscript remain confidential to protect the integrity of the deliberative process. We wish to thank the following individuals for their review of this report:

Linda S. Birnbaum, Ph.D., U.S. Environmental Protection Agency
Mark R. Cullen, M.D., Yale University
John Doull, Ph.D., University of Kansas Medical Center
Howard M. Kippen, M.D., M.P.H., Rutgers University
David Kriebel, Ph.D., University of Massachusetts Lowell
Paul Lioy, Ph.D. Environmental and Occupational Health Sciences Institute

Although the reviewers listed above have provided many constructive comments and suggestions, they were not asked to endorse the conclusions or recommendations nor did they see the final draft of the report before its release. The review of this report was overseen by Kristine Gebbie, Dr.P.H., R.N., Columbia University, who was responsible for making certain that an independent examination of this report was carried out in accordance with institutional procedures and that all review comments were carefully considered. Responsibility for the final content of this report rests entirely with the authoring committee and the institution.

Preface

In response to the concerns voiced by Vietnam veterans and their families, Congress called upon the National Academy of Sciences (NAS) to review the scientific evidence on the possible health effects of exposure to Agent Orange and other herbicides (Public Law 102-4, enacted on February 6, 1991). The creation of the first NAS Institute of Medicine committee, in 1992, underscored the critical importance of approaching these questions from a non-partisan scientific standpoint. The original Committee to Review the Health Effects in Vietnam Veterans of Exposure to Herbicides realized from the beginning that it could not conduct a credible scientific review without a full understanding of the experiences and perspectives of veterans. Thus, to supplement its standard scientific process, the committee opened several of its meetings to the public in order to allow veterans and other interested individuals to voice their concerns and opinions, to provide personal information about individual exposure to herbicides and associated health effects, and to educate committee members on recent research results and studies still under way. This information provided a meaningful backdrop for the numerous scientific articles that the committee considered.

Veterans and Agent Orange: Health Effects of Herbicides Used in Vietnam (abbreviated as *VAO* in this report) reviewed and evaluated the available scientific evidence regarding the association between exposure to dioxin or other chemical compounds contained in herbicides used in Vietnam and a wide range of health effects. The report provided information for the Secretary of Veterans Affairs to consider as the Department of Veterans Affairs carried out its responsibilities to Vietnam veterans. It also described areas in which the available scientific data were insufficient to determine whether an association exists and provided the committee's recommendations for future research.

Public Law 102-4 also tasked the NAS to conduct biennial updates that would review newly published scientific literature regarding statistical associations between health outcomes and exposure to dioxin and other chemical compounds in these herbicides. The first of these, *Veterans and Agent Orange: Update 1996* (*Update 1996*) was published in March of that year. The second, *Veterans and Agent Orange: Update 1998* (*Update 1998*) was published in 1999. The focus of this third updated review is on scientific studies published since the release of *Update 1998*. To conduct the review, the IOM established a committee of 10 members representing a wide range of expertise to take a fresh look at the studies reviewed in *VAO*, *Update 1996*, and *Update 1998* along with the newest scientific evidence. In order to provide a link to the experience and expertise developed by the previous committees, four of the members of the committee responsible for this report were recruited from the committee responsible for *Update 1998*. All committee members were selected because they are leading experts in their fields, have no conflicts of interest with regard to the matter under study, and have taken no public positions concerning the potential health effects of herbicides in Vietnam veterans or related aspects of herbicide or dioxin exposure. Biographical sketches of committee members and staff appear in Appendix C.

The committee worked on several fronts in conducting this updated review, always with the goal of seeking the most accurate information and advice from the widest possible range of knowledgeable sources. Consistent with procedures of the NAS, the committee met in a series of closed sessions and working group meetings in which members could freely examine, characterize, and weigh the strengths and limitations of the evidence. It also convened an open meeting in May 2000 to provide the opportunity for veterans and veterans service organizations, researchers, policymakers, and other interested parties to present their concerns, review their research, and exchange information directly with committee members. The oral presentations and written statements submitted to the committee are described in Appendix A. The committee thanks these individuals who provided valuable insights into the health problems experienced by Vietnam veterans.

In addition to its formal meetings, the committee actively and continuously sought information from, and explained its mission to, a broad array of individuals and organizations with interest or expertise in assessing the effects of exposure to herbicides. The committee also heard from the public through telephone calls, letters, and emails.

David A. Butler served as the study director for this project. The committee would also like to acknowledge the excellent work of IOM staff members James Bowers, Michelle Catlin, Jennifer Cohen, Marjan Najafi, and Anna Staton. Thanks are also extended to Melissa French, who handled the finances for the project; Florence Poillon who provided excellent editorial skills; Susan Fourt, who conducted database searches; Paige Baldwin, Michael Edington, and Sarah Schlosser, who supervised the report through the editorial and publication phases; and Rita Gaskins, who provided administrative support to the project.

PREFACE

The committee also benefited from the assistance of several scientists and researchers who generously lent their time and expertise to help give committee members insight on particular issues, provide copies of newly-released research, or answer queries concerning their work. Special thanks are extended to Drs. Keith Horsley (Commonwealth Department of Veterans' Affairs, Australia) and Joel Michalek (Air Force Research Laboratory, Brooks Air Force Base, Texas).

Irva Hertz-Picciotto, *Chair*

Contents

1 EXECUTIVE SUMMARY   1
Organization and Framework, 2
Toxicology Summary, 3
Exposure Assessment, 5
Conclusions About Health Outcomes, 5
Increased Risk of Disease Among Vietnam Veterans, 12
Observations and Research Recommendations, 13

2 VETERANS AND AGENT ORANGE: PREVIOUS IOM REPORTS   15
Background, 15
Conclusions About Health Outcomes, 17
Increased Risk of Disease Among Vietnam Veterans, 20
Existence of a Plausible Biologic Mechanism or Other Evidence of a
    Causal Relationship, 20
Research Recommendations, 21

3 TOXICOLOGY   22
Lay Summary, 23
Overview of the Scientific Literature in *Update 2000*, 27
Toxicity Profile Updates, 33
Issues in Evaluating the Evidence, 85

4	**METHODOLGICAL CONSIDERATIONS IN EVALUATING THE EVIDENCE**	**103**

Questions to Be Addressed, 103
Issues in Evaluating the Evidence, 106

5	**EXPOSURE ASSESSMENT**	**110**

Occupational and Environmental Exposures to Herbicides and Dioxin, 110
Military Use of Herbicides in Vietnam, 117
Exposure Assessment in Studies of Vietnam Veterans, 122

6	**EPIDEMIOLOGIC STUDIES**	**132**

Occupational Studies, 134
Environmental Studies, 147
Vietnam Veteran Studies, 150
Observations and Research Recommendations, 160

7	**CANCER**	**248**

Gastrointestinal Tract Tumors, 250
Hepatobiliary Cancers, 267
Nasal and Nasopharyngeal Cancer, 273
Laryngeal Cancer, 277
Lung Cancer, 281
Bone Cancer, 287
Soft-Tissue Sarcomas, 291
Skin Cancers—All Types, 299
Skin Cancer—Melanoma, 302
Skin Cancer—Basal and Squamous Cell (Nonmelanoma), 308
Breast Cancer, 314
Cancers of the Female Reproductive System, 320
Prostate Cancer, 326
Testicular Cancer, 335
Urinary Bladder Cancer, 339
Renal Cancer, 345
Brain Tumors, 350
Non-Hodgkin's Lymphoma, 355
Hodgkin's Disease, 364
Multiple Myeloma, 371
Leukemia, 377
Summary, 383

8 REPRODUCTIVE EFFECTS — 399
Introduction, 399
Birth Defects, 400
Fertility, 405
Spontaneous Abortion, 409
Stillbirth, Neonatal Death, and Infant Death, 412
Low Birthweight and Preterm Birth, 413
Childhood Cancers, 417
Sex Ratio, 429
Summary, 431

9 NEUROBEHAVIORAL DISORDERS — 440
Introduction, 440
Cognitive and Neuropsychiatric Effects, 441
Motor/Coordination Dysfunction, 443
Chronic Persistent Peripheral Neuropathy, 454
Acute and Subacute Transient Peripheral Neuropathy, 457
Conclusions for Neurobehaviorial Disorders, 457

10 OTHER HEALTH EFFECTS — 463
Introduction, 463
Chloracne, 463
Porphyria Cutanea Tarda, 466
Respiratory Disorders, 468
Immune System Disorders, 475
Diabetes, 481
Lipid and Lipoprotein Disorders, 492
Gastrointestinal and Digestive Disease, Including Liver Toxicity, 498
Circulatory Disorders, 505
Amyloidosis, 511
Summary, 513

APPENDIXES

A SUMMARY OF WORKSHOP — 523

B ICD-9 CODES FOR CANCER OUTCOMES — 524

C COMMITTEE AND STAFF BIOGRAPHIES — 527

INDEX — 533

Veterans and Agent Orange

Update 2000

1

Executive Summary

Because of continuing uncertainty about the long-term health effects of exposure to the herbicides used in Vietnam, Congress passed Public Law 102-4 (P.L. 102-4), the "Agent Orange Act of 1991." This legislation directed the Secretary of Veterans Affairs to request the National Academy of Sciences (NAS) to conduct a comprehensive review and evaluation of scientific and medical information regarding the health effects of exposure to Agent Orange, other herbicides used in Vietnam, and the various chemical components of these herbicides, including dioxin. A committee convened by the Institute of Medicine (IOM) of the NAS conducted this review and in 1994 published a comprehensive report entitled *Veterans and Agent Orange: Health Effects of Herbicides Used in Vietnam* (hereafter referred to as *VAO*) (IOM, 1994).

P.L. 102-4 also called for NAS to conduct subsequent reviews at least every 2 years for a period of 10 years from the date of the first report. NAS was instructed to conduct a comprehensive review of the evidence that had become available since the previous IOM committee report and to reassess its determinations and estimates of statistical association, risk, and biological plausibility. Committees were formed that produced *Veterans and Agent Orange: Update 1996* (hereafter, *Update 1996*) (IOM, 1996) and *Veterans and Agent Orange: Update 1998* (hereafter, *Update 1998*) (IOM, 1999). In 1999, in response to a request from the Department of Veterans Affairs (DVA), IOM convened a committee to conduct a focused review of the scientific evidence regarding Type 2 (adult-onset) diabetes. Although limited to one health outcome, its report, *Veterans and Agent Orange: Herbicide/Dioxin Exposure and Type 2 Diabetes* (hereafter, *Type 2 Diabetes*), otherwise adhered to the format of the *Veterans and Agent Orange* series (IOM, 2000).

The present report is the third comprehensive review and evaluation of the newly published scientific evidence regarding associations between health outcomes and exposure to dioxin and other chemical compounds in herbicides used in Vietnam. In accordance with P.L. 102-4, the committee was asked to determine, to the extent that available data permitted meaningful determinations, (1) whether a statistical association with herbicide exposure exists, taking into account the strength of the scientific evidence and the appropriateness of the statistical and epidemiologic methods used to detect the association; (2) the increased risk of the disease among those exposed to herbicides during Vietnam service; and (3) whether there is a plausible biologic mechanism or other evidence of a causal relationship between herbicide exposure and the disease.

DVA also asked the committee to examine the possible association between the herbicides of concern in this report and AL-type primary amyloidosis, a condition not examined in previous *Veterans and Agent Orange* reports.

In conducting its study, the IOM committee operated independently of the DVA and other government agencies. The committee was not asked to and did not make judgments regarding specific cases in which individual Vietnam veterans have claimed injury from herbicide exposure. Rather, the study provides scientific information for the Secretary of Veterans Affairs to consider as the DVA exercises its responsibilities to Vietnam veterans.

ORGANIZATION AND FRAMEWORK

Chapter 2 provides an overview of the methods and conclusions of the previous *Veterans and Agent Orange* series reports. Chapter 3 updates the experimental toxicology data on the effects of the herbicides and 2,3,7,8-TCDD (2,3,7,8-tetrachlorodibenzo-*p*-dioxin, commonly referred to as TCDD, or "dioxin"), a compound found as a contaminant in the herbicide 2,4,5-trichlorophenoxyacetic acid (2,4,5-T). These data contribute to the biologic plausibility of potential health effects in human populations. Chapter 4 briefly describes the methodological considerations that guided the committee's review and its evaluation. Chapter 5 addresses exposure assessment issues. Chapter 6 provides a general review of the epidemiologic studies used to assess the potential association between herbicides and specific health outcomes. The chapter is organized to reflect similarities and differences in the nature of exposure among three types of study populations: occupationally exposed, environmentally exposed, and Vietnam veterans. Health outcomes are addressed in the remaining chapters: Chapter 7 focuses on cancer outcomes; Chapter 8, on reproductive effects; Chapter 9, on neurobehavioral disorders; and Chapter 10, on other (noncancer) health effects including respiratory, immune system, metabolic, digestive, and circulatory disorders. Many epidemiologic studies assess multiple health outcomes. These chapters provide detailed information on and citations for the research discussed below.

TOXICOLOGY SUMMARY

The results of cellular and animal studies published since the release of *Update 1998* that investigate the toxicokinetics, mechanism of action, and disease outcomes of the herbicides and TCDD are reviewed in Chapter 3. Although effects in such experiments cannot be translated directly to effects in humans at the same doses, these experiments provide important information on the biologic plausibility of toxic effects and the underlying mechanisms by which these effects occur.

TCDD is considered more toxic than the uncontaminated components of the herbicides used in Vietnam. TCDD elicits a diverse spectrum of sex-, strain-, age-, and species-specific effects, including carcinogenicity, immunotoxicity, reproductive and developmental toxicity, hepatotoxicity, neurotoxicity, chloracne, and loss of body weight. Most species studied experimentally develop a "wasting syndrome," characterized by a loss of body weight and fatty tissue, from acutely toxic doses. Liver necrosis (i.e., cell death) was seen at lethal doses. Effects on the morphology and function of the liver are seen at lower doses. TCDD affects the endocrine system of animals. Some experiments indicate that treating animals with TCDD alters thyroid hormone levels, but others do not, making the interpretation of effects on thyroid hormones difficult. In utero TCDD exposure decreased performance on certain learning and memory tasks in the offspring of rats and monkeys but improved performance on other tasks. However, animal studies to date suggest that the adult nervous system is sensitive to the effects of TCDD only at high doses.

In experimental animals, one of the most sensitive systems to TCDD toxicity is the immune system. Recent studies have demonstrated that TCDD can alter the number and activity of immune cells and the ability of animals to fight off infection. Effects on the immune system, however, appear to be dependent on the species and strain of animal studied.

Reproductive and developmental effects have been seen in animals exposed to TCDD. Effects on sperm counts, sperm production, and seminal vesicle weights have been seen in male offspring of rats and hamsters treated with TCDD during pregnancy. Effects on the female reproductive system have also been seen following in utero exposure to TCDD. Effects on the male and female reproductive systems, however, are not always accompanied by effects on reproductive outcomes. It is possible that effects on the reproductive system are secondary to effects on reproductive hormones. In recent studies, TCDD did not affect surgically induced endometrial lesions in rats, although effects were seen in earlier studies. Pre- and postnatal exposure of mice to TCDD increased sensitivity to endometrial lesion growth.

TCDD is an extremely potent tumor promoter in laboratory rats. In a recent study there was an increase in hepatic foci at doses as low as 0.01 ng/kg/day. This is the lowest dose of TCDD to promote tumors to date. Recent data also suggest that promotion of liver tumors by TCDD in female rats depends on continuous exposure to TCDD.

Over the past 10 years, much has been learned about the mechanisms by which the dioxins exert their toxic effects. Most information published to date is consistent with the hypothesis that TCDD produces its biological and toxic effects by binding to a protein that regulates gene expression, the aryl hydrocarbon receptor (AhR). The binding of TCDD to the AhR triggers a sequence of cellular events that involve interactions with numerous other cellular components. The actual biochemical and cellular events that follow the initial binding of these chemicals to the AhR and lead to particular toxic end points, however, have yet to be defined. Thus, although the presence of the AhR appears to be necessary for toxicity to occur, it alone is not sufficient. The findings that many AhR-modulated genes and responses are regulated in a cell-, tissue-, developmental stage-, and species-specific pattern suggest that the molecular and cellular pathways leading to any particular toxic event are extremely complex and probably involve multiple events, genes, and signal transduction pathways. Further definition of the pathways regulated by the AhR in a tissue-specific fashion will help to clarify the understanding of the relationships between the dose of TCDD that reaches the tissue and the events leading to specific toxic end points.

Several publications have documented the presence of the AhR and associated proteins in a variety of tissues from different animal species and strains. Detailed analysis of variant forms has associated structure and levels of expression with function. Experiments in species and strains expressing different forms of the AhR suggest that differences in specific regions of the receptor also may be responsible in part for differential sensitivity to TCDD. Humans express the AhR, but differences in the levels of AhR among species and cell types preclude direct extrapolation of effects from one animal to another. Evidence continues to indicate that the sequence of the AhR in humans is highly conserved across individuals; therefore, expression of different forms of the AhR is not likely to explain differential responses to TCDD among individuals. Although structural differences in the AhR have been identified, it operates in a similar manner in animals and humans, and a connection between TCDD exposure and human health effects is, in general, considered biologically plausible. However, as mentioned previously, animals differ greatly in their susceptibility to TCDD-induced effects. Controversy still exists over whether the effects of TCDD are threshold dependent, that is, whether some exposure levels may be too low to induce any effect. Investigations into the endogenous ligand for the AhR (i.e., the compound in the body that normally binds to the receptor) continue. Although several endogenous compounds that bind to the AhR have been described, it is not yet clear whether these have any physiological significance.

Recent experiments demonstrate that 2,4-dichlorophenoxyacetic acid (2,4-D) can cause behavioral effects, muscle weakness, and incoordination in animals, but these effects are seen only at high doses. 2,4-D affects neuron function and some hormones, including reproductive hormones. Reproductive and developmental effects have been seen in animals following 2,4-D exposure, but also only at high doses. A precursor of 2,4-D, 2,4-dichlorophenoxybutyric acid (2,4-DB), did not cause an immunotoxic or carcinogenic response in rodents or dogs. 2,4-D does not appear to be genotoxic except at very high concentrations, and it has very low oncogenic (i.e., tumor-forming) activity.

Little recent work has been conducted on 2,4,5-T. One study, which investigated its myelotoxicity, found that it had relatively weak potency to produce toxic effects on blood components. No new studies were identified that investigate disease outcomes associated with 2,4,5-T exposure in animals.

Cacodylic acid (dimethylarsinic acid, DMA) has been shown to cause bladder tumors in rats and lung cancer in mice, and to promote skin cancer in mice sensitized by genetic manipulation or by exposure to ultraviolet B radiation.

One recent report was found in which the toxic effects of picloram were investigated. In that study, a herbicide mixture was used and the observed effects were attributed to ingredients other than picloram.

Researchers continue to investigate the actions of 2,4-D, 2,4,5-T, and cacodylic acid at the molecular and cellular levels to determine the mechanisms that underlie the toxicity of these compounds. No one mechanism has been established that explains their toxicity.

EXPOSURE ASSESSMENT

Assessment of individual exposures to herbicides and dioxin is a key element in determining whether specific health effects are linked to these compounds. The committee that produced *VAO* found that the definition and quantification of exposure are the weakest methodologic aspects of the epidemiologic studies. Although different approaches have been used to estimate exposure among Vietnam veterans, each approach is limited in its ability to determine precisely the intensity and duration of individual exposure.

Another IOM committee is facilitating the development and evaluation of models of herbicide exposure for use in studies of Vietnam veterans. That committee authored and disseminated a Request for Proposals (RFP) for exposure assessment research in 1997 (IOM, 1997) and is performing scientific oversight of the research. Work funded under this RFP began in 1998 and was still under way at the end of 2000.

CONCLUSIONS ABOUT HEALTH OUTCOMES

Chapters 7, 8, 9, and 10 provide a detailed evaluation of the epidemiologic studies reviewed by the committee and their implications for cancer, reproductive effects, neurobehavioral effects, and other health effects. As detailed in Chapter 4, the committee weighed the strengths and limitations of the epidemiologic evidence in previous *Veterans and Agent Orange* reports as well as the newly published scientific data and reached its conclusions by interpreting the new evidence in the context of the whole of the literature. It assigned each health outcome being considered to one of the four categories listed in Table 1-1. The definitions of the categories and the criteria for assigning a particular health outcome to them are described in the table, and the specific rationale for each of the findings is detailed in the appropriate chapter. Since this update is intended to supplement rather than replace earlier reports, much of the information on studies reviewed in those reports has not been repeated. The reader is referred to relevant sections of the previous reports for additional detail and explanation.

Consistent with the mandate of P.L. 102-4, the distinctions between categories are based on "statistical association," not on causality, as is common in scientific reviews. Thus, standard criteria used in epidemiology for assessing causality (Hill, 1971) do not strictly apply. The committee was charged with reviewing the scientific evidence, rather than making recommendations regarding DVA policy, and the findings reported in Table 1-1 are not intended to imply or suggest any policy decisions; these must rest with the Secretary of Veterans Affairs.

TABLE 1-1 Updated (2000) Summary of Findings in Occupational, Environmental, and Veterans Studies Regarding the Association Between Specific Health Outcomes and Exposure to Herbicides

Sufficient Evidence of an Association
Evidence is sufficient to conclude that there is a positive association. That is, a positive association has been observed between herbicides and the outcome in studies in which chance, bias, and confounding could be ruled out with reasonable confidence. For example, if several small studies that are free from bias and confounding show an association that is consistent in magnitude and direction, there may be sufficient evidence for an association. There is sufficient evidence of an association between exposure to herbicides and the following health outcomes:
        Soft-tissue sarcoma
        Non-Hodgkin's lymphoma
        Hodgkin's disease
        Chloracne

Limited/Suggestive Evidence of an Association
Evidence is suggestive of an association between herbicides and the outcome but is limited because chance, bias, and confounding could not be ruled out with confidence. For example, at least one high-quality study shows a positive association, but the results of other studies are inconsistent. There is limited/suggestive evidence of an association between exposure to herbicides and the following health outcomes:
        Respiratory cancers (lung/bronchus, larynx, trachea)
        Prostate cancer
        Multiple myeloma
        Acute and subacute transient peripheral neuropathy
        Porphyria cutanea tarda
        Type 2 diabetes (category change from Update 1998*)*

Spina bifida in the children of veterans
Acute myelogenous leukemia (AML) in the children of veterans (category change from Update 1998)

Inadequate/Insufficient Evidence to Determine Whether an Association Exists
The available studies are of insufficient quality, consistency, or statistical power to permit a conclusion regarding the presence or absence of an association. For example, studies fail to control for confounding, have inadequate exposure assessment, or fail to address latency. There is inadequate or insufficient evidence to determine whether an association exists between exposure to herbicides and the following health outcomes:

Hepatobiliary cancers
Nasal/nasopharyngeal cancer
Bone cancer
Skin cancers (melanoma, basal, and squamous cell)
Breast cancer
Female reproductive cancers (cervical, uterine, ovarian)
Testicular cancer
Urinary bladder cancer
Renal cancer
Leukemia
Spontaneous abortion
Birth defects (other than spina bifida)
Neonatal/infant death and stillbirths
Low birthweight
Childhood cancer in offspring, other than acute myelogenous leukemia
Abnormal sperm parameters and infertility
Cognitive and neuropsychiatric disorders
Motor/coordination dysfunction
Chronic peripheral nervous system disorders
Gastrointestinal, metabolic and digestive disorders (changes in liver enzymes, lipid abnormalities, ulcers)
Immune system disorders (immune suppression and autoimmunity)
Circulatory disorders
Respiratory disorders
AL-type primary amyloidosis (new health outcome)

Limited/Suggestive Evidence of *No* Association
Several adequate studies, covering the full range of levels of exposure that human beings are known to encounter, are mutually consistent in not showing a positive association between exposure to herbicides and the outcome at any level of exposure. A conclusion of "no association" is inevitably limited to the conditions, level of exposure, and length of observation covered by the available studies. *In addition, the possibility of a very small elevation in risk at the levels of exposure studied can never be excluded.* There is limited/suggestive evidence of *no* association between exposure to herbicides and the following health outcomes:

Gastrointestinal tumors (stomach cancer, pancreatic cancer, colon cancer, rectal cancer)
Brain tumors

NOTE: "Herbicides" refers to the major herbicides used in Vietnam: 2,4-D (2,4-dichlorophenoxyacetic acid), 2,4,5-T (2,4,5-trichlorophenoxyacetic acid) and its contaminant TCDD (2,3,7,8-tetrachlorodibenzo-*p*-dioxin), cacodylic acid, and picloram. The evidence regarding association is drawn from occupational and other studies in which subjects were exposed to a variety of herbicides and herbicide components.

Health Outcomes with Sufficient Evidence of an Association

In *Update 1998*, the committee found sufficient evidence of an association between exposure to herbicides and/or TCDD and soft-tissue sarcoma, non-Hodgkin's lymphoma, Hodgkin's disease (HD), and chloracne. Recent scientific literature continues to support the classification of these diseases in this category. Based on the recent literature, there are no additional diseases that satisfy this category's criteria. The evidence that supports the committee's conclusions for the three cancers is detailed in Chapter 7 and for chloracne in Chapter 10.

The studies reviewed for this report continue a pattern of mixed findings regarding the evidence of an association between soft-tissue sarcoma (STS) and herbicide or dioxin exposure. No new cases were observed in the latest update of ongoing studies of U.S. and Dutch chemical workers. A study of Danish paper mill workers found some excess of STS, but the possible link with dioxin exposure was not well established. Updates of the Air Force Health Study and Seveso populations did not add any new information on STS. An investigation of cancers in the vicinity of a solid waste incinerator in France found a statistically significant spatial cluster, although methodologic concerns lessen confidence in these findings.

Several new studies of non-Hodgkin's lymphoma incidence and mortality have been published since *Update 1998*. Of the three with the largest sample populations, two—studies of a population living near a solid waste incinerator and of male Vietnam veterans from Australia—reported elevated incidence rates. The third—a mortality study in areas where chlorophenoxy herbicides may have been used—observed rates similar to those expected in the general population.

Three new reports of males occupationally exposed to chlorinated organic compounds indicated either elevated HD incidence or mortality. Elevated rates for men and women were also observed in the "medium-exposure" zone for the environmentally exposed Seveso cohort.

A new study found that despite the high frequency of skin disorders reported during service in Vietnam, there were no cases of chloracne and no evidence for an increased risk of acne among Ranch Hand participants compared to other theater veterans either during the Vietnam conflict or subsequently. Nonetheless, there is abundant evidence that TCDD exposure causes chloracne.

Health Outcomes with Limited/Suggestive Evidence of an Association

In *Update 1998*, the committee found limited/suggestive evidence of an association for three cancers—respiratory (larynx, lung or bronchus, and trachea) cancer, prostate cancer, and multiple myeloma—and three other health outcomes—spina bifida in the children of veterans, acute and subacute (transient) peripheral neuropathy, and porphyria cutanea tarda. The recent scientific literature continues to support the classification of these diseases in the limited/suggestive category of evidence.

In 2000, the committee responsible for *Type 2 Diabetes* found that there was limited/suggestive evidence of an association between exposure to the herbicides used in Vietnam or the contaminant dioxin and that health outcome. Evidence reviewed in this report continues to support that finding.

The committee also found that one additional condition satisfies the criteria necessary for inclusion in this category: acute myelogenous leukemia (AML)[1] in the children of veterans. Two studies, in particular, support this conclusion. One is a case-control study of AML (Wen et al., 2000) in which self-reported service in Vietnam or Cambodia was associated with an elevated risk after adjustment for numerous potentially confounding life-style and sociodemographic factors. The second, a study of the children of Australian Vietnam veterans (AIHW, 2000), found a greater than fourfold risk although confounding factors other than age and gender were not controlled. While direct measures of exposure are lacking, the committee found the following characteristics of these studies to be particularly persuasive: (1) both were conducted in Vietnam veteran populations; (2) the association was specific for AML, with no excess risk found for other forms of leukemia; (3) one study adjusted for numerous confounders, while the other had an association of sufficiently large magnitude to reduce the likelihood of being completely due to confounding; and (4) the strongest association was seen in children diagnosed at the youngest ages—cases that are considered the strongest candidates for an etiology of parental origin. These characteristics diminish the likelihood that the outcomes were unrelated to service in Vietnam. A third study (Buckley et al., 1989), which reported a 2.7-fold increased risk of AML in the children of fathers with self-reported exposure of more than 1,000 days to pesticides or weed killers, adds to the plausibility that herbicide exposure could be related to the higher risk observed among those who served in Vietnam.

Recently published research on lung and bronchus cancer in U.S. chemical production workers and Ranch Hand veterans continues to support the finding that there is limited/suggestive evidence for an association between the herbicides of concern in this report and the risk of these outcomes. Evidence for an exposure–response relationship has been slightly strengthened since *Update 1998* but still does not support a conclusion of sufficient evidence. Although the latest data on the Seveso cohort do not show an excess, it remains early in the follow-up of this cohort for the characterization of cancers with latencies of decades. Studies also continue to support the conclusion that there is limited/suggestive evidence of an association between laryngeal cancer and exposure to the herbicides of concern in this report. The conclusion that there is sufficient evidence cannot be reached at this time because the most important risk factors for cancer of the larynx are not controlled in any of these studies and may confound the

---

[1] *Acute myelogenous leukemia* (ICD·9 205) is referred to by other names as well, including acute myeloid leukemia and acute nonlymphocytic leukemia. There are also numerous subtypes of the disease.

relationship to the extent that they could produce the slight elevation observed in most positive studies.

The new data on prostate cancer are not entirely consistent. Excess incidence was reported in studies of pesticide appliers in Sweden and Florida, but the exposure of both cohorts is not well defined and the studies do not provide direct evidence that dioxin is carcinogenic to the prostate. The clear excess observed in Australia's Vietnam veterans supports an association between prostate cancer and service in Vietnam, under the assumption that the veterans are not receiving better health surveillance than the general population of the same age in that country. The null findings among Ranch Hand personnel run counter to this conclusion. Among the three newly reviewed mortality studies of prostate cancer, the two cohorts showing nonsignificant excesses of about 20 percent had the highest-quality exposure information. Although the results for this outcome are mixed, it should be kept in mind that most Vietnam veterans have not yet reached the age at which prostate cancer tends to appear.

Among the newly reviewed studies of multiple myeloma (MM), only the National Institute of Occupational Safety and Health cohort of chemical production workers has both a relatively large number of subjects and data that clearly point to exposure to the herbicides and contaminants most relevant to Vietnam veterans. This study found a twofold increased mortality risk.

The committee is aware of no new publications that investigate the association between exposure to the compounds of interest and acute or subacute transient peripheral neuropathy, and knows of no evidence that new cases of these conditions that develop long after service in Vietnam would be associated with wartime herbicide exposure.

Since *Update 1998* was published, a validation study found a significant excess of spina bifida cases in the children born to Australian Vietnam veterans. A study of occupational exposure to pesticides and selected congenital malformations in Spain did not find an increased risk where there had been paternal exposure to organophosphates or organochlorines pesticides, although there were a small number of exposed cases and the statistical power and precision of the study were poor.

A new study of a group of Austrian chemical workers exposed to TCDD in herbicide production in the 1970s reported that urinary porphyrins remained abnormal, although not clinically characteristic of porphyria cutanea tarda (PCT). Coproporphyrinogen levels were within the normal range, but there was a reversal in the normal ratio of isomer I to isomer III in almost half of the subjects. The authors inferred that this indicated persistent liver injury and abnormal porphyrin metabolism due to TCDD, and implied that exposed workers may be at risk for related conditions including PCT.

Several new studies of herbicide or dioxin exposure and Type 2 diabetes were published after the completion of *Update 1998*. As detailed in *Type 2*

Diabetes, no one paper or study was determinative in reaching the finding that there was limited/suggestive evidence of an association. Instead, the committee found that the information accumulated over years of research met the definition established for this category. Positive associations were reported in many mortality studies, which may underestimate the incidence of diabetes, and in most of the morbidity studies identified by the committee. Since the completion of *Type 2 Diabetes*, an updated review of the Seveso cohort has been published that found an excess incidence of this condition among women but not men in the high- and medium-exposure zones.

Health Outcomes with Inadequate/Insufficient Evidence to Determine Whether an Association Exists

The scientific data for many of the cancers and other diseases reviewed by the committee were inadequate or insufficient to determine whether an association exists. This group includes hepatobiliary cancers (cancers of the liver and intrahepatic bile duct), nasal and nasopharyngeal cancer, bone cancer, skin cancers (including melanoma, basal or squamous cell carcinoma and nonmelanocytic skin cancers), breast cancer, cancers of the female reproductive system (including cervix, endometrium, and ovaries), testicular cancer, urinary bladder cancer, renal cancer (cancers of the kidney and renal pelvis), and leukemias. The scientific evidence regarding each of these cancers is detailed in Chapter 7.

Several reproductive effects are classified in this category, including spontaneous abortion, birth defects other than spina bifida, neonatal or infant death and stillbirths, low birthweight, childhood cancer in offspring (other than acute myelogenous leukemia), and abnormal sperm parameters and infertility. The scientific evidence for reproductive effects is detailed in Chapter 8. Evidence for the neurobehavioral effects classified in this category—cognitive and neuropsychiatric disorders, motor or coordination dysfunction, and chronic peripheral nervous system disorders—is detailed in Chapter 9.

Other health effects that are classified in the inadequate/insufficient category include metabolic and digestive disorders, immune system disorders, circulatory disorders, respiratory disorders, and AL-type primary amyloidosis. The scientific evidence underlying these findings is detailed in Chapter 10.

Health Outcomes with Limited/Suggestive Evidence of *No* Association

In *VAO*, the committee found a sufficient number and variety of well-designed studies to conclude that there is limited/suggestive evidence of *no* association between a small group of cancers and exposure to TCDD or herbicides. This group includes gastrointestinal tumors (colon, rectal, stomach, and pancreatic) and brain tumors. Recent scientific evidence continues to support the classification of such cancers in this category and is detailed in Chapter 7. Based on the recent literature, there are no additional diseases that satisfy the criteria necessary for this category.

A conclusion of "no association" is inevitably limited to the conditions, level of exposure, and length of observation covered by the available studies. In addition, the possibility of a very small elevation in risk at the levels of exposure studied can never be excluded.

INCREASED RISK OF DISEASE AMONG VIETNAM VETERANS

Although there have been numerous health studies of Vietnam veterans, most have been hampered by relatively poor measures of exposure to herbicides or TCDD, in addition to other methodological problems. Most of the evidence on which the findings regarding disease association are based comes from studies of people exposed to dioxin or herbicides in occupational and environmental settings, rather than from studies of Vietnam veterans. The committee found this body of evidence sufficient for reaching the conclusions about statistical associations between herbicides and the health outcomes. However, the lack of adequate data on Vietnam veterans per se complicates the quantification of any increased risk of disease among individuals exposed to herbicides during service in Vietnam. Given the large uncertainties that remain about the magnitude of potential risk from exposure to herbicides in the epidemiologic studies reviewed (Chapters 7–10), the inadequate control for other important risk factors in many studies, and uncertainty about the nature and magnitude of exposure to herbicides in Vietnam (Chapter 5), the necessary information to undertake a quantitative risk assessment is lacking.

Thus, the committee cannot quantify the degree of risk likely to be experienced by those exposed to herbicides during service in the Republic of Vietnam during the Vietnam era. For those outcomes in the "sufficient" and "limited/suggestive" categories, what can be said is that too little is known about the herbicide exposure of veterans to make a meaningful determination of the increased risk, if any, of these outcomes among Vietnam veterans. Where there is inadequate/insufficient evidence to determine whether an association exists between herbicide exposure and a particular health outcome, there is also inadequate/insufficient information to assess the increased risk, if any, of that outcome. Finally, a finding of "limited/suggestive evidence of *no* association" between herbicide exposure and a health outcome means that the evidence suggests there is no increased risk of that outcome among Vietnam veterans. These conclusions are inevitably limited to the conditions, level of exposure, and length of observation covered by the studies reviewed by the committee. There are certain diseases about which the committee can draw more specific conclusions, and this information is related in the discussion of those diseases.

OBSERVATIONS AND RESEARCH RECOMMENDATIONS

Although great strides have been made over the past several years in understanding the health effects of exposure to the herbicides used in Vietnam and dioxin, and in elucidating the mechanisms underlying these effects, there are still important gaps in our knowledge. Subsequent chapters of this report contain recommendations for further work addressing some specific research needs identified in the course of this study. Additional observations on one major research effort are offered below.

The Air Force Health Study (AFHS) is an epidemiologic study whose purpose is to determine whether exposure to the herbicides used in Vietnam may be responsible for any adverse health conditions observed in a cohort of Air Force personnel responsible for conducting aerial spray missions (the Ranch Hands). A baseline morbidity study of the Ranch Hands and a matched comparison cohort was conducted in 1982, with follow-up assessments in 1985, 1987, 1992, and 1997. In accordance with the study protocol, one additional assessment is planned for 2002, after which a final report will be issued.

Because this study represents one of the few primary sources of information on the health of Vietnam veterans and is coming close to its scheduled end, the committee believes it is timely to offer some observations and recommendations about it.

The AFHS cohorts represent an unusually thoroughly studied population. Some of the data generated in the course of the study are already or soon will be available to the public. However, there are also medical records and biological specimens that are not amenable to such public disclosure. The committee believes there is scientific merit in retaining and maintaining these medical records and samples, so that—with proper respect for the privacy of the study participants—they could be available for future research. It therefore recommends that the federal government examine whether and how the various forms of data and specimens collected in the course of the Air Force Health Study could be retained and maintained, and what form of oversight should be established for their future use. The committee further recommends that consideration be given to whether it is appropriate to continue the study past its planned completion date. It notes that the AFHS cohorts are only now reaching the age where several health outcomes of interest may be expected to manifest. The committee cannot draw a conclusion on whether or not a continuation of research on the AFHS cohorts will inform specific questions regarding the health effects of exposure to the herbicides used in Vietnam. However, the committee's judgment is that continued research on the health of the Ranch Hand and comparison veterans is likely to yield important information on the determinants of health and disease in males who served in the military during the Vietnam era and perhaps their offspring. If the records were to be retained and maintained and/or the research continued, this would have to be done with the full knowledge and consent of the AFHS population and be subject to controls that would respect the privacy of the participants.

REFERENCES

AIHW (Australian Institute of Health and Welfare). 2000. Morbidity of Vietnam veterans. Adrenal gland cancer, leukaemia and non-Hodgkin's lymphoma: Supplementary report No. 2. (AIHW cat. No. PHE 28). Canberra: AIHW.

Buckley JD, Robison LL, Swotinsky R, Garabrant DH, LeBeau M, Manchester P, Nesbit ME, Odom L, Peters JM, Woods WG, Hammond GD. 1989. Occupational exposures of parents of children with acute nonlymphocytic leukemia: a report from the Children's Cancer Study Group. Cancer Research 49:4030–4037.

Hill, AB. 1971. Principles of Medical Statistics, 9th Ed. New York: Oxford University Press.

IOM (Institute of Medicine). 1994. Veterans and Agent Orange: Health Effects of Herbicides Used in Vietnam. Washington, DC: National Academy Press.

IOM. 1996. Veterans and Agent Orange: Update 1996. Washington, DC: National Academy Press.

IOM. 1997. Characterizing Exposure of Veterans to Agent Orange and Other Herbicides Used in Vietnam: Scientific Considerations Regarding a Request for Proposals for Research. Washington, DC: National Academy Press.

IOM. 1999. Veterans and Agent Orange: Update 1998. Washington, DC: National Academy Press.

IOM. 2000. Veterans and Agent Orange: Herbicide/Dioxin Exposure and Type 2 Diabetes. Washington, DC: National Academy Press.

Wen WQ, Shu XO, Steinbuch M, Severson RK, Reaman GH, Buckley JD, Robison LL. 2000. Paternal military service and risk for childhood leukemia in offspring. American Journal of Epidemiology 151(3):231–240.

2

Veterans and Agent Orange: Previous IOM Reports

BACKGROUND

Public Law 102-4, the "Agent Orange Act of 1991," was enacted on February 6, 1991. This legislation, codified as 38 USC Sec. 1116, directed the Secretary of Veterans Affairs to request that the National Academy of Sciences conduct a comprehensive review and evaluation of scientific and medical information regarding the health effects of exposure to Agent Orange, other herbicides used in Vietnam, and their components, including dioxin. In February 1992, the Institute of Medicine (IOM) of the National Academy of Sciences signed an agreement with the Department of Veterans Affairs (DVA) to review and summarize the strength of the scientific evidence concerning the association between herbicide exposure during Vietnam service and each disease or condition suspected to be associated with such exposure. The IOM was also asked to make recommendations concerning the need, if any, for additional scientific studies to resolve areas of continuing scientific uncertainty and to comment on four particular programs mandated in the law. Finally, P.L. 102-4 called for subsequent reviews of newly available information to be completed every 2 years after the initial report for a period of 10 years.

To carry out the mandate, the IOM established the Committee to Review the Health Effects in Vietnam Veterans of Exposure to Herbicides. The results of the original committee's work were published in 1994 as *Veterans and Agent Orange: Health Effects of Herbicides Used in Vietnam* (hereafter referred to as *VAO*) (IOM, 1994). Successor committees of the same name were formed to fulfill the requirement for subsequent reviews. These committees produced *Vet-*

erans and Agent Orange: Update 1996 (IOM, 1996) and *Update 1998* (IOM, 1999). In 1999, in response to a request from DVA, IOM called together a committee to conduct an interim review of the scientific evidence regarding one of the conditions addressed in the *Veterans and Agent Orange* series of reports: Type 2 diabetes. The committee, which consisted of individuals responsible for the *Update 1998* report plus recognized experts in the field of Type 2 diabetes, focused on information published since the deliberations of the *Update 1998* committee. This effort resulted in the report *Veterans and Agent Orange: Herbicide/Dioxin Exposure and Type 2 Diabetes* (hereafter, *Type 2 Diabetes*) (IOM, 2000). Although limited to one health outcome, this report otherwise adhered to the format of the *VAO* series.

In conducting their work, the committees responsible for these reports operated independently of the DVA and other government agencies. They were not asked to and did not make judgments regarding specific cases in which individual Vietnam veterans have claimed injury from herbicide exposure; this was not part of the congressional charge. Rather, the studies provide scientific information for the Secretary of Veterans Affairs to consider as the DVA exercises its responsibilities to Vietnam veterans.

To fulfill their charge of judging whether each of a set of human health effects is associated with exposure to herbicides or dioxin, the committees concentrated on reviewing and interpreting human epidemiologic studies, as well as experimental investigations that may contribute to biologic plausibility. The committees began their evaluation presuming neither the presence nor the absence of association. They sought to characterize and weigh the strengths and limitations of the available evidence. These judgments have both quantitative and qualitative aspects. They reflect the nature of the exposures, health outcomes, and populations exposed; the characteristics of the evidence examined; and the approach taken to evaluate this evidence. To facilitate independent assessment of the committee's conclusions, Chapter 5 of *VAO* describes as explicitly as possible the methodological considerations that guided the original committee's review and its process of evaluation. This methodology was subsequently adopted by successor committees. It is briefly summarized in Chapter 4 of this report.

To obtain additional information pertinent to the evaluation of possible health effects of herbicide exposure, the committees decided to review studies of other groups potentially exposed to the herbicides used in Vietnam (2,4,5-trichlorophenoxyacetic acid [2,4,5-T], 2,4-dichlorophenoxyacetic acid [2,4-D], cacodylic acid, and picloram), 2,3,7,8-tertachlorodibenzo-*p*-dioxin (2,3,7,8-TCDD, TCDD, or dioxin), phenoxy herbicides, chlorophenols, and other compounds. These groups include chemical production and agricultural workers; people possibly exposed heavily to herbicides or dioxins as a result of residing near the site of an accident or near areas used to dispose of toxic waste; and residents of Vietnam. The committees felt that considering studies of other groups could help address the issue of whether these compounds might be associated with particular health outcomes, even though the results would have only an indirect bearing on the increased risk of disease in veterans themselves. Some of these studies, especially those of workers in chemical production plants, provide stronger evidence about health effects than studies of veterans because exposure was generally more easily quantified and measured. Furthermore, the general levels and duration of exposure to the chemicals were greater, and the studies were of sufficient size to examine the health risks among people with varying levels of exposure.

Because of the great differences among studies, the committee concluded that it was inappropriate to use a quantitative technique such as meta-analysis to combine individual results into a single summary measure of statistical association. Using such a summary measure would also inappropriately focus attention on one piece of information used by the committee when, in fact, all the factors discussed above are important in evaluating the literature.

CONCLUSIONS ABOUT HEALTH OUTCOMES

VAO, *Update 1996*, and *Update 1998* provide detailed reviews of the scientific studies evaluated by the committee and their implications for cancer, reproductive problems, neurobehavioral problems, and other health effects. The original report summarized the literature available in 1993; *Update 1996* focused on research through mid-1995; and *Update 1998* focused on work published through the fall of 1998. *Type 2 Diabetes* evaluated the evidence available through mid-2000 for that outcome only. This report focuses on research published since the *Update 1998* committee's work was completed and is current through the fall of 2000.

The original committee addressed the statutory mandate to determine whether there is a statistical association between the suspect diseases and herbicide use by assigning each of the health outcomes under study to one of four categories on the basis of the epidemiologic evidence reviewed. The categories used by that committee were adapted from those used by the International Agency for Research on Cancer (IARC) in evaluating evidence for the carcinogenicity of various agents (IARC, 1977). Successor committees have adopted these categorizations in their evaluations. The definitions of the categories and the criteria for assigning a particular health outcome to them are discussed below.

Health Outcomes with Sufficient Evidence of an Association

The original committee found sufficient evidence of an association with herbicides and/or TCDD for three cancers—soft-tissue sarcoma, non-Hodgkin's lymphoma, and Hodgkin's disease—and two other health outcomes, chloracne and porphyria cutanea tarda (PCT). After reviewing the whole of the literature available in 1995, the committee responsible for the first update concluded that the statistical evidence still supported this classification for the three cancers and chloracne. However, new data regarding porphyria cutanea tarda combined with the studies reviewed in *VAO* justified moving PCT to the category of limited/ suggestive evidence of an association with herbicide exposure. Chapter 11 of *Update 1996* details this decision. No changes were made to this category in *Update 1998* or this report.

For diseases in this category, a positive association between herbicides and the outcome must be observed in studies in which chance, bias, and confounding can be ruled out with reasonable confidence. The committee regarded evidence from several small studies that are free from bias and confounding, and show an association that is consistent in magnitude and direction, as sufficient evidence for an association.

Health Outcomes with Limited/Suggestive Evidence of an Association

The committee responsible for *VAO* found limited/suggestive evidence of an association for three cancers: respiratory cancers, prostate cancer, and multiple myeloma. The *Update 1996* committee added three health outcomes to this list: PCT (explained above), acute and subacute transient peripheral neuropathy, and spina bifida in children of veterans. Transient peripheral neuropathies had not been addressed in *VAO* since, because of their transient nature, they were not amenable to epidemiologic study. In response to a request from DVA, the *Update 1996* committee added them to the list of reviewed health outcomes and made its determination on the basis of evidence available from case histories. This classification is addressed in Chapter 10 of the 1996 report. A 1995 analysis of birth defects among the offspring of Ranch Hand veterans, in combination with earlier studies of neural tube defects in the children of Vietnam veterans published by the Centers for Disease Control and Prevention, led the *Update 1996* committee to distinguish spina bifida from other adverse reproductive outcomes and classify it in the limited/suggestive category. Chapter 9 of *Update 1996* discusses this decision in detail.

Based on its evaluation of newly available scientific evidence as well as the cumulative findings of research reviewed in previous *Veterans and Agent Orange* reports, the committee responsible for the *Type 2 Diabetes* report found there was limited/suggestive evidence of an association between exposure to the herbicides used in Vietnam or the contaminant dioxin and that health outcome. Evidence reviewed in this report continues to support that finding. As detailed in Chapter 8 of the report, the present committee has added acute myelogenous leukemia in the children of veterans to this category.

For diseases in this category, the evidence must be suggestive of an association between herbicides and the outcome considered, but the association may be limited because chance, bias, or confounding could not be ruled out with confidence. Typically, at least one high-quality study indicates a positive association, but the results of other studies may be inconsistent.

Health Outcomes with Inadequate/Insufficient Evidence to Determine Whether an Association Exists

Scientific data for many of the cancers and other diseases reviewed by the *VAO*, *Update 1996*, and *Update 1998* committees were inadequate or insufficient to determine whether any association exists. There was one change in the health outcomes in this category between the first two reports: skin cancer was moved into this category in *Update 1996* when available evidence no longer supported its classification as a condition with limited/suggestive evidence of no association.

Based on an evaluation of all the epidemiologic evidence, including studies published since the release of *Update 1996*, the *Update 1998* committee felt that urinary bladder cancer should be added to this category. Although there is no evidence that exposure to herbicides or dioxin is related to this cancer, newly available evidence weakened the committees' prior conclusion that there was positive evidence of no association.

The present committee has not made any changes to the list of health outcomes in this category.

For diseases in this category, the available studies are of insufficient quality, consistency, or statistical power to permit a conclusion regarding the presence or absence of an association. For example, studies may fail to control for confounding or have inadequate exposure assessment.

Health Outcomes with Limited/Suggestive Evidence of *No* Association

For a small group of cancers, the *VAO* committee found a sufficient number and variety of well-designed studies to conclude that there is limited/suggestive evidence of *no* association between these cancers and TCDD or the herbicides under study. This group included gastrointestinal tumors (colon, rectal, stomach, and pancreatic), skin cancer, brain tumors, and bladder cancer. As noted above, the *Update 1996* committee removed skin cancer from this category and the *Update 1998* committee removed urinary bladder cancer because the evidence no longer supported a no-association classification for these health outcome. No further changes to the categorizations were made for this report.

For outcomes in this category, several adequate studies covering the full range of levels of exposure that human beings are known to encounter are mutually consistent in not showing a positive association between exposure to herbicides and the outcome at any level of exposure, and have relatively narrow confidence intervals. A conclusion of "no association" is inevitably limited to the conditions, levels of exposure, and length of observation covered by the available studies. In addition, the possibility of a very small elevation in risk at the levels of exposure studied can never be excluded.

INCREASED RISK OF DISEASE AMONG VIETNAM VETERANS

The second of the committee's three statutory mandates calls on it to determine, to the extent that available scientific data permit meaningful determinations, the increased risk of disease among individuals exposed to herbicides during service in Vietnam. Although there have been numerous health studies of Vietnam veterans, many have been hampered by relatively poor measures of exposure to herbicides or TCDD, in addition to other methodological problems. Most of the evidence on which the findings regarding associations are based comes from studies of people exposed to dioxin or herbicides in occupational and environmental settings, rather than from studies of Vietnam veterans. The *VAO, Update 1996*, and *Update 1998* committees found this body of evidence sufficient for reaching their conclusions about statistical associations between herbicides and health outcomes. However, the lack of adequate data on Vietnam veterans per se complicates consideration of the second part of the statutory charge. To estimate the magnitude of risk for a particular health outcome among herbicide-exposed Vietnam veterans, quantitative information about the dose–time–response relationship for each health outcome in humans, information on the extent of herbicide exposure among Vietnam veterans, and estimates of individual exposure are needed. The large uncertainties that remain about the magnitude of potential risk from exposure to herbicides in the studies that have been reviewed, the sometimes-inadequate control for important confounders, and uncertainty about the nature and magnitude of exposure to herbicides in Vietnam—all combine to make quantitative risk assessments problematic. Thus, the committees have found that in general, it is not possible to quantify the degree of risk likely to be experienced by veterans because of their exposure to herbicides in Vietnam. The existing evidence about herbicide exposure among various groups studied does suggest that most Vietnam veterans (except those with documented high exposures, such as participants in Operation Ranch Hand) had lower exposure to herbicides and TCDD than did the subjects in many occupational and environmental studies. However, individual veterans who had very high exposures to herbicides could have risks approaching those described in the occupational and environmental studies. The committees do offer observations regarding increased risk in specific veteran populations where data are available.

EXISTENCE OF A PLAUSIBLE BIOLOGIC MECHANISM OR OTHER EVIDENCE OF A CAUSAL RELATIONSHIP

Toxicological information forms the basis of the committee's response to the third part of the statutory charge—to determine whether there is a plausible biologic mechanism or other evidence of a causal relationship between herbicide exposure and a disease. This information is summarized in general terms in separate toxicology chapters in previous reports: Chapter 4 of *VAO* and Chapter 3 of *Update 1996, Update 1998*, and this report. Specific findings for each health outcome are also given in the chapters that review the epidemiologic literature.

RESEARCH RECOMMENDATIONS

The IOM was also asked to make recommendations concerning the need, if any, for additional scientific studies to resolve areas of continuing scientific uncertainty concerning the health effects of the herbicides used in Vietnam. Based on its review of the epidemiologic evidence and a consideration of the quality of exposure information available in existing studies, especially of Vietnam veterans, the committee responsible for *VAO* concluded that a series of epidemiologic studies of veterans could yield valuable information if a new, valid exposure reconstruction model could be developed. The original committee also saw value in continuing the existing Ranch Hand study and expanding it to include Army Chemical Corps veterans. The committee's research recommendations emphasized studies of Vietnam veterans, rather than general toxicologic or epidemiologic studies of occupationally or environmentally exposed populations. A substantial amount of research on the toxicology and epidemiology of herbicides and herbicide components is under way in the United States and abroad. Indeed, many of the studies on which the committee's conclusions are based have been published since 1991. Although this research is not targeted specifically to Vietnam veterans, it probably will also contribute to the knowledge of potential health effects in this population.

The committees responsible for *VAO, Update 1996, Update 1998, Type 2 Diabetes,* and this report have also made observations on research needs and opportunities regarding specific health outcomes and have offered advice on the conduct of future studies. The reports detail the committees' comments on these topics.

REFERENCES

IARC (International Agency for Research on Cancer). 1977. Some Fumigants, the Herbicides 2,4-D and 2,4,5-T, Chlorinated Dibenzodioxins and Miscellaneous Industrial Chemicals. IARC Monographs on the Evaluation of the Carcinogenic Risk of Chemicals to Man, Vol. 15. Lyon, France: World Health Organization, IARC.
IOM (Institute of Medicine). 1994. Veterans and Agent Orange: Health Effects of Herbicides Used in Vietnam. Washington, DC: National Academy Press.
IOM. 1996. Veterans and Agent Orange: Update 1996. Washington, DC: National Academy Press.
IOM. 1999. Veterans and Agent Orange: Update 1998. Washington, DC: National Academy Press.
IOM. 2000. Veterans and Agent Orange: Herbicide/Dioxin Exposure and Type 2 Diabetes. Washington, DC: National Academy Press.

3

Toxicology

As in *Veterans and Agent Orange: Health Effects of Herbicides Used in Vietnam* (IOM, 1994; hereafter referred to as *VAO*), *Veterans and Agent Orange: Update 1996* (IOM, 1996; hereafter, *Update 1996*) and *Veterans and Agent Orange: Update 1998* (IOM, 1999; hereafter, *Update 1998*), this review summarizes the experimental data that serve as a scientific basis for assessment of the biologic plausibility of health outcomes reported in epidemiologic studies. Efforts to establish the biologic plausibility of effects due to herbicide exposure in the laboratory strengthen the evidence for the herbicide effects suspected to occur in humans. Differences in chemical levels, frequency of administration, single or combined exposures, including exposures to chemicals other than herbicides, preexisting health status, genetic factors, and routes of exposure significantly influence toxicity outcomes. Thus, any attempt to extrapolate from experimental studies to human exposure must carefully consider such variables before conclusions are made.

Multiple chemicals were used for various purposes in Vietnam. Four herbicides documented in military records were of particular concern and are addressed here: 2,4-dichlorophenoxyacetic acid (2,4-D), 2,4,5-trichlorophenoxyacetic acid (2,4,5-T), picloram, and cacodylic acid. In addition, the toxicologic properties of 2,3,7,8-tetrachlorodibenzo-*p*-dioxin (TCDD or dioxin), a contaminant of 2,4,5-T, are discussed. This chapter focuses to a large extent on the toxicological effects of TCDD because considerably more information is available on TCDD than on the herbicides. Most of the experimental studies of these chemicals, unless otherwise noted, are conducted with pure chemical. This is in contrast to the epidemiologic studies discussed in later chapters in which exposures are often to mixtures of chemicals. Some studies of herbicides are conducted using herbicide mixtures and are noted as such in the text.

This chapter begins with a brief summary of major conclusions derived from the literature reviews in *VAO*, *Update 1996*, and *Update 1998*. This is followed by a summary of toxicological research findings as they relate to human health, and then an overview of the scientific literature published since release of *Update 1998*, reviewed in detail in this chapter. Note that these more general summaries do not include references to the scientific literature because they are intended to provide background for the nonspecialist.

The "Toxicity Profile Updates" section then provides details of the relevant scientific studies, with references, that have been conducted on 2,4-D, 2,4,5-T, picloram, cacodylic acid, and TCDD since *Update 1998*. The toxicity profile update for TCDD includes a section that discusses the issues involved in estimating potential health risk and factors influencing toxicity. That subsection includes a discussion of the toxic equivalency factor approach to estimating the toxicity of TCDD. It is important, when evaluating the experimental data for all of the compounds, to keep in mind the advantages, disadvantages, and limitations of various types of studies. These considerations are discussed in the final section of the chapter, "Issues in Evaluating the Evidence."

LAY SUMMARY

Highlights of Previous Reports

Chapter 4 of *VAO* and Chapter 3 of both *Update 1996* and *Update 1998* review the results of animal and in vitro studies published through 1997 that investigate the toxicokinetics, mechanism of action, and disease outcomes of TCDD and herbicides. According to these earlier reviews, TCDD elicits a diverse spectrum of biological sex-, strain-, age-, and species-specific effects, including carcinogenicity, immunotoxicity, reproductive and developmental toxicity, hepatotoxicity, neurotoxicity, chloracne, and loss of body weight. The scientific consensus is that TCDD is not directly genotoxic and that its ability to influence the carcinogenic process is mediated via epigenetic events such as effects on enzyme induction, cell proliferation, apoptosis, and intracellular communication. The toxicity of the herbicides used in Vietnam has been poorly studied. In general, the herbicides 2,4-D, 2,4,5-T, cacodylic acid, and picloram have not been identified as particularly toxic substances since high concentrations are often required to modulate cellular and biochemical processes. A comprehensive description of the toxicological literature published through 1997 can be found in *VAO*, *Update 1996*, and *Update 1998*.

Toxicokinetics

The distribution of toxicants within the body, or toxicokinetics, can determine the amounts of a particular chemical reaching potential target organs or cells. Earlier data indicate that all four of the herbicides can be absorbed into the body. No data have been published on the toxicokinetics of 2,4-D, 2,4,5-T, or picloram since *Update 1998*. Since *Update 1998*, some research has been conducted that is relevant to the distribution of cacodylic acid, an organic form of arsenic, in the body. The distribution in the body and excretion out of the body of organic arsenicals were shown to be minimally affected by the dose administered. Data also indicate that some organic forms of arsenic are transferred to the fetus, and it was seen following a human poisoning that organic arsenicals preferentially distribute to organs that are high in lipids.

Studies conducted in veterans of Operation Ranch Hand since *Update 1998* have refined estimates of how long it takes for half of the TCDD in the body to be eliminated (i.e., its half-life); the average half-life in humans is 7.6 years. Other studies demonstrate that the distribution of TCDD can be affected by several variables; lipoidal additives in the diet may enhance TCDD excretion, the half-life of TCDD can vary between individuals, and the half-life can vary with dietary modification. Research has also been conducted on how to estimate initial exposure levels using blood measurements of TCDD years after the exposure occurred.

Mechanisms of Toxic Action

There is still little known about the way that herbicides produce toxic effects in animals. Since *Update 1998* the ability of 2,4-D to induce mutations has been investigated using a number of assays. Mutations were seen only in one study and there only at very high concentrations of 2,4-D in vivo. 2,4-D did affect the levels of some hormones and cellular components involved in the development and functioning of brain cells. Both 2,4-D and 2,4,5-T inhibited mitochondrial benzoyl coenzyme A (benzoyl-CoA) synthetase and an organic acid transporter. 2,4,5-T also affected Neu tyrosine kinase, a tyrosine kinase receptor that has been shown in other experiments to be correlated with an increased incidence of breast cancer. The relevance of the effects of 2,4,5-T on that enzyme to the toxic effects of 2,4,5-T is unknown. Cacodylic acid can affect microtubule networks at particular points in mitosis. Research on cacodylic acid indicates that it can cause bladder hyperplasia and tumors in rats, lung cancer in mice, and promote skin cancer in mice sensitized by genetic manipulation or exposure to ultraviolet B radiation. One study in mice has demonstrated that it can cause chromosomal abnormalities.

Data published to date are consistent with the hypothesis that TCDD produces most of its biological and toxic effects by binding to a protein that regulates gene expression, the aryl hydrocarbon receptor (AhR). The binding of TCDD to the AhR triggers a sequence of cellular events that involve interactions with numerous other cellular components. Research in animals that have been engineered not to express the AhR, and in animals with slightly different forms of the receptor, supports a role of the AhR in the toxicity of TCDD. Modulation of genes by AhR may have species-, cell-, and developmental stage-specific patterns, suggesting that the molecular and cellular pathways that lead to any particular toxic event are complex.

Additional research demonstrates that the biochemical and biological outcomes of TCDD exposure can be modulated by numerous other proteins with which the AhR interacts. It is plausible, for example, that the AhR could divert other proteins and transcription factors from other signaling pathways; the disruption of these other pathways could have serious consequences for a number of cell and tissue processes.

With respect to the mechanism underlying the carcinogenic effects of TCDD, it still appears that TCDD does not act directly on the genetic material. Effects on enzymes or hormones could be involved in the carcinogenicity of TCDD.

Disease Outcomes

Recent experiments demonstrated that 2,4-D can cause behavioral effects, muscle weakness, and incoordination in animals, but these effects are seen only at high doses. Reproductive and developmental effects have been seen in animals, but also only at high doses. Furthermore, a precursor of 2,4-D, 4-(2,4-dichlorophenoxy)butyric acid (2,4-DB), did not cause an immunotoxic or carcinogenic response in rodents or dogs. Evidence suggests that cacodylic acid can act as a tumor promoter in mice and rats.

Many effects have been observed in animals following exposure to TCDD, and this contaminant is considered more toxic than the pure components of the herbicides used in Vietnam. Sensitivity to TCDD varies among species and strains, but most species studied develop a "wasting syndrome" from acutely toxic doses. This syndrome is characterized by a loss of body weight and fatty tissue. One target of TCDD is the liver, where lethal doses of TCDD cause necrosis, but the effect is dependent on the animal species exposed. Effects on the morphology and function of the liver are seen at lower doses. A recent study demonstrated that TCDD inhibits the ability of the liver to accumulate vitamin A.

TCDD may affect, directly or indirectly, many organs of the endocrine system in a species-specific manner. For example, thyroid hormone levels are altered by treatment of animals with TCDD. Some of the results in different studies of thyroid hormones are contradictory, however, making interpretation of these results difficult.

The adult nervous system has been shown to be sensitive to the effects of TCDD only at high doses. After in utero exposure, however, even these high-dose effects are not straightforward, with in utero TCDD exposure decreasing performance on certain learning and memory tasks, but improving performance on other tasks.

In animals, one of the most sensitive systems to TCDD toxicity is the immune system. Recent studies have demonstrated that TCDD can alter the levels of immune cells, the measured activity of these cells, and the ability of animals to fight off infection. Effects on the immune system, however, appear to depend on the species, strain, and developmental stage of animal studied.

Reproductive and developmental effects have been seen in animals exposed to TCDD. For example, effects on sperm counts, sperm production, and seminal vesicle weights have been seen in male offspring of rats treated with TCDD during pregnancy. Effects on the female reproductive system have also been seen following developmental exposure to TCDD. In some recent studies, however, the effects on the male and female reproductive system were not accompanied by effects on reproductive outcomes. The mechanism underlying the reproductive effects is not known, but it is possible that they are secondary to effects on reproductive hormones. In recent studies, TCDD did not affect surgically induced endometrial lesions in rats, although effects were seen in earlier studies. Pre- and postnatal exposure of mice to TCDD increased sensitivity to endometrial lesion growth.

TCDD is an extremely potent promoter of neoplasia in laboratory rats. In a recent study, there was an increase in hepatic foci at doses as low as 0.01 ng/kg/day. This is the lowest dose of TCDD to promote tumors to date. Recent data also suggest that promotion of liver tumors by TCDD in female rats is dependent on continuous exposure to TCDD.

Relevance to Human Health

As indicated above, exposure to 2,3,7,8-TCDD has been associated with both cancer and noncancer end points in animals, and most TCDD effects are mediated through the AhR. Although structural differences in the AhR have been identified, it operates in a similar manner in animals and humans, and a connection between TCDD exposure and human health effects is, in general, considered biologically plausible. Animal research indicates that TCDD can cause both cancers and benign tumors, and also enhance the incidence of certain cancers or tumors in the presence of known carcinogens. However, experimental animals differ greatly in their susceptibility to TCDD-induced effects; the sites at which tumors are induced also vary from species to species. Other noncancer health effects vary according to dose and to the animal exposed. Controversy still exists over whether the effects of TCDD and other exposures are threshold dependent, that is, whether some exposure levels may be too low to induce any effect.

Limited information is available on the biologic plausibility that health effects caused by Agent Orange occur through chemicals other than TCDD. Although concerns have been raised about nondioxin contaminants of herbicides, far too little is known about the distribution and concentration of these compounds in the formulations used in Vietnam to draw conclusions concerning their impact.

Considerable uncertainty remains about how to apply mechanistic information from non-human studies to an evaluation of the potential health effects in Vietnam veterans of herbicide or dioxin exposure. Therefore, scientists disagree over the extent to which information derived from animal and cellular studies predicts human health outcomes and the extent to which health effects resulting from high-dose exposure are comparable to those resulting from low-dose exposure. A great deal of research on biological mechanisms has been and continues to be conducted, especially on TCDD. No single mechanism has been established as underlying the toxic effects of TCDD, and with the many different effects seen, more than a single mechanism might exist. It is hoped that as the cellular mechanisms of these compounds are discovered, subsequent *VAO* updates will have better information on which to base conclusions and to aid in determining the relevance of experimental data to effects in humans.

OVERVIEW OF THE SCIENTIFIC LITERATURE IN *UPDATE 2000*

Toxicokinetics

Since *Update 1998*, no data have been published that add to the information available on the toxicokinetics of 2,4-D, 2,4,5-T, or picloram. Research has been conducted on the distribution of cacodylic acid, an organic form of arsenic that was used as an herbicide in small quantities in Vietnam. Research in mice demonstrates that the administered dose minimally affects the distribution and excretion of organic arsenicals. In humans it was observed that at least some organic forms of arsenic are transferred to the fetus and that organic arsenicals are distributed more to organs that are high in lipids.

In contrast, a great deal of research conducted since *Update 1998* improves the understanding of the processes that affect the distribution of TCDD to different parts of the body. Studies continue to demonstrate that an enzyme, cytochrome P450 1A2 (CYP1A2), plays an important role in the distribution of TCDD. CYP1A2 is expressed at high levels in the liver and binds TCDD. Because of this binding, the levels of TCDD in the liver are more dependent on CYP1A2 levels than on liver lipid content, but this is highly dependent on the concentration of TCDD. Experiments in mice that do not express the *Cyp1A2* gene (*Cyp1A2* knockout mice) in the liver further demonstrate the importance of CYP1A2 protein in the distribution of TCDD. A greater amount of TCDD is distributed to other organs, and urinary excretion is increased in knockout animals. In addition to CYP1A2 levels, other polyhalogenated aromatic hydrocarbons (PHAHs) can affect the toxicokinetics of TCDD; there is decreased retention of TCDD in the presence of other PHAHs.

Studies have been conducted investigating the length of time that TCDD remains in the body and the factors that can influence this. Follow-up examinations in Operation Ranch Hand veterans indicate that TCDD has a mean half-life of 7.6 years and elimination is inversely proportional to bodyfat content, but that age does not have an observable effect on elimination. A study in non-Ranch Hand Vietnam veterans, however, shows that age has a weak effect on the elimination rate of TCDD, and a study in an occupationally exposed cohort also indicates that the elimination rate changes with age, but this may, in part, reflect changes in body composition with age. These studies converge on a consistent estimate of half-life but are inconsistent on the effect of age.

TCDD is also excreted in breast milk, causing both a decrease in maternal TCDD levels and the transfer of TCDD to breast-fed infants. Recent studies show that the volume of breast milk produced can affect the rate at which TCDD is eliminated from the mother. In addition, the concentration of TCDD in breast milk decreases over time with continued breast feeding. Modeling the residue kinetics in infants indicates that the TCDD initially accumulated in infants following exposure from breast feeding is substantially decreased by 2 years of age.

Dietary factors also can affect the absorption and excretion of TCDD. The amount of fat in the diet can greatly affect absorption and excretion. Ingestion of a nonabsorbed dietary fat substitute (olestra) increased the fecal excretion of a very high dose of TCDD.

It is important to know whether the TCDD levels measured in blood are representative of levels in target tissues because TCDD is often measured in blood in human studies. Autopsy studies of human tissues indicate that there is a correlation between the levels of TCDD measured in the blood lipids and the levels measured in adipose, kidney, spleen, liver, and brain tissue, but not in muscle and lung tissue. A study in rodents demonstrates that concentrations of TCDD in the fetal compartment are comparable to the levels in maternal blood.

Mechanisms of Toxic Action

Since *Update 1998*, the actions of 2,4-D, 2,4,5-T, cacodylic acid, and TCDD at the molecular and cellular level have been investigated. These studies enhance our understanding of the actions of these chemicals, particularly TCDD, but the exact mechanisms by which these chemicals are toxic still are not established. No new research has been published that provides data on the mechanisms underlying the toxic effects of picloram.

2,4-D has previously been shown to have low oncogenic potential, with genotoxic effects seen only at high concentrations. Recent evidence is consistent with these earlier data. Only a high concentration of 2,4-D was genotoxic in a wing spot test. There was no evidence of genotoxicity in assays testing for recombination; bacterial gene mutation; chromosomal aberrations; forward mutations in the hypoxanthine-guanine phosphoribosyl transferase gene (*HGPRT*) locus; and induction of DNA damage, repair, and unscheduled synthesis, as well as in tests of the frequency of micronucleated polychromatic erythrocytes in mice.

Research continues to demonstrate effects of 2,4-D on hormone levels and the function of the nervous system. 2,4-D decreased serum thyroxine concentrations, testosterone concentrations in serum and gonads, and serum concentrations of lutenizing hormone, follicle-stimulating hormone, prostaglandin I_2, and prostaglandin E_2. 2,4-D also inhibited neurite extension in primary cultures of cerebellar granule cells. This effect is accompanied by a reduction in cellular microtubules, disorganization of the Golgi apparatus, and inhibition of ganglioside synthesis. It also inhibits the polymerization of purified tubulin. Although the biological relevance of these affects is not established, it is possible that the effects on hormones and the nervous system are involved in the reproductive and neurological toxicity seen at high doses of 2,4-D.

Both 2,4-D and 2,4,5-T have inhibitory effects on the formation and renal transport of benzylglycine. These compounds inhibit the mitochondrial enzyme benzoyl-CoA synthetase and competitively inhibit an organic acid transporter, inhibiting the secretion of benzoylglycine. 2,4,5-T also activated Neu tyrosine kinase in a cell-free system, stimulated the enzyme in MCF-7 cells, and stimulated foci formation of MCF-7 cells. Although activation of Neu tyrosine kinase has been found to be correlated with an increased incidence of breast cancer in animal models, how these cellular and biochemical effects are related to any toxic end point is unknown.

Most research indicates that cacodylic acid can act as a promoter in the carcinogenic process, and one study has demonstrated that it can cause aneuploidy. It also can disrupt cell growth by affecting the microtubule network. Evidence indicates that it decreases liver glutathione levels, as well as pulmonary and hepatic ornithine decarboxylase levels.

Studies published since *Update 1998* are consistent with the hypothesis that TCDD produces its biological and toxic effects by binding to the AhR. For example, recent data indicate that TCDD has only minimal teratogenicity, if any, in *AhR* knockout mice compared to wild-type mice. Data from knockout mice also suggest that the AhR plays an important, but as yet unknown, developmental and physiological role. Many of the recent data published are consistent also with the notion that cellular processes involving growth, maturation, and differentiation are sensitive to TCDD-induced effects. Findings in animals indicating that reproductive, developmental, and oncogenic end points appear to be sensitive to TCDD are consistent with this notion, and the cellular data provide biologic plausibility for similar end points of toxicity in exposed humans. However, many of the responses to TCDD are tissue- and species-specific and the mechanistic basis for these differences is not completely understood.

The presence of the AhR and ARNT in a variety of tissues from different animal species and strains is well documented. Detailed analysis of variant forms has provided much information associating structure and expression levels with function. Furthermore, experiments in species and strains expressing different forms of the AhR suggest that differences in specific regions of the AhR may be in part responsible for differential sensitivity to TCDD. Evidence continues to indicate that the sequence of the AhR in humans is highly conserved among different individuals.

Research has shown that the association of several proteins with newly synthesized AhR may modulate AhR function. For example, association with 90 kDa heat shock protein (HSP90) is important to maintain the AhR in a conformation that can bind ligand. Recent data are consistent with a mechanism in which HSP90 is released from the ligand-bound AhR following nuclear localization concomitant with ARNT–AhR dimerization. One study, however, demonstrated that dissociation of HSP90 is not required for nuclear translocation of the AhR but is essential for dimerization with ARNT.

Many of the more recent investigations have focused on identifying and characterizing factors that may modulate, by either activation or repression, the ability of the activated AhR–ARNT complex to alter gene expression. In addition, several studies have noted the ability of a variety of AhR ligands to act as receptor antagonists. Studies have investigated the roles of immunophilin proteins, nuclear accessory proteins or coactivators, repression by as yet unidentified cellular factors specific to certain cell types, nuclear factor κB (NF-κB), and histone acetylators and deacetylators.

Investigations into the endogenous ligand for the AhR continue. Although several endogenous compounds which bind to the AhR have been described, it is not yet clear whether any of these have any physiological significance. Naturally occurring ligands for the receptor include resveratrol, curcumin, tryptophan metabolites, galangin, the dietary flavonols quercetin and kaempferol, lipoxin A4, and products of heme metabolism.

Details of the many studies investigating the cellular and molecular effects of TCDD are summarized later in this chapter.

Disease Outcomes

Studies published since *Update 1998* are consistent with the previous view that 2,4-D is relatively nontoxic and has weak oncogenic potential. Decreased motor activity, muscle weakness, motor incoordination, decreased weight gain, and serum alterations were seen only at doses greater than 100 mg/kg. Reversible and permanent behavioral alterations have also been seen in rats following treatment with high doses of 2,4-D from gestational day 16 to postnatal day 23. These observations are consistent with previous studies suggesting that 2,4-D could have neurotoxic effects. Exposure to 2,4-D had no effect on lymphocyte blastogenesis, immunoglobulin M (IgM) antibody production in response to sheep red blood cells, expression of lymphocyte cell surface markers, or phagocytic function of peritoneal macrophages. Only mild, reversible effects on the skin were observed following 2,4-D treatments. Developing fetuses appear to be the most sensitive to the effects of 4-(2,4-2,4-dichlorophenoxy)butyric acid (2,4-DB), of which 2,4-D is the major metabolite, but even these effects occur at relatively high concentrations. There was no evidence of an oncogenic response in studies of rodents and dogs treated with 2,4-DB.

The ability of 2,4,5-T to produce myelotoxicity was examined using the mouse granulocyte–macrophage (GM) colony-forming unit (CFU) assay and the 3-[4,5-dimethylthiazol-2-yl]-2,5-diphenyl tetrazolium bromide (MTT) test for inhibition of proliferation. The concentration that caused a 50 percent inhibition in the assays (i.e., the IC_{50}) was at least 202 µM, indicating a relatively weak potency of 2,4,5-T to produce myelotoxicity. No other studies were found that investigate disease outcomes following exposure to 2,4,5-T.

The pulmonary carcinogenic activity of cacodylic acid (dimethylarsinic acid, DMA) was examined in mice; treated mice developed more pulmonary neoplasms (number per mouse) than untreated mice. Exposure to DMA for 2 years produced bladder hyperplasia and tumors in rats. In other studies, DMA acted as a skin cancer promoter in transgenic mice sensitive to carcinogens and in hairless mice irradiated with ultraviolet B radiation.

There are no recent studies investigating toxic effects following exposure to picloram; one study looking at oxidative functions showed effects of Tordon 75D (a mixture of the triisopropanolamine salts of 2,4-D and picloram) and attributed these effects to the surfactant in the mixture, not picloram.

Many effects have been observed in animals following exposure to TCDD. The classic symptoms of the "wasting syndrome" (i.e., extreme loss of body weight, decreased food consumption with an increase in consumption prior to death, and bloody stool) were observed in female mink treated with TCDD.

Thermoregulatory control is affected by TCDD. A study in rats indicates that the thermoregulatory centers in the hypothalamus are not permanently altered by TCDD.

Neurotoxic effects have been observed after developmental exposure to TCDD, with some learning and memory tasks being affected in rats.

Of the many organ systems affected by TCDD, one of the most sensitive is the immune system. Increased parasitic larval burdens occurred in rats following TCDD exposure; there was some indication that age increased the sensitivity of humoral immunity to TCDD exposure. TCDD has been shown to decrease delayed-type hypersensitivity responses, decrease the total percentage of $CD4^+$ cells and the percentage of the $CD4^+$ cells cycling following repeated exposure, and stimulate the production of interleukin-2 (IL-2) and increase the percentage of $CD4^+$ and $CD8^+$ cells in the S and $G2^M$ phase of lymphocyte cycling in primed rats. Although there are considerable species and strain differences in immune responses to TCDD, some evidence indicates that TCDD compromises (suppresses) the immune system of laboratory animals.

Developmental effects on the male reproductive system have been seen following exposure to TCDD. Male offspring of rats gavaged on gestational day 15 with TCDD had significantly decreased body and seminal vesicle weights, and decreased epithelial branching and differentiation in the seminal vesicles. In another study, the number of sperm per cauda epididymis and daily sperm production were decreased, and sperm transit rate was affected at puberty and adulthood in male offspring of female rats treated with TCDD. In the highest-TCDD-exposure group, serum testosterone concentration was decreased at adulthood. In this study, however, reproductive outcomes of those males were not affected. Similarly, female offspring of pregnant female hamsters treated with TCDD on gestational day 15 showed effects on the reproductive system, but reproductive outcomes in female progeny were not reported.

In recent studies TCDD did not affect surgically induced endometrial lesions in rats, although effects were seen in earlier studies. The lesions were increased in mice only with a combination of perinatal and adult exposure to TCDD. Some researchers suggest that TCDD blocks the ability of progesterone to prevent experimental endometriosis, which correlates with its ability to inhibit progesterone-associated transforming growth factor-β_2 (TGF-β_2) expression and endometrial matrix metalloproteinase suppression.

In utero and lactational exposure of rats to TCDD decreased prostate weight without inhibiting testicular androgen production or decreasing serum androgen concentrations. Additional studies showed that the prostatic epithelial budding process was impaired, suggesting that in utero and lactational TCDD exposure interferes with prostate development by decreasing early epithelial growth, delaying cell differentiation, and producing alterations in epithelial and stromal cell histological arrangement and the spatial distribution of androgen receptor expression.

Data are conflicting as to whether TCDD induces cellular apoptosis. This may be highly dependent on cell type. TCDD failed to induce apoptosis in Fas-deficient and Fas-ligand-defective mice at the lower doses tested, compared to control wild-type mice, suggesting that Fas–Fas ligand interactions may play a role in the TCDD-mediated induction of apoptosis.

TCDD is an extremely potent promoter of neoplasia in laboratory rats. TCDD significantly increased the volume fraction and number of altered hepatic foci at the highest dose. Increases in the number of guanosine 5'-triphosphatase (GTPase) and adenosine 5'-triphosphatase (ATPase) deficient altered hepatic foci per cubic centimeter also occurred at doses as low as 0.01 ng/kg/day. This is the lowest dose of TCDD to promote tumors to date. Recent data also suggest that promotion of liver tumors by TCDD in female rats is dependent on continuous exposure to TCDD.

TOXICITY PROFILE UPDATES

This section updates the toxicity profiles of the five substances discussed in *VAO*, *Update 1996*, and *Update 1998*: (1) 2,4-D, (2) 2,4,5-T, (3) picloram, (4) cacodylic acid, and (5) TCDD (dioxin). The chemical nature of these substances is discussed in more detail in Chapter 6 of *VAO*.

Each profile update contains a review of experimental studies published during 1998–2000. Information in this literature update is organized under the following topics: (1) toxicokinetics, (2) mechanisms of toxic action, (3) disease outcomes, and if applicable, (4) estimating potential health risks and factors influencing toxicity.

Toxicity Profile Update of 2,4-D

Toxicokinetics

No toxicokinetic studies were identified for the reference period.

Mechanisms of Toxic Action

In *Update 1998*, several studies supported the view that the mechanism of toxic action of 2,4-D involved disruption of thiol homeostasis. No new studies have been published regarding this aspect.

Several studies, using in vitro and in vivo model systems, published since *Update 1998* are consistent with the relatively weak genotoxic potential of 2,4-D. Using the *Drosophila melanogaster* wing spot test, which assesses somatic mutation and recombination events, a slight, but significant, increase in the frequency of total spots was observed only at the highest concentration (10 mM) of 2,4-D tested. To determine recombinagenic activity, the frequency of *Mwh* (multiple wing hairs) clones was also evaluated. No increases were observed with any concentration of 2,4-D (Kaya et al., 1999). Another study examined the potential genetic toxicity of 2,4-D and seven of its salts and esters by examining their ability to produce gene mutations in bacteria (Ames test) and their ability to induce DNA damage, repair, and unscheduled DNA synthesis in rat hepatocytes. For all assays, there were no indications of genotoxicity (Charles et al., 1999a). Similarly, no evidence for the genotoxicity of 2,4-D was observed using assays in which the induction of chromosomal aberrations in primary cultures of rat lymphocytes and forward mutations at the *HGPRT* locus of Chinese hamster ovary cells were examined (Gollapudi et al., 1999). The ability of 2,4-D and its derivatives to induce cytogenetic abnormalities in vivo was also investigated by examining the frequency of micronucleated polychromatic erythrocytes (MN-PCEs) in mice treated with these chemicals by oral gavage. There were no increases in MN-PCE for single doses of 2,4-D up to 400 mg/kg (Charles et al., 1999b).

Notably, all of the above results are consistent with recent data indicating the lack of oncogenic response to 2,4-dichlorophenoxybutyric acid, of which 2,4-D is the major metabolite, following chronic exposure of rats, mice, and dogs (Charles and Leeming, 1998a,b) (see below).

Investigations by Gregus et al. (1999) indicate that both 2,4-D and 2,4,5-T may interfere with the biotransformation and renal elimination of small aromatic carboxylic acids. The effect of these herbicides on glycine conjugation and excretion of benzoic acid was examined. The inhibition of benzoylglycine formation by 2,4-D was demonstrated in the rat following a single intraperitoneal treatment with 110.5 mg/kg. It was found that 2,4-D acted as an inhibitor, but not a substrate, of mitochondrial benzoyl-CoA synthetase. 2,4-D also inhibited the renal secretion of benzoylglycine, apparently by acting as a competitive substrate of the organic acid transporter. 2,4,5-T was approximately equipotent in producing those same effects.

Several studies suggest effects of 2,4-D on hormones and hormone-regulated functions. Prior to *Update 1998*, investigations reported effects of 2,4-D on serum concentrations of thyroid hormones, particularly, thyroxine. Similarly, Rawlings et al. (1998) observed that two oral doses of 2,4-D of 10 mg/kg/week for 43 days to ewes resulted in significant decreases in serum thyroxine concentrations. No overt signs of toxicity were observed, and there were no significant effects on blood concentrations of luteinizing hormone (LH), follicle-stimulating hormone (FSH), progesterone, estradiol, cortisol, or insulin. Treating male rats with 5 and 50 mg/kg/day for a month, however, led to decreased testosterone levels in serum and gonads. In addition, these dosages produced decreased serum concentrations of LH, FSH, prostaglandin I_2, and prostaglandin E_2 (Galimov et al., 1998).

A study by Oakes and Pollak (1999) evaluated the toxicity of the components of Tordon 75D (a mixture of the triisopropanolamine salts of 2,4-D and picloram) on the oxidative functions of submitochondrial particles (SMPs). Notably, the concentrations that caused a 50 percent inhibition of oxidative functions (i.e., the effective concentration$_{50}$, EC_{50}) were in the low micromolar range for 2,4-D and picloram in the presence of other components of Tordon 75D (triisopropanolamine, diethylene glycol monoethyl ether, a silicone defoamer, and a proprietary surfactant). However, in the absence of the other components, the EC_{50} values for these chemicals were approximately 136 times higher. The results indicate that the toxic effects of Tordon 75D on SMPs and intact rat liver mitochondria were caused mainly, if not solely, by the proprietary surfactant.

Rosso and coworkers (2000) examined the effects of 2,4-D on primary cultures of cerebellar granule cells. A 24-hour exposure to concentrations up to 2 mM produced a dose-dependent inhibition of neurite extension. This inhibition was accompanied by a reduction in the cellular content of microtubules, disorganization of the Golgi apparatus, and inhibition of ganglioside synthesis. They also observed that 2,4-D inhibited the polymerization of purified tubulin in vitro.

Disease Outcomes

Studies published since *Update 1998* are consistent with the previous view that 2,4-D is relatively nontoxic and has weak oncogenic potential. Developing fetuses appear to be the most sensitive to the effects of 2,4-D for a number of toxic end points.

Lethality

Morgulis et al. (1998) studied the acute oral toxicity of 2,4-D in chicks. A number of signs of toxicity were observed, but only at doses higher than 100 mg/kg. Those effects included decreased motor activity, muscle weakness, motor incoordination, and decreased weight gain. Serum alterations included increased serum uric acid, creatinine and total protein, and serum creatine kinase and alkaline phosphatase activities. These changes were time dependent and reversible at the lower doses. The dose that causes death in 50 percent of the animals (i.e., LD_{50}) was 420 mg/kg. Histopathological postmortem examination indicated vacuolar degeneration of hepatocytes, renal tubular necrosis, and intestinal hemorrhages.

Barile and Cardona (1998) examined 30 different chemicals in cytotoxicity assays using human fetal lung fibroblasts and human skin fibroblasts in culture to evaluate the methods as screens for cytotoxicity and as potential predictors of human toxicity. IC_{50} values of 2,4-D in these cell lines ranged from 0.87 to 1.3 mg/ml. Evaluation of data for the other chemicals suggests that the experimental IC_{50} values are as accurate predictors of human toxicity as equivalent blood concentrations derived from rodent LD_{50} studies.

Bracco and Favre (1999) described an acute fatal case of 2,4-D self-poisoning. A plasma concentration of 2,4-D of 720 µg/kg was measured. Clinical and hemodynamic data indicated the failure of multiple organ systems, supporting an uncoupling of oxidative phosphorylation as a predominant mechanism of 2,4-D toxicity in this case.

Neurotoxicity

Studies by Bortolozzi et al. (1999) examined whether exposure of rats to 2,4-D during pre- and postnatal development induces behavioral alterations. Pregnant rats were exposed to 70 mg/kg/day from gestational day 16 to postnatal day 23. This exposure produced no overt signs of toxicity, but several types of neurobehavioral alterations were observed. Some of the effects were reversible, others were permanent, and others were seen only after pharmacological challenges. Although the exact mechanism of these effects is unknown, some of the results suggest that alterations in the serotonergic and dopaminergic systems might be involved.

Immunotoxicity

Blakley et al. (1998) examined the effects of a commercial formulation of 2,4-D on immune function in male rats. 2,4-D was administered orally twice per week for 28 days at a dosage of 10 mg/kg. No effect on body weight was observed. Exposure to 2,4-D had no effect on lymphocyte blastogenesis, IgM antibody production in response to sheep red blood cells, expression of lymphocyte cell surface markers, or phagocytic function of peritoneal macrophages.

Dermatotoxicity

Kimura et al. (1998) examined the dermatotoxicity of several chemicals with or without ultraviolet (UV) irradiation in hairless descendants of Mexican hairless dogs. Each agent was applied daily for 7 days as a 0.1 percent solution in ethanol:propylene glycol:distilled water (2:1:2 volume per volume [v/v]) to a 3 cm × 3 cm test site at a concentration of 4 µl/cm^2. One day after cessation of the 2,4-D treatment only mild histological changes (i.e., slight epidermal thickening) were observed. At 14 days after treatment, no significant lesions were observed that were different from controls at sites treated with 2,4-D with or without UV exposure.

Reproductive or Developmental Toxicity

Charles et al. (1999c) performed developmental toxicity studies in rats and rabbits and a two-generation reproduction toxicity study in rats using 2,4-DB, whose major metabolite is 2,4-D. The maximum tolerated dose (MTD) was exceeded at 125 mg/kg/day as evidenced by maternal body weight loss and resorption of fetuses in several dams. The no-observable-adverse-effect level (NOAEL) for maternal toxicity in rats was 31.25 mg/kg/day based on decreased body weight gain. The NOAEL for embryonic or fetal toxicity was also 31.25 mg/kg/day based on fetal skeletal anomalies. For rabbits, the MTD was exceeded at 60 mg/kg/day based on decreased body weight gain, abortions in two does, and moribund conditions of two does. The NOAEL for maternal toxicity in rabbits was 30 mg/kg/day based on decreased body weight gain, and the NOAEL for embryonic or fetal toxicity was 60 mg/kg/day. For the two-generation study in rats, maternal performance, fertility rate, and pregnancy were unimpaired at concentrations of 60 and 300 parts per million (ppm). A NOAEL for reproductive toxicity was 1,500 ppm (111.8 mg/kg/day for males and 110.6 mg/kg/day for females), but severe postnatal toxicity was produced at this level. The NOAEL for postnatal toxicity based on litter size, decreased weight gain, and pup mortality was 22.5–32.6 mg/kg/day in males and 26.4–36.7 mg/kg/day in females. Notably, these NOAEL values are similar to the values obtained for 2,4-D and indicate the relatively low reproductive and developmental toxicity of these chemicals.

Carcinogenicity

An investigation by Charles and Leeming (1998a) evaluated the chronic (2-year) dietary toxicity and oncogenicity of 2,4-DB in rodents. Concentrations of 2,4-DB in food were as high as 1,800 ppm. A NOAEL of 2.48 mg/kg/day for male rats and 3.23 mg/kg/day for female rats was observed based on decreased body weight gain. Minor histopathological lesions were thought to be due to decreased body weight gain. There was no evidence of increased tumors at any dose level. Likewise, no oncogenic effect was observed in an 18-month chronic feeding study in mice. The highest dosages were 128.7 and 100.4 mg/kg/day for 66 weeks in female and male mice, respectively, and 110.6 mg/kg/day for 104 weeks in male rats. A similar 1-year study was conducted with 2,4-DB in dogs (Charles and Leeming, 1998b). The highest dosages for male and female dogs were 12.94 mg/kg/day and 14.16 mg/kg/day for 52 weeks, respectively. Treatment-related findings include reductions in body weight gain and food consumption, and small increases in serum levels of inorganic phosphorus, blood urea nitrogen, creatinine, aspartate aminotransferase, and alanine aminotransferase. Most of these values, except for aspartate aminotransferase, returned to normal in a group allowed a 4-week recovery period following cessation of treatment. Histopathological changes related to treatment were seen predominantly in the liver and kidney. These changes were less marked in animals after the 4-week recovery period. There was no evidence for any immunotoxic or oncogenic response. A NOAEL of 75 ppm 2,4-DB (2.39 and 2.15 mg/kg/day for males and females, respectively) was seen. All three studies were consistent with the generally low toxicity and weak oncogenic potential of 2,4-DB.

Toxicity Profile Update of 2,4,5-T

Toxicokinetics

No toxicokinetic studies of 2,4,5-T were identified for the reference period.

Mechanisms of Toxic Action

Studies summarized in *Update 1998* indicate that 2,4,5-T enters cells and disrupts cellular pathways involving acetylcoenzyme A. It was suggested that this might be the mechanism for altered cholinergic transmission and the mechanism for neurotoxicity.

As reported for 2,4-D, 2,4,5-T was found to interfere with both the formation and the renal transport of benzylglycine, the glycine conjugate of benzoic acid, in the rat. Reported data suggest that these effects were due to the inhibition of mitochondrial benzoyl-CoA synthetase by 2,4,5-T and the ability of this chemical to act as a competitive substrate of the renal organic acid transporter. 2,4,5-T was approximately equipotent with 2,4-D for these effects (Gregus et al., 1999).

Activation of the Neu tyrosine kinase has been found to be highly correlated with an increased incidence of breast cancer and may have prognostic value in predicting overall survival and time to breast cancer relapse. Hatakeyama and Matsumura (1999) examined the ability of several organochlorine compounds to activate Neu tyrosine kinase and promote foci formation in human MCF-7 breast tumor cells. 2,4,5-T, at a concentration of 1 nM, was found to significantly activate Neu tyrosine kinase in a cell-free system and stimulate this enzyme at 100 nM in intact MCF-7 cells. A concentration of 100 nM 2,4,5-T also stimulated foci formation of MCF-7 cells to approximately 56 percent the level induced by 100 nM estradiol. Notably, there was a reasonable correlation between the ability of the individual organochlorine compounds to activate Neu tyrosine kinase in the cell-free system and to induce foci formation. The exact mechanism by which 2,4,5-T modulates Neu tyrosine kinase activity is not known. It is also not clear how these effects are related to any toxic end point observed in vivo.

Disease Outcomes

Update 1998 focused on the ability of 2,4,5-T to acutely affect neuronal and muscular function by altering cholinergic transmission. Also, the ability of 2,4,5-T to alter xenobiotic metabolizing enzymes was indicated. No further research has been published in these areas.

Gribaldo et al. (1998) examined several environmental contaminants, including 2,4,5-T, for their ability to produce myelotoxicity using the mouse CFU-GM assay and the MTT test for inhibition of proliferation. The IC_{50} for the ability of 2,4,5-T to inhibit CFU-GM was >391 µM. For the MTT assay, the IC_{50} values were 202 and >391 µM for two different cell lines. Those data suggest that 2,4,5-T has a relatively weak potency to produce myelotoxicity.

Toxicity Profile Update of Cacodylic Acid

Cacodylic acid (dimethylarsinic acid, DMA; Chemical Abstracts Service [CAS] registry number 75-60-5) was present (4.7 percent) in an herbicide that was used in Vietnam in defoliation and crop destruction missions. As discussed in *VAO*, cacodylic acid is a metabolite of inorganic arsenic, but it is very resistant to hydrolysis and no demethylation of cacodylic acid to inorganic arsenic has been observed in any species. Therefore, only studies relevant to organic arsenic, not the entire literature on inorganic arsenic, are reviewed in this toxicity profile.

Toxicokinetics

Arsenic forms reactive metabolites that affect cellular respiration and nearly every organ system in the body. The potency of the arsenical compounds (organic and inorganic), however, depends on absorption rates. Soluble forms are more readily absorbed than the more insoluble preparations. Methylation of inorganic arsenic to monomethylarsonic acid (MMA) and dimethylarsinic acid (DMA) is a pathway of inorganic biotransformation. It remains to be determined whether inorganic arsenic, and/or its methylated metabolites or other reactive intermediates formed in the methylation process mediate arsenic toxicity. The primary route of excretion is via the urine.

Hughes et al. (1999) evaluated the differences in inorganic arsenic disposition (methylation) between three strains of mice to determine whether there are strain differences in the methylation of arsenic. There were no overall differences in arsenic disposition between the strains of mice. Hughes and Kenyon (1998) injected mice with radioactive MMA and DMA to determine whether dose affects the excretion and tissue deposition of these two organic arsenicals. It was determined that dose had a minimal effect on excretion and tissue disposition of these compounds. More recently, however, Hughes et al. (2000) found that retention of DMA in the lung increased with increased doses of DMA.

In a study to evaluate transfer of arsenic to the fetus and suckling infant, it was found that the concentration of arsenic in cord blood (9 µg/l) was similar to maternal blood (11 µg/l) (Concha et al., 1998). Essentially all of the arsenic in the blood of both newborns and their mothers was in the form of DMA, an end product of metabolism of inorganic arsenic. Approximately 90 percent of urinary arsenic in both the newborns and their mothers during late gestation was present as DMA. Therefore, the authors suggested that methylation of arsenic is increased during pregnancy and that DMA is the major form of arsenic transferred to the fetus.

Human organs were examined for the distribution of arsenic species following fatal acute intoxication by arsenic trioxide (Benramdane et al., 1999). The liver and kidneys contained the highest concentrations of total arsenic. The total concentration in the blood was up to 350 times less than in organs. Arsenic(III) was the predominant species, while MMA was more concentrated than DMA. MMA and DMA were more prevalent in organs high in lipids compared to other organs.

Mechanisms of Toxic Action

Most evidence indicates that DMA acts in the carcinogenic process as a promoter. A recent study demonstrated that DMA could cause aneuploidy in bone marrow cells following a single intraperitoneal injection in mice.

Kato et al. (1999) investigated the mechanism underlying the suppression of apoptosis by DMA. A heat shock protein (HSP79) was induced by 3-hour exposure to 10 mM DMA. The authors suggest that the induction could mediate DMA's suppression of apoptosis.

Ochi et al. (1998, 1999) investigated the effects of DMA in Chinese hamster V79 cells. DMA decreased growth and caused morphological changes in these cells by disrupting the microtubule network during the transition from interphase to mitosis.

Disease Outcomes

Sakurai et al. (1998) showed that methylated arsenicals, including DMA, have lower cytotoxicity in mouse macrophage cells than inorganic arsenicals. Using three different cytotoxicity assays, Petrick et al. (2000) found that DMA has a higher LD_{50} in Chang human hepatocytes than monomethylarsonic acid, monomethylarsonous acid, and arsenite.

Ahmad et al. (1999) observed decreases in liver glutathione concentration, evidence of hepatic DNA damage, and reduced pulmonary and hepatic ornithine decarboxylase in mice gavaged once with 720 mg DMA/kg. The authors indicate that mice are less responsive to the toxicity of DMA than rats.

Several recent investigations have focused on the carcinogenic properties of arsenicals in mice and rats. The pulmonary carcinogenic activity of DMA was examined in A/J mice fed 400 ppm DMA for 50 weeks (Hayashi et al., 1998). Treated mice developed more pulmonary neoplasms (number per mouse) than untreated mice. In another study, DMA fed to F344 rats for 2 years produced bladder hyperplasia and tumors at 40 and 100 ppm; more effects were seen in females than in males (Arnold et al., 1999). Using scanning electron microscopy to evaluate urothelial toxicity and hyperplasia after 10 weeks of exposure, it was determined that the urothelial effects of DMA were reversible, that the toxicity is probably not due to urinary solids, and that the toxicity and regeneration are produced in a dose-responsive manner in female rats. In a similar study (M. Wei et al., 1999), urinary bladder tumors were produced in male rats administered 50 or 200 ppm DMA in drinking water for 104 weeks. The authors proposed that DMA may be related to the human carcinogenicity of arsenicals. DMA also promoted urinary bladder neoplasms in $\alpha 2\mu$-globulin-deficient rats, the NCI-Black-Reiter rat (Li et al., 1998), and (Lewis x F344) F_1 rats (Chen et al., 1999).

Morikawa et al. (2000) demonstrated that DMA can promote skin carcinogenesis. Transgenic mice with ornithine decarboxylase targeted to hair follicle keratinocytes have an increased sensitivity to carcinogens. These mice were initiated with 7,12-dimethylbenz[a]anthracene and treated topically once with 3.6 mg DMA. Induction of skin tumors was significantly accelerated in mice treated with DMA. Yamanaka et al. (2000) also demonstrated that DMA can be a skin cancer promoter. Hairless mice irradiated with UVB and dosed with DMA (100 ppm in drinking water) had more malignant tumors with severe atypism than irradiated mice not dosed with DMA.

Toxicity Profile Update of Picloram

Since *Update 1998*, only one study has been published that is relevant to the toxicity of picloram. Oakes and Pollak (1999) evaluated the toxicity of the components of Tordon 75D (a mixture of the triisopropanolamine salts of 2,4-D and picloram) on the oxidative functions of submitochondrial particles. Details of that study are discussed further in the section on 2,4-D. Results indicate that the toxic effects of Tordon 75D on SMPs and intact rat liver mitochondria were caused mainly, if not solely, by the proprietary surfactant.

Toxicity Profile Update of TCDD

Toxicokinetics

The distribution of planar halogenated aromatic hydrocarbons, including specific congeners of the polychlorinated dibenzo-*p*-dioxins (PCDDs), polychlorinated dibenzofurans (PCDFs), and polychlorinated biphenyls (PCBs), has been examined extensively in animal models and to a lesser extent in humans. These chemicals are all hydrophobic and thus tend to be absorbed readily across cell membranes. Properties of the chemicals, properties of the organs and cells, and route of exposure affect the partitioning, absorption, and accumulation of these chemicals. Lipid content is a major factor in the accumulation of TCDD and other PHAHs in different organs and in the body as a whole. Biological processes, especially metabolism, subsequently can affect the distribution and elimination of these chemicals. The concentration of chemical in a given tissue thus depends on the dose as well as the absorption, lipid content, metabolism, and excretion within the organ of concern and in other organs. In addition, binding proteins in some organs may influence the accumulation of TCDD in extrahepatic organs. For example, proteins present in the liver can bind TCDD causing it to accumulate there rather than other organs.

The toxicokinetics of TCDD are discussed in *VAO, Update 1996*, and *Update 1998*. These reports indicate that TCDD is distributed to all compartments of the body. Since *Update 1998* there have been several findings that improve our understanding of processes affecting this distribution. Earlier, Wang et al. (1997) identified parameters important in modeling the pharmacokinetic (or toxicokinetic) behavior of TCDD. Santostefano et al. (1998) tested the model as related to cytochrome P450 gene expression in rats. The model was further evaluated by Wang et al. (2000) across doses, gender, strain, and species. Those studies and the results of Evans and Anderson (2000) assessing available physiologically-based pharmacokinetic (PBPK) models indicate that PBPK models can validly predict the distribution of TCDD in animals.

DeVito et al. (1998) have addressed further the role of inducible proteins, especially cytochrome P450 1A2, in sequestering TCDD and related PHAHs in liver. CYP1A2 continues to be established as a determining factor in this sequestration. The planar halogenated compounds examined by DeVito et al. (1998), including PCDDs, PCDFs, and PCBs, showed increased concentrations in liver relative to the concentrations in adipose tissue or skin, a condition not seen with the noncoplanar compounds. Thus, these chemicals do not distribute solely on the basis of lipid solubility. However, an examination of dose–accumulation relationships for TCDD and other dioxin-like compounds in mice showed that TCDD was sequestered in liver to a lesser extent than some other PHAHs. For example, the liver–adipose ratio at a high dose of TCDD was about 3, while for 2,3,4,7,8-pentachlorodibenzofuran (PeCDF) at the same dose, the ratio was about 10. The structure–activity relationships for sequestration are not the same as those determined previously for binding to the AhR (Safe, 1990).

The issue of chemical absorption when the exposure is to mixtures is an important consideration because environmental exposures almost always involve mixtures. In a study in rats, van der Plas et al. (1998) examined possible interactions between dioxin-like and non-dioxin-like compounds and found that combined exposures can alter the toxicokinetics and patterns of elimination of specific compounds. The retention of TCDD is decreased by the presence of other PHAHs. These researchers showed that liver lipid content was positively correlated with retention of non-AhR agonists but that no such correlation was observed with TCDD or TCDF; the authors suggested that the lack of correlation results from CYP1A2 binding of the latter compounds.

The importance of CYP1A2 in influencing the pharmacokinetic behavior of TCDD was emphasized further in rodent studies by Diliberto et al. (1999). The tissue distributions of TCDD, another potent AhR agonist PeCDF, and a PCB congener (PCB 153) that is not bound by CYP1A2, were examined in mice lacking the gene for *Cyp1A2* (*Cyp1A2* knockout mice). Comparing the distributions in *Cyp1A2* knockouts to the distributions in parental strains confirmed that CYP1A2, expressed primarily in the liver, can strongly affect the concentrations of TCDD in other organs. In mice lacking *Cyp1A2* expression in the liver, the concentrations of TCDD accumulating in most other organs or tissues examined (lungs, kidneys, spleen, thymus, skin, adipose tissue, and blood) were greater than the concentrations in organs of mice given the same dose that did express hepatic *Cyp1A2*. Similar results were obtained for 2,3,4,7,8-PeCDF, but not for 2,2',4,4',5,5'-hexachlorobiphenyl, which is not an AhR agonist and does not bind to CYP1A2. In *Cyp1A2* knockout mice, the ratio of TCDD in liver to TCDD in fat was 0.07, and in the wild type, the liver–fat ratio was 2.49. Notably, the absence of CYP1A2 in knockout mice also was associated with greatly increased urinary excretion of TCDD or PeCDF (Diliberto et al., 1999).

CYP1A2 is expressed in human liver. However, DeVito et al. (1998) comment that although evidence exists for PHAH sequestration in human liver, there are not good data concerning the amounts of the putative human binding protein (CYP1A2) in studies of TCDD distribution in humans. Nevertheless, studies in rodents have implications for understanding the distribution and half-life of TCDD in humans.

Studies of TCDD levels in humans have continued, especially studies of

Vietnam era veterans. In a follow-up study of Ranch Hand veterans, the mean half-life of TCDD was estimated from concentrations in serum collected from 97 of these veterans (Michalek and Tripathi, 1999). Samples were collected in 1982, 1987, 1992, and 1997. The TCDD half-life was estimated as 7.6 years, with a 95 percent confidence interval (95% CI) of 7.0 to 8.2 years. The elimination rate of TCDD decreased significantly with increases in the percentage of body fat, but the rate of elimination did not appear to change with age in this study.

A statistical analysis of serum TCDD levels also was carried out with samples from 1,302 Air Force veterans who were controls for the Agent Orange-exposed group (Michalek et al., 1998). The strength of this study is that it involved the largest single cohort of male Vietnam veterans not known to be exposed to Agent Orange and that all analyses were done in a single laboratory. In this cohort, the mean concentration of TCDD in serum was 4.23 ± 2.53 pg/g (parts per trillion), and the upper bound of the confidence limit was 10.2 pg/g. The statistical analysis supported a weak positive effect of age and a somewhat stronger positive effect of body mass index (BMI, the ratio of weight to square of height) on the levels of TCDD in serum. There was no association between BMI and age. The age effect was suggested to reflect a gradual accumulation of TCDD, which could reflect its long half-life and continual exposure via other sources.

Related to this are estimates of TCDD elimination rates. Van der Molen et al. (1998) employed models to reevaluate the *specific* elimination rates of TCDD in Vietnam veterans and concluded that TCDD half-life may actually change with age. With the model employed, they predicted half-lives for TCDD in humans ranging from 5.5 years in young adults to 11 years in older adult males. Although this prediction appears to be at variance with the results of Michalek and Tripathi (1999), they emphasize that the mechanism of TCDD elimination in humans is not known, and the model of Van de Molen et al. (1998) does not include hepatic sequestration due to inducible binding to CYP1A2.

Blood and excreta, in addition to milk, are the media in which TCDD residues most often are measured in human subjects. An important concern in toxicology is how the levels of a chemical in blood relate to levels that may occur in other organs. In studies of blood and human tissues taken from eight individuals at autopsy, Iida et al. (1999) found a correlation between the levels of selected chemicals in blood and the levels in some tissues (all expressed as picogram/gram of tissue lipid). The correlations differed for different congeners of PCDDs and PCBs. TCDD levels in blood were correlated with levels in adipose tissue, kidney, spleen, liver, and brain. However, there was no correlation between blood levels of TCDD and the levels in muscle or lung. Octachlorodibenzo-*p*-dioxin (OCDD) showed similar correlation between blood and organs except for muscle. PCB 126 showed blood–tissue correlation in fat, kidney, spleen, and liver, while PCB 77, which is rapidly metabolized and does not persist, did not show a good correlation between levels in the blood and any tissue.

In a study of postmortem tissues of 25 humans, Bachour et al. (1998) evaluated the distribution of different PCB congeners in brain, liver, lung, and muscle. They observed that the lower-chlorinated congeners showed a relatively higher degree of accumulation in lung than the higher-chlorinated congeners. Although the distribution to lung may be important in considering the effects of PCBs, this finding may not bear on patterns of distribution of TCDD.

In studies of distribution of TCDD to fetal and embryonic tissues in rodents, Hurst et al. (1998) reported that at selected doses, the amounts of TCDD reaching the fetal compartment were comparable to those measured in maternal blood. A dose of 1.15 µg/kg on gestation day 8 produced fetal body burdens of 18.1 to 39.6 ng/kg, depending on the time of gestation. The authors note that the doses used were in the range of body burdens of 2,3,7,8-TCDD toxicity equivalents (TEQs) estimated to occur in humans exposed through accidents. This suggests that concentrations able to cause effects in developing rodents could potentially accumulate in humans in utero.

Excretion of TCDD in the milk of nursing women has been established as an important route of elimination. Recent studies continue to increase the knowledge of partitioning and elimination in milk. In a study of five women, Schecter et al. (1998a) analyzed PCDDs and PCDFs in predelivery blood, placenta and cord blood, and post-partum blood and milk. They reported a positive relationship between levels in blood, milk, placenta, and cord blood. A further study by Schecter et al. (1998b) showed that total PCDDs, PCDFs, and PCBs in milk and in maternal blood decreased substantially over 2 years in a woman nursing twins. The TCDD levels in milk decreased from 2.7 pg/g milk lipid to <0.4 pg/g in 2.5 years; the TCDD in maternal blood decreased from 2.5 to 1.1 pg/g lipid in just under 2 years. Declines were observed in the other chemicals, and total TEQ in blood declined as well. These results suggest that the volumes of milk expressed may be a factor in the degree of elimination of chemicals from the mother, and that the exposure rate of infants via milk may decline with time.

LaKind et al. (2000) employed a model in an effort to develop reliable estimates of incremental body burden in infants who are exposed to TCDD via nursing. This model considered parameters including chemical absorption, infant growth, TCDD half-life in infants, lipid content of milk, and others. The authors point out that both the progressive depuration from the mother via lactation and the half-life of chemicals in the infant should be considered. They indicate that incremental body burdens of TCDD in infants who are breast-fed initially increase, but the body burdens decrease thereafter as the levels in milk decline over time. They calculate that there is a substantial loss of the initially accumulated TCDD by 2 years and that nursing does not result in a long-term elevation of TCDD body burdens. On the other hand, Patandin et al. (1999) calculated that 12–14 percent of TEQ in adults at age 25 could derive from the TEQ consumed during nursing. However, this is based only on TEQ in breast milk, and does not incorporate a physiologically based model.

Few studies have examined both TCDD intake and elimination in adult humans. Schlummer et al. (1998) examined the mass balance of PCDDs, PCDFs, PCBs, and hexachlorobenzene (HCB) in seven volunteers, measuring the daily intake by analysis of TCDD in the food consumed and the amount excreted by measuring TCDD in feces. They compared the levels in food and excreta to the levels of TCDD in blood as well. The difference between ingested and excreted TCDD was defined as net absorption. Negative differences were interpreted as net excretion. There were differences in net absorption for different chemicals, including different PCDD, PCDF, and PCB congeners. Interestingly, older subjects showed a greater tendency toward net excretion (greater amounts excreted than ingested) of some compounds than younger subjects. The fat in the diet was found to be a factor affecting absorption and excretion of the compounds, and the authors speculate that distinct processes occur in different parts of the gut, with absorption occurring in the duodenum and jejunum and net excretion back into the gut lumen in the large intestine and particularly the colon.

In a mass balance study of PCDDs and PCDFs in German volunteers, Schrey et al. (1998) measured the dietary intake and fecal excretion of 14 adults, age 24–64 years. These investigators reported that the measured amounts of TCDD and OCDD excreted, paradoxically, exceeded the amounts consumed in the diet. The intake of TCDD in picograms per day averaged 6.6, while the fecal excretion rate averaged 11.0. The ranges were 3.3–14 pg/day intake and 3.1–20 pg/day excreted. These investigators also reported that the excretion rate of PCDD or PCDF increased with the age of the participants. These authors concluded that there must be missing sources of PCDD for these subjects and that the diet did not reveal total exposure. They also suggested the possibility of formation of PCDDs in vivo, perhaps in the intestine. PCDDs and PCDFs formed in vitro from peroxidase-catalyzed reactions with chlorophenol substrates (Wittsiepe et al., 1999). Such results raise questions about interpretations regarding exposure levels or body burdens based on analysis of excreted residues. On the other hand, this might be explained, in part, if the later dioxin exposure levels were lower than the earlier ones.

Rohde et al. (1999) examined uptake and elimination of TCDD and other PCDDs and PCDFs in men in Germany who had previously accumulated high levels of TCDD in the workplace. Their studies show that concentrations of TCDD in feces had a high positive correlation with blood levels of TCDD (picograms per gram of blood lipid), indicating that fecal excretion contributes to clearance and that fecal PCDD and PCDF may be determined by body burden. The authors also calculate that an amount of TEQ equivalent to that in about 1.7 g of blood lipids is cleared daily through fecal excretion. The results of Rohde et al. (1999) also show that the amounts of TCDD, as well as other congeners, are greater in the excreta than in the food consumed. The excess amount of chemical excreted could be due to the initially high body burdens of these subjects.

Increasing fecal excretion of TCDD may help to increase clearance from the body. Recent studies have reported that ingestion of a nonabsorbed dietary fat substitute (olestra) can increase the fecal excretion of TCDD. In one study (Geusau et al., 1999), patients with chloracne who had very high blood levels of TCDD were fed olestra, and the rate of intestinal excretion of TCDD was increased up to tenfold, substantially decreasing the half-life, from about 7 years to less than 2 years. In a similar study (Moser and McLachlan, 1999), the excretion of PCDDs, PCDFs, PCBs, and HCB was monitored in three volunteers, first while they were fed a normal diet and then when they were fed a diet supplemented with a fat substitute (olestra). The chemical excretion rates were 1.5 to 11 times greater, depending on the compound, on the supplemented diet. The exact mechanism underlying the increased excretion is not presently understood, although it may simply be due to the increase in the total amount of fat (dietary plus olestra) excreted via the feces (Geusau et al., 1999).

Accurately assessing the risk of TCDD or other PHAH exposures above background levels may require knowledge of the levels accumulated at the time(s) of greatest exposure. Estimating these levels usually requires back-extrapolation from current blood levels in exposed subjects. Heederik et al. (1998) carried out such modeling of TCDD levels in a cohort exposed to TCDD during work at a plant that manufactured chlorophenoxy herbicides. They grouped workers according to several variables, including the category and location of work in the plant during herbicide production, whether they had been employed at the time of an accident in 1963 that caused a release of PCDD, and whether they did or did not have chloracne. Levels of PCDDs, PCDFs, and PCBs were measured in serum drawn in 1993. TCDD levels in serum ranged from 7.6 pg/g serum lipid in nonexposed workers to 105 pg/g in workers exposed to the accident who had chloracne. The back-extrapolation employed a one-compartment first-order model, for which the authors varied assumptions concerning half-life, using three values that have been derived largely from studies of Vietnam veterans: 5.8, 7.1, and 11.3 years. The model assumes that half-lives do not vary between individuals. As expected, the predictions of serum levels at the time of last exposure were strongly dependent on the half-life chosen. This results in differences in levels at which elevated risk occurs, although risk groups did not change. The range in predicted levels might be expected to encompass the real values.

To summarize, studies since *Update 1998* have refined estimates of TCDD half-life, suggesting further that the internal distribution of TCDD can be affected by several variables and that excretion rates can be enhanced by lipoidal additives to the diet. There have been refinements in the effort to calculate earlier exposure levels from later measurement of blood levels. The half-life of TCDD can vary between individuals and with dietary modification.

There are a number of controversies surrounding the use of these models. A detailed discussion of the models can be found in EPA's draft dioxin risk assessment document (U.S. EPA, 2000).

Mechanisms of Toxic Action

Studies published since *Update 1998* are consistent with the hypothesis that TCDD produces its biological and toxic effects by binding to a gene regulatory protein, the aryl hydrocarbon receptor. Several earlier studies had suggested that some immunological effects might occur via a non-AhR-mediated mechanism, but now, based on data in AhR-defective animals, these effects are thought to be related to pharmacokinetic factors rather than AhR-related factors. The model indicates that the binding of TCDD to the AhR, dimerization of the AhR with the ARNT protein, binding of this complex to specific DNA sequences (called aryl hydrocarbon-responsive elements [AhREs] or dioxin-responsive elements) present in the 5'-promoter regions of responsive genes, and inappropriate modulation of gene expression represent the initial steps in a series of biochemical, cellular, and tissue changes that result in the toxicity observed. Much of our current understanding of the mechanism of TCDD action is based on analysis of the induction of particular genes, (e.g., *cytochrome P4501A1 [CYP1A1]*), by TCDD. This hypothesis is supported by numerous studies published evaluating structure–activity relationships of various AhR ligands, the genetics of mutant *AhR* genes, AhR-deficient mice, and the molecular events contributing to and regulating expression of the AhR and its activity. Although the promoter regions of many genes, including *CYP1A1*, contain DREs, only a few of these are known to be directly regulated by the AhR–ARNT complex (reviewed by Denison et al., 1998). However, the modulated expression of these genes does not completely explain (at least not as yet) the diversity of toxic effects elicited by TCDD in numerous animal species. By analogy, it is predicted that other genes have inappropriate expression (or repression) directly related to particular toxic events. The findings that many AhR-modulated genes are regulated in a species-, cell-, and developmental stage-specific pattern suggest that molecular and cellular pathways leading to any particular toxic event are complex.

Additional research has shown that the biochemical and biological outcomes of TCDD exposure can be modulated by numerous other proteins with which the AhR interacts. Thus, it is now considered possible that TCDD could modulate gene expression by pathways that do not involve the interaction of the AhR with either ARNT or DREs. In fact, to date there are no data proving that Arnt is required for any toxic effects elicited by TCDD. It is plausible, for example that the AhR (and/or the AhR–ARNT complex) could divert other proteins and transcription factors from other signaling pathways; whose disruption could have serious consequences on a number of cell and tissue processes.

Studies summarized below report on the structural and functional aspects of the AhR and ARNT, processes regulating DNA binding and transcriptional events, biochemical and biological processes associated with AhR activation, interactions of the AhR with several cellular signaling processes, evidence for different mechanisms of toxicity, and interactions with other chemicals. Many of these data are consistent with the notion that cellular processes involving growth, maturation, and differentiation are most sensitive to TCDD-induced modulation as mediated by the AhR. The findings in animals indicating that reproductive, developmental, and oncogenic end points appear to be most sensitive to this chemical are consistent with that notion. These data support a biologic plausibility for similar end points of toxicity that may occur in exposed humans. However, it is clear that many of these responses are tissue and species specific. The mechanistic basis for these differences is not completely understood.

It is important to consider exposure levels when discussing animal data, because experimental studies are often conducted at much higher levels than humans are exposed to, even in intense occupational settings. A discussion of the level of TCDD in the herbicides used in Vietnam and the possible levels of exposure of U.S. military personnel is found in *Update 1998* and in Chapter 5 of this report.

Structural and Functional Aspects of AhR and ARNT

Several publications have documented the presence of the AhR and ARNT in a variety of tissues from different animal species and strains. Detailed analysis of variant forms has provided much information associating structure and expression levels with function. Jana et al. (1998) observed a good correlation between the steady-state level of AhR expression and the relative inducibility of CYP1A1 in eight different rat strains. Analysis of ARNT demonstrated the presence of a wild-type form and an alternatively spliced variant in all strains. The expressed levels of both ARNT forms were equal in five strains, but the presence of the wild-type form predominated in the other three strains. Data on the tissue-specific expression of both forms suggested that their relative expression could contribute to differential induction of CYP1A1.

The Han/Wistar (H/W) rat strain has been shown to be at least a thousand-fold less sensitive to the acute lethal effects of TCDD than most other rat strains. However, the H/W strain appears to be just as sensitive to other biological effects of TCDD, including CYP1A1 induction. Genetic analysis has shown that two genes, the *Ahr* gene and an additional unknown gene, contribute to this resistance. However, the *Ahrhw* allele appears to be the major determinant (Tuomisto et al., 1999). It was found that the apparent mass of the AhR from the H/W rats (~98 kDa) is lower than that of the receptor of other rat strains (~106 kDa) (Pohjanvirta et al., 1999). This difference is due to a deletion–insertion-type change at the 3'-end of exon 10 in the receptor cDNA resulting from a single point mutation at the first nucleotide at intron 10 and subsequent altered mRNA splicing (Pohjanvirta et al., 1998). The mutation leads to a loss of 38 to 43 amino acids within the transactivation domain of the AhR. Although the functional consequences of this loss remain to be characterized, the data suggest that this region may provide differential selectivity in the responses elicited by TCDD.

Korkalainen et al. (2000) recently reported the sequence of the *AhR* contained in the hamster. Hamsters are highly resistant to the acute toxicity of TCDD. The amino terminal was found to be highly conserved with other species. However, the glutamine-rich C-terminal region known to be involved in transactivation is substantially expanded. The functional significance is not known, but the authors hypothesized that it may account for the selective responsiveness of this species.

Several different forms of the AhR have been identified in fish. Two forms of the AhR were characterized in rainbow trout (Abnet et al., 1999). These forms demonstrated significant sequence homology with AhRs cloned from mammalian species, especially in the basic helix–loop–helix (bHLH) and the PAS domain. The glutamine-rich sequence found in the transactivation domain of mammalian AhR, however, was absent. Both forms bound TCDD with high affinity but demonstrated tissue-specific differences in expression and distinct preferences for different enhancer DNA sequences. The data suggest that the two AhR forms may regulate different genes and contribute to tissue-specific responses to AhR agonists. Similarly, two divergent AhR forms have been characterized in the teleost *Fundulus heteroclitus* (Karchner et al., 1999). Although both possess bHLH and PAS domains related to mammalian AhR, the two forms were found to be highly divergent in other domains. In particular, the transactivation domain in one form lacks the glutamine-rich region. Furthermore the two genes displayed different tissue-specific patterns of expression. The authors suggested that one form represents a novel subfamily of bHLH–PAS proteins within the vertebrate AhR family. Notably, the glutamine-rich region found in the transactivation domain of mammalian AhR was also found to be lacking in zebrafish AhR (Tanguay et al., 1999).

The hepatic binding affinity of the AhR for TCDD was compared between the beagle dog and cynomolgus monkey. The AhR from both species possessed a low binding affinity for TCDD (K_d values of 17.1 and 16.5 nM, respectively) similar to that previously reported for humans (Sandoz et al., 1999). Wanner et al. (1999) also demonstrated high conservation of the *Ahr* gene sequence in humans by an analysis for polymorphisms in 14 chemical workers involved in a trichlorophenol accident. Only one amino acid-exchanging polymorphism was identified (arginine–lysine at codon 554); this polymorphism did not appear to influence susceptibility to induced chloracne. Human AhR and ARNT were found to be transcriptionally active in response to TCDD when they were expressed in yeast; yeast possess no natural counterpart to the AhR pathway (Miller, 1999). Different AhR agonists displayed additive responses within this system. The author indicated that this may provide a useful model for further study and characterization of AhR agonists and AhR-dependent signal transduction pathways. It should be pointed out that although only one AhR sequence polymorphism has been identified and this has no apparent influence on the susceptibility to induced chloracne, other data suggest some heterogeneity of AhR concentrations and characteristics in the human population (Perdew and Hollenback, 1995; Roberts et al., 1990, 1991). In addition, because as indicated above there are a number of factors and pathways regulating AhR activity, it is possible that although the AhR in humans might have lower affinity for TCDD than other species, differences in other regulatory factors might actually increase the relative responsiveness under certain conditions. At present, there are no clear data on the molecular properties of the AhR to conclude whether humans would be more or less susceptible to TCDD as compared to other species.

Research has shown that the association of newly synthesized AhR with a 90 kDa heat shock protein is important to maintain the AhR in a conformation that can bind ligand. Much of this work has been performed using AhR isolated from mice and rats. Recent investigations using AhR from the guinea pig and rabbit suggest some species differences in ligand binding-initiated stability of the AhR. Using AhR in which HSP90 dissociation was induced by increased salt content, these studies indicated that, at least for some species, HSP90 is not absolutely required to maintain the AhR in a ligand binding conformation (Phelan et al., 1998). Association with HSP90 is also thought to regulate nuclear uptake by blocking an N-terminal nuclear localization sequence (see below). However, it is not clear whether ligand binding-elicited dissociation of HSP90 occurs prior to or following nuclear localization. Additional work has shown the unliganded and unchaperoned AhR to be extremely labile in cells (Lees and Whitelaw, 1999). These data are consistent with a mechanism in which HSP90 is released from ligand-bound AhR following nuclear localization and concomitant with ARNT dimerization. Further studies by Heid et al. (2000) demonstrated that dissociation of HSP90 is not required for nuclear translocation of the AhR but is essential for dimerization with ARNT.

Hahn (1998) recently compared the AhR signal transduction pathway in mammalian and nonmammalian species. Together the information suggests that the AhR is an ancient protein and that its development stemmed from functions not related to regulation of *CYP1A* genes and divergent from the ability of the mammalian AhR to bind TCDD and related xenobiotics.

A number of publications have demonstrated that mammalian AhR and ARNT are expressed in a tissue-specific manner. Furthermore, a number of factors including developmental and differentiation stage, presence and activation of other transcription factors, and prior exposure to AhR ligands have been found to have a significant influence on the relative expression of the AhR. Garrison and Denison (2000) characterized the 5'-flanking region of the mouse *Ahr* gene. Putative binding sites for several transcription factors, such as stimulatory *protein* 1 (Sp1), were identified.

TCDD exposure elicits developmental alterations in many species and induces cleft palate in the mouse embryo. Abbott et al. (1999a) examined the expression of AhR, ARNT, and CYP1A1 mRNAs in embryonic craniofacial tissues during their development. CYP1A1 mRNA was found to be expressed in developing craniofacial tissue and was highly induced by TCDD exposure. AhR and ARNT mRNAs were upregulated during early palatogenesis. ARNT mRNA expression was about five- to sixfold lower than that of AhR. Note that these data might support a hypothesis that TCDD may act by activating the AhR and diverting ARNT away from other normal functions of this protein. This study also observed a decreased expression of ARNT mRNA following TCDD treatment. Abbott et al. (1999b) also compared AhR and ARNT expression in cultured human embryonic palate with mouse palate. Palate from human embryos expressed approximately 350 times less AhR mRNA and 135 times less Arnt mRNA than the mouse palate. Within the 18 different human palatal tissues examined, there was a strong correlation between TCDD-induced CYP1A1 mRNA and AhR content. However, it was previously observed that human palates required about 200 times more TCDD to produce the same changes in cellular differentiation and proliferation and affect changes in growth factor (i.e., epidermal growth factor [EGF] and transforming growth factor) compared to mouse palatal tissue exposed under the same conditions in vitro (Abbott et al., 1998, 1999b). Together these data suggest that the embryonic human palate may not be as susceptible to altered growth and differentiation effects as the mouse palate and that the relative expression of the AhR and ARNT in these tissues may influence their responsiveness.

In the male rat, in utero and lactational TCDD exposure impairs development of the accessory sex organs, including the prostate, and alters sexual behavior (see below). Sommer et al. (1999) examined the effects of stage of development and TCDD treatment on AhR protein, ARNT protein, and mRNA concentrations in rat prostate. AhR protein in developing ventral and dorsolateral prostate decreased with age between postnatal day (pnd) 1 and 21. A similar decrease in ARNT protein was seen in the dorsolateral prostate. These changes were associated with decreases in AhR and ARNT mRNA. Exposure of the adult male rat to TCDD decreased AhR but not ARNT protein in prostate tissue, vas deferens, and epididymis. In utero and lactational exposure to TCDD reduced prostate AhR protein levels on pnd 7 and delayed the developmental decrease in AhR protein. These data indicate that prostatic AhR and ARNT levels are regulated during development in the rat. AhR and ARNT were also found to be expressed in normal human fetal prostate, with the most intense reactivity found in smooth muscle cells followed by epithelial cells and fibrocytes (Kashani et al., 1998). Decreased AhR expression was observed in benign hyperplastic tissue, but increased expression was frequently observed in carcinomatous prostate tissue from adult subjects.

Exposure of experimental animals to TCDD during pregnancy has been shown to cause in utero death and a variety of developmental abnormalities. Studies by Robles et al. (2000) examined AhR expression in mouse ovary. AhR protein was present at relatively high concentrations in oocytes and granulosa cells of follicles at all stages of development. Other studies detected AhR mRNA,

ARNT mRNA, and AhR protein in preimplantation rabbit embryos (Tscheudschilsuren et al., 1999a) and during early gestation in the rabbit uterus (Tscheudschilsuren et al., 1999b). In contrast, very low levels of AhR mRNA were found in the preimplantation uterus. In addition, Kuchenhoff et al. (1999) demonstrated cycle- and age-dependent AhR expression in the human endometrium, with maximal receptor levels observed near the time of ovulation. Together these data suggest that AhR and ARNT have some functional role in fetomaternal interactions during early gestation. Additional data obtained using *Ahr* null-allele animals are consistent with this hypothesis (see below).

TCDD exposure has been shown to elicit a wide variety of immune system alterations in all experimental animals examined. Stromal cells in bone marrow play an essential role in the support and direction of hematopoiesis, and it is possible that TCDD may exert its effects through alterations in stromal cell support capacity. Lavin et al. (1998) demonstrated the presence and functionality of AhR and ARNT in three mouse bone marrow stromal cell lines and in primary bone marrow cell cultures. These data demonstrate that the molecular machinery necessary for mediating TCDD-dependent alterations is present and functional in bone marrow stromal cells.

It has been demonstrated previously by many investigators that nuclear uptake of ligand-bound AhR is an essential event leading to transcriptional alterations of TCDD-responsive genes. A recent study by Ikuta et al. (2000) suggests that the shuttling of the AhR from nucleus to cytosol is also essential for the inducible expression of the *CYP1A1* gene. Although the exact mechanisms responsible for these events are not clear, an additional study by Ikuta et al. (1998) demonstrates that the AhR contains both nuclear localization and export signals in the N-terminal region. The minimum AhR nuclear localization signal was contained in residues 13–39 of the human AhR, while the minimal nuclear export signal was contained in residues 55–75.

Several investigations utilizing whole animals and cells in culture demonstrated that TCDD treatment elicits a sustained depletion of AhR protein, without an effect on AhR mRNA, in a variety of tissues (Giannone et al., 1998; Pollenz et al., 1998; Roman et al., 1998a). Additional research has shown this induced degradation to involve TCDD-elicited nuclear uptake of the ligand-bound receptor, subsequent nuclear export and ubiquination, and proteasomal degradation (Davarinos and Pollenz, 1999; Roberts and Whitelaw, 1999; Ma and Baldwin, 2000). These data suggest a novel mechanism for the regulatory control of activated AhR and cellular AhR content. Notably, Shimba et al. (1998) reported that AhR protein levels decreased with ongoing adipose differentiation in 3T3-L1 cells and that cellular responsiveness to TCDD was concomitantly decreased. Whether the regulation of AhR levels in the latter case is related to TCDD-elicited degradation via proteasomes has yet to be determined. Nevertheless, these data indicate that normal cellular processes regulate AhR protein and the responsiveness of its signal transduction pathway.

As indicated in *Update 1998*, the resistance of *Ahr* null-allele (knockout) mice to the enzyme-inductive and toxic effects of even very high doses of TCDD further corroborates the role of this protein in these responses. Recent data from Peter et al. (1999) demonstrating only minimal teratogenicity of TCDD in knockout mice compared to wild-type mice are consistent with this. Previous data from investigations with *Ahr* null-allele mice also suggested that the AhR plays an important, but as yet unknown, developmental and physiological role. Data published by Abbott et al. (1999c) demonstrated a number of adverse reproductive outcomes in *Ahr* null-allele mice. Null-allele females had difficulty maintaining the conceptus, surviving pregnancy and lactation, and rearing pups to weaning. Null-allele pups demonstrated poor survival during lactation and after weaning. However, across different genotypes, the sex ratios and genotypic frequencies were comparable. A recent study by Robles et al. (2000) examined the ovarian germ cell dynamics in *Ahr* null-allele and wild-type mice. An analysis of serial ovarian sections revealed a twofold greater number of primordial follicles in *Ahr* null-allele animals at day 4 postpartum. Additional investigations suggested that this may result from a decrease in the death rate of the developing germ cell line because AhR deficiency attenuated oocyte apoptosis in fetal ovaries cultured in vitro. It was hypothesized that the AhR may have some role in regulating the size of the oocyte reserve by affecting germ cell death. These data are consistent with those published by Benedict et al. (2000), who provide evidence to suggest that the AhR may be involved in regulation of the number of antral follicles in postnatal life. Because antral follicles are necessary for the secretion of several reproductive hormones, it is possible that these results could explain the reproductive abnormalities observed in *Ahr* null-allele animals by Abbott et al. (1999c). Recently, data reported by Thurmond et al. (2000) in chimeric *Ahr*+/+ and *Ahr*–/– animals also suggested that the AhR may have some role in B-lymphocyte maturation processes. Finally, Lahvis et al. (2000) recently observed alterations in vascular development in AhR-deficient mice. It should be noted that although the knockout mice generated by several laboratories have shown many similar characteristics, distinct phenotypes have also been observed (Lahvis and Bradfield, 1998). Whether these differences occur because of local environmental effects or different genetic backgrounds has yet to be determined.

DNA Binding and Transcriptional Interference

As indicated above, the ability of TCDD to directly modulate gene expression depends on: (1) its ability to activate the AhR to a form that can dimerize with ARNT; (2) the ability of this complex to bind to specific DNA sequences located in the regulatory regions of certain genes; (3) and the alteration of transcriptional events regulating the expression of those genes. DNA binding and transactivation domains have been identified in both the AhR and ARNT. However, it is clear that the ability of this activated complex to induce particular genes and alter cell morphology and/or function is very tissue and species specific. It seems likely that the relative presence of tissue-specific factors may play a large role in regulating these responses to AhR ligands. Many of the more recent investigations have focused on identifying and characterizing factors that may modulate, by either activation or repression, the ability of the activated AhR–ARNT complex to alter gene expression. In addition, several studies have noted the ability of a variety of AhR ligands to act as receptor antagonists.

The AhR has been shown to associate with several proteins. One of these is known to be a member of the immunophilin family. The presence of this protein has been shown to enhance the transcriptional activity of the AhR–ARNT complex in several different cellular systems (Carver et al., 1998; Meyer et al., 1998). The exact function of this protein is not clear, but some evidence suggests that although it is not required for the interaction of HSP90 with the AhR, it increases the level of active AhR by regulating the rate of AhR turnover (Meyer and Perdew, 1999; La Pres et al., 2000). In contrast, a 23 kDa protein has been shown to associate with the ligand-binding form of the AhR and is thought to play a role in stabilizing the complex containing HSP90 (Kazlauskas et al., 1999).

Nuclear accessory proteins, or coactivators, have been shown to act as bridging factors between enhancer-binding proteins, such as the estrogen receptor, and the basal transcription complex. For example, RIP140 has been found to interact with several nuclear receptors to enhance transcriptional activity. Similarly, Kumar et al. (1999) demonstrated that in several cell lines the presence of RIP140 enhanced TCDD-mediated, AhR-dependent transcriptional activity. Mapping of the interactions sites indicated that the AhR recruits RIP140 via the glutamine-rich region within the transactivation domain. Nguyen et al. (1999) also found that the coactivator ERAP140 immunoprecipitates with the AhR–ARNT complex, enhances AhR–ARNT binding to DREs, and increases AhR-mediated gene expression.

Several publications have suggested the repression of AhR-mediated signal transduction by cellular factors. Gradin et al. (1999) identified the presence of a factor in human fibroblasts that is able to repress the activity of the AhR. Within these cells, genes controlled by the activated AhR–ARNT complex have been shown to be nonresponsive to TCDD. The repressor was shown to act by binding with ARNT to form an inactive complex able to bind to the DRE. Using mouse hepatoma cells, Eltom et al. (1999) identified the presence of an ARNT-like protein that may act as a selective suppressor of *CYP1B1* gene expression. The presence of this factor may account for the selective expression of *CYP1A1* over *CYP1B1* in some cell types with and without TCDD exposure. Studies by Mimura et al. (1999) identified and characterized an AhR repressor (AhRR) in mice that acts by competing with the AhR for dimerization with ARNT. The gene for this repressor was activated by the TCDD–AhR–ARNT complex. The encoded sequence exhibited a great degree of similarity to the *AhR*. However, the PAS-A domain is variable and the PAS-B sequence, which functions in ligand binding and interaction with HSP90, is missing. This is thought to represent a novel regulatory mechanism of AhR function.

The mouse AhR has been shown to physically associate with the pleiotropic transcription factor NF-κB, and this interaction appears to produce a mutual functional repression of their actions (Tian et al., 1999). These authors suggest that the ability of the TCDD-activated AhR to interact with NF-κB and divert it from other actions may provide a possible mechanistic explanation for some of the toxic responses elicited by TCDD. Similarly, AhR and ARNT proteins were found to coimmunoprecipitate with SMRT (silencing mediator for retinoic acid and thyroid hormone receptor), and this interaction was found to block both AhR–ARNT DRE binding and AhR-mediated gene expression (Nguyen et al., 1999). The actual mechanism by which these interactions occur and their relative importance in the gene- and tissue-specific responses elicited by TCDD are unknown.

Histone acetylation and deacetylation have been demonstrated to be highly specific regulatory processes that control the activation and repression of some genes. Several coactivators and repressors possess histone acetylase and deacetylase activities. Garrison et al. (2000) reported that the treatment of cells in culture with histone deacetylase inhibitors increased the constitutive activity of an AhR-dependent DRE-driven gene reporter construct. Cotransfection with a protein having histone acetylase activity decreased the activity of this promoter. These studies provide evidence that histone acetylation–deacetylation may regulate AhR-responsive genes.

As indicated above, several lines of evidence suggest a normal functional role of the AhR. However, an endogenous ligand that has clear functionality under physiological conditions has not been identified. Previous reports have indicated stimulation of AhR-dependent processes in the absence of added ligand. A recent report by Chang and Puga (1998) found that CYP1A1-deficient mouse hepatoma c37 cells possess transcriptionally active AhR–ARNT complexes in the absence of exogenous ligands. A similar finding was observed following treatment of Hepa-1 cells with an inhibitor of CYP1A1 activity. Likewise the expression of a DRE-responsive reporter gene in CV-1 cells leads to high levels of reporter gene expression. These data suggest that a CYP1A1 substrate that accumulates in cells lacking this enzyme activity is an endogenous ligand for the AhR. This ligand has yet to be identified.

There have been several reports of naturally occurring high-affinity ligands for the receptor. Many of these exist in plants that are consumed by humans. These include resveratrol (Ciolino et al., 1998a; Casper et al., 1999; Ciolino and Yeh, 1999), curcumin (Ciolino et al., 1998b), tryptophan metabolites (Heath-Pagliuso et al., 1998; Y.D. Wei et al., 1999), galangin (Ciolino and Yeh, 1998; Quadri et al., 2000), the dietary flavonols quercetin and kaempferol (Ciolino et al., 1999), lipoxin A4 (Schaldach et al., 1999), and products of heme metabolism (Sinal and Bend, 1997). Several of these, such as the tryptophan metabolites, lipoxin A4, appear primarily to have AhR agonist activity. Galangin, quercetin, kaempferol, and curcumin have concentration-dependent agonist and antagonist activity, whereas resveratrol appears to act mainly as an AhR antagonist. Under certain conditions, several of these compounds have been shown to have some anticancer activity, but a role of the AhR in that activity has not yet been demonstrated. Although there are good data available on the structure–activity relationships for AhR agonists, the structural requirements and mechanisms of AhR antagonists are poorly understood. A study by Henry et al. (1999) examined certain flavone derivatives for their ability to produce AhR antagonist activity in mouse hepatoma cells. Overall, the data indicate that particular substituent groups, such as a 3'-methoxy group or one possessing terminal atoms with high electron density that can form hydrogen bonds or interact electrostatically with receptor amino acids, promote antagonist activity. Additional studies indicate that these chemicals act as antagonists by binding the same site on the AhR as TCDD but fail to elicit a conformational change resulting in nuclear translocation, dissociation of HSP90, and ARNT dimerization. Recently, Ashida et al. (2000a) suggested that dietary levels of certain flavones and flavanols may act as AhR antagonists.

As indicated above, the AhR and ARNT have been localized to a variety of different tissues at various stages of development. This information, although useful, does not indicate when and where the AhR–ARNT complex might be activated in vivo by various agonists. This information could be used to determine tissues that are sensitive to TCDD and to explore the physiological function of the AhR. Willey et al. (1998) developed a transgenic mouse model that can be used to indicate the temporal and spatial context of transcriptionally active AhR following agonist exposure in vivo. Transgenic mice containing a TCDD-responsive *lacZ* reporter gene construct demonstrated TCDD-inducible β-galactosidase activity in several tissues following adult and in utero exposure. These tissues included palate, liver, lung, genital tubercle, paws, tooth buds, intestine, brain, and developing ear. These data indicate that TCDD can initiate altered gene expression in these tissues, thereby identifying potential targets of toxicity.

Biological Consequences of Activation

Many toxic effects of TCDD have been described in experimental animals and exposed human populations. The exact mechanisms responsible for most, if not all, of these species- and tissue-specific effects are not known. Although there is information about particular genes that may be altered under certain conditions, the relationships between altered gene expression and more complex biological responses such as altered growth, differentiation, developmental effects, and neoplasia are not understood. A major obstacle to clarifying these issues has been the lack of understanding of the actual direct cell targets and the developmental stage of greatest sensitivity. Since *Update 1998*, several investigations have been conducted to identify both cellular and gene targets for TCDD.

In animals lethally intoxicated with TCDD, a wasting syndrome characterized by decreased food intake and body weight loss is most often observed. The biochemical pathways responsible for this syndrome are not understood, but reduced gluconeogenesis has been thought to play a role in the process. Work by Viluksela et al. (1999) demonstrated a dose-dependent decrease in hepatic phosphoenolpyruvate carboxykinase (PEPCK) activity, the rate-limiting enzyme of gluconeogenesis, following the exposure of TCDD-resistant H/W rats to TCDD. This decrease was not observed in TCDD-sensitive Long-Evans (L-E) rats. However, TCDD treatment attenuated the increase in PEPCK activity observed in pair-fed controls. Although the change in PEPCK activity alone could not explain the difference in sensitivity between the two rat strains, the gluconeogenic response following TCDD treatment appeared to be altered. Unkila et al. (1998) also compared these two rat strains for the effects of TCDD on tryptophan homeostasis. In L-E rats, TCDD treatment produced an elevation in brain tryptophan and plasma free tryptophan concentrations and a decrease in hepatic tryptophan pyrrolase. Much smaller or no effects were seen in the H/W animals. Although there appeared to be some correlation between the relative sensitivity of these strains to TCDD-induced body weight loss and alterations in tryptophan metabolism, the analysis of other dioxin congeners did not demonstrate the same relationships. CAAT-enhancer binding proteins (C-EBP) have been suggested to play a role in the coordination of energy homeostasis. Liu et al. (1998) examined the effect of TCDD treatment (100 µg/kg) on C-EBPβ and C-EBPβ expression and function in mice. There was a time- and dose-dependent decrease in the amount of C-EBPβ mRNA in adipose tissue and liver and an increase in C-EBPβ mRNA. These changes were also reflected in the protein–C-EBP recognition element complexes formed using hepatic nuclear extracts from control and TCDD-treated mice. Induced changes in the expression of these transcription factors may have a role in the mechanism by which TCDD treatment causes a wasting syndrome in animals.

Gao et al. (1998) reported the induction of an ecto-ATPase in mouse hepatoma cells that is AhR dependent and is regulated at the transcriptional level. Ecto-ATPases influence several physiological processes including the metabolism of nucleic acids. However, their exact role in induced toxicity is not understood.

Liver lesions have been reported in several animal species following exposure to TCDD, and this chemical is a potent tumor promoter in the liver of male and female mice, as well as female rats. Two recent studies evaluated the relative contributions of different cell types to the hepatic lesions observed in rats. Using a chimeric *Ahr* null-allele model, Thurmond et al. (1999) found that hematopoietic cells contribute to the hepatic lesions induced by TCDD. More specifically, the presence of the AhR in hepatic parenchyma alone was sufficient for TCDD-elicited hepatic necrosis. An inflammatory response is secondary to this damage but depends on the presence of the AhR in immune cells. Riebniger and Schrenk (1998) examined the expression of TGF-β_1 in fat-storing cells isolated from rat liver. TGF-β_1 is an inhibitor of hepatocellular proliferation but is synthesized predominantly in nonparenchymal hepatic cells. Exposure of these cells to TCDD either in vivo or in vitro had no effect on *TGF-β_1* gene expression. In addition, no effect on *CYP1A1* expression was observed in these cells. This was likely due to the absence of a detectable amount of the AhR. Increased portal fibrosis and small liver size have been reported in *Ahr* null-allele mice. Zaher et al. (1998) examined the relationship between TGF-β expression and apoptosis in this mouse line. Livers from *Ahr* null-allele animals had increased expression of TGF-β_1 and TGF-β_3 proteins and increased numbers of hepatocytes undergoing apoptosis compared to wild-type animals. These parameters were especially increased in the portal areas. Primary hepatocytes from null-allele animals exhibited increased numbers of cells in apoptosis and increased secretion of TGF-β_3 into the media. Conditioned media from null-allele cells stimulated apoptosis in hepatocytes from wild-type mice. These data suggest that abnormal liver morphology in *Ahr* null-allele animals may be mediated by abnormal levels of TGF-β and increased apoptosis of hepatocytes. The AhR may have a normal function in regulating these processes. Puga et al. (2000a) observe that exposure of human hepatoma HepG2 cells to 10 nM TCDD resulted in the altered expression of 310 known genes; 30 of these were upregulated and 78 were downregulated. The significance of this information to the specific toxic responses in the liver is not clear.

Several reports on exposed animal and human populations suggest that halogenated aromatic hydrocarbons, such as TCDD, may alter cognitive function and learning, especially when exposure occurs during critical periods of brain development. Hong et al. (1998) examined the effect of TCDD on evoked excitatory postsynaptic potentials (EPSPs) using hippocampal slices from adolescent and adult male rats. The hippocampus has been shown to have a role in learning and memory. A TCDD concentration of 100 nM was shown to decrease EPSPs in ventral slices but not in slices from the middle third of the hippocampus. The calcium channel blocker nifedipine blocked the inhibition of EPSPs by TCDD but not by 2,2',5,5'-tetrachlorobiphenyl. These data suggest that the effect of TCDD is mediated by L-type calcium channels and is congener specific.

Newborn infants are often susceptible to vitamin K deficiency, which may lead to hemorrhagic disorders. Bouwman et al. (1999) investigated whether TCDD exposure might affect vitamin K-dependent blood coagulation. Single oral doses up to 10 µg/kg to adult female and male rats caused a dose-dependent reduction in vitamin K-dependent coagulation factor VII. This was negatively correlated with an induction of CYP1A1 activity. The greatest reduction achieved was 44 percent in female rats. No effect on male rats was observed. Sex-dependent differences in vitamin K-dependent carboxylase and vitamin K 2,3-epoxide reductase were also observed. The carboxylase was greatly induced in female rats. Further studies in newborns are needed.

TCDD has been shown to induce the expression of various cytokines in a variety of cell types. Lang et al. (1998) examined the expression of various cytokine genes in human airway epithelial cells, alveolar macrophages, and peripheral blood monocytes and lymphocytes. CYP1A1 activity and mRNA were increased in a concentration-dependent manner in brochoepithelial cells and blood lymphocytes, with epithelial cells being the most inducible (EC_{50} of 30 pM). TCDD treatment did not affect the expression or production of IL-6 or IL-8 in these cells.

Perinatal exposure to TCDD has been shown to alter thermoregulatory control in hamsters and rats. Gordon and Miller (1998) examined behavioral thermoregulation, ability to develop fever, and thermoregulatory stability in rats exposed perinatally at gestational day (gd) 15 to 1 µg TCDD/kg. Although the data confirmed that TCDD induced nocturnal hypothermia in males up to 11 months of age, the hypothalamic thermoregulatory centers did not appear to be permanently altered. Accentuated fever in TCDD-treated animals in response to lipopolysaccharide was also observed. These data suggest that there are functional alterations in the hypothalamic–pituitary–thyroid axis. Whether these findings relate to previously reported alterations in blood thyroid hormone levels in response to TCDD is unknown. Using primary rat anterior pituitary cells in culture, Bestervelt et al. (1998) assessed whether TCDD exposure directly affected pituitary function. Maximal effects of TCDD on adrenocorticotropic hormone (ACTH) secretion occurred at media concentrations between 10^{-11} and 10^{-15} M after 24-hour exposure. Alterations in secretion were observed as early as 6 hours and persisted up to 10 days. Decreased pituitary responsiveness to corticotropin-releasing hormone and arginine-8-vasopressin was also observed. These data support the hypothesis that TCDD might directly interfere with anterior pituitary gland function, and this might occur at very low cellular concentrations.

It has been known for some time that TCDD alters the expression of several types of cytochrome P450 isozymes. Although the effect of these changes on the metabolism of drugs and xenobiotics has been widely documented, the relationship of these alterations to the complex biological and toxic effects of TCDD is not understood. Walker et al. (1999) investigated the dose-dependent expression of CYP1A1, CYP1A2, and CYP1B1 in the livers of female rats exposed for 30 weeks to doses of TCDD up to 125 ng/kg/day. There was a dose-dependent induction of all three isozymes by TCDD. However, at the highest levels of exposure, the protein levels of CYP1A1 and CYP1A2 induced were between forty- and a hundredfold higher than those of CYP1B1. The authors suggested that if CYP1B1 is involved in TCDD-induced hepatocarcinogenesis, its function is unique and does not overlap with that of CYP1A1 or CYP1A2. Mahajan and Rifkind (1999) observed differential induction of CYP1A4 and CYP1A5 in a variety of tissues from the chick embryo following TCDD exposure. The data suggest that the ability of

TCDD to induce CYP1A isozymes is very tissue and species specific because of differences in the function of these isozymes and that these differences may contribute to differential sensitivity of animal species to TCDD.

AhR Signaling Interactions

Since *Update 1998*, additional evidence has been published indicating that the AhR affects and is affected by other signal transduction pathways. Furthermore, it seems likely that the ability of the TCDD-activated AhR to interact with these pathways results in the altered regulation of processes involving tissue development, growth, and differentiation that is observed following exposure of animals to TCDD. There is also additional evidence that the AhR may have some role in the normal regulation of the cell cycle. The newest data on AhR interactions with growth and differentiation processes, redox signaling, kinase activities, and hormone receptor signaling are discussed below.

Growth and Differentiation Signaling

TCDD has been demonstrated to be a potent tumor promoter in several types of initiation–promoter models. Its ability to induce cell proliferation and altered differentiation is believed to be an important factor in the mechanism of TCDD-induced carcinogenesis. A study by Walker et al. (1998) investigated the time course and reversibility of cell proliferation in control and diethylnitrosamine-initiated female rats exposed biweekly to an average daily dose of 125 ng TCDD/kg/day for up to 60 weeks. Cell proliferation, as determined by the incorporation of 5-bromo-2′-deoxyuridine into DNA, was not increased until after 30 weeks of exposure. In contrast, CYP1A1 activity was increased at all times examined after 14 weeks. Even 16 weeks after the cessation of TCDD treatment, cell proliferation remained significantly elevated over controls. Proliferation was not increased, however, 30 weeks after withdrawal of treatment. Notably, dosimetric analysis suggested that the rat liver tissue burden of TCDD was predictive of CYP1A1 expression but not of cell proliferation. The measurement of total dose over time was not predictive of CYP1A1 expression or cell proliferation. Therefore, tissue burden correlated with a simple reversible response (i.e., CYP1A1 activity), but not with a more complex response.

The regulation of and balance between cellular differentiation, proliferation and cell death (apoptosis) are essential components of a tissue's ability to succumb to or escape chemical-induced developmental abnormalities or carcinogenesis. The proto-oncogene *c-myc* is an important factor in apoptosis regulation and has been shown to be increased in human and rodent liver neoplasia. A study by Christensen et al. (1999) examined whether apoptosis is altered in hepatocytes that overexpress *c-myc* and whether TCDD alters that apoptosis. Concentrations of TCDD up to 1 nM did not affect *c-myc*-induced apoptosis in hepatocytes.

Reiners and Clift (1999) examined the relationship between AhR content of mouse hepatoma cells and susceptibility to ceramide-induced apoptosis. Ceramide exposure caused a concentration-dependent inhibition of cell proliferation and induction of apoptosis. In variant cells that possess approximately 10 percent of the AhR content of wild-type cells, ceramide also arrested growth but did not induce apoptosis. Furthermore, modulation of the AhR content confirmed the relationship between AhR content and susceptibility to ceramide-induced apoptosis. This relationship appears to be relatively specific for ceramide-affected pathways because AhR content did affect apoptosis induced by other agents. Ceramide, however, was able to induce apoptosis in a cell line possessing AhR but lacking ARNT, suggesting that the AhR modulates ceramide-induced apoptosis by a mechanism that does not require ARNT protein and exogenous AhR ligands.

Dioxin-like chemicals have profound effects on the immune system of experimental animals. The direct cell targets that mediate these responses in vivo have not been unequivocally identified, in part because of the multicellular nature of the immune system, conflicting data from in vivo and in vitro studies, and the possibility that immune responses may be mediated indirectly through an action on other tissue systems (e.g., endocrine effects). Several studies have examined whether TCDD-induced changes in the immune system are caused by altered differentiation and maturation processes that lead to cellular arrest, proliferation, or apoptosis. Based on previous publications indicating that TCDD induces thymic atrophy through its ability to elicit apoptosis in thymocytes, Kamath et al. (1998) examined phenotypic changes in thymocytes from animals treated with 50 μg TCDD/kg and compared these changes to cells undergoing spontaneous apoptosis in vitro. Similar phenotypic changes were observed in both populations. Therefore, phenotypic alteration in the density of thymocyte surface molecules might be a biomarker of apoptosis. Such a biomarker would be useful because detection of apoptosis in vivo is often difficult. Pryputniewicz et al. (1998) examined whether resting or activated T cells are more susceptible to TCDD exposure. T cells isolated from the popliteal lymph nodes of mice treated with 50 μg TCDD/kg had a decreased proliferative response to anti-CD3 antibody compared to cells from control animals. Freshly isolated cells from TCDD-treated animals did not show increased apoptosis. However, activated cells that were cultured for 24 hours alone or with anti-CD3 antibody demonstrated increased apoptosis compared to resting lymph node T cells. These data suggest that TCDD elicits differential effects on activated and resting T cells. This same group of researchers also determined that Fas-deficient and Fas ligand-defective mice were resistant to TCDD-induced thymic atrophy and apoptosis. TCDD treatment resulted in increased FasL protein but not Fas mRNA (Kamath et al., 1999). Fas ligand is a cytokine belonging to the tumor necrosis factor family, and it appears to be involved in controlling pathways that lead to activation of caspases and subsequent cell death. The data from Kamath et al. (1999) suggest that Fas ligand may play an important role in TCDD-mediated immune effects through its ability to control apoptotic events. A study by Hart et al. (1999) demonstrated an increased number of apoptotic cells in the lymphoid regions of the spleen and pronephros from fish (*Tilapia*) treated with 5 µg/kg/day TCDD for 5 days. No significant effect was observed at a dosage of 1 µg/kg/day TCDD. Finally, another study found that TCDD concentrations of 1–40 nM induced apoptosis in two cultured human leukemic lymphoblastic T cell lines. However, two other AhR ligands, 2,3,7,8-tetrachlorodibenzofuran and β-naphthoflavone failed to elicit apoptosis even at concentrations up to 20 µM. Cell death was not observed in a cell line containing a dominant-negative mutant of c-Jun N-termal kinase (JNK). Those data suggest that the AhR may not be involved in TCDD-induced apoptosis and that the JNK signal transduction pathway may play a role.

In contrast to the studies cited above, other investigations in mice indicate that apoptosis is not involved in TCDD-induced thymic atrophy. Overexpression of the antiapoptotic oncogene *Bcl-2* in the thymus did not prevent atrophy induced by 30 µg TCDD/kg. Although distinct phenotypic changes in thymocytes were observed, no signs of apoptosis were detected using several different methods (Staples et al., 1998a). However, apoptosis was detected in animals treated with dexamethasone, and the overexpression of *Bcl-2* prevented that apoptosis. In another publication, Staples et al. (1998b) demonstrated that thymic alterations induced by TCDD were strictly dependent on the presence of the AhR in hematopoietic cells. These studies were performed using chimeric animals with either TCDD-responsive (*Ahr*+/+) stromal components and TCDD-unresponsive (*Ahr*–/–) hematopoietic components, or the reverse. Thymic atrophy was not observed in animals with *Ahr*+/+ stroma and *Ahr*–/– hematopoietic cells, or in animals with *Ahr*–/– in both components. However, the same degree of atrophy was observed in animals with *Ahr*–/– stroma and *Ahr*+/+ hematopoietic cells as in animals *Ahr*+/+ in both components. These results indicate that the targets for TCDD-induced atrophy are in the hematopoietic compartment. Nohara et al. (2000) examined phenotypic changes in thymus and lymph nodes following treatment of rats with 1 or 2 µg TCDD/kg. Similar phenotypic changes in thymocytes were observed as previously reported, with the exception that a reduction in $CD4^+CD8^+$ cells did not occur. However, the phenotype of lymph node cells indicated that the number of recent thymic emigrants was decreased. Based on this observation, the authors suggest that TCDD might result in immunosuppression, in part, through its ability to alter differentiation of T cells and cause a subsequent reduction in the peripheral T-cell repertoire. Prell et al. (2000) report a hyporesponsive cytotoxic T-cell response in TCDD-treated mice because of a disruption of precursor activation. This was found not to be caused by insufficient IL-2 or apoptotic deletion $CD8^+$ T cells. On the other hand, in mice exposed to TCDD and infected with influenza virus, the number of $CD8^+$ mediastinal lymph node cells was reduced, these cells failed to develop cytolytic activity, and the production of IL-2 and interferon-γ (IFN-γ) was suppressed. Exposure to TCDD also decreased the production of virus-specific antibodies, the recruitment of $CD8^+$ cells to the lung, and the percentage of cells bearing a cytotoxic T-lymphocyte (CTL) phenotype (Warren et al., 2000). The cytolytic activity of lung lavage cells from TCDD- and vehicle-treated mice, however, was equivalent in this study.

Much evidence indicates that TCDD exposure during development results in altered tissue growth and differentiation processes. Several studies demonstrate that in utero and lactational exposure of male rats to TCDD impairs prostate development. Pregnant rats were treated with 1 µg TCDD/kg at gd 15, and male pups were examined between gd 20 and pnd 32. At gd 20 an impairment of the prostatic epithelial budding process was observed. Cell proliferation of the ventral prostate was decreased on pnd 1 but was not altered at later periods. There were delays in the differentiation of the prostate periductal smooth muscle cells and luminal epithelial cells. In addition, there were alterations in the arrangement of cell types in the ventral prostate characterized by hyperplastic epithelium, increased density or continuous layer of basal epithelial cells, and thickened periductal smooth muscle sheaths (Roman et al., 1998b). These effects may be related to an observed transient downregulation in the expression of androgen-regulated prostatic mRNAs used as markers of differentiated ductal epithelium. Increased expression of CYP1A1 mRNA, however, was also seen (Roman and Peterson, 1998). Hamm et al. (2000) demonstrated that treatment of rats with 1 µg TCDD/kg at gd 15 resulted in decreased seminal vesicle weights in offspring 8–11 months of age. Decreased seminal vesicle epithelial branching and differentiation were also observed.

Developmental effects on female offspring of in utero exposure to TCDD have been observed in several other studies. A single oral dose of 2 µg TCDD/kg to pregnant hamsters at gd 11.5 altered reproductive tissue and function in female offspring (Wolf et al., 1999). Body weights were reduced, vaginal opening was delayed, and vaginal estrous cycles were altered. In addition, there was increased incidence of external urogenital malformations characterized by clefting of the phallus, which has also been observed in the rat. More recently, Dienhart et al. (2000) reported that a single dose of 1 µg TCDD/kg at gd 15 to pregnant rats results in abnormal vaginal development in female fetuses by inhibiting regression of the Wolffian ducts, increasing the size of the interductal mesenchyme, and preventing fusion of the Mullerian ducts. Cummings et al. (1999) report that exposure of mice at gd 8 to TCDD (3 µg/kg), supplemented by adult exposure, resulted in increased sensitivity to the promotion of surgically-induced endometrial lesion growth; no effects were observed in the rat. It is not clear if this growth is related to previous reports of increased incidence of endometriosis in exposed monkeys. A recent publication by Yang et al. (2000), however, indicates that TCDD exposure of cynomolgus monkeys exerted a bimodal effect on survival and growth of endometrial implants. This study is of particular interest because the dose levels used (1–25 ng/kg, 5 days per week for 12 months) resulted in tissue dioxin levels representative of dioxin concentrations in human adipose tissue. Exposure of pregnant rats to 1 μg TCDD/kg at gd 15 reduced the number of ovarian antral and preantral follicles of certain size classes in female offspring examined at pnd 21–22 (Heimler et al., 1998). The loss of these follicles did not appear to be due to apoptotic events.

Two studies suggest that TCDD and the AhR may have effects on the developing mammary gland. Brown et al. (1998) investigated whether prenatal exposure to TCDD predisposes rats to mammary cancer. The exposure of pregnant rats to 1 μg TCDD/kg at gd 15 resulted in significantly more terminal end buds and fewer lobules in 50-day-old female offspring. There were also increased numbers of 7,12-dimethylbenz[a]anthracene (DMBA) induced mammary adenocarcinomas in rats prenatally treated with TCDD. The alterations in mammary gland differentiation were correlated with increased susceptibility to mammary cancer from prenatal TCDD exposure. Hushka et al. (1998) examined the actions of 2,3,7,8-tetrachlorodibenzofuran (TCDF) and AhR presence on AhR signal transduction pathways in the developing mouse mammary gland. In untreated 6- to 8-week-old *Ahr* null-allele littermates, there were reductions of terminal end buds and increased numbers of blunt-ended terminal ducts. Treatment of mammary glands in vitro with TCDF suppressed lobule development and DNA synthesis. These data suggest that normal mammary gland development may be dependent on the presence of the AhR and that exposure to TCDF during this period may alter normal AhR function to suppress development.

Previous studies suggest that the presence of dioxin-like compounds in mother's milk may affect the mineralization of children's permanent first molars. Developmental dental defects have also been reported in monkeys and rats exposed to TCDD, and in humans exposed in utero following the accidental contamination of cooking oil with PCBs and dibenzofurans in Taiwan (Rogan et al., 1988). To examine the role of EGF in the actions of TCDD on tooth development, Partanen et al. (1998) cultured embryonic teeth from mice with TCDD in the absence or presence of EGF. Exposure to 0.5–1.0 μM TCDD caused depolarization of ondontoblasts and ameloblasts and improper mineralization and deposition of enamel matrix. The presence of EGF attenuated many of the effects of TCDD. These results suggest that interference of TCDD with mouse molar development in vitro involves EGF receptor (EGFR) signaling. Studies by Willey et al. (1998) suggest the presence of transcriptionally active AhR in developing mouse tooth buds exposed to TCDD in vivo.

Hurst et al. (2000) examined the embryonic concentrations of TCDD that were associated with developmental defects. Pregnant rats received a single oral dose of radiolabeled TCDD on gd 15, and fetal concentrations were measured at gd 16 and 21. In an animal that was administered 0.2 μg TCDD/kg, at gd 16 there were 13.2 pg TCDD/g present in an individual fetus. This concentration has been previously associated with delayed puberty, decreased epididymal sperm counts in male pups, and malformations in the external genitalia of females.

Several groups have investigated the signal transduction pathways that are altered by TCDD exposure and that may be responsible for altered tissue development and cellular differentiation. Kolluri et al. (1999) demonstrated that TCDD-induced activation of the AhR induces the p27Kip1 cyclin/cdk inhibitor by altering *Kip1* transcription in hepatoma cells and in cultured fetal thymus glands. Hepatoma cells expressing Kip1 antisense RNA are resistant to TCDD-induced suppression of proliferation and delay of cell cycle through the G_1 phase. In addition, Kip1-deficient thymic glands are less sensitive to the inhibition of proliferation by TCDD. Because Kip1 appears to act as a tumor suppressor gene, at present it seems unlikely that the effects of TCDD on this gene could underlie some of TCDD's carcinogenicity and tumor-promoting activity.

It has been shown that TCDD induces a G_1 cell cycle arrest in rat 5L hepatoma cells via the AhR (Ma and Whitlock, 1996). In addition, retinoblastoma (RB) protein is known to control cell cycle progression through G_1, and to promote cell differentiation (Goodrich and Lee, 1992; Richon et al., 1992; Sehy et al., 1992). Two publications have implicated an interaction of the AhR with the RB protein in the ability of TCDD to mediate cell cycle arrest via the AhR. Ge and Elferink (1998) demonstrated that the RB protein and the AhR interact directly, that the interaction occurs through two distinct regions in the AhR, and that the RB preferentially associates with ligand-bound AhR. Puga et al. (2000b) also verified this interaction using both the yeast two-hybrid system and human breast carcinoma MCF-7 cells. They also demonstrated that the AhR acts in synergy with the RB to repress E2 promoter binding factor (E2F)-dependent transcription and induce cell cycle arrest. The AhR has also been shown to interact with p300, an important coactivator in the regulation of the cell cycle (Tohkin et al., 2000).

Arachidonic acid and its metabolites modulate cell growth and differentiation and may be involved in the multistep process of carcinogenesis (Tsunamoto et al., 1987; Gaillard et al., 1989). Work by Lee et al. (1998) examining the profile of CYP1A isozymes in different tissues from mice and chicks treated with TCDD suggest that species-specific differences in the catalytic activities of these isozymes and subsequent differences in arachidonic acid metabolism may contribute to species differences in sensitivity to TCDD. Using inhibitors of cyclooxygenase (COX) and lipoxygenase activities, Wolfle et al. (2000) examined the potential role of arachidonic acid metabolism in the promotion of malignant transformation of mouse fibroblasts by TCDD. The promoting effects of 1.5 pM TCDD were blocked by cotreatment with COX inhibitors. However, selective inhibition of COX-2 did not abolish the effect of TCDD. Long-term treatment with TCDD induced both COX-1 and COX-2 mRNA and protein, and this resulted in the accumulation of PGE_2 and 6-keto-$PGF_{1\alpha}$. The data suggest that the stimulation of arachidonic acid metabolism by COX induction may be a critical event in the promotional actions of TCDD in mouse fibroblasts. In contrast, exposure of mice to a single dose of 15 µg TCDD/kg did not alter COX mRNA or protein in the spleen (Lawrence and Kerkvliet, 1998). Furthermore, several inhibitors blocked arachidonic acid metabolism but did not affect either TCDD-induced suppression of the cytotoxic T-lymphocyte response to tumor cells or antibody formation in response to sheep red blood cells.

Several previous reports indicated that TCDD modulates the expression of prostaglandin endoperoxide H synthase 2 (PGHS-2) in different cell lines. A study by Vogel et al. (1998) further examined whether this activity is altered in TCDD-exposed mice and whether any alteration was mediated by the AhR. A single dose of 10 μg TCDD/kg to C57BL/6J mice did not alter PGHS-1 in any tissue examined. However, TCDD treatment increased PGHS-2 mRNA in the lung and spleen, but not in the liver and kidney. A nearly hundredfold higher dose of TCDD was necessary to produce the same response in lungs of DBA/2J mice, which possess a defective AhR that has a lower affinity for TCDD. These studies indicate that TCDD modulates PGHS-2 activity in selected tissues by a mechanism involving the AhR.

A study by J.H. Yang et al. (1999) examined the relationships between the malignant transformation of human epidermal keratinocyte cells in culture by TCDD and the expression of several growth regulatory factors. Concentrations of TCDD up to 100 nM altered the expression of TGF-β_1, plasminogen activator inhibitor-2 (PAI-2), and TNF-α in the transformed cells compared to the parental cells. There was a concentration-dependent increase in PAI-2 mRNA in the parental cells but not in the transformed cells. Although there were significant differences in TGF-β_1 and TNF-α mRNA expression between the transformed and parental cells, TCDD exposure did not produce a change in the expression of these growth factors. There was also a concentration-dependent increase in expression of IL-β1 and PAI-2 mRNA in immortalized human endometrial stromal cells following TCDD treatment (Yang, 1999). Expression of PAI-2 mRNA appeared to be altered by TCDD at the posttranscriptional level.

Abbott et al. (1998) examined the expression of several growth factors in nine separate samples of human embryonic palate placed in culture following their exposure to 10 nM TCDD. AhR protein levels were increased in five individuals. This increase was accompanied by increased expression of TGF-β, EFG, glucocorticoid receptor (GR), and/or TGF-β_2. EGF was increased in tissues where there was either no change in or decreased expression of the AhR. TGF-β expression was increased in six of nine samples. The effect of TCDD on the expression of TGF-β_2 was dependent on the age of the tissue; younger tissue demonstrated decreased expression, while older tissue had increased expression. The authors suggest that differences in the patterns of expression between human and mouse palates exposed to TCDD, as well as genetic variability, may provide a partial explanation for the relative insensitivity of human palatal cells to TCDD in culture.

Enan et al. (1998a) demonstrated, in cynomolgus macaques that had an increased incidence of endocervical squamous metaplasia approximately 1 year after a single doses of 2 or 4 μg TCDD/kg, that the expression of several growth factors was altered in endocervical cells from these monkeys. EGFR binding activity, Cdk4 protein levels, and DNA binding activity of AP-1 were significantly decreased, whereas H-ras, p53, wafl/p21, and Cdc2p34 protein levels increased. Significant alterations were also observed in c-Src kinase, protein tyrosine kinase, and casein kinase II (see below).

The mutational activation of the *K-ras* oncogene often occurs in human and mouse lung adenocarcinomas. TCDD treatment (1.6 μg/kg) increased the expression of K-ras p21 in the lungs of several strains of mice and altered the membrane–cytosol ratio of this protein (Ramakrishna and Anderson, 1998). Those effects were strain dependent and also depended on the *Ahr* genotype expressed. Treatment of immortalized alveolar type 2 E10 cells with 10 nM TCDD increased K-ras p21 levels in the membrane fraction approximately fourfold. It is not known how these data are related to proposed mechanisms underlying human lung cancer.

Urokinase plasminogen activator (*uPA*) is one of the genes shown to be altered by TCDD exposure. This protein is a serine protease that is involved in matrix turnover and growth of tumor cells. Unlike many other genes that are affected by TCDD at the transcriptional level, *uPA* is upregulated by TCDD due to mRNA stabilization. The mechanism of this regulation is still poorly understood. Shimba et al. (2000) demonstrated that a liver cytoplasmic protein of approximately 50 kDa recognizes the 3′-untranslated region of uPA mRNA in a TCDD-dependent manner. Additional work suggests that the effect is mediated by a protein phosphorylation cascade, not by de novo protein synthesis. These data indicate that TCDD alters uPA expression by a mechanism that apparently does not alter gene expression at the transcriptional level, suggesting that the binding of the AhR–ARNT complex to DREs is not involved in the process.

Redox Signaling

As discussed in *Update 1998*, exposure to TCDD might affect cellular redox (oxidation-reduction) status and associated signaling pathways through several mechanisms. Since *Update 1998,* more evidence has accumulated suggesting that cross-talk occurs between the AhR and hypoxia inducible factor (HIF) signaling pathways. Chan et al. (1999) investigated whether competition for ARNT or other cellular factors in rat hepatoma cells is involved in the cross-talk between the signaling pathways, because some HIFs complex with ARNT to bind with hypoxia responsive enhancers (HREs). In transfection assays, hypoxia inhibited DRE-driven transcription (i.e., induction of *CYP1A1*). AhR agonists inhibited activation of the HRE and induction of *erythropoietin* (*EPO*), a gene that regulates adaptation to low oxygen. Using endogenous loci activation of hypoxia pathways still inhibited *CYP1A1* upregulation; however, AhR activation enhanced the induction of *EPO*. Because of this result, the investigators looked at the promoter region of *EPO* and discovered that it contains DREs. Therefore, *EPO* appears to be an AhR-regulated gene. In addition, they found that the DREs present in the *EPO* promoter region can compensate for the inhibitory effects that TCDD has on HRE-mediated transcription. These are novel mechanisms for multiple levels of reciprocal cross-talk. Studies by Kim and Sheen (2000) also demonstrated that hypoxia inhibits TCDD-induced *CYP1A1* expression in hepatoma cells.

TCDD is known to induce a number of enzyme systems, through the AhR, that are involved in either the generation or the metabolism of oxidative intermediates. An imbalance of these intermediates could have profound effects on the cellular signaling pathways that regulate growth control and differentiation. In mice, treatment with 5 µg TCDD/kg three times daily produced an oxidative stress response characterized by increased hepatic oxidized glutathione levels and increased urinary levels of 8-hydroxydeoxyguanosine, a product of DNA base oxidation and excision repair (Shertzer et al., 1998). The latter persisted up to 8 weeks following treatment. In a recent study by Slezak et al. (2000) oxidative stress was characterized in several tissues following oral subchronic (0.15–150 ng/kg; 5 days/week for 13 week) or acute (0.001–100 µg/kg) exposure to TCDD. Acute treatment with doses of 10 and 100 µg/kg resulted in increases in hepatic superoxide anion production and lipid peroxidation. These were also increased at a subchronic dose of 150 ng/kg/day with a liver TCDD concentration of only 12 ng/kg. Subchronic doses as low as 0.15 ng/kg/day decreased glutathione concentrations in lung and kidney, but this was not observed at higher doses of TCDD.

Hassoun et al. (1998) examined the ability of subchronic exposure to TCDD to produce oxidative stress in the brains of mice. Exposure to 0.45 to 150 ng/kg/day for 5 days per week for 13 weeks resulted in a dose-dependent increase in the production of superoxide anion and lipid peroxidation in brain tissues. Similarly, Bagchi et al. (2000) noted dose-dependent increases in mouse brain and liver lipid peroxidation, DNA fragmentation, and production of superoxide anion. Notably, these effects of TCDD were exacerbated in mice deficient in the tumor suppressor p53. Machala et al. (1998) found that TCDD induced the activity of microsomal glutathione S-transferase (GST) in trout liver. Using TCDD and a variety of other chemicals, these investigators determined that induction of microsomal GST might be an early biochemical indicator of oxidative stress. Several previous investigations suggest that reactive oxygen species (ROS) might be generated by the increased presence of several of the cytochrome P450 isozymes known to be induced by TCDD and related halogenated aromatic hydrocarbons. More recently Schlezinger et al. (1999) demonstrated, using tissue microsomes from humans and in vitro expressed enzymes of other species, that the slowly metabolized AhR agonist 3,3',4,4'-tetrachlorobiphenyl stimulates the release of ROS by an uncoupling of the CYP1A1 enzyme reaction.

Investigations by Smith et al. (1998) indicate that iron potentiates the hepatic porphyria and toxicity of TCDD in AhR-responsive mouse strains. The administration of iron prior to a single dose of 75 μg TCDD/kg increased the formation of hydroxylated and peroxylated uroporphyrin derivatives and the induction of GST compared to animals treated with vehicle or TCDD alone. Iron overload, however, resulted in a reduction of TCDD-induced CYP1A activities. These data suggest that iron may potentiate an oxidative process elicited by TCDD.

Protein Kinases

Research continues to support the hypothesis that TCDD modulates cellular function in part through an alteration of kinase activities. How these changes relate to specific end points of TCDD toxicity, however, has yet to be determined. Evidence also suggests that phosphorylation–dephosphorylation processes regulate the activity of the AhR–ARNT complex, but where the phosphorylation sites are located or how they regulate AhR function has yet to be determined.

Ashida et al. (2000b) studied the effects of TCDD treatment on nuclear protein kinases and phosphatases that affect the transcription factors c-myc and AP-1 in guinea pig liver. A single TCDD treatment of 1 μg/kg resulted in an increase in nuclear protein tyrosine kinase within 1 day after treatment. The activity had returned to near control levels by day 40. There was a reduction in casein kinase II (CKII) activity, however, at all times studied up to 40 days. A similar effect on CKII activity was also seen in this study following TCDD treatment of liver explants in culture. DNA binding of AP-1 was increased, but a biphasic effect on protein binding to the *c-myc* response element occurred, with an initial increase in binding followed by a suppression of binding. Additional studies demonstrated that changes in phosphorylation were responsible for TCDD-induced changes in DNA binding of these transcription factors and that CKII played an important role in transducing the actions of TCDD.

The p53 protein is a key mediator of apoptosis after genotoxic stress, and inhibition of apoptosis of preneoplastic cells is thought to be a major mechanism of action of tumor promoters. The activity of p53 is controlled primarily at the posttranslational level by hyperphosphorylation which decreases the ability of p53 to activate transcription (see review by Colman et al., 2000). Exposure of primary rat hepatocytes to TCDD at concentrations up to 10 nM resulted in a concentration-dependent suppression of apoptosis induced by UV light and an increase in p53 phosphorylation (Worner and Schrenk, 1998). This effect of TCDD on p53 was also observed in hepatocyte extracts in the same study. Treatment of the extracts with anti-src antibodies almost completely eliminated the effect of TCDD on p53 phosphorylation, suggesting a key role of c-src in these effects of TCDD. It is of interest that recent investigations suggest that low levels of p53 are associated with the resistance of certain mouse strains to TCDD toxicity and that this resistance is additive to that associated with the Ah^{dd} locus, which encodes a defective AhR protein (A.L. Yang et al., 1999).

The results of several studies suggest a role of c-src kinase in the toxicity induced by TCDD. Some of these investigations further suggest that c-src might directly interact with the AhR. Enan et al. (1998b) report that treatment of guinea pigs with 1 µg TCDD/kg increases src kinase activity in adipose tissue from males but not females and that the increase is associated with an increased phosphorylation of cytosolic protein that occurs in males but not females. This and other publications by the same group also report that treatment of guinea pigs with the tyrosine kinase inhibitors geldanamycin and quercetin and src deficiency in mice partially protect against some effects of TCDD-induced toxicity, including the excess fatty deposits and mottled appearance of liver (Matsumura et al., 1997; Enan et al., 1998c; Dunlap et al., 1999). Kohle et al. (1999) examined the effects of TCDD on c-src activity and membrane translocation and cell contact inhibition in WB-F344 cells. Exposure to 1 nM TCDD decreased cytosolic c-src and increased c-src in the plasma membrane. EGFR tyrosine phosphorylation was also enhanced by TCDD treatment. Pretreatment of cells with geldanamycin, which also disrupts HSP90 protein complexes, abolished the TCDD-induced translocation of src to the membrane and the TCDD-mediated reduction of cell contact inhibition. The increase in membrane src did not depend on de novo protein synthesis. These data suggest that the membrane translocation of c-src and altered cell contact inhibition are mediated by activation of the cytosolic AhR–HSP90 complex.

Investigations by El-Sabeawy et al. (1998) indicate that exposure of rats to TCDD during pubertal development affects kinase activities and EGFR binding in the testis, as well as sperm motility. Doses of TCDD up to 10 µg/kg were administered to 21-day-old male rats, and tissues were examined up to 90 days of age. Treatment with 10 µg/kg caused testicular atrophy, a decrease in the diameter of the seminiferous tubules, and an absence of spermatogonia cells. Doses as low as 1 µg/kg decreased testicular sperm numbers, affected sperm motility, and affected acrosome reactions. Decreases in EGFR were found in rat testicular tissue from 34 to 90 days. TCDD significantly increased c-src kinase activity but decreased the activities of protein tyrosine kinase, mitogen-activated kinase, and protein kinase C. Pretreatment with genedanamycin blocked the testicular atrophy observed with the 10 µg/kg dose of TCDD. These data suggest the involvement of src kinase and EGFR in TCDD-induced effects on testicular development.

Several lines of evidence indicate that phosphorylation of the AhR and/or ARNT contributes to both the DNA binding and the transactivation functions of the complex. The actual sites of phosphorylation on these proteins and their role in regulating the action of these transcription factors are unknown. Several reports by Long and coworkers (Long et al., 1998, 1999; Long and Perdew, 1999) demonstrate that protein kinase C activity is required for AhR-mediated transactivation function. This activity, however, does not affect AhR or ARNT protein levels, nuclear localization, or AhR–ARNT dimerization. Additional work indicates that the action of protein kinase C is not dependent on the transactivation domains present in the AhR or ARNT, further suggesting that coactivators recruited by these domains are not affected by protein kinase C activity.

Hormone Receptor Signaling

During the past 2 years, considerable research has continued to focus on the interactions among hormone receptor signaling pathways that might play a role in TCDD toxicity, especially on interactions between the estrogen receptor and the AhR. Several groups have investigated the mechanisms by which these pathways might interact. Proposed mechanisms include altered hormone metabolism, effects on receptor expression, competition for accessory transcription factors, and binding to overlapping response elements in responsive genes.

As discussed in *Update 1998*, TCDD is a more potent hepatocarcinogen in female rats than in male rats or ovariectomized female rats, suggesting a role of ovarian hormones in the mechanism of TCDD-induced hepatocarcinogenesis. Wyde et al. (2000) studied the effects of cotreatment with TCDD and 17β-estradiol in diethylnitrosamine (DEN) initiated ovariectomized rats. Rats were initiated with DEN and treated with TCDD at 100 ng/kg/day for 20 or 30 weeks with and without 17β-estradiol treatment using constant-release pellets. Hepatotoxicity was observed in the TCDD-treated groups, but no excess hepatotoxicity was associated with 17β-estradiol supplementation in the ovariectomized animals. Notably, liver TCDD concentrations were similar between intact rats and ovariectomized rats supplemented with 17β-estradiol but were higher in ovariectomized rats not supplemented with 17β-estradiol. A study by Petroff et al. (2000) investigated whether estrogens increased the toxic effects of TCDD on growth and ovarian function in the rat. Immature rats were treated with estradiol followed by a single dose of 10 µg TCDD/kg. Follicular development was induced with equine chorionic gonadotropin followed by an ovulator dose of human chorionic gonadotropin. TCDD treatment inhibited ovulation; this inhibition was potentiated by estradiol treatment in hypophysectomized but not intact animals. Only hypophysectomized rats exposed to both TCDD and estradiol showed weight loss. Inhibition of ovulation by TCDD was alleviated by estradiol treatment into the ovarian bursa. This treatment, however, increased the body weight loss elicited by TCDD. These data demonstrate the complex interactions between TCDD, estrogen, and other hormonal systems in intact animals and suggest that the interactions occur systemically and in the ovary. Gao et al. (2000) demonstrated that several AhR agonists blocked ovulation in gonadotropin-primed immature female rats.

Chaffin et al. (2000) investigated the regulation of AhR and ARNT mRNAs in liver and ovarian tissues during the rat estrous cycle. Hepatic AhR mRNA was increased on the morning of proestrus and decreased dramatically by the evening of proestrus. Hepatic ARNT mRNA decreased between diestrus and the morning of proestrus and between the evening of proestrus and the morning of estrus.

Ovarian AhR mRNA did not change between diestrus and proestrus but decreased on the evening of proestrus. Changes in ovarian ARNT mRNA were similar to those seen in the liver. Treatment with estradiol or an estradiol antagonist did not affect AhR mRNA in the liver. This study suggests that changes in the reproductive cycle also regulate the expression of both AhR and ARNT, although estradiol levels may not play a major role in those changes.

Enan et al. (1998d) investigated the effect of TCDD treatment on the ability of estradiol to alter kinase activities in adipose tissues of immature and mature female rats. In mature females, estradiol treatment (15 µg/kg) increased tyrosine kinase (TK) and protein kinase A (PKA) activities and decreased mitogen-activated protein 2 kinase (MAP2K) activity. TCDD treatment at doses of 10–115 µg/kg blocked the stimulatory effect of estradiol on TK and PKA activities. In immature females, estradiol treatment decreased TK and PKA activities, and TCDD exposure potentiated these effects. TCDD treatment also decreased binding of radiolabeled estradiol to estrogen receptors (ERs) in both mature and immature females and blocked the stimulatory effect of estradiol on ER binding activity. Geldanamycin treatment abolished most of the effects of TCDD. These data indicate the ability of TCDD to disrupt estrogen-dependent signal transduction pathways in female rats.

Several other studies have demonstrated the ability of TCDD to disrupt estrogen signaling processes in cultured cells. Smeets et al. (1999) demonstrated that several AhR agonists, including TCDD, suppress estradiol-induced secretion of the yolk protein vitellogenin in carp hepatocytes. This was not correlated with the induction of CYP1A1 activity by TCDD, since induction of this enzyme occurred at lower concentrations of TCDD. Exposure of human endometrial cells to TCDD reduced the ER level by 40 percent and reduced ER-mediated transcription by 50 percent (Ricci et al., 1999a).

Estrogen treatment has also been shown to affect the AhR-mediated signal transduction pathway. Sarkar et al. (2000) demonstrated that estradiol (5 µg/kg) enhances the induction by TCDD (0.3 µg/kg) of *CYP1A1* in female rat livers. The increase in nuclear AhR content resulting from TCDD treatment, however, was not altered by estradiol treatment, suggesting that estrogen affects the induction of the *CYP1A1* gene after formation of the active AhR–ARNT complex. In contrast, estradiol treatment decreased *CYP1A1* expression (constitutive and TCDD induced) in cultured human endometrial cells (Ricci et al., 1999b). The authors suggested that the activated pathways were competing for available transcription factors. Studies by Schuur et al. (1998) demonstrated that thyroid status did not affect the induction of CYP1A1 activity by TCDD.

Using GST-pulldown assays and immunoprecipitation, Klinge et al. (2000) demonstrated that the AhR directly interacts with ERα, COUP-TF (an orphan nuclear receptor expressed in estrogen target tissues), and ERRα1 (an estrogen-related receptor) in vitro. Agonist-bound AhR showed a stronger interaction than antagonist-bound AhR. These receptors do not appear to interact with ARNT.

COUP-TF1 was found to bind the DRE in vitro, and overexpression of this protein in MCF-7 breast cancer cells inhibited TCDD-induced reporter gene activity. TCDD treatment inhibited estradiol-activated reporter genes, but COUP-TF did not block the antiestrogenic effect of TCDD. COUP-TF may regulate AhR-dependent responses by direct protein–protein interaction and by DRE binding competition.

Data from Jana et al. (1999a) suggest that ERα acts as a positive modulator in the regulation of AhR-responsive genes. The relationship between ERα activity and TCDD responsiveness was examined using human uterine endometrial carcinoma cells. RL95-2 cells were highly responsive to TCDD, but KLE cells were not, despite the fact that KLE cells express higher levels of the AhR. Nuclear translocation of ERα, however, was shown to be defective in KLE cells. Transient expression of ERα in KLE cells restored the cells' responsiveness to estradiol and TCDD. Caruso et al. (1999) investigated the role of HSP90 in mediating cross-talk between ER and AhR-regulated pathways. Overexpression of HSP90 in human breast cancer cells inhibited TCDD responsiveness, but had no effect on estrogen responsiveness. Expression of an ER deletion mutant that does not bind DNA or the ligand binding domain of the AhR increased basal and TCDD-inducible CYP1A1 expression. Notably, HSP90 mainly localized to the cytoplasm in ER-positive cell lines, whereas in ER-negative cells, HSP90 was equally distributed between cytosol and nucleus. These data suggest that cellular ER content may regulate AhR responsiveness by a mechanism that involves HSP90.

Tian et al. (1998) demonstrated that TCDD causes tissue-specific down-regulation of ER mRNA. Treatment of mice with 5 µg TCDD/kg resulted in decreased ER mRNA in the ovaries, uterus, liver, and lungs. The most pronounced changes occurred in the ovaries and uterus. No changes were observed in the kidney and brain. These data suggest that the ovary and uterus may be the most sensitive organs to the antiestrogenic effects of TCDD.

TCDD treatment (10 nM) of MCF-7 cells blocked estradiol induced *c-fos* protooncogene mRNA levels (Duan et al., 1999). This inhibitory response was not observed in the presence of an AhR antagonist and in variant Ah-nonresponsive cells, indicating that the AhR was required for the effect of TCDD. Further studies indicated that the activated AhR complex bound to a DRE sequence that overlapped with an estradiol-responsive site rich in guanine and cytosine. The data suggest that TCDD acts by activating the AhR, which then binds to an inhibitory DRE complex, thus blocking ER/Sp1 DNA complex formation and subsequent activation of the *c-fos* gene. Additional work by Klinge et al. (1999) suggests that the activated AhR–ARNT complex inhibits estrogen action by inhibiting ER binding to imperfect estrogen responsive elements (ERE) sites that are adjacent to or overlap DRE sites.

Jana et al. (1999b) demonstrated an interaction between the AhR and testosterone signal transduction pathways. Normal and testosterone-stimulated growth of LNCaP prostate cancer cells were inhibited by 10–100 nM TCDD, and testosterone treatment inhibited the induction of CYP1A1 mRNA by TCDD in a concentration-dependent manner. TCDD inhibited testosterone-dependent transcriptional activity and testosterone-regulated prostate-specific antigen expression. Treatment of porcine preovulatory follicles with 10 nM TCDD decreased the number of proliferating cells, reduced testosterone secretion, and increased estradiol secretion (Grochowalski et al., 2000). The exposure of isolated porcine luteal cells to 10 nM TCDD also resulted in decreased progesterone secretion by these cells (Gregoraszczuk et al., 2000).

Exposure to TCDD has been shown to produce hyperkeratosis of the skin in humans and several other species. The characteristics of this response resemble those of vitamin A deficiency. Krig and Rice (2000) reported that TCDD suppressed retinoid-induced transglutaminase mRNA in a human squamous carcinoma cell line.

Significant Interactions

Research has identified other groups of chemicals that may either interact directly with the AhR or affect AhR function indirectly. When exposure to such chemicals and TCDD occurs, the toxicological consequences of TCDD exposure can be modified. Likewise, exposure to TCDD and AhR ligands may modify the toxicity of other chemicals.

Loeffler and Peterson (1999) investigated the effects of in utero and lactational exposure of rats to mixtures of TCDD and p,p'-dichlorodiphenyldichloroethylene (DDE). Rats were treated with 0.25 µg TCDD/kg on gd 15 and 100 mg/kg DDE on gd 14–18, or with 0.25 µg TCDD/kg on gd 15 and 100 mg/kg DDE on gd 14–18. Male offspring were examined on pnd 21 through 63. Treatment with TCDD or DDE alone decreased prostate weights in a time-dependent manner. Coexposure appeared to potentiate these effects at pnd 21 but not at later periods. Individual exposures reduced epididymal sperm numbers, but cotreatment did not further reduce sperm numbers. Roman et al. (1998b) demonstrated that TCDD treatment produced a hyperplastic and disorganized pattern of androgen receptor staining, and Loeffler and Peterson (1999) found that DDE treatment alone decreased epithelial androgen receptor staining in ventral prostate. Androgen receptor staining following cotreatment exhibited a pattern that was characteristic of the effects of the individual compounds.

Several studies have examined the effect of exposure to both PCBs and dioxins. Wolfle (1998) studied the interactions between these compounds in an in vitro promotion assay that measures malignant transformation of carcinogen-initiated mouse fibroblasts. PCB 126 (a coplanar AhR agonist) (1 and 0.3 pM) and TCDD (0.15 pM) produced an additive effect in this assay system, but PCB 153 (a diortho-substituted compound) (3 or 30 nM) antagonized the TCDD (1.5 pM) mediated promotion. Smialowicz et al. (1997) examined the effect of cotreatment with 2,2′,4,4′,5,5′-hexachlorobiphenyl (PCB153) and TCDD on the antibody plaque-forming cell (PFC) response to sheep red blood cells in B6C3F1 mice. While exposure to TCDD alone resulted in a dose-related suppression of the PFC response, exposure to PCB153 alone resulted in an enhanced response at 358 mg/kg. Combined exposure did not change the response relative to PCB treatment alone. However, the PFC response was enhanced at combined exposures with low concentrations of TCDD, but suppressed with combined exposures with a higher concentration of TCDD. The data suggested that PCB153 acts as a functional antagonist rather than an AhR antagonist, but the effect may be concentration dependent. Some of these interactions with PCBs and their implications are discussed further in the section on toxic equivalency factors (TEFs).

Studies by Kim et al. (1999) suggest that compounds present in ginseng extracts may protect against some end points of TCDD-induced toxicity. Treatment of guinea pigs with a single dose of 1 μg TCDD/kg produced decreased body weight gain and decreased testicular weight (there was no effect on testes weight, however, when the data were expressed as percentage of body weight). Light and electron microscopic examination of the testes showed smaller tubules and maturation arrest of spermatogonia, dissolution of germinal epithelium, and disruption of tight junctions between Sertoli cells. Cotreatment with extracts from *Panax ginseng* protected against the effects of TCDD on testes weight and the morphological alterations.

Humans are exposed to both cigarette smoke and diesel exhaust. Publications by Meek and Finch (1999) and Meek (1998) indicate that both mainstream cigarette smoke and diesel exhaust particles contain chemicals that bind to the AhR and ER and regulate AhR- and ER-responsive genes. Additional work by Dertinger et al. (1998) indicated that cigarette smoke contains chemicals that transform the AhR to an active transcription factor. These investigators also demonstrated that the genotoxic effect of cigarette smoke condensate, as determined by reticulocyte micronuclei formation, was potentiated in mouse hepatoma cells pretreated with 1 nM TCDD. This effect was attenuated in hepatoma cells that contained approximately tenfold lower levels of AhR. Furthermore, while the cigarette smoke condensate increased the incidence of micronucleated reticulocytes in *Ahr*+/+ mice, no increase was observed in *Ahr* null-allele mice. The data suggest that AhR-regulated enzyme induction plays an important role in mediating the genotoxicity of chemicals found in cigarette smoke. A study by Chang et al. (1999) examined the differential response of human lung adenocarcinoma cell lines to benzo[*a*]pyrene and demonstrated that a variation in AhR-mediated *CYP1A1* induction contributes to the differential susceptibility of different cell lines to benzo[*a*]pyrene metabolite–DNA adduct formation. The above data are consistent with recent work by Shimizu et al. (2000) showing that *Ahr*-positive mice develop tumors in response to benzo[*a*]pyrene treatment, but *Ahr* null-allele animals do not develop tumors. The latter study provides direct evidence that AhR-regulated signaling pathways are involved in carcinogenesis induced by certain chemicals. Together these data are consistent with the proposed hypothesis that exposure to TCDD or other AhR agonists, some of which are found in tobacco smoke, results in the induction of cytochrome P450 isozymes that are further responsible for the metabolic activation of polycyclic aromatic hydrocarbons in smoke or other pro-carcinogens to genotoxic intermediates. However, the exact quantitative relationships between the level of enzyme induction, metabolic activation of pro-carcinogens, and increased tumor incidence have yet to be determined.

Disease Outcomes

Lethality There is considerable variation in species susceptibility to the lethal effects of TCDD. Sensitivity among strains of rats can vary as much as one thousandfold. The LD_{50} values between species range from 0.6 µg/kg for guinea pig to more than 5 mg/kg for hamster (U.S. EPA, 1985). Most species, however, commonly develop a wasting disease that follows exposure to acute toxic doses of TCDD, which is characterized by loss of body weight and fatty tissue. The mechanism responsible for this syndrome remains unclear.

A study conducted to assess the toxicity of dietary TCDD in female mink identified "$LD_{50}s$" of approximately 0.264 and 0.047 µg TCDD/kg body weight per day for 28 and 125 days of exposure, respectively (Hochstein et al., 1998). In this study, mink were fed diets supplemented with 0.001, 0.01, 0.1, 1.0, 10, or 100 parts per billion (ppb) TCDD for up to 125 days. Mortality occurred in the 1, 10, and 100 ppb groups, and these mink displayed the classic symptoms of the wasting syndrome (i.e., extreme loss of body weight, decreased food consumption with an increase in consumption prior to death, and bloody stool). The mink remained content and alert until they became moribund. This phenomenon has been widely accepted as a manifestation of TCDD toxicity.

Dermal Toxicity There have not been any studies the past 2 years demonstrating significant health effects of TCDD on the skin of animals. Although chloracne is a hallmark of TCDD toxicity in humans, the skin of most animals is not as sensitive to the condition.

Cardiovascular Toxicity Very little attention has been given recently to the cardiovascular effects of TCDD in animals. Although prior to *Update 1998* there were reports of developmental defects in the cardiovascular system of TCDD-treated animals suggesting that the cells lining the blood vessels can be a target of TCDD toxicity, to date there is little information available regarding the potential for TCDD to act as a cardiovascular toxicant following postnatal exposure (acute or chronic). Therefore, the cardiovascular system does not appear to be a primary target organ of TCDD toxicity in animals.

Renal Toxicity The kidney does not appear to be a primary target organ of TCDD toxicity in animals. Significant lesions are not reported in the kidney, even at doses of TCDD that induce major effects on other organs. A recent report indicates, however, that halogenated aromatic hydrocarbons can interfere with the mitochondrial function and glutathione homeostasis of renal tissue (Parrish et al., 1998).

Hepatotoxicity As discussed in *Update 1998*, the liver is a primary target organ of halogenated aromatic hydrocarbons. The severity of damage varies considerably between species. Alterations in the liver are usually associated with the *Ah* locus. Hepatomegaly occurs at sublethal doses and is a result of hyperplasia and hypertrophy of hepatocytes. Lethal doses of TCDD result in necrosis of hepatocytes. Alterations in liver morphology are accompanied by impaired hepatobiliary function, including increased microsomal monooxygenase activity, liver enzyme leakage, impaired plasma membrane function, porphyria, hyperlipidemia, hyperbilirubinemia, hyperproteinemia, and increased regenerative DNA synthesis. TCDD can also inhibit DNA synthesis of liver cells, decrease receptors in liver cell membranes, and inhibit liver enzymes. It has been recently confirmed that TCDD can also inhibit normal hepatic accumulation of dietary vitamin A (Kelley et al., 1998).

Endocrine Effects TCDD affects the levels of thyroid hormone. Those effects appear to be species dependent and may reflect both the dose and duration of exposure. For example, in one study discussed there, serum total thyroxine (T_4) levels were dose dependently decreased, whereas serum total triiodothyronine (T_3) levels were unaffected by TCDD when female rats were killed 4 days after dosing. However, at 90 days, postdosing, serum T_3 and T_4 were both dose dependently elevated (Fan and Rozman, 1995). In other studies, when rats and mice were exposed to multiple doses of TCDD, T_3 (in mice) and T_4 (in mice and rats) were decreased dose dependently. Follicular hyperplasia and hypertrophy of the thyroid gland occurred in rats gavaged biweekly for 30 weeks with 0.1–125 ng/kg/day of TCDD. Thyroid-stimulating hormone (TSH) was elevated in these animals, and there was increased excretion of T_3 glucuronide (Sewall et al., 1995). These contrasting results confuse direct interpretation of the effects of TCDD on the production and activity of thyroid hormones.

Other endocrine effects of TCDD focus on reproduction, and these effects are discussed below in "Reproductive and Developmental Toxicity."

Neurotoxicity Although some early studies indicated that TCDD can be neurotoxic (see *Update 1998*), many acute toxicity studies have been conducted with TCDD without noted signs of neurotoxicity. Intravenous injections of 8 μg/kg, resulting in total brain concentrations of 356 ppb TCDD, were not associated with systemic toxicity or neurotoxicity in rats (Stahl and Rozman, 1990). Rats administered 1,000 μg/kg TCDD intraperitoneally had significant decreases in body weight but no significant neurological impairment (Sirkka et al., 1992). The nervous system does not appear to be a sensitive target organ for TCDD toxicity, at least in adult animals.

Prenatal exposure of L-E rats to 1 µg TCDD/kg (per os) on gd 15 reduced the nocturnal core temperature in male offspring (Gordon and Miller, 1998). At some ages, however, the diurnal core temperature of TCDD-treated rats was elevated. No effect on behavioral thermoregulation was seen. The ability to develop a fever following administration of a lipopolysaccharide (LPS) endotoxin was also increased in the TCDD group. Although prenatal exposure to TCDD led to dysfunction in temperature control, the authors concluded that the normal behavioral regulation of core temperature suggests that hypothalamic thermoregulatory centers are not permanently altered.

Seo et al. (1999) gavaged pregnant Sprague-Dawley rats with 0 and 1 µg/kg/day of TCDD on gestational days 10–16. Male and female offspring were assessed beginning on day 80 for three spatial learning and memory tasks (radial arm maze [RAM], Morris water maze [MWM], and spatial discrimination-reversal learning [RL]), as well as a nonspatial learning task (visual RL). Both male and female TCDD-exposed rats showed a deficit in learning on the visual RL task, but male rats exposed during gestation and lactation showed a facilitation of task-specific spatial learning and memory. These data concurred with data from monkeys showing that perinatal exposure to TCDD facilitated certain spatial tasks but impaired visual RL tasks.

Immunotoxicity Of the many organs and systems affected by TCDD, one of the most sensitive is the immune system. Many immunotoxicological studies involving TCDD have been conducted over the past two decades in mice. It has been demonstrated by many investigators that the consequences of TCDD exposure include suppression of the antibody plaque-forming cell (PFC) response to T-cell-dependent antigens, inhibition of T-cell helper function, and inhibition of cytotoxic T-lymphocyte activity. In addition, in general, TCDD suppresses the production of cytokines (IL-1, IL-2, IFN-γ, and TNF); prevents maturation of thymocytes to mature T cells; inhibits B-lymphocyte differentiation; skews thymocyte subsets toward $CD4^-CD8^+$ cells; and increases the expression of CYP1A1 in selected immune cells. Most of these effects appear to be mediated by specific binding to the AhR. TCDD does not appear to alter many macrophage activities such as phagocytosis, tumor cytolysis and cytostasis, or antigen presentation, but it may stimulate macrophage-generated inflammatory cytokines and reactive oxygen species (IOM, 1994, 1999).

Since *Update 1998*, a study has been conducted to determine whether TCDD affects the resistance of mice and rats to parasitic infection with comparison of effects between exposures in the young and aged (Luebke et al., 1999). Mice and rats were gavaged with a single dose of 1, 10, or 30 µg TCDD/kg for 7 days before being infested with *Trichinella spiralis* (Ts). Eleven days later, young controls eliminated a greater proportion of the original parasite burden from the intestine than did aged control animals; this TCDD effect was not seen in aged rodents. Rats in the experiment were also evaluated for larval burdens. Increased larval burdens occurred in young rats at 30 µg/kg and in aged rats at 10 and 30 µg/kg doses. In addition, parasite-specific splenocyte and lymph node cell proliferation was suppressed by TCDD in young mice. The authors concluded that age-related immunosuppression did not exacerbate TCDD-induced suppression of T-cell-mediated expulsion of adult parasites and, in fact, provided some degree of protection. However, a lower dose of TCDD in aged rats suppressed humoral and cellular responses that limited the burden of encysted larvae, suggesting that age increases the sensitivity of humoral immunity to TCDD exposure.

The effects of TCDD on cytotoxic T lymphocytes in the lungs of mice were evaluated by Warren et al. (2000). The number of $CD8^+$ mediastinal lymph node (MLN) cells was reduced by 60 percent in mice exposed to a single dose of TCDD (10 µg/kg) and infected with influenza virus compared to vehicle-treated mice. The cytolytic activity of lavaged cells from lung in both TCDD- and vehicle-treated mice, however, was equivalent, and interferon levels in the lungs of TCDD-treated mice were tenfold higher than those in control mice. The authors indicated that the link between these effects remains unclear.

Since arachidonic acid metabolites are potent immunoregulatory molecules, Lawrence and Kerkvliet (1998) examined the effects of TCDD on the production of AA metabolites. Mice (C57BL/6) exposed to 15 µg/kg TCDD (intrapentoneally) had a 2-fold increase in the release of AA from spleen cell membranes, a 1.4-fold enhancement of leukotriene B_4 (LTB_4) and prostaglandin E_2 (PGE_2) production in the spleen, and 3-fold higher levels of PGE_2 in the peritoneal cavity during the immune response to allogenic p815 tumor cells. Metabolic inhibitors did not affect TCDD-induced suppression of the cytotoxic T-lymphocyte response and antibody formation. TCDD, however, did not alter the message or protein levels of COX-1, COX-2, or IL-1. The investigators, therefore, concluded that AA metabolites most likely do not mediate TCDD immunotoxicity.

It has been suggested that the proliferation and/or differentiation of hematopoietic stem cells is affected by TCDD, contributing to a reduced capacity of bone marrow to generate pro-T lymphocytes (Murante and Gasiewicz, 2000). In addition, data from a recent study suggest that TCDD exerts its effect on those cells entering and/or within the mature B-lymphocyte subpopulation and that effects noted in the earlier stages of B-lymphocyte maturation are a compensatory response to the effect on the mature cells (Thurmond and Gasiewiez, 2000).

TCDD also appears to interfere with normal physiological cell death (apoptosis) and to induce apoptosis in most laboratory mice (Kamath et al., 1998, 1999). However, TCDD failed to induce apoptosis in Fas-deficient and Fas ligand-defective mice at a lower dose than in control wild-type mice. These studies suggest that Fas–Fas ligand interactions may play a role in the TCDD-mediated induction of apoptosis. However, other investigations suggested that TCDD exposure does not induce apoptosis in T cells (Staples et al., 1998a). These effects may be highly dependent on both dose and specific maturation stage.

TCDD suppresses the response of cytotoxic-T-lymphocytes (CTL) to allogeneic tumor cells in mice; this suppression is accompanied by a decrease in expression of CD86 and suppression of IL-2 and IFN-γ production. In a series of experiments to determine the role of IL-2, IFN-γ, and CD8$^+$ cells in this process, data indicated that TCDD induces an early defect in CTL precursor activation and that the defect is not due to insufficient IL-2 production or deletion of CD8$^+$ cells (Prell et al., 2000). The authors suggest that ligands of the AhR may disrupt CTL precursor activation.

The immune system of laboratory rodents appears to be highly sensitive to in utero exposure to TCDD. Rats (F344) exposed on gd 14 to TCDD (3 μg/kg) had significantly decreased delayed-type hypersensitivity responses up to 4 months (female) and 19 months (male) of age (Gehrs and Smialowicz, 1999). The lowest maternal dose of TCDD that produced DTH suppression in offspring at 14 months of age was 0.1 μg TCDD/kg for males and 0.3 μg TCDD/kg for females. Cell phenotype analysis was performed on thymus and lymph node suspensions, but no correlations were established between altered phenotypes and suppressed DTH responses. The authors concluded that suppression of the DTH response following perinatal TCDD exposure is persistent through late adulthood, occurs at a low dose to the dam (0.1 μg/kg), and is most pronounced in male offspring.

Many investigators have evaluated immune effects following exposure to a single dose of TCDD. Huang and Koller (1999) compared the effects of single and repeated dosing of TCDD on splenic T-cell subpopulations in L-E rats. They demonstrated that repeated dosing of TCDD decreased the total percentage of CD4$^+$ cells and the percentage of the CD4$^+$ cells cycling 9 days, postexposure, while an analogous single dose of TCDD failed to affect the CD4$^+$ cell subpopulation. The authors suggest that the disease pattern of TCDD toxicity could differ between single and equivalent multiple (cumulative) exposures. This is consistent with results indicating that the immunotoxic effects of TCDD are associated with the length and repetitive nature of exposure.

In a study to determine if TCDD alters (suppresses) the activation events that follow exposure to a superantigen, it was concluded that TCDD further stimulated the production of IL-2, as well as increased the percentage of CD4$^+$ and CD8$^+$ cells in the S and G2^M phase of lymphocyte cycling in rats primed with a superantigen (Huang and Koller, 1998). In this investigation, IL-6, TNF, IL-2R, IL-1, and T-cell receptor (TCR) expression were basically unaffected by TCDD exposure. Although reduced body weight gain and histopathology confirmed that a single 25 μg/kg oral dose of TCDD caused morbidity but not mortality in L-E rats, the effect on the immune system was one of stimulation or no effect in an activated (TCDD + superantigen) versus nonactivated (TCDD) immune system, respectively.

These studies collectively demonstrate that there are considerable species differences between rats and mice, as well as strain differences, in their immune responses following exposure to TCDD. Nevertheless, TCDD appears to compromise (suppresses) the immune system of laboratory animals and the developmental period appears to be extremely sensitive to the immunosuppressive effects of TCDD in multiple species.

Reproductive and Developmental Toxicity As discussed in *Update 1998*, low doses of TCDD can affect reproductive development and fertility of progeny. Recently, considerable interest has been focused on "endocrine disrupters," that is, chemicals in the environment that affect the endocrine system and its target organs, especially the endocrine-associated developmental effects of TCDD. In one study (Faqi et al., 1998), the male offspring of female rats treated with TCDD 2 weeks prior to mating, and throughout mating, pregnancy, and lactation were evaluated for developmental effects. The number of sperm per cauda epididymis was decreased in the TCDD groups at puberty and adulthood. Daily sperm production was permanently decreased, as was the sperm transit rate. TCDD-exposed groups showed an increased number of abnormal sperm at adulthood. In the highest TCDD exposure group, serum testosterone concentration was decreased at adulthood. The authors concluded that sperm parameters were more susceptible than other end points investigated. Nevertheless, all TCDD-exposed males were able to impregnate unexposed female rats that yielded viable fetuses. In addition, mating, pregnancy, and fertility indices were not affected, and the number of implantations, resorption rates, number of viable and dead fetuses, fetal weights, and sex ratios were similar among groups. Female offspring from this study (Faqi and Chahoud, 1998) had a delay in vaginal opening (1 day) and reduced uterine weight. The authors regarded these effects as antiestrogenic. Since "endocrine-related" effects occurred only at the highest dose of TCDD in the female, it was concluded that male offspring are more susceptible to TCDD than female progeny when exposure occurs throughout pregnancy and lactation. Additional studies have shown that when pregnant female rats were administered a single oral dose of TCDD (10 µg/kg) on gd 15, TCDD interfered with vaginal development in female fetuses by impairing regression of the Wolffian ducts, increasing the size of interductal mesenchyme, and preventing fusion of the Mullerian ducts (Dienhart et al., 2000).

When pregnant female hamsters were dosed orally with 2 µg TCDD/kg body weight on gd 15, material viability, body weight, fertility, and F_1 litter size did not differ between treated and control groups (Wolf et al., 1999). In the offspring, body weight was permanently reduced by about 30 percent, vaginal opening was delayed, and the vaginal estrous cycle was altered by TCDD, but the regular 4-day estrous cycle in female progeny was not disrupted. In this study, 20 percent of the female offspring did not become pregnant, 38 percent of pregnant F_1 females from the TCDD group died near term, and the number of implants and live births was reduced by TCDD treatment. Effects in the progeny occurred at a dosage nearly four orders of magnitude below the toxic level for adult hamsters.

To evaluate the effects of TCDD on endometriosis, rats and mice were treated on gd 8 with 1 and 3 µg TCDD/kg, respectively (Cummings et al., 1999). Female offspring were reared to adulthood, and endometriosis was surgically induced. All animals were treated with 0, 3, or 10 µg TCDD/kg 3 weeks prior to surgery; at the time of surgery; and 3, 6, and 9 weeks after surgery. When the animals were killed 12 weeks after surgery, TCDD was seen not to affect the surgically induced endometrial lesions in the rats, although effects were seen in rats in an earlier study (Cummings et al., 1996). In mice, the lesions were increased only with a combination of perinatal and adult exposure to TCDD. A similar protocol in rhesus monkeys revealed that TCDD facilitated the survival of endometrial implants but had no effect on circulating gonadal steroid levels or on the menstrual cycle (Yang et al., 2000). Other researchers (Bruner-Tran et al., 1999) suggest that TCDD blocks the ability of progesterone to prevent experimental endometriosis, which correlates with its ability to inhibit progesterone-associated TGF-β_2 expression and endometrial matrix metalloproteinase suppression.

In utero and lactational exposure of Holtzman rats to TCDD decreased prostate weight without inhibiting testicular androgen production or decreasing serum androgen concentrations (Roman et al., 1998a). Additional studies (Roman et al., 1998b) showed that the prostatic epithelial budding process was impaired, suggesting that in utero and lactational TCDD exposure interferes with prostate development by decreasing early epithelial growth, delaying cytodifferentiation, and altering epithelial and stromal cell histological arrangement and the spatial distribution of androgen receptor expression.

Pregnant L-E rats were gavaged on gd 15 with 1.0 µg/kg TCDD, and their male offspring were necropsied at intervals up to 120 days postnatally to observe the effects of TCDD on seminal vesicles (Hamm et al., 2000). TCDD treatment significantly decreased body and seminal vesicle weights in male rats 49–120 days postnatally. Epithelial branching and differentiation were decreased in the seminal vesicles of TCDD-treated rats. It was concluded that TCDD decreases seminal vesicle growth by impairing development of the epithelium.

During the past few years, reproductive and developmental TCDD research has focused on exposure of pregnant females. As discussed in previous reports, the reproductive systems of adult male laboratory animals are considered to be relatively insensitive to TCDD because high doses are required to elicit effects.

Carcinogenicity TCDD is considered to be a carcinogen in animals and humans. TCDD is not directly genotoxic and acts as a promoter in multistage models of carcinogens. The carcinogenic activity of TCDD depends on the presence of the AhR, and involves multiple pathways in regulating cell proliferation and differentiation; the multiple site specificity suggests multiple mechanisms of action. Two possible mechanisms of tumor promotion by TCDD may involve oxygen radicals and interference of gap junction intercellular communication. TCDD is a known hepatocarcinogen in rats and mice (IOM, 1999).

In a two-stage model of hepatocarcinogenesis, TCDD significantly increased the volume fraction and number of altered hepatic foci at the highest dose (10 ng/kg/day) (Teeguarden et al., 1999). Increases in the number of GTPase- and ATPase-deficient altered hepatic foci per cubic centimeter occurred at doses as low as 0.01 ng/kg/day. This is the lowest dose of TCDD to promote tumors to date and indicates that TCDD is an extremely potent promoter of neoplasia in laboratory rats.

When female Sprague-Dawley rats were administered 1.75 μg/kg TCDD biweekly continuously for 60 weeks via oral gavage, an increase (nonsignificant) in liver tumors occurred in these rats compared to corn oil controls (Walker et al., 2000). The incidence of hepatocellular adenomas and carcinomas, however, was significantly decreased in rats treated with 1.75 μg/kg TCDD for 30 weeks followed by no TCDD treatment for an additional 30 weeks, compared to the TCDD continuously treated and vehicle control groups. Although there may be several other explanations, such as differences in total dosage delivered, the authors interpreted these data to suggest the possibility that the promotion of liver tumors by TCDD in female rats is dependent upon continuous exposure to TCDD.

Estimating Potential Health Risk and Factors Influencing Toxicity

Several approaches have been used to estimate the potential health risks associated with TCDD exposures. These include the use of toxic equivalency factors, quantitative structure–activity relationship (QSAR) models, in vitro screening methods, and toxicity equivalent concentrations (TECs).

TEF Approach   In recent years the TEF methodology for comparing the relative toxicity of dioxin-like chemicals has been used by several government agencies around the world. Although it is considered one of the best approaches for assessing the relative risk of complex mixtures of these contaminants, it is an interim approach and there are several inherent uncertainties with this procedure.

TEFs are determined by inspection of the available congener-specific biological and biochemical data and assignment of an "order-of-magnitude" estimate of relative toxicity when compared to 2,3,7,8-TCDD. TEF values are by no means precise; scientific judgment and expert opinion, based on all the available data, form the basis of these values. The actual scientific data upon which these values are based may vary considerably, often by several orders of magnitude depending on the different biological end points chosen for a particular dioxin-like chemical. Therefore, considerable uncertainty exists about the use of these values, and it is often difficult to quantify that uncertainty. Although the recent World Health Organization TEF values (van den Berg et al., 1998) are most often cited and generally accepted, the TEF values used can differ slightly depending on the state, country, and particular health organization, as well as the classification schemes accepted by an agency. Nevertheless, most agencies in the United States, including the U.S. Environmental Protection Agency, support the basic approach as a "reasonable estimate" of relative toxicity. Furthermore, numerous countries and several international organizations have adopted this approach although, again, the accepted values may differ.

The basic TEF concept is based on the premise that the toxic and biologic responses of all of these chemicals are mediated through the AhR. Although all of the data to date support this concept, the set of data for each particular chemical considered to be "dioxin-like" is incomplete. One possible limitation of the approach is that it does not consider synergistic or antagonistic interactions among these chemicals. In addition, this approach does not consider possible actions or interactions of these chemicals that are not mediated by the AhR. Indeed, little research has been done in this area.

For a chemical mixture such as PCBs, another limitation of the TEF methodology is that the risk from non-dioxin-like chemicals (i.e., noncoplanar PCBs) is not evaluated.

Furthermore, the actual kinetics and metabolism for each dioxin-like chemical differ considerably. Data are often available only on tissue concentrations at any given time and not necessarily on the original exposure of the organism. Sometimes tissue concentrations are not available. Extrapolation to a meaningful dose may add considerable uncertainty to calculation of the 2,3,7,8-TCDD toxicity equivalent (TEQ) to which an individual may have been exposed.

QSAR Models   As discussed in *Update 1998*, quantitative structure–activity relationship (QSAR) models have been used to estimate the binding affinity of multiple chemical classes. The predictive nature of these approaches has been largely unsuccessful due to a focus on minimum energy conformations to predict the activity of molecules. Some QSAR models have shown good utility across multiple classes of halogenated aromatic compounds.

In Vitro Screening Methods   As discussed in *Update 1998*, techniques such as the use of H411E-luc cells have been developed for the detection of AhR agonists in environmental samples. Since *Update 1998*, other methods have been proposed for detecting TCDD and assaying TEQs. Li et al. (1999) concluded that enzyme immunoassay could be used as a rapid and sensitive screening tool in many circumstances. Bovee et al. (1998) concluded that a chemical-activated luciferase gene expression bioassay is promising for detecting dioxins in milk. Smeets et al. (1999) demonstrated that vitellogenin secretion from primary carp hepatocytes can indicate the presence of compounds with estrogenic or antiestrogenic activity, including TCDD.

ISSUES IN EVALUATING THE EVIDENCE

For an animal model to be valid in the study of a human disease, the model must reproduce with some consistency the manifestations of the disease in humans. Whole-animal studies or animal-based experimental systems are used to study herbicide toxicity because they allow for rigid control of chemical exposures and close monitoring of health outcomes. Because many of the chemical exposures presently associated with certain diseases in humans have been confirmed in experimental studies (Huff, 1993; Huff et al., 1994), data derived from such studies are generally accepted as a valuable guide in the assessment of biological plausibility.

As discussed in this chapter, many of the toxic effects of the herbicides used in Vietnam have been ascribed to 2,3,7,8-tetrachlorodibenzo-p-dioxin, a contaminant of some of the herbicides. This has not, however, simplified the risk assessment process because the toxicologic profile of TCDD is rather complex. In general, there is consensus that most of the toxic effects of TCDD involve interaction with the AhR, a protein that binds TCDD and other aromatic hydrocarbons with high affinity. The development of AhR knockout mice has helped to establish a definitive association between the AhR and TCDD-mediated toxicity. Formation of an active complex involving the receptor, ligand (the TCDD molecule), and other protein factors is followed by interaction of the activated complex with specific sites on DNA. This interaction results in DNA changes that alter the expression of genes involved in the regulation of cellular processes. Furthermore, it is possible that TCDD, via the AhR, may modulate signal transduction pathways by mechanisms not involving the interaction of the AhR with DNA. Regardless of the specific mechanism, TCDD and other AhR ligands modulate target cells and presumably exert toxic effects.

Establishing a correlation between the effects of TCDD in experimental systems and in humans, however, is particularly problematic because species differences in susceptibility to TCDD have been documented. Humans may actually be more resistant than other species to the toxic effects of this chemical (Dickson and Buzik, 1993), however, there are data suggesting that for certain end points humans may be at least as sensitive as some experimental animals (DeVito et al., 1995). Differences in susceptibility involve a toxicokinetic component, since elimination rates in humans are slower than in rodents (Ahlborg and Hanberg, 1992). Toxicodynamic interactions are also important because the affinity of TCDD for the AhR is species and strain specific (Lorenzen and Okey, 1991) and responses to occupancy of the receptor vary among different cell types and during different developmental stages. The drug-metabolizing enzymes induced in humans are different from those induced in rodents (Neubert, 1992), suggesting that the impact of different genetic backgrounds on AhR function is not yet completely understood. It is generally accepted that genetic susceptibility plays a key role in determining the adverse effects of environmental chemicals.

This issue is particularly central to the assessment of biologic plausibility, because polymorphisms of the *AhR* in humans similar to those in laboratory animals would place some individuals at greater risk for the toxic and carcinogenic effects of TCDD.

Ultimately however, the challenge in the assessment of the biologic plausibility of the toxicity of herbicides and TCDD is not restricted to understanding receptor-mediated events. The dose–response relationships that arise from multiple toxicokinetic and toxicodynamic interactions must also be considered. Gene regulation models described to date do not consider the intricacies of the many interactions between the AhR and other proteins. Future attempts to define the quantitative relationship between receptor occupancy and biologic response to TCDD must consider that multiple biochemical changes may influence the overall cellular response.

Although studying AhR biology in transformed human cell lines minimizes the inherent error associated with species extrapolations, caution must be exercised because the extent to which transformation itself influences toxicity outcomes has yet to be fully defined.

REFERENCES

Abbott BD, Probst MR, Perdew GH, Buckalew AR. 1998. AH receptor, ARNT, glucocorticoid receptor, EGF receptor, TGFα, TGFβ$_1$, TGFβ$_2$, and TGFβ$_3$ expression in human embryonic palate, and effects of 2,3,7,8-tetrachlorodibenzo-*p*-dioxin (TCDD). Teratology 58(2):30–43.

Abbott BD, Schmid JE, Brown JG, Wood CR, White RD, Buckalew AR, Held GA. 1999a. RT–PCR quantification of AHR, ARNT, GR, and CYP1A1 mRNA in craniofacial tissues of embryonic mice exposed to 2,3,7,8-tetrachlorodibenzo-*p*-dioxin and hydrocortisone. Toxicological Sciences 47(1):76–85.

Abbott BD, Held GA, Wood CR, Buckalew AR, Brown JG, Schmid J. 1999b. AhR, ARNT, and CYP1A1 mRNA quantitation in cultured human embryonic palates exposed to TCDD and comparison with mouse palate in vivo and in culture. Toxicological Sciences 47(1):62–75.

Abbott BD, Schmid JE, Pitt JA, Buckalew AR, Wood CR, Held GA, Diliberto JJ. 1999c. Adverse reproductive outcomes in the transgenic Ah receptor-deficient mouse. Toxicology and Applied Pharmacology 155(1):62–70.

Abnet CC, Tanguay RL, Hahn ME, Heideman W, Peterson RE. 1999. Two forms of aryl hydrocarbon receptor type 2 in rainbow trout (*Oncorhynchus mykiss*). Evidence for differential expression and enhancer specificity. Journal of Biological Chemistry 274(21):15159–15166.

Ahlborg UG, Hanberg A. 1992. Toxicokinetics of PCDDs and PCDFs of importance to the development of human risk assessment. Toxic Substances Journal 12(2-4):197–211.

Ahmad S, Anderson WL, Kitchin KT. 1999. Dimethylarsinic acid effects on DNA damage and oxidative stress related biochemical parameters in B6C3F1 mice. Cancer Letters 139(2):129–135.

Arnold LL, Cano M, St John M, Eldan M, van Gernert M, Cohen SM. 1999. Effects of dietary dimethylarsinic acid on the urine and urothelium of rats. Carcinogenesis 20(11):2171–2179.

Ashida H, Fukuda I, Yamashita T, Kanazawa K. 2000a. Flavones and flavonols at dietary levels inhibit a transformation of aryl hydrocarbon receptor induced by dioxin. FEBS Letters 476:213–217.

Ashida H, Nagy S, Matsumura F. 2000b. 2,3,7,8-Tetrachlorodibenzo-*p*-dioxin (TCDD)-induced changes in activities of nuclear protein kinases and phosphatases affecting DNA binding activity of c-Myc and AP-1 in the livers of guinea pigs. Biochemical Pharmacology 59(7):741–751.

Bachour G, Failing K, Gerogii S, Elmadfa I, Brunn H. 1998. Species and organ dependence of PCB contamination in fish, foxes, roe deer and humans. Archives of Environmental Contamination and Toxicology 35(4):666–673.

Bagchi D, Balmorri J, Bagchi M, Ye X, Williams CB, Stohs SJ. 2000. Role of p53 tumor suppressor gene in the toxicity of TCDD, endrin, naphthalene, and chromium(VI) in liver and brain tissues of mice. Free Radical Biology and Medicine 28:895–903.

Barile FA, Cardona M. 1998. Acute cytotoxicity testing with cultured human lung and dermal cells. In Vitro Cellular and Developmental Biology 34(8):631–635.

Benedict JC, Lin TM, Loeffler IK, Peterson RE, Flaws JA. 2000. Physiological role of the aryl hydrocarbon receptor in mouse ovary development. Toxicological Sciences 56(2):382–388.

Benramdane L, Accominotti M, Fanton L, Malicier D, Vallon JJ. 1999. Arsenic speciation in human organs following fatal arsenic trioxide poisoning—a case report. Clinical Chemistry 45(2):301–306.

Bestervelt LL, Pitt JA, Nolan CJ, Cai Y, Piper DW, Dybowski JA, Dayharsh GA, Piper WN. 1998. In vitro 2,3,7,8-tetrachlorodibenzo-*p*-dioxin interferes with the anterior pituitary hormone adrenocorticortropin. Toxicological Sciences 44(2):107–115.

Blakley BR, Yole MJ, Brousseau P, Boermans H, Fournier M. 1998. Effect of 2,4-dichlorophenoxyacetic acid, trifluralin and triallate herbicides on immune function. Veterinary and Human Toxicology 40(1):5–10.

Bortolozzi AA, Duffard RO, Evangelista De Duffard AM. 1999. Behavioral alterations induced in rats by a pre- and postnatal exposure to 2,4-dichlorophenoxyacetic acid. Neurotoxicology and Teratology 21(4):451–465.

Bouwman CA, Van Dam E, Fase KM, Koppe JG, Seinen W, Thijssen HHW, Vermeer C, Van den Berg M. 1999. Effects of 2,3,7,8-tetrachlorodibenzo-*p*-dioxin or 2,2',4,4',5,5'-hexachlorobiphenyl on vitamin K-dependent blood coagulation in male and female WAG/RIJ-rats. Chemosphere 38(3):489–505.

Bovee TF, Hoogenboom LA, Hamers AR, Traag WA, Zuidema T, Aarts JM, Brouwer A, Kuiper HA. 1998. Validation and use of the CALUX-bioassay for the determination of dioxins and PCBs in bovine milk. Food Additives and Contaminants 15(8):863–875.

Bracco D, Favre JB. 1999. Lethal intoxication with the hormone weedkiller 2,4-dichlorophenoxyacetic acid. Reanimation Urgences 8:55–58.

Brown NM, Manzolillo PA, Zhang JX, Wang J, Lamartiniere CA. 1998. Prenatal TCDD and predisposition to mammary cancer in the rat. Carcinogenesis 19(9):1623–1629.

Bruner-Tran KL, Rier SE, Eisenberg E, Osteen KG. 1999. The potential role of environmental toxins in the pathophysiology of endometriosis. Gynecologic and Obstetric Investigation 48(Suppl 1):45–56.

Caruso JA, Laird DW, Batist G. 1999. Role of HSP90 in mediating cross-talk between the estrogen receptor and the Ah receptor signal transduction pathways. Biochemical Pharmacology 58(9):1395–1403.

Carver LA, LaPres JJ, Jain S, Dunham EE, Bradfield CA. 1998. Characterization of the Ah receptor-associated protein, ARA9. Journal of Biological Chemistry 273(50):33580–33587.

Casper RF, Quesne M, Rogers IM, Shirota T, Jolivet A, Milgrom E, Savouret JF. 1999. Resveratrol has antagonist activity on the aryl hydrocarbon receptor: implications for prevention of dioxin toxicity. Molecular Pharmacology 56(4):784–790.

Chaffin CL, Trewin AL, Hutz RJ. 2000. Estrous cycle-dependent changes in the expression of aromatic hydrocarbon receptor (AHR) and AHR-nuclear translocator (ARNT) mRNAs in the rat ovary and liver. Chemico-Biological Interactions 124(3):205–216.

Chan WK, Yao G, Gu YZ, Bradfield CA. 1999. Cross-talk between the aryl hydrocarbon receptor and hypoxia inducible factor signaling pathways. Demonstration of competition and compensation. Journal of Biological Chemistry 274(17):12115–12123.

Chang CY, Puga A. 1998. Constitutive activation of the aromatic hydrocarbon receptor. Molecular and Cellular Biology 18(1):525–535.

Chang KW, Lee H, Wang HJ, Chen SY, Lin P. 1999. Differential response to benzo[a]pyrene in human lung adenocarcinoma cell lines: the absence of aryl hydrocarbon receptor activation. Life Sciences 65(13):1339–1349.

Charles JM, Leeming NM. 1998a. Chronic dietary toxicity/oncogenicity studies on 2,4-dichlorophenoxybutric acid in rodents. Toxicological Sciences 46(1):21–30.

Charles JM, Leeming NM. 1998b. Chronic dietary toxicity study of 2,4-dichlorophenoxybutyric acid in the dog. Toxicological Sciences 46(1):134–142.

Charles JM, Cunny HC, Wilson RD, Bus JS, Lawlor TE, Cifone MA, Fellows M, Gollapudi, B. 1999a. Ames assays and unscheduled DNA synthesis assays on 2,4-dichlorophenoxyacetic acid and its derivatives. Mutation Research 444(1):207–216.

Charles JM, Cunny HC, Wilson RD, Ivett JL, Murli H, Bus JS, Gollapudi B. 1999b. In vivo micronucleus assays on 2,4-dichlorophenoxyacetic acid and its derivatives. Mutation Research 444(1): 227–234.

Charles JM, Henwood SM, Leeming NM. 1999c. Developmental toxicity studies in rats and rabbits and two-generation reproduction study in rats on 4-(2,4-dichlorophenoxy)butyric acid. International Journal of Toxicology 18:177–189.

Chen T, Na Y, Wanibuchi H, Yamamoto S, Lee CC, Fukushima S. 1999. Loss of heterozygosity in (Lewis x F344) F_1 rat urinary bladder tumors induced with N-butyl-N-(4-hydroxybutyl) nitrosamine followed by dimethylarsinic acid or sodium L-ascorbate. Japanese Journal of Cancer Research 90(8):818–823.

Christensen JG, Goldsworthy TL, Cattley RC. 1999. Dysregulation of apoptosis by c-myc in transgenic hepatocytes and effects of growth factors and nongenotoxic carcinogens. Molecular Carcinogenesis 25(4):273–284.

Ciolino HP, Yeh GC. 1998. The flavonoid galangin is an inhibitor of CYP1A1 activity and an agonist/antagonist of the aryl hydrocarbon receptor. British Journal of Cancer 79(9–10):1340–1346.

Ciolino HP, Yeh GC. 1999. Inhibition of aryl hydrocarbon-induced cytochrome P-450 1A1 enzyme activity and CYP1A1 expression by resveratrol. Molecular Pharmacology 56(4):760–767.

Ciolino HP, Daschner PJ, Yeh GC. 1998a. Resveratrol inhibits transcription of CYP1A1 in vitro by preventing activation of the aryl hydrocarbon receptor. Cancer Research 58(24):5707–5712.

Ciolino HP, Daschner PJ, Wang TTY, Yeh GC. 1998b. Effect of curcumin on the aryl hydrocarbon receptor and cytochrome P450 1A1 in MCF-7 human breast carcinoma cells. Biochemical Pharmacology 56(2):197–206.

Ciolino HP, Daschner PJ, Yeh GC. 1999. Dietary flavonols quercetin and kaempferol are ligands of the aryl hydrocarbon receptor that affect CYP1A1 transcription differentially. Biochemical Journal 34(Pt. 3):715–722.

Colman MS, Afshari CA, Barrett JC. 2000. Regulation of p53 stability and activity in response to genotoxic stress. Mutation Research 462(2–3):179–188.

Concha G, Vogler G, Lezeano D, Lezcano D, Nermell B, Vahter M. 1998. Exposure to inorganic arsenic metabolites during early human development. Toxicological Sciences 44(2):185–190.

Cummings AA, Metcalf JL, Birnbaum LS. 1996. Promotion of endometriosis by 2,3,7,8-tetrachlorodibenzo-p-dioxin in rats and mice: time-dose dependence and species comparison. Toxicology and Applied Pharmacology 138:131–139.

Cummings AM, Hedge JM, Birnbaum LS. 1999. Effect of prenatal exposure to TCDD on the promotion of endometriotic lesion growth by TCDD in adult female rats and mice. Toxicological Sciences 52(1):45–49.

Davarinos NA, Pollenz RS. 1999. Aryl hydrocarbon receptor imported into the nucleus following ligand binding is rapidly degraded via the cytoplasmic proteasome following nuclear export. Journal of Biological Chemistry 274(40):28708–28715.

Denison MS, Phelan D, Elferink CJ. 1998. The Ah receptor signal transduction pathway. In: Denison MS and Helferich WG (eds.), Toxicant–Receptor Interactions. Bristol, PA: Taylor & Francis, pp. 3–33.

Dertinger SD, Silverstone AE, Gasiewicz TA. 1998. Influence of aromatic hydrocarbon receptor-mediated events on the genotoxicity of cigarette smoke condensate. Carcinogenesis 19(11): 2037–2042.

DeVito MJ, Birnbaum LS, Farland WH, Gasiewicz TA. 1995. Comparisons of estimated human body burdens of dioxin-like chemicals and 2,3,7,8-tetrachlorodibenzo-p-dioxin body burdens in experimentally exposed animals. Environmental Health Perspectives 103(9):820–830.

DeVito MJ, Ross DG, Dupuy, AE Jr, Ferrario J, McDaniel D, Birnbaum LS. 1998. Dose–response relationships for disposition and hepatic sequestration of polyhalogenated dibenzo-p-dioxins, dibenzofurans, and biphenyls following subchronic treatment in mice. Toxicological Sciences 46(2):223–234.

Dickson LC, Buzik SC. 1993. Health risks of "dioxins": a review of environmental and toxicological considerations. Veterinary and Human Toxicology 35(1):68–77.

Dienhart MK, Sommer RJ, Peterson RE, Hirshfield AN, Silbergeld EK. 2000. Gestational exposure to 2,3,7,8-tetrachlorodibenzo-p-dioxin induces developmental defects in the rat vagina. Toxicological Sciences 56(1):141–149.

Diliberto JJ, Burgin DE, Birnbaum LS. 1999. Effects of CYP1A2 on disposition of 2,3,7,8-tetrachlorodibenzo-p-dioxin, 2,3,4,7,8-pentachlorodibenzofuran, and 2,2',4,4',5,5'-hexachlorobiphenyl in CYP1A2 knockout and parental (C57BL/6N and 129/Sv) strains of mice. Toxicology and Applied Pharmacology 159(1):52–64.

Duan R, Porter W, Samudio I, Vyhlidal C, Kladde M, Safe S. 1999. Transcriptional activation of c-fos protooncogene by 17β-estradiol: mechanism of aryl hydrocarbon receptor-mediated inhibition. Molecular Endocrinology 13(9):1511–1521.

Dunlap DY, Moreno-Aliaga MJ, Wu Z, Matsumura F. 1999. Differential toxicities of TCDD in vivo among normal, c-src-knockout, geldanamycin- and quercetin-treated mice. Toxicology 135(2–3):95–107.

El-Sabeawy F, Wang S, Overstreet J, Miller M, Lasley B, Enan E. 1998. Treatment of rats during pubertal development with 2,3,7,8-tetrachlorodibenzo-p-dioxin alters both signaling kinase activities and epidermal growth factor receptor binding in the testis and the motility and acrosomal reaction of sperm. Toxicology and Applied Pharmacology 150(2):427–442.

Eltom SE, Zhang L, Jefcoate CR. 1999. Regulation of cytochrome P-450 (CYP) 1B1 in mouse Hepa-1 variant cell lines: a possible role for aryl hydrocarbon receptor nulcear translocator (ARNT) as a suppressor of CYP1B1 gene expression. Molecular Pharmacology 55(3):594–604.

Enan E, El-Sabeawy F, Scott M, Overstreet J, Lasley B. 1998a. Alterations in the growth factor signal transduction pathways and modulators of the cell cycle in endocervical cells from Macaques exposed to TCDD. Toxicology and Applied Pharmacology 151(2):283–293.

Enan E, El-Sabeawy F, Overstreet J, Matsumura F, Lasley B. 1998b. Mechanisms of gender-specific TCDD-induced toxicity in guinea pig adipose tissue. Reproductive Toxicology 12(3): 357–369.

Enan E, Dunlap DY, Matsumura F. 1998c. Use of c-src and c-fos knockout mice for the studies on the role of c-src signaling in the expression of toxicity of TCDD. Journal of Biochemical and Molecular Toxicology 12(5):263–274.

Enan E, El-Sabeawy F, Moran F, Overstreet J, Lasley B. 1998d. Interruption of estradiol transduction by 2,3,7,8-tetrachlorodibenzo-*p*-dioxin (TCDD) through disruption of the protein phosphorylation pathway in adipose tissue from immature and mature female rats. Biochemical Pharmacology 55(7):1077–1090.

Evans MV, Andersen ME. 2000. Sensitivity analysis of a physiological model for 2,3,7,8-tetrachlorodibenzo-*p*-dioxin (TCDD): assessing the impact of specific model parameters on sequestration in liver and fat in the rat. Toxicological Sciences 54(1):71–80.

Fan F, Rozman KK. 1995. Short- and long-term biochemical effects of 2,3,7,8-tetrachlorodibenzo-*p*-dioxin in female Long-Evans rats. Toxicology Letters 75(1-3):209–216.

Faqi AS, Chahoud I. 1998. Antiestrogenic effects of low doses of 2,3,7,8-tetrachlorodibenzo-*p*-dioxin in offspring of female rats exposed throughout pregnancy and lactation. Bulletin of Environmental Contamination Toxicology 61(4):462–469.

Faqi AS, Dalsenter PR, Merker HJ, Chahoud I. 1998. Reproductive toxicity and tissue concentration of low doses of 2,3,7,8-tetrachlorodibenzo-*p*-dioxin in male offspring rats exposed throughout pregnancy and lactation. Toxicology and Applied Pharmacology 150(2):383–392.

Gaillard D, Negrel R, Lagarde M, Ailhaud G. 1989. Requirement and role of arachidonic acid in the differentiation of pre-adipose cells. Journal of Biological Chemistry 257(2):389–397.

Galimov SH, Kamilov FH, Davletov EG. 1998. Pituitary–testicular tissue relationships and blood levels of some prostaglandins in the experimental poisoning with organochlorine compounds. Problemy Endokrinologii 44:38–40.

Gao L, Dong L, Whitlock JP Jr. 1998. A novel response to dioxin. Induction of ecto-ATPase gene expression. Journal of Biological Chemistry 273(25):15358–15365.

Gao X, Terranove PF, Rozman KK. 2000. Effects of polychlorinated dibenzofurans, biphenyls, and their mixture with dibenzo-*p*-dioxins on ovulation in the gonadotropin-primed immature rat: support for the toxic equivalency concept. Toxicology and Applied Pharmacology 163(2):115–124.

Garrison PM, Denison MS. 2000. Analysis of the murine AhR gene promoter. Journal of Biochemical and Molecular Toxicology 14(1):1–10.

Garrison PM, Rogers JM, Brackney WR, Denison MS. 2000. Effects of histone deacetylase inhibitors on the Ah receptor gene promoter. Archives of Biochemistry and Biophysics 374(2):161–171.

Ge NL, Elferink CJ. 1998. A direct interaction between the aryl hydrocarbon receptor and retinoblastoma protein. Journal of Biological Chemistry 273:22708–22713.

Gehrs BC, Smialowicz RJ. 1999. Persistent suppression of delayed type hypersensitivity in adult F344 rats after perinatal exposure to 2,3,7,8-tetrachlorodibenzo-*p*-dioxin. Toxicology 134(1):79–88.

Geusau A, Tschachler E, Meixner M, Sandermann S, Papke O, Wolf C, Valic E, Stingl G, McLachlan M. 1999. Olestra increases faecal excretion of 2,3,7,8-tetrachlorodibenzo-*p*-dioxin. Lancet 354(9186):1266–1267.

Giannone JV, Li W, Probst M, Okey AB. 1998. Prolonged depletion of AH receptor without alteration of receptor mRNA levels after treatment of cells in culture with 2,3,7,8-tetrachlorodibenzo-*p*-dioxin. Biochemical Pharmacology 55(4):489–497.

Gollapudi BB, Charles JM, Linscombe VA, Day SJ, Bus JS. 1999. Evaluation of the genotoxicity of 2,4-dichlorophenoxyacetic acid and its derivatives in mammalian cell cultures. Mutation Research 444(1):217–225.

Goodrich DW, Lee WH. 1992. Abrogation by c-myc of G1 phase arrest induced by RB protein but not by p53. Nature 360(6400):177–179.

Gordon CJ, Miller DB. 1998. Thermoregulation in rats exposed perinatally to dioxin: core temperature stability to altered ambient temperature, behavioral thermoregulation, and febrile response to lipopolysaccharide. Journal of Toxicology and Environmental Health 54(8):647–662.

Gradin K, Toftgard R, Poellinger L, Berghard A. 1999. Repression of dioxin signal transduction in fibroblasts. Identification of a putative repressor associated with ARNT. Journal of Biological Chemistry 274(19):13511–13518.

Gregoraszczuk EL, Worriwicz AK, Grochowalski A. 2000. Dose- and time-dependent effect of 2,3,7,8-tetrachlorodibenzo-p-dioxin (TCDD) on progesterone secretion by porcine luteal cells cultured in vitro. Journal of Physiology and Pharmacology 51:127–135.

Gregus Z, Halaszi E, Klaassen CD. 1999. Effect of chlorophenoxyacetic acid herbicides on glycine conjugation of benzoic acid. Xenobiotica 29(6):547–559.

Gribaldo L, Casati S, Figliuzzi L, Marafante E. 1998. In vitro myelotoxicity of environmental contaminants. Environmental Toxicology and Pharmacology 6:135–141.

Grochowalski A, Pieklo R, Gasiriska A, Chrzaszcz R, Gregoraszczuk EL. 2000. Accumulation of 2,3,7,8-tetrachlorodibenzo-p-dioxin (TCDD) in porcine preovulatory follicles after in vitro exposure to TCDD: effects on steroid secretion and cell proliferation. Cytobios 102:21–31.

Hahn ME. 1998. The aryl hydrocarbon receptor: a comparative perspective. Comparative Biochemistry and Physiology. Part C, Pharmacology, Toxicology and Endocrinology 121(1-3):23–53.

Hamm JT, Sparrow BR, Wolf D, Birnbaum LS. 2000. In utero and lactational exposure to 2,3,7,8-tetrachlorodibenzo-p-dioxin alters postnatal development of seminal vesicle epithelium. Toxicological Sciences 54:424–430.

Hart LJ, Gogal RM Jr, Smith SA, Smith BJ, Robertson J, Holladay SD. 1999. Leukocyte hypocellularity in the spleen and pronephros of tilapia (*Oreochromis niloticus*) exposed to 2,3,7,8-tetrachlorodibenzo-p-dioxin (TCDD) may result from antiproliferative effects and enhanced apoptosis. Toxic Substance Mechanisms 18:21–38.

Hassoun EA, Wilt SC, DeVito MJ, van Birgelen A, Alsharif NZ, Birnbaum LS, Stohs SJ. 1998. Induction of oxidative stress in brain tissues of mice after subchronic exposure to 2,3,7,8-tetrachlorodibenzo-p-dioxin. Toxicological Sciences 42(1):23–27.

Hatakeyama M, Matsumura F. 1999. Correlation between the activation of Neu tyrosine kinase and promotion of foci formation induced by selected organochlorine compounds in the MCF-7 model system. Biochemical and Molecular Toxicology 13(6):296–302.

Hayashi H, Kanisawa M, Yamanaka K, Ito T, Udaka N, Ohji H, Okudela K, Okada S, Kitamura H. 1998. Dimethylarsinic acid, a main metabolite of inorganic arsenics, has tumorigenicity and progression effects in the pulmonary tumors of A/J mice. Cancer Letters 125(1–2):83–88.

Heath-Pagliuso S, Rogers WJ, Tullis K, Seidel SD, Cenijn PH, Brouwer A, Denison MS. 1998. Activation of the Ah receptor by tryptophan and tryptophan metabolites. Biochemistry 37(33):11508–11515.

Heederik D, Hooiveld M, Bueno de Mesquita HB. 1998. Modelling of 2,3,7,8-tetrachlorodibenzo-p-dioxin levels in a cohort of workers with exposure to phenoxy herbicides and chlorophenols. Chemosphere 37(9–12):1743–1754.

Heid SE, Pollenz RS, Swanson HI. 2000. Role of heat shock protein 90 dissociation in mediating agonist-induced activation of the aryl hydrocarbon receptor. Molecular Pharmacology 57(1):82–92.

Heimler I, Trewin AL, Chaffin CL, Rawlins RG, Hutz RJ. 1998. Modulation of ovarian follicle maturation and effects on apoptotic death in Holtzman rats exposed to 2,3,7,8-tetrachlorodibenzo-p-dioxin (TCDD) in utero and lactationally. Reproductive Toxicology 12(1):69–73.

Henry EC, Kende AS, Rucci G, Totleben MJ, Willey JJ, Dertinger SD, Pollenz RS, Jones JP, Gasiewicz TA. 1999. Flavone antagonists bind competitively with 2,3,7,8-tetrachlorodibenzo-p-dioxin (TCDD) to the aryl hydrocarbon receptor but inhibit nuclear uptake and transformation. Molecular Pharmacology 55(4):716–725.

Hochstein JR, Bursian SJ, Aulerich RJ. 1998. Effects of dietary exposure to 2,3,7,8-tetrachlorodibenzo-p-dioxin in adult female mink (*Mustela vision*). Archives of Environmental Contamination and Toxicology 35(2):348–353.

Hong SJ, Grover CA, Safe SH, Tiffany-Castiglioni E, Frye GD. 1998. Halogenated aromatic hydrocarbons suppress CA1 field excitatory postsynaptic potentials in rat hippocampal slices. Toxicology and Applied Pharmacology 148(1):7–13.

Huang W, Koller LD. 1998. 2,3,7,8-Tetrachlorodibenzo-p-dioxin co-stimulates staphylococcal enterotoxin b (SEB) cytokine production and phentype cell cycling in Long-Evans rats. International Journal of Immunopharmacology 20(1–3):39–56.

Huang W, Koller LD. 1999. Effects of a single or repeated dose of 2,3,7,8-tetrachlorodibenzo-p-dioxin (TCDD) on T-cell subpopulations in the Long-Evans rat. Toxicology Letters 109(1–2):97–104.

Huff J. 1993. Chemicals and cancer in humans: first evidence in experimental animals. Environmental Health Perspectives 100:201–210.

Huff J, Lucier G, Tritscher A. 1994. Carcinogenicity of TCDD: experimental, mechanistic, and epidemiologic evidence. Annual Review of Pharmacology and Toxicology 34:343–372.

Hughes MF, Kenyon EM. 1998. Dose-dependent effects on the disposition on monomethylarsonic acid and dimethylarsinic acid in the mouse after intravenous administration. Journal of Toxicology and Environmental Health 53(2):95–112.

Hughes MF, Kenyon EM, Edwards BC, Mitchell CT, Thomas D. 1999. Strain-dependent disposition of inorganic arsenic in the mouse. Toxicology 137(2):95–108.

Hughes MF, Del Razo LM, Kenyon EM. 2000. Dose-dependent effects on tissue distribution and metabolism of dimethylarsinic acid in the mouse after intravenous administration. Toxicology 143(2):155–166.

Hurst CH, Abbott BD, DeVito MJ, Birnbaum LS. 1998. 2,3,7,8-Tetrachlorodibenzo-p-dioxin in pregnant Long Evans rats: disposition to maternal and embryo/fetal tissues. Toxicological Sciences 45(2):129–136.

Hurst CH, DeVito MJ, Setzer RW, Birnbaum LS. 2000. Acute administration of 2,3,7,8-tetrachlorodibenzo-p-dioxin (TCDD) in pregnant Long Evans rats: association of measured tissue concentrations with developmental effects. Toxicological Sciences 53(2):411–420.

Hushka LJ, Williams JS, Greenlee WF. 1998. Characterization of 2,3,7,8-tetrachlorodibenzfuran-dependent suppression and AH receptor pathway gene expression in the developing mouse mammary gland. Toxicology and Applied Pharmacology 152(1):200–210.

Iida T, Hirakawa H, Matsueda T, Nagayama J, Nagata T. 1999. Polychlorinated dibenzo-p-dioxins and related compounds: correlations of levels in human tissues and in blood. Chemosphere 38(12):2767–2774.

Ikuta T, Egushi H, Tachibana T, Yoneda Y, Kawajiri K. 1998. Nuclear localization and export signals of the human aryl hydrocarbon receptor. Journal of Biological Chemistry 273(5):2895–2904.

Ikuta T, Tachibana T, Watanabe J, Yoshida M, Yoneda Y, Kawajiri K. 2000. Nucleocytoplasmic shuttling of the aryl hydrocarbon receptor. Journal of Biochemistry 127(3):503–509.

IOM (Institute of Medicine). 1994. Veterans and Agent Orange: Health Effects of Herbicides Used in Vietnam. Washington, DC: National Academy Press.

IOM. 1996. Veterans and Agent Orange: Update 1996. Washington, DC: National Academy Press.

IOM. 1999. Veterans and Agent Orange: Update 1998. Washington, DC: National Academy Press.

Jana NR, Sarkar S, Yonemoto J, Tohyama C, Sone H. 1998. Strain differences in cytochrome P450 1A1 gene expression caused by 2,3,7,8-tetrachlorodibenzo-p-dioxin in the rat liver: role of the aryl hydrocarbon receptor and its nuclear translocator. Biochemical and Biophysical Research Communications 248(3):554–558.

Jana NR, Sarkar S, Ishizuka M, Yonemoto J, Tohyama C, Sone H. 1999a. Role of estradiol receptor-a in differential expression of 2,3,7,8-tetrachlorodibenzo-p-dioxin-inducible genes in the RL95-2 and KLE human endometrial cancer cell lines. Archives of Biochemistry and Biophysics 368(1):31–39.

Jana NR, Sarkar S, Ishizuka M, Yonemoto J, Tohyama C, Sone H. 1999b. Cross-talk between 2,3,7,8-tetrachlorodibenzo-*p*-dioxin and testosterone signal transduction pathways in LNCaP prostate cancer cells. Biochemical and Biophysical Research Communications 256(3):462–468.

Kamath AB, Nagarkatti PS, Nagarkatti M. 1998. Characterization of phenotypic alterations induced by 2,3,7,8-tetrachlorodibenzo-*p*-dioxin on thymocytes in vivo and its effect on apoptosis. Toxicology and Applied Pharmacology 150(1):117–124.

Kamath AB, Camacho I, Nagarkatti PS, Nagarkatti M. 1999. Role of Fas-Fas ligand interactions in 2,3,7,8-tetrachlorodibenzo-*p*-dioxin (TCDD)-induced immunotoxicity: increased resistance of thymocytes from Fas-deficient (lpr) and Fas ligand-defective (gld) mice to TCDD-induced toxicity. Toxicology and Applied Pharmacology 160(2):141–155.

Karchner SI, Powell WH, Hahn, ME. 1999. Identification and functional characterization of two highly divergent aryl hydrocarbon receptors (AHR1 and AHR2) in the teleost *Fundulus heteroclitus*. Evidence for a novel subfamily of ligand-binding basic helix loop helix-per-ARNT-Sim (bHLH-PAS) factors. Journal of Biological Chemistry 274(47):33814–33824.

Kashani M, Steiner G, Haitel A, Schaufler K, Thalhammer T, Amann G, Kramer G, Marberger M,Scholler A. 1998. Expression of the aryl hydrocarbon receptor (AhR) and the aryl hydrocarbon receptor nuclear translocator (ARNT) in fetal, benign hyperplastic, and malignant prostate. Prostate 37(2):98–108.

Kato K, Yamanaka K, Hasegawa A, Okada S. 1999. Dimethylarsinic acid exposure causes accumulation of Hsp72 in cell nuclei and suppresses apoptosis in human alveolar cultured (L-132) cells. Biological and Pharmaceutical Bulletin 22(11):1185–1188.

Kaya B, Yanikoglu A, Marcos R. 1999. Genotoxicity studies on the phenoxyacetates 2,4-D and 4-CPA in the *Drosophila* wing spot test. Teratogenesis, Carcinogenesis, and Mutagenesis 19(4): 305–312.

Kazlauskas A, Poellinger L, Pongratz I. 1999. Evidence that the co-chaperone p23 regulates ligand responsiveness of the dioxin (aryl hydrocarbon) receptor. Journal of Biological Chemistry 274(19):13519–13524.

Kelley SK, Nilsson CB, Green MH, Green JB, Hakansson H. 1998. Use of model-based compartmental analysis to study effects of 2,3,7,8-tetrachlorodibenzo-*p*-dioxin on vitamin A kinetics in rats. Toxicological Sciences 44(1):1–13.

Kim JE, Sheen YY. 2000. Inhibition of 2,3,7,8-tetrachlorodibenzo-*p*-dioxin (TCDD)-stimulated Cyp1a1 promoter activity by hypoxic agents. Biochemical Pharmacology 59(12):1549–1556.

Kim W, Hwang S, Lee H, Song H, Kim S. 1999. *Panax ginseng* protects the testis against 2,3,7,8-tetrachlorodibenzo-*p*-dioxin induced testicular damage in guinea pigs. BJU International 83(7): 842–849.

Kimura T, Kuroki K, Doi K. 1998. Dermatotoxicity of agricultural chemicals in the dorsal skin of hairless dogs. Toxicologic Pathology 26(3):442–447.

Klinge CM, Bowers, JL, Kulakosky PC, Kamboj KK, Swanson HI. 1999. The aryl hydrocarbon receptor (AHR)/AHR nuclear translocator (ARNT) heterodimer interacts with naturally occurring estrogen response elements. Molecular and Cellular Endocrinology 157(1–2):105–119.

Klinge CM, Kaur K, Swanson HI. 2000. The aryl hydrocarbon receptor interacts with estrogen receptor alpha and orphan receptors COUP-TF1 and ERRalpha1. Archives of Biochemistry and Biophysics 373(1):163–174.

Kohle C, Gschaidmeier H, Lauth D, Topell S, Zitzer H, Bock KW. 1999. 2,3,7,8-Tetrachlorodibenzo-*p*-dioxin (TCDD)-mediated membrane translocation of c-Src protein kinase in liver WB-F344 cells. Archives of Toxicology 73(3):152–158.

Kolluri SK, Weiss C, Koff A, Gottlicher M. 1999. p27Kip1 induction and inhibition of proliferation by the intracellular Ah receptor in developing thymus and hepatoma cells. Genes and Development 13(13):1742–1753.

Korkalainen M, Tuomisto J, Pohjanvirta R. 2000. Restructured transactivation domain in hamster AH receptor. Biochemical and Biophysical Research Communications 273(1):272–281.

Krig SR, Rice RH. 2000. TCDD suppression of tissue transglutaminase stimulation by retinoids in malignant human keratinocytes. Toxicological Sciences 56(2):357–364.

Kuchenhoff A, Seliger G, Klonisch T, Tscheudschilsuren G, Kaltwasser P, Seliger E, Buchmann J, Fischer B. 1999. Arylhydrocarbon receptor expression in the human endometrium. Fertility and Sterility 71(2):354–360.

Kumar MB, Tarpey RW, Perdew GH. 1999. Differential recruitment of coactivator RIP140 by Ah and estrogen receptors. Absence of a role for LXXLL motifs. Journal of Biological Chemistry 274(32):22155–22164.

Lahvis GP, Bradfield CA. 1998. Ahr null alleles: distinctive or different? Biochemical Pharmacology 56(7):781–787. Review.

Lahvis GP, Lindell SL, Thomas RS, McCuskey RS, Murphy C, Glover E, Bentz M, Southard J, Bradfield CA. 2000. Portosystemic shunting and persistent fetal vascular structures in aryl hydrocarbon receptor-deficient mice. Proceedings National Academy of Sciences USA 97:10442–10447.

LaKind JS, Berlin CM, Park CN, Naiman DQ, Gudka NJ. 2000. Methodology for characterizing distributions of incremental body burdens of 2,3,7,8-TCDD and DDE from breast milk in North American nursing infants. Journal of Toxicology and Environmental Health 59(8):605–639.

Lang DS, Becker S, Devlin RB, Koren HS. 1998. Cell-specific differences in the susceptibility of potential cellular targets of human origin derived from blood and lung following treatment with 2,3,7,8-tetrachlorodibenzo-p-dioxin (TCDD). Cell Biology and Toxicology 14(1):23–38.

La Pres JJ, Glover E, Dunham EE, Bunger MK, Bradfield CA. 2000. ARA9 modifies agonist signaling through an increase in cytosolic aryl hydrocarbon receptor. Journal of Biological Chemistry 275(9):6153–6159.

Lavin AL, Hahn DJ, Gasiewicz TA. 1998. Expression of functional aromatic hydrocarbon receptor and aromatic hydrocarbon nuclear translocator proteins in murine bone marrow stromal cells. Archives of Biochemistry and Biophysics 352(1):9–18.

Lawrence BP, Kerkvliet NI. 1998. Role of altered arachidonic acid metabolism in 2,3,7,8-tetrachlorodibenzo-p-dioxin-induced immune suppression of C57Bl/6 mice. Toxicological Sciences 42(1):13–22.

Lee CA, Lawrence BP, Kerkvliet NI, Rifkind AB. 1998. 2,3,7,8-Tetrachlorodibenzo-p-dioxin induction of cytochrome P450-dependent arachidonic acid metabolism in mouse liver microsomes: evidence for species-specific differences in responses. Toxicology and Applied Pharmacology 153(1):1–11.

Lees MJ, Whitelaw ML. 1999. Multiple roles of ligand in transforming the dioxin receptor to an active basic helix-loop-helix/PAS transcription factor complex with the nuclear protein Arnt. Molecular and Cellular Biology 19(18):5811–5822.

Li W, Wanibuchi H, Salim EI, Yamamoto S, Yoshida K, Endo G, Fokushima S. 1998. Promotion of NCI-Black-Reiter male rat bladder carcinogenesis by dimethylarsinic acid on organic compound. Cancer Letters 134(1):24–36.

Li W, Wu WZ, Barbara RB, Schramm KW, Kettrup A. 1999. A new enzyme immunoassay for PCDD/F TEQ screening in environmental samples: comparison to micro-EROD assay and to chemical analysis. Chemosphere 38(14):3313–3318.

Liu PCC, Dunlap DY, Matsumura F. 1998. Suppression of C/EBPalpha and induction of C/EBPbeta by 2,3,7,8-tetrachlorodibenzo-p-dioxin in mouse adipose tissue and liver. Biochemical Pharmacology 55(10):1647–1655.

Loeffler IK, Peterson RE. 1999. Interactive effects of TCDD and p,p'-DDE on male reproductive tract development in in utero and lactationally exposed rats. Toxicology and Applied Pharmacology 154(1):28–39.

Long WP, Perdew GH. 1999. Lack of an absolute requirement for the native aryl hydrocarbon receptor (AhR) and AhR nuclear translocator transactivation domains in protein kinase C-mediated modulation of the AhR pathway. Archives of Biochemistry and Biophysics 371(2): 246–259.

Long WP, Pray-Grant M, Tsai JC, Perdew GH. 1998. Protein kinase C activity is required for aryl hydrocarbon receptor pathway-mediated signal transduction. Molecular Pharmacology 53(4): 691–700.

Long WP, Chen X, Perdew GH. 1999. Protein kinase C modulates aryl hydrocarbon receptor nuclear translocator protein-mediated transactivation potential in a dimer context. Journal of Biological Chemistry 274(18):12391–12400.

Lorenzen A, Okey AB. 1991. Detection and characterization of Ah receptor in tissue and cells from human tonsils. Toxicology and Applied Pharmacology 107:203–214.

Luebke RW, Copeland CB, Andrews DL. 1999. Effects of aging on resistance to *Trichinella spiralis* infection in rodents exposed to 2,3,7,8-tetrachlorodibenzo-*p*-dioxin. Toxicology 136(1):15–26.

Ma Q, Baldwin KT. 2000. 2,3,7,8-Tetrachlorodibenzo-*p*-dioxin-induced degradation of aryl hydrocarbon receptor (AhR) by the ubiquitin–proteasome pathway. Role of the transcription activation and DNA binding of AHR. Journal of Biological Chemistry 275(12):8432–8438.

Ma Q, Whitlock JP Jr. 1996. The aromatic hydrocarbon receptor modulates the Hepa 1c1c7 cell cycle and differentiated state independently of dioxin. Molecular and Cellular Biology 16(5): 2144–2150.

Machala M, Drabek P, Neca J, Kolarova J, Svobodova Z. 1998. Biochemical markers for differentiation of exposures to nonplanar polychlorinated biphenyls, organochlorine pesticides or 2,3,7,8-tetrachlorodibenzo-*p*-dioxin in trout liver. Ecotoxicology and Environmental Safety 41(1):107–111.

Mahajan SS, Rifkind AB. 1999. Transcriptional activation of avian CYP1A4 and CYP1A5 by 2,3,7,8-tetrachlorodibenzo-*p*-dioxin: differences in gene expression and regulation compared to mammalian CYP1A1 and CYP1A2. Toxicology and Applied Pharmacology 155(1):96–106.

Matsumura F, Enan E, Dunlap DY, Pinkerton KE, Peake J. 1997. Altered in vivo toxicity of 2,3,7,8-tetrachlorodibenzo-*p*-dioxin (TCDD) in C-SRC deficient mice. Biochemical Pharmacology 53(10):1397–1404.

Meek MD. 1998. Ah receptor and estrogen receptor-dependent modulation of gene expression by extracts of diesel exhaust particles. Environmental Research 79(2):114–121.

Meek MD, Finch GL. 1999. Diluted mainstream cigarette smoke condensates activate estrogen receptor and aryl hydrocarbon receptor-mediated gene transcription. Environmental Research 80(1):9–17.

Meyer BK, Perdew GH. 1999. Characterization of the AhR-hsp90-XAP2 core complex and the role of the immunophilin-related protein XAP2 in AhR stabilization. Biochemistry 38(28):8907–8917.

Meyer BK, Pray-Grant MG, Vanden Heuvel JP, Perdew GH. 1998. Hepatitis B virus X-associated protein 2 is a subunit of the unliganded aryl hydrocarbon receptor core complex and exhibits transcriptional enhancer activity. Molecular and Cellular Biology 18(2):978–988.

Michalek JE, Tripathi RC. 1999. Pharmacokinetics of TCDD in veterans of Operation Ranch Hand: 15-year follow-up. Journal of Toxicology and Environmental Health 57(6):369–378.

Michalek JE, Rahe AJ, Kulkarni PM, Tripathi RC. 1998. Levels of 2,3,7,8-tetrachlorodibenzo-*p*-dioxin in 1,302 unexposed Air Force Vietnam-era veterans. Journal of Exposure Analysis and Environmental Epidemiology 8(1):59–64.

Miller, CA III. 1999. A human aryl hydrocarbon receptor signaling pathway constructed in yeast displays additive responses to ligand mixtures. Toxicology and Applied Pharmacology 160(3): 297–303.

Mimura J, Ema M, Sogawa K, Fujii-Kuriyama Y. 1999. Identification of a novel mechanism of regulation of Ah (dioxin) receptor function. Genes and Development 13(1):20–25.

Morgulis MS, Oliveira GH, Dagli ML, Palermo-Neto J. 1998. Acute 2,4-dichlorophenoxyacetic acid intoxication in broiler chicks. Poultry Science 77(4):509–515.

Morikawa T, Wanibuchi H, Morimura K, Ogawa M, Fukushima S. 2000. Promotion of skin carcinogenesis by dimethylarsinic acid in keratin (K6)/ODC transgenic mice. Japanese Journal of Cancer Research 91(6): 579–581.

Moser GA, McLachlan MS. 1999. A non-absorbable dietary fat substitute enhances elimination of persistent lipophilic contaminants in humans. Chemosphere 39(9):1513–1521.

Murante FG, Gasiewicz TA. 2000. Hemopoietic progenitor cells are sensitive targets of 2,3,7,8-tetrachlorodibenzo-p-dioxin in C57BL/6J mice. Toxicological Sciences 54(2):374–383.

Neubert D. 1992. Evaluation of toxicity of TCDD in animals as a basis for human risk assessment. Toxic Substances Journal 12:237–276.

Nguyen TA, Hoivik D, Lee JE, Safe S. 1999. Interactions of nuclear receptor coactivator/corepressor proteins with the aryl hydrocarbon receptor complex. Archives of Biochemistry and Biophysics 367(2):250–257.

Nohara K, Ushio H, Tsukumo S, Kobayashi T, Kijima M, Tohyama C, Fujimaki H. 2000. Alterations of thymocyte development, thymic emigrants and peripheral T cell population in rats exposed to 2,3,7,8-tetrachlorodibenzo-p-dioxin. Toxicology 145(2–3):227–235.

Oakes DJ, Pollack JK. 1999. Effects of a herbicide formulation, Tordon 75D®, and its individual components on the oxidative functions of mitochondria. Toxicology 136(1):41–52.

Ochi T, Nakajima F, Fukumori N. 1998. Different effects of inorganic and dimethylated arsenic compounds on cell morphology, cytoskeletal organization, and DNA synthesis in cultured Chinese hamster V79 cells. Archives of Toxicology 72(9):566–573.

Ochi T, Nakajima F, Nasui M. 1999. Distribution of gamma-tubulin in multipolar spindles and multinucleated cells induced by dimethylarsinic acid, a methylated derivative of inorganic arsenics, in Chinese hamster V79 cells. Toxicology 136(2-3):79–88.

Parrish AR, Alejandro NF, Bowes RC, Ramos KS. 1998. Cytotoxic response profiles of cultured renal epitheial and mesenchymal cells to selected aromatic hydrocarbons. Toxicology in Vitro 12:219–232.

Partanen AM, Alaluusua S, Miettinen PJ, Thesleff I, Tuomisto J, Pohjanvirta R, Lukinmaa PL. 1998. Epidermal growth factor receptor as a mediator of developmental toxicity of dioxin in mouse embryonic teeth. Laboratory Investigation 78(12):1473–1481.

Patandin S, Dagnelie PC, Mulder PG, Op de Coul E, van der Veen JE, Weisglas-Kuperus N, Sauer PJ. 1999. Dietary exposure to polychlorinated biphenyls and dioxins from infancy until adulthood: A comparison between breast-feeding, toddler, and long-term exposure. Environmental Health Perspectives 107(1):45–51.

Perdew GH, Hollenback CE. 1995. Evidence for two functionally distinct forms of the human Ah receptor. Journal of Biochemical Toxicology 10(2):95–102.

Petrick JS, Ayala-Fierro F, Cullen WR, Carter DE, Vasken Aposhian H. 2000. Monomethylarsonous acid (MMA(III)) is more toxic than arsenite in Chang human hepatocytes. Toxicology and Applied Pharmacology 163(2):203–207.

Petroff BK, Gao X, Rozman KK, Terranova PF. 2000. Interaction of estradiol and 2,3,7,8-tetrachlorodibenzo-p-dioxin (TCDD) in an ovulation model: evidence for systemic potentiation and local ovarian effects. Reproductive Toxicology 14(3):247–255.

Phelan DM, Brackney WR, Denison MS. 1998. The Ah receptor can bind ligand in the absence of receptor-associated heat-shock protein 90. Archives of Biochemistry and Biophysics 353(1):47–54.

Pohjanvirta R, Wong JMY, Li W, Harper PA, Tuomisto J, Okey AB. 1998. Point mutation in intron sequence causes altered carboxyl-terminal structure in the aryl hydrocarbon receptor of the most 2,3,7,8-tetrachlorodibenzo-p-dioxin-resistant rat strain. Molecular Pharmacology 54(1): 86–93.

Pohjanvirta R, Viluksela M, Tuomisto JT, Unkila M, Karasinska J, Franc MA, Holowenko M, Giannone JV, Harper PA, Tuomisto J, Okey AB. 1999. Physicochemical differences in the AH receptors of the most TCDD-susceptible and the most TCDD-resistant rat strains. Toxicology and Applied Pharmacology 155(1):82–95.

Pollenz RS, Santostefano MJ, Klett E, Richardson VM, Necela B, Birnbaum LS. 1998. Female Sprague-Dawley rats exposed to a single oral dose of 2,3,7,8-tetrachlorodibenzo-*p*-dioxin exhibit sustained depletion of aryl hydrocarbon receptor protein in liver, spleen, thymus, and lung. Toxicological Sciences 42(2):117–128.

Prell RA, Dearstyne E, Steppan LG, Vella AT, Kerkvliet NI. 2000. CTL hyporesponsiveness induced by 2,3,7,8-tetrachlorodibenzo-*p*-dioxin: role of cytokines and apoptosis. Toxicology and Applied Pharmacology 166(3):214–221.

Pryputniewicz SJ, Nagarkatti M, Nagarkatti PS. 1998. Differential induction of apoptosis in activated and resting T cells by 2,3,7,8-tetrachlorodibenzo-*p*-dioxin (TCDD) and its repercussion on T cell responsiveness. Toxicology 129(2-3):211–226.

Puga A, Maier A, Medvedovic M. 2000a. The transcriptional signature of dioxin in human hepatoma HepG2 cells. Biochemical Pharmacology 60:1129–1142.

Puga A, Barnes SJ, Dalton TP, Chang C, Knudsen ES, Maier MA. 2000b. Aromatic hydrocarbon receptor interaction with the retinoblastoma protein potentiates repression of E2F-dependent transcription and cell cycle arrest. Journal of Biological Chemistry 275(4):2943–2950.

Quadri SA, Quadri AN, Hahn ME, Mann KK, Sherr DH. 2000. The bioflavonoid galangin blocks aryl hydrocarbon receptor activation and polycyclic aromatic hydrocarbon-induced pre-B cell apoptosis. Molecular Pharmacology 58:515–525.

Ramakrishna G, Anderson LM. 1998. Levels and membrane localization of the c-K-ras p21 protein in lungs of mice of different genetic strains and effects of 2,3,7,8-tetrachlorodibenzo-*p*-dioxin (TCDD) and Aroclor 1254. Carcinogenesis 19(3):463–470.

Rawlings NC, Cook SJ, Waldbillig D. 1998. Effects of the pesticides carbofuran, chlorpyrifos, dimethoate, lindane, triallate, trifluralin, 2,4-D, and pentachlorophenol on the metabolic endocrine and reproductive endocrine system in ewes. Journal of Toxicology and Environmental Health 54(1):21–36.

Reiners JJ Jr., Clift RE. 1999. Aryl hydrocarbon receptor regulation of ceramide-induced apoptosis in murine hepatoma 1c1c7 cells. A function independent of aryl hydrocarbon receptor nuclear translocator. Journal of Biological Chemistry 274(4):2502–2510.

Ricci MS, Toscano DG, Toscano WA Jr. 1999a. ECC-1 human endometrial cells as a model system to study dioxin disruption of steroid hormone function. In Vitro Cellular and Developmental Biology 35(4):183–189.

Ricci MS, Toscano DG, Mattingly CJ, Toxcano WA Jr. 1999b. Estrogen receptor reduces CYP1A1 induction in cultured human endometrial cells. Journal of Biological Chemistry 274(6):3430–3438.

Richon VM, Rifkind RA, Marks PA. 1992. Expression and phosphorylation of the retinoblastoma protein during induced differentiation of murine erythroleukemia cells. Cell Growth and Differentiation 3(7):413–420.

Riebniger D, Schrenk D. 1998. Nonresponsiveness to 2,3,7,8-tetrachlorodibenzo-*p*-dioxin of transforming growth factor beta1 and CYP 1A1 gene expression in rat liver fat-storing cells. Toxicology and Applied Pharmacology 152(1):251–260.

Roberts EA, Johnson KC, Harper PA, Okey AB. 1990. Characterization of the Ah receptor mediating aryl hydrocarbon hydroxylase induction in the human liver cell line Hep G2. Archives of Biochemistry and Biophysics 276(2):442–450.

Roberts EA, Johnson KC, Dippold WG.1991. Ah receptor mediating induction of cytochrome P450IA1 in a novel continuous human liver cell line (Mz-Hep-1). Detection by binding with [3H]2,3,7,8-tetrachlorodibenzo-*p*-dioxin and relationship to the activity of aryl hydrocarbon hydroxylase. Biochemical Pharmacology 42(3):521–528.

Roberts BJ, Whitelaw ML. 1999. Degradation of the basic helix-loop-helix/Per-ARNT-Sim homology domain dioxin receptor via the ubiquitin/proteasome pathway. Journal of Biological Chemistry 274(51):36351–36356.

Robles R, Morita Y, Mann KK, Perez GI, Yang S, Matikainen T, Sherr DH, Tilly JL. 2000. The aryl hydrocarbon receptor, a basic helix-loop-helix transcription factor of the PAS gene family, is required for normal ovarian germ cell dynamics in the mouse. Endocrinology 141(1):450–453.

Rogan WJ, Gladen BC, Hung KL, Koong SL, Shih LY, Taylor JS, Wu YC, Yang D, Ragan NB, Hsu CC. 1988. Congenital poisoning by polychlorinated biphenyls and their contaminants in Taiwan. Science 241(4863):334–336.

Rohde S, Moser GA, Popke O, McLachlan MS. 1999. Clearance of PCDD/Fs via the gastrointestinal tract in occupationally exposed persons. Chemosphere 38(14):3397–3410.

Roman BL, Peterson RE. 1998. In utero and lactational exposure of the male rat to 2,3,7,8-tetrachlorodibenzo-p-dioxin impairs prostate development. 1. Effects on gene expression. Toxicology and Applied Pharmacology 150(2):240–253.

Roman BL, Pollenz RS, Peterson RE. 1998a. Responsiveness of the adult male rat reproductive tract to 2,3,7,8-tetrachlorodibenzo-p-dioxin exposure: Ah receptor and ARNT expression, CYP1A1 induction, and Ah receptor down-regulation. Toxicology and Applied Pharmacology 150(2): 228–239.

Roman BL, Timms BG, Prins GS, Peterson RE. 1998b. In utero and lactational exposure of the male rat to 2,3,7,8-tetrachlorodibenzo-p-dioxin impairs prostate development. 2. Effects on growth and cytodifferentiation. Toxicology and Applied Pharmacology 150(2):254–270.

Rosso SB, Caceres AO, de Duffard AM, Duffard RO, Quiroga S. 2000. 2,4-Dichlorophenoxyacetic acid disrupts the cytoskeleton and disorganizes the Golgi apparatus of cultured neurons. Toxicological Sciences 56(1):133–140.

Safe S. 1990. Polychlorinated biphenyls (PCBs), dibenzo-p-dioxins (PCDDs), dibenzofurans (PCDFs), and related compounds: environmental and mechanistic considerations which support the development of toxic equivalency factors (TEFs). Critical Reviews in Toxicology 21(1):51–88.

Sakurai T, Kaise T, Matsubara C. 1998. Inorganic and methylated arsenic compounds induce cell death in murine macrophages via different mechanisms. Chemical Research and Toxicology 11(4):273–283.

Sandoz C, Lesca P, Narbonne JF. 1999. Hepatic Ah receptor binding affinity for 2,3,7,8-tetrachlorodibenzo-p-dioxin: similarity between beagle dog and cynomolgus monkey. Toxicology Letters 109(1–2):115–121.

Santostefano MJ, Wang X, Richardson VM, Ross DG, DeVito MJ, Birnbaum LS. 1998. A pharmacodynamic analysis of TCDD-induced cytochrome P-450 gene expression in multiple tissues: dose- and time-dependent effects. Toxicology and Applied Pharmacology 151:294–310.

Sarkar S, Jana NR, Yonemoto J, Tohyama C, Sone H. 2000. Estrogen enhances induction of cytochrome P-4501A1 by 2,3,7,8-tetrachlorodibenzo-p-dioxin in liver of female Long-Evans rats. International Journal of Oncology 16(1):141–147.

Schaldach CM, Riby J, Bjeldanes LF. 1999. Lipoxin A4: a new class of ligand for the Ah receptor. Biochemistry 38(23):7594–7600.

Schecter A, Kassis I, Popke O. 1998a. Partitioning of dioxins, dibenzofurans, and coplanar PCBs in blood, milk, adipose tissue, placenta and cord blood from five American women. Chemosphere 37(9–12):1817–1823.

Schecter A, Ryan JJ, Popke O. 1998b. Decrease in levels and body burden of dioxins, dibenzofurans, PCBs, DDE, and HCB in blood and milk in a mother nursing twins over a thirty-eight month period. Chemosphere 37(9–12):1807–1816.

Schlezinger JJ, White RD, Stegeman JJ. 1999. Oxidative inactivation of cytochrome P-450 1A (CYP1A) stimulated by 3,3',4,4'-tetrachlorobiphenyl: production of reactive oxygen by vertebrate CYP1As. Molecular Pharmacology 56(3):588–597.

Schlummer M, Moser GA, McLachlan MS. 1998. Digestive tract absorption of PCDD/Fs, PCBs, and HCB in humans: mass balances and mechanistic considerations. Toxicology and Applied Pharmacology 152(1):128–137.

Schrey P, Wittsiepe J, Mackrodt P, Selenka F. 1998. Human fecal PCDD/F excretion exceeds the dietary intake. Chemosphere 37(9-12):1825–1831.

Schuur AG, Tacken PJ, Visser TJ, Brouwer A. 1998. Modulating effects of thyroid state on the induction of biotransformation enzymes by 2,3,7,8-tetrachlorodibenzo-p-dioxin. Environmental Toxicology and Pharmacology 5:7–16.

Sehy DW, Shao LE, Yu AL, Tsai WM, Yu J. 1992. Activin A-induced differentiation in K562 cells is associated with a transient hypophosphorylation of RB protein and the concomitant block of cell cycle at G_1 phase. Journal of Cellular Biochemistry 50(3):255–265.

Seo BW, Sparks AJ, Medora K, Amin S, Schantz SL. 1999. Learning and memory in rats gestationally and lactationally exposed to 2,3,7,8-tetrachlorodibenzo-p-dioxin (TCDD). Neurotoxicology and Teratology 21(3):231–239.

Sewall CH, Flagler N, Heuvel J PV, Clark GC, Tritshcer AM, Maronpot RM, Lucier GW. 1995. Alterations in thyroid function in female Sprague-Dawley rats following chronic treatment with 2,3,7,8-tetrachlorodibenzo-p-dioxin. Toxicology and Applied Pharmacology 132 (2):237–244.

Shertzer HG, Nebert DW, Puga A, Ary M, Sonntag D, Dixon K, Robinson LJ, Cianciolo E, Dalton TP. 1998. Dioxin causes a sustained oxidative stress response in the mouse. Biochemical and Biophysical Research Communications 253(1):44–48.

Shimba S, Todoroki K, Aoyagi T, Tezuka M. 1998. Depletion of arylhydrocarbon receptor during adipose differentiation in 3T3-L1 cells. Biochemical and Biophysical Research Communications 249(1):131–137.

Shimba S, Hayashi M, Sone H, Yonemoto J, Tezuka M. 2000. 2,3,7,8-Tetrachlorodibenzo-p-dioxin (TCDD) induces binding of a 50 kDa protein on the 3' untranslated region of urokinase-type plasminogen activator mRNA. Biochemical and Biophysicals Research Communications 272(2):441–448.

Shimizu Y, Nakatsura Y, Ichinose M, Takahashi Y, Kume H, Mimura J, Fujii-Kuriyama Y, Ishikawa T. 2000. Benzo[a]pyrene carcinogenicity is lost in mice lacking the aryl hydrocarbon receptor. Proceeding of the National Academy of Sciences 97:779–782.

Sinal CJ, Bend JR. 1997. Aryl hydrocarbon receptor-dependent induction of Cyp1a1 by bilirubin in mouse hepatoma Hepa 1c1c7 cells. Molecular Pharmacology 52(4):590–599.

Sirkka U, Pohjanvirta R, Nieminen SA, Tuomisto J, Ylitalo P. 1992. Acute neurobehavioural effects of 2,3,7,8 tetrachlorodibenzo-p-dioxin (TCDD) in Han/Wistar rats. Pharmacology and Toxicology 71(4): 284–288.

Slezak BP, Hatch GE, DeVito MJ, Diliberto JJ, Slade R, Crissman K, Hassoun E, Birnbaum LS. 2000. Oxidative stress in female B6C3F1 mice following acute and subchronic exposure to 2,3,7,8-tetrachlorodibenzo-p-dioxin (TCDD). Toxicological Sciences 54(2):390–398.

Smeets JMW, van Holsteijn I, Giesy JP, van den Berg M. 1999. The anti-estrogenicity of Ah receptor agonists in carp (*Cyprinus carpio*) hepatocytes. Toxicological Sciences 52(2):178–188.

Smialowicz RJ, DeVito MJ, Riddle MM, Williams WC, Birnbaum LS. 1997. Opposite effects of 2,2',4,4',5,5'-hexachlorobiphenyl and 2,3,7,8-tetrachlorodibenzo-p-dioxin on the antibody response to sheep erythrocytes in mice. Fundamental and Applied Toxicology 37(2):141–149.

Smith AG, Clothier B, Robinson S, Scullion MJ, Carthew P, Edwards R, Luo J, LIm CK, Toledano M. 1998. Interaction between iron metabolism and 2,3,7,8-tetrachlorodibenzo-p-dioxin in mice with variants of the Ahr gene: a hepatic oxidative mechanism. Molecular Pharmacology 53(1): 52–61.

Sommer RJ, Sojka KM, Pollenz RS, Cooke PS, Peterson RE. 1999. Ah receptor and ARNT protein and mRNA concentrations in rat prostate: effects of stage of development and 2,3,7,8-tetrachlorodibenzo-p-dioxin treatment. Toxicology and Applied Pharmacology 155(2):177–189.

Stahl BU, Rozman K. 1990. 2,3,7,8-Tetrachlorodibenzo-*p*-dioxin (TCDD)-induced appetite suppression in the Sprague-Dawley rat is not a direct effect on feed intake regulation in the brain. Toxicology and Applied Pharmacology 106:158–162.

Staples JE, Fiore NC, Frazier DE Jr, Gasiewicz TA, Silverstone AE. 1998a. Overexpression of the anti-apoptotic oncogene, bcl-2, in the thymus does not prevent thymic atrophy induced by estradiol or 2,3,7,8-tetrachlorodibenzo-*p*-dioxin. Toxicology and Applied Pharmacology 151(1): 200–210.

Staples JE, Murante FG, Fiore NC, Gasiewicz TA, Silverstone AE. 1998b. Thymic alterations induced by 2,3,7,8-tetrachlorodibenzo-*p*-dioxin are strictly dependent on aryl hydrocarbon receptor activation in hemopoietic cells. Journal of Immunology 160(8):3844–3854.

Tanguay RL, Abnet CC, Heideman W, Peterson RE. 1999. Cloning and characterization of the zebrafish (*Danio rerio*) aryl hydrocarbon receptor. Biochimica et Biophysica Acta 1444:35–48.

Teeguarden JG, Dragan YP, Singh J, Vaughan J, Xu YH, Goldsworthy T, Pitot HC. 1999. Quantitative analysis of dose- and time-dependent promotion of four phenotypes of altered hepatic foci by 2,3,7,8-tetrachlorodibenzo-*p*-dioxin in female Sprague-Dawley rats. Toxicological Sciences 51:211–223.

Thurmond TS, Gasiewiez TA, 2000. A single dose of 2,3,7,8-tetrachlorodibenzo-*p*-dioxin produces a time-and dose-dependent alteration in the murine bone marrow B-lymphocyte maturation profile. Toxicological Sciences 58:88–95.

Thurmond TS, Silverstone AE, Baggs RB, Quimby FW, Staples JE, Gasiewicz TA. 1999. A chimeric aryl hydrocarbon receptor knockout mouse model indicates that aryl hydrocarbon receptor activation is hematopoietic cells contributes to the hepatic lesions induced by 2,3,7,8-tetrachlorodibenzo-*p*-dioxin. Toxicology and Applied Pharmacology 158:33–40.

Thurmond TS, Staples JE, Silverstone AE, Gasiewicz TA. 2000. The aryl hydrocarbon receptor has a role in the in vivo maturation of murine bone marrow B lymphocytes and their responses to 2,3,7,8-tetrachlorodibenzo-*p*-dioxin. Toxicology and Applied Pharmacology 165:227–236.

Tian Y, Ke S, Thomas T, Meeker RJ, Gallo MA. 1998. Regulation of estrogen receptor mRNA by 2,3,7,8-tetrachlorodibenzo-*p*-dioxin as measured by competitive RT–PCR. Journal of Biochemical and Molecular Toxicology 12:71–77.

Tian Y, Ke S, Denison MS, Rabson AB, Gallo MA. 1999. Ah receptor and NF-kB interactions, a potential mechanism for dioxin toxicity. Journal of Biological Chemistry 274:510–515.

Tohkin M, Fukuhara M, Elizondo G, Tomita S, Gonzalez FJ. 2000. Aryl hydrocarbon receptor is required for p300-mediated induction of DNA synthesis by adenovirus E1A. Molecular Pharmacology 58:845–851.

Tscheudschilsuren G, Kuchenhoff A, Klonisch T, Tetens F, Fischer B. 1999a. Induction of arylhydrocarbon receptor (AhR) expression in embryoblast cells of rabbit preimplantation blastocysts upon degeneration of Rauber's polar trophoblast. Toxicology and Applied Pharmacology 157:125–133.

Tscheudschilsuren G, Hombach-Klonsich S, Kuchenhoff A, Fischer B, Klonisch T. 1999b. Expression of the arylhydrocarbon receptor and the arylhydrocarbon receptor nuclear translocator during early gestation in the rabbit uterus. Toxicology and Applied Pharmacology 160:231–237.

Tsunamoto K, Todo S, Imashuku S. 1987. Effects of 5-bromo-2'-deoxyuridine on arachidonic acid metabolism of neuroblastoma and leukemia cells in culture: a possible role of endogenous prostaglandins in tumor cell proliferation and differentiation. Prostaglandins, Leukotrienes and Medicine 26(2):157–169.

Tuomisto JT, Viluksela M, Pohjanvirta R, Tuomisto J. 1999. The AH receptor and a novel gene determine acute toxic responses to TCDD: segregation of the resistant alleles to different rat lines. Toxicology and Applied Pharmacology 155:71–81.

U.S. EPA (U.S. Environmental Protection Agency). 2000. Draft Exposure and Human Health Reassessment of 2,3,7,8-Tetrachlorodibenzo-*p*-Dioxin (TCDD) and Related Compounds. Office of Research and Development. U.S. Environmental Protection Agency. [Online]. Available: http://www.epa.gov/ncea/pdfs/dioxin/dioxreass.htm. (Last updated Nov. 14, 2000).

U.S. EPA. 1985. Health Assessment Document for Polychlorinated Dibenzo-*p*-Dioxins. Washington, DC. EPA/600/3-84/014F.

Unkila M, Pohjanvirta R, Tuomisto J. 1998. Body weight loss and changes in tryptophan homeostasis by chlorinated dibenzo-*p*-dioxin congeners in the most TCDD-susceptible and the most TCDD-resistant rat strain. Archives of Toxicology 72:769–776.

van den Berg M, Birnbaum LS, Bosveld BTC, Brunström B, Cook P, Feeley M, Giesy JP, Hanberg A, Hasegawa R, Kennedy SW, Kubiak T, Larsen JC, van Leeuwen FXR, Liem AKD, Nolt C, Peterson RE, Poellinger L, Safe S, Schrenk D, Tillitt D, Tysklind M, Younces M, Waern F, Zacharewski T. 1998. Toxic equivalency factors (TEFs) for PCBs, PCDDs, PCDFs for humans and wildlife. Environmental Health Perspectives 106(12):775–792.

Van der Molen GW, Kooijman S, Michalek JE, Slob W. 1998. The estimation of elimination rates of persistent compounds: a re-analysis of 2,3,7,8-tetrachlorodibenzo-*p*-dioxin levels in Vietnam veterans. Chemosphere 37:1833–1844.

Van der Plas SA, de Jongh J, Faassen-Peters M, Scheu G, van den Berg M, Brouwer A. 1998. Toxicokinetics of an environmentally relevant mixture of dioxin-like PHAHs with or without a non-dioxin-like PCB in a semi-chronic exposure study in female Sprague-Dawley rats. Chemosphere 37:1941–1955.

Viluksela M, Unkila M, Pohjanvirta R, Tuomisto JT, Stahl BU, Rozman KK, Tuomisto J. 1999. Effects of 2,3,7,8-tetrachlorodibenzo-*p*-dioxin (TCDD) on liver phosphoenolpyruvate carboxykinase (PEPCK) activity, glucose hemeostasis and plasma amino acid concentrations in the most TCDD-susceptible and the most TCDD-resistant rat strains. Archives of Toxicology 73:323–336.

Vogel C, Schuhmacher US, Degen GH, Bolt HM, Pineau T, Abel J. 1998. Modulation of prostaglandin H synthase-2 mRNA expression by 2,3,7,8-tetrachlorodibenzo-*p*-dioxin in mice. Archives of Biochemistry and Biophysics 351:265–271.

Walker NJ, Miller BD, Kohn MC, Lucier GW, Tritscher AM. 1998. Differences in kinetics of induction and reversibility of TCDD-induced changes in cell proliferation and CYP1A1 expression in female Sprague-Dawley rat liver. Carcinogenesis 19:1427–1435.

Walker NJ, Portier CJ, Lax SF, Crofts FG, Li Y, Lucier GW, Sutter TR. 1999. Characterization of the dose–response of CYP1B1, CYP1A1, and CYP1A2 in the liver of female Sprague-Dawley rats following chronic exposure to 2,3,7,8-tetrachlorodibenzo-*p*-dioxin. Toxicology and Applied Pharmacology 154:279–286.

Walker NJ, Tritscher AM, Sills RC, Lucier GW, Portier CJ. 2000. Hepatocarcinogenesis in female Sprague-Dawley rats following discontinuous treatment with 2,3,7,8-tetrachlorodibenzo-*p*-dioxin. Toxicological Sciences 54:330–337.

Wang X, Santostefano MJ, Evans MV, Richardson VM, Diliberto JJ, Birnbaum LS. 1997. Determination of parameters responsible for pharmacokinetic behavior of TCDD in female Sprague-Dawley rats. Toxicology and Applied Pharmacology 147:151–168.

Wang X, Santostefano MJ, DeVito MJ, Birnbaum LS. 2000. Extrapolation of a PBPK model for dioxin across dosage regimen, gender, strain and species. Toxicological Sciences 56(1):49–60.

Wanner R, Zober A, Abraham K, Kleffe J, Henz BM, Wittig B. 1999. Polymorphism at codon 554 of the human Ah receptor: different allelic frequencies in Caucasians and Japanese and no correlation with severity of TCDD- induced chloracne in chemical workers. Pharmacogenetics 9:777–780.

Warren TK, Mitchell KA, Lawrence BP. 2000. Exposure to 2,3,7,8-tetrachlorodibenzo-*p*-dioxin (TCDD) suppresses the humoral and cell-mediated immune responses to influenze A virus without affecting cytolytic activity in the lung. Toxicological Sciences 56:114–123.

Wei M, Wanibuchi H, Yamamoto S, Li W, Fukushima S. 1999. Urinary bladder carcinogenicity of dimethylarsinic acid in male F344 rats. Carcinogenesis 20:1873–1876.

Wei YD, Rannug U, Rannug A. 1999. UV-induced CYP1A1 gene expression in human cells is mediated by tryptophan. Chemico-Biological Interactions 118:127–140.

Willey JJ, Stripp BR, Baggs RB, Gasiewicz TA. 1998. Aryl hydrocarbon receptor activation in genital tubercle, palate and other embryonic tissue in 2,3,7,8-tetrachlorodibenzo-p-dioxin-responsive lacZ mice. Toxicology and Applied Pharmacology 151:33–44.

Wittsiepe J, Kullmann Y, Schrey P, Selenka F, Wilhelm M. 1999. Peroxidase-catalyzed in vitro formation of polychlorinated dibenzo-p-dioxins and dibenzofurans from chlorophenols. Toxicology Letters 106:191–200.

Wolf CJ, Ostby JS, Gray LE Jr. 1999. Gestational exposure to 2,3,7,8-tetrachlorodibenzo-p-dioxin (TCDD) severely alters reproductive function of female hamster offspring. Toxicological Sciences 51:259–264.

Wolfle D. 1998. Interactions between 2,3,7,8-TCDD and PCBs as tumor promoters: limitations of TEFs. Teratogenesis, Carcinogenesis, and Mutagenesis. 17:217–224.

Wolfle D, Marotzki S, Dartsch D, Schafer W, Marquardt H. 2000. Induction of cyclooxygenase expression and enhancement of malignant cell transformation by 2,3,7,8-tetrachlorodibenzo-p-dioxin. Carcinogenesis 21:15–21.

Worner W, Schrenk D. 1998. 2,3,7,8-Tetrachlorodibenzo-p-dioxin suppresses apoptosis and leads to hyperphosphorylation of p53 in rat hepatocytes. Environmental Toxicology and Pharmacology 6:239–247.

Wyde ME, Seely J, Lucier GW, Walker NJ. 2000. Toxicity of chronic exposure to 2,3,7,8-tetrachlorodibenzo-p-dioxin in diethylnitrosamine-initiated ovariectomized rats implanted with subcutaneous 17β-estradiol pellets. Toxicological Sciences 54:493–499.

Yamanaka K, Katsumata K, Ikuma K, Hasegawa A, Nakano M, Okada S. 2000. The role of orally administered dimethylarsinic acid, a main metabolite of inorganic arsenics, in the promotion and progression of UVB-induced skin tumorigenesis in hairless mice. Cancer Letters 152(1):79–85.

Yang AL, Smith AG, Akhtar R, Clothier B, Robinson S, MacFarlane M, Festing MFW. 1999. Low levels of p53 are associated with resistance to tetrachlorodibenzo-p-dioxin toxicity in DBA/2 mice. Pharmacogenetics 9:183–188.

Yang JH. 1999. Expression of dioxin-responsive genes in human endometrial cells in culture. Biochemical and Biophysical Research Communications 257:259–263.

Yang JH, Vogel C, Abel J. 1999. A malignant transformation of human cells by 2,3,7,8-tetrachlorodibenzo-p-dioxin exhibits altered expressions of growth regulatory factors. Carcinogenesis 20:13–18.

Yang JZ, Agarwal SK, Foster WG. 2000. Subchronic exposure to 2,3,7,8-tetrachlorodibenzo-p-dioxin modulates the pathophysiology endometriosis in the cynomolgus monkey. Toxicological Sciences 56:374–381.

Zaher H, Fernandez-Salguero PM, Letterio J, Sheikh MS, Fornace AJ Jr, Roberts AB, Gonzalez FJ. 1998. The involvement of aryl hydrocarbon receptor in the activation of transforming growth factor-beta and apoptosis. Molecular Pharmacology 54(2):313–321.

4

Methodological Considerations in Evaluating the Evidence

QUESTIONS TO BE ADDRESSED

The committee was charged with the task of summarizing the strength of the scientific evidence concerning the association between herbicide exposure during Vietnam service and each of a set of diseases or conditions suspected to be associated with such exposure. Public Law 102-4 (codified as 38 USC Sec. 1116) specifies three scientific determinations concerning diseases that must be made. It charges the committee to determine (to the extent that available scientific data permit meaningful determinations) the following:

1. whether a statistical association with herbicide exposure exists, taking into account the strength of the scientific evidence and the appropriateness of the statistical and epidemiologic methods used to detect the association;

2. the increased risk of each disease among those exposed to herbicides during service in the Republic of Vietnam during the Vietnam era; and

3. whether there exists a plausible biologic mechanism or other evidence of a causal relationship between herbicide exposure and the disease.

P.L. 102-4 did not provide a specific list of diseases and conditions suspected to be associated with herbicide exposure. The committee staff and members responsible for the 1994 report *Veterans and Agent Orange: Health Effects of Herbicides Used in Vietnam* (hereafter referred to as *VAO*) (IOM, 1994) developed such a list based on diseases and conditions that had been mentioned in the scientific literature or in other documents that came to their attention through extensive literature searches. The *VAO* list has been supplemented over time in response to developments in the literature.

The information used by the committee was developed through a comprehensive search of relevant data bases. Public and commercial data bases covering biological, medical, toxicological, chemical, historical, and regulatory information were examined. The majority of these data bases were bibliographic, providing citations to scientific literature. Committee staff examined the reference lists of major review articles, books, and reports for relevant citations. Reference lists of individual articles were also scanned for pertinent citations. Search engines were used to scan for information posted on the Internet. Literature identification continued through September 30, 2000. The input received both in written and oral form from veterans and other interested persons at public hearings and in written submissions served as a valuable source of additional information.

This third biennial update concentrates on evaluating the evidence published following the completion of work on *Veterans and Agent Orange: Health Effects of Herbicides Used in Vietnam* (IOM, 1994), *Veterans and Agent Orange: Update 1996* (IOM, 1996), *Veterans and Agent Orange: Update 1998* (IOM, 1999), and *Veterans and Agent Orange: Herbicide/Dioxin Exposure and Type 2 Diabetes* (IOM, 2000). For each health outcome, the new evidence is reviewed in detail. Conclusions are based on the totality of accumulated evidence, not just on recently published studies. In other words, new evidence is not interpreted alone but is put in the context of evidence addressed in previous reports.

The committee's judgments have both quantitative and qualitative aspects; they reflect both the evidence examined and the approach taken to evaluate it. In *VAO*, the committee delineated how it approached its task so that readers would be able to assess and interpret the committee's findings. By offering this information, the committee wished to make the report useful to those seeking to update its conclusions as new information was obtained. The committees responsible for subsequent reports have adopted the original committee's approach.

The remainder of this chapter delineates the primary considerations underlying the evaluation process. A more complete description of methodological issues may be found in Chapter 5 of *VAO* and in Chapter 4 of *Update 1996* and *Update 1998*.

Is Herbicide Exposure Statistically Associated with the Health Outcome?

The committee necessarily focused on a pragmatic question: What is the nature of the relevant evidence for or against a statistical association between exposure and the health outcome? The evidentiary base that the committee found to be most helpful derived from epidemiologic studies of populations—that is, investigations in which large groups of people are studied to determine the association between the occurrence of particular diseases and exposure to the substances at issue. To determine whether an association exists, epidemiologists estimate the magnitude of an appropriate quantitative measure (such as the relative risk or the odds ratio) that describes the relationship between exposure and disease in defined populations or groups. However, the use of terms such as "relative risk," "odds ratio," or "estimate of relative risk" is not consistent in the literature. In this report, the committee intends *relative risk* to refer to the results of cohort studies and *odds ratio* (an estimate of relative risk) to refer to the results of case-control studies. Values of relative risk greater than 1 may indicate a positive or direct association—that is, a harmful association—whereas values between 0 and 1 may indicate a negative or inverse association—that is, a protective association. A "statistically significant" difference is one that, under the assumptions made in the study and the laws of probability, would be unlikely to occur if there were no true difference and no biases.

Determining whether an observed statistical association between exposure and a health outcome is "real" requires additional scrutiny because there may be alternative explanations for the observed association. These include: *error* in the design, conduct, or analysis of the investigation; *bias*, or a systematic tendency to distort the measure of association so that it may not represent the true relation between exposure and outcome; *confounding*, or distortion of the measure of association because another factor related to both exposure and outcome has not been recognized or taken into account in the analysis; and *chance*, the effect of random variation, which produces spurious associations that can, with a known probability, sometimes depart widely from the true relation.

Therefore, in deciding whether an association between herbicide exposure and a particular outcome exists, the committee examined the quantitative estimates of risk and evaluated whether these estimates might be due to error, bias, confounding, or chance or were likely to represent a true association.

In pursuing the question of statistical association, the committee recognized that an absolute conclusion about the absence of association may never be attained. As in science generally, studies of health outcomes following herbicide exposure are not capable of demonstrating that the purported effect is impossible or could never occur. Any instrument of observation, including epidemiologic studies, has a limit to its resolving power. Hence, in a strict technical sense, the committee could not prove the absolute absence of a health outcome associated with herbicide or dioxin exposure.

What Is the Increased Risk of the Outcome in Question Among Those Exposed to Herbicides in Vietnam?

This question, which is pertinent principally (but not exclusively) if there is evidence for a positive association between exposure and a health outcome, concerns the likely magnitude of the association in Vietnam veterans exposed to herbicides. The most desirable evidence in answering this type of question involves knowledge of the rate of occurrence of the disease in those Vietnam veterans who were actually exposed to herbicides, the rate in those who were not exposed (the "background" rate of the disease in the population of Vietnam veterans), and the degree to which any other differences between the exposed and unexposed groups of veterans influence the difference in rates. When exposure levels among Vietnam veterans have not been adequately determined, which has been the case in most studies, this question is very difficult to answer. The committees have found the available evidence sufficient for drawing conclusions about the association between herbicide exposure and a number of health outcomes. However, the lack of good data on Vietnam veterans per se, especially with regard to herbicide exposure, complicates the assessment of the increased risk of disease among individuals exposed to herbicides during service in Vietnam. Indeed, most of the evidence on which the findings in this and other reports are based comes from studies of people exposed to dioxin or herbicides in occupational and environmental settings rather than from studies of Vietnam veterans.

Is There a Plausible Biologic Mechanism?

Chapter 3 details the cellular and animal experimental evidence that provides the basis for the assessment of biologic plausibility, that is, the extent to which a statistical association is consistent with existing biological or medical knowledge. As with the epidemiologic evidence, the chapter concentrates on studies published during 1999–2000 but considers all relevant studies in drawing conclusions. The issue of whether a given chemical exposure–health outcome relationship reflects a true association in humans is addressed in the context of research regarding the mechanism of interaction between the chemical and biological systems, evidence in animal studies, evidence of an association between exposure and the occurrence of a health outcome in humans, and/or evidence that a given outcome is associated with occupational or environmental chemical exposures. It must be recognized, however, that lack of data in support of a plausible biologic mechanism does not rule out the possibility that a causal relationship does exist.

ISSUES IN EVALUATING THE EVIDENCE

Toxicologic Studies

A valid surrogate animal model for the study of a human disease must reproduce with some degree of fidelity the manifestations of the disease in humans. Whole-animal studies or animal-based experimental systems continue to be used to study herbicide toxicity because they allow for rigid control of chemical exposures and close monitoring of health outcomes. Because many of the chemical exposures presently associated with certain diseases in humans have been confirmed in experimental studies, data derived from such studies are generally accepted as a valuable guide in the assessment of biologic plausibility.

As discussed in Chapter 3, many of the toxic effects of the herbicides used in Vietnam have been ascribed to 2,3,7,8-tetrachlorodibenzo-*p*-dioxin (TCDD), a contaminant of some of these herbicides. This has not, however, simplified the risk assessment process because the toxicologic profile of TCDD is rather complex. There is consensus that most of the toxic effects of TCDD involve interaction with the aryl hydrocarbon receptor (AhR), a protein that binds TCDD and other aromatic hydrocarbons with high affinity. Attempts to establish correlations between the effects of TCDD in experimental systems and in humans are particularly problematic, because species-, gender-, and endpoint-specific differences in susceptibility to TCDD have been documented. Although studies in which transformed human cell lines are employed to study AhR biology minimize the inherent error associated with species extrapolations, caution must be exercised because the extent to which transformation itself influences toxicity outcomes has yet to be fully defined. In addition, while it is generally accepted that genetics plays a key role in determining the adverse effects of environmental chemicals, the impact of different genetic backgrounds on AhR function is not yet well understood.

Epidemiologic Studies

Environmental and/or occupational exposures to herbicides or TCDD provide data on human responses that can be compared directly to data obtained in experimental studies. Higher-than-background body burdens of dioxin have been documented in many of these groups, and details describing the major findings from these studies are reviewed in Chapters 7–10 of this report. In general, the elevated risks of cancers at various sites reported in epidemiologic studies are consistent with the known biological actions of the agents present in herbicide formulations. Although its full potential has yet to be realized, the application of molecular and cellular measurements to epidemiologic research promises to increase our understanding of the association between herbicide exposure and disease occurrence. This may provide a significant advantage in the assessment of biologic plausibility, because biologically based epidemiologic data allow more accurate identification and quantification of exposures. For instance, the analytical data available from individuals known to have been exposed to herbicides during the Vietnam War constitute a valuable resource for the study of TCDD-related disease, with documented TCDD body burdens providing a quantitative bridge between experimental studies and human epidemiology. Taken together, experimental studies and epidemiologic investigations provide complementary perspectives from which to view human health effects of exposure to herbicides. However, it must be recognized that the ultimate test of associations between exposure and disease occurrence lies in data obtained from human populations.

To obtain additional information pertinent to evaluation of the potential effects of herbicide exposure of veterans, this and previous committees decided to review studies of other groups potentially exposed to the herbicides contained in Agent Orange, to other herbicides, and to dioxin, the contaminant believed to cause many of the purported adverse effects of Agent Orange. These study populations include industrial and agricultural workers, Vietnamese citizens, and people exposed environmentally as a result of residing near the site of an accident or a toxic waste dump. The committee felt that reviewing the studies of such groups would help in determining (1) whether these compounds could be associated with particular health outcomes in veterans and (2) the nature of any dose–response relationships, although the committee acknowledged that such findings may have only an indirect bearing on the association in veterans themselves. It is also important to note that the categories of association described below relate to the association between exposure to chemicals and health outcomes in human populations, not to the likelihood that any individual's health problem is associated with or caused by the herbicides in question.

With the exception of acute and subacute transient peripheral neuropathy, the committee did not specifically consider case studies or other published studies lacking a control or comparison group. The committee elected to consider case histories when evaluating the association between exposure and these conditions because their transient nature precluded using case-control and other types of studies with comparison populations.

Publication Bias

It has been well documented (Song et al., 2000) in biomedical research that studies with a statistically significant finding are more likely to be published than studies with nonsignificant results. Thus, evaluations of disease–exposure associations that are based solely on the published literature could be biased in favor of a positive association. In general, however, for reports of overall associations with exposure, the committee did not consider the risk of publication bias to be high among studies of herbicide exposure and health risks. The committee took this position because there are numerous published studies showing no positive association; because it examined a substantial amount of unpublished material; and because the committee felt that publicity surrounding the issue of exposure to herbicides, particularly regarding Vietnam veterans, has been so intense that any studies showing no association would be unlikely to be viewed as unimportant by the investigators. In short, the pressure to publish such "negative" findings would be considerable.

The Role of Judgment

The evaluation of evidence to reach conclusions about statistical associations goes beyond quantitative procedures at several stages: assessing the relevance and validity of individual reports; deciding on the possible influence of error, bias, confounding, or chance on the reported results; integrating the overall evidence within and across diverse areas of research; and formulating the conclusions themselves. These aspects of the committee's review required thoughtful consideration of alternative approaches at several points. They could not be accomplished by adherence to a narrowly prescribed formula.

Rather, the approach described here evolved throughout the process of review and was determined in important respects by the nature of the evidence, exposures, and health outcomes at issue. Both the quantitative and the qualitative aspects of the process that could be made explicit were important to the overall review. Ultimately, the conclusions about association expressed in this report are based on the committee's collective judgment. The committee has endeavored to express its judgments as clearly and precisely as the data allowed.

REFERENCES

IOM (Institute of Medicine). 1994. Veterans and Agent Orange: Health Effects of Herbicides Used in Vietnam. Washington, DC: National Academy Press.

IOM. 1996. Veterans and Agent Orange: Update 1996. Washington, DC: National Academy Press.

IOM. 1999. Veterans and Agent Orange: Update 1998. Washington, DC: National Academy Press.

IOM. 2000. Veterans and Agent Orange: Herbicide/Dioxin Exposure and Type 2 Diabetes. Washington, DC: National Academy Press.

Song F, Eastwood AJ, Gilbody S, Duley L, Sutton AJ. 2000. Publication and related biases. Health Technology Assessment 4(10):1–115.

5

Exposure Assessment

Assessment of individual exposure to herbicides and dioxin is a key element in determining whether specific health outcomes are linked to these compounds. This chapter briefly reviews information on occupational and environmental dioxin exposures, and herbicide spraying in Vietnam and exposure of veterans. More complete discussions of the occupational and environmental exposures, and the U.S. military's wartime use of herbicides in Vietnam and of herbicide and dioxin exposure assessment in epidemiologic studies may be found in Chapters 3 and 6 of *Veterans and Agent Orange: Health Effects of Herbicides Used in Vietnam* (IOM, 1994) and in Chapter 5 of *Veterans and Agent Orange: Update 1996* (IOM, 1996) and *Update 1998* (IOM, 1999). Reviews of the most recent studies of the absorption, distribution, and passage of herbicides and dioxin through the body may be found under the discussions of toxicokinetics in Chapter 3 of this report.

OCCUPATIONAL AND ENVIRONMENTAL EXPOSURES TO HERBICIDES AND DIOXIN

The committee reviewed a large number of epidemiologic studies of occupationally or environmentally exposed groups for evidence of an association between health risks and exposure to TCDD and herbicides used in Vietnam, especially the phenoxy herbicides 2,4-D and 2,4,5-T, chlorophenols, and other compounds. In reviewing these studies, two types of exposure were explicitly considered: exposure to TCDD per se and exposure to the various herbicides used, particularly 2,4-D and 2,4,5-T. This separate consideration is necessary because of the possibility that, for example, some health effects may be associated with exposure to 2,4-D in agriculture and forestry. The herbicide 2,4-D does not contain TCDD, although small quantities of other dioxins are present.

For TCDD-exposed populations, serum measures of TCDD concentrations can be collected from a representative sample of those exposed. Serum biomarkers of TCDD exposure are sometimes used to estimate the degree of prior exposure of individuals; however, there are limitations to their use.

The available information on occupational and environmental exposures to dioxin, the contaminant found in 2,4,5-T includes studies of residents living in and around Seveso, Italy, who were exposed during industrial accidents; chemical plant workers who were occupationally or accidentally exposed to TCDD during the production of 2,4,5-T or other phenoxy herbicides or chlorophenols such as hexachlorophene or trichlorophenol; sawmill workers exposed to higher chlorinated dioxins from contaminated wood preservatives; and pulp and paper workers exposed to dioxin through the pulp bleaching process.

Occupational Studies

Production Workers

One of the most extensive sets of data on workers engaged in the production of chemicals potentially contaminated with TCDD has been compiled by NIOSH. From 12 chemical companies, more than 5,000 workers were identified from personnel and payroll records indicating whether the worker had been involved in production or maintenance processes associated with TCDD contamination (Fingerhut et al., 1991). In an update, Steenland (1999) constructed an exposure matrix for a subcohort of the workers, and attempted to evaluate the relationship between estimated TCDD exposures and mortality.

A multisite study by the International Agency for Research on Cancer (IARC) involved 18,390 production workers and herbicide sprayers from 10 countries (Saracci et al., 1991). Exposure was estimated from a combination of factory records, work histories, spraying data, and questionnaires. Several other occupational studies of workers involved in chemical production plants have relied upon job titles as recorded on individual work histories and company personnel records to classify exposure (Ott et al., 1980; Zack and Gaffey, 1983; Coggon et al., 1986, 1991; Cook et al., 1986; Zober et al., 1990). Similarly, exposure in chemical plant workers has been characterized by worker involvement in various production processes such as synthesis, packaging, waste removal, shipping, and plant supervision (Manz et al., 1991; Bueno de Mesquita et al., 1993). Flesch-Janys et al. (1995) did an update of this cohort and added quantitative exposure assessment based on blood or adipose measurements of polychlorinated dibenzo-p-dioxin and furan (PCDD/F). Using a first-order kinetics model, half-lives from an elimination study in 48 workers from this cohort, and background levels for the German population, the authors estimated PCDD/F levels for the 190 workers with serum or adipose measurements of PCDD/F. Then regressing the estimated PCDD/F level of these workers at the end of their exposure against the time they worked in each production department in the plant, the authors estimated the contribution of the working time in each production department to the PCDD/F level at the end of exposure. These production department working time "weights" were then used, along with the work histories of the remainder of the cohort, to estimate the PCDD/F level for each cohort member at the end of the person's exposure. The epidemiologic analysis used these estimated TCDD doses.

Becher et al. (1996) report an analysis of several German cohorts including the Boehringer-Ingelheim cohort described above, a cohort from the BASF Ludwigshafen plant that did not include those involved in the 1953 accident, and a cohort from a Bayer plant in Uerdingen and a Bayer plant in Dormagen. All of the plants were involved in the production of phenoxy herbicides or chlorophenols. Exposure assessment involved the estimation of duration of employment from the start of work in a department with suspected exposure until the end of employment at the plant. This may include some periods without exposure. Analysis was based upon time since first exposure. Hooiveld et al. (1998) reported on an update of a mortality study of workers at two chemical factories in the Netherlands. This study included analysis by estimated maximum TCDD serum level. This was estimated for each member of the cohort by measuring serum TCDD levels for 144 subjects, including production workers known to be exposed to dioxins, workers in herbicide production, nonexposed production workers, and workers known to be exposed as a result of an accident that occurred in 1963. Assuming first-order TCDD elimination with an estimated half-life of 7.1 years, $TCDD_{max}$ was extrapolated for a group of 47 workers, then a regression model was constructed to estimate the effect of exposure as a result of the accident, duration of employment in main production department, time of first exposure before (or after) 1970 on the estimated $TCDD_{max}$ for each cohort member.

Agricultural/Forestry/Outdoor Workers

Occupational studies of agricultural workers have estimated exposure to herbicides or TCDD using a variety of methods. In the simplest method, data on an individual's occupation are derived from death certificates, cancer registries, or hospital records (Burmeister, 1981). Although this information is relatively easy to obtain, it is not possible to estimate duration or intensity of exposure, or to determine the specific type of herbicide or chemical a worker was exposed to. Some studies of agricultural workers have attempted to investigate differences in occupational practices to identify subsets of workers who were likely to have had higher levels of herbicide exposure (Vineis et al., 1986; Wiklund and Holm, 1986; Musicco et al., 1988; Wiklund et al., 1988a; Hansen et al., 1992; Ronco et al., 1992). Other studies have used county of residence as a surrogate of exposure, relying upon agricultural censuses of farm production and chemical use to characterize exposure in individual counties (Gordon and Shy, 1981; Cantor, 1982; Blair and White, 1985). Still other studies attempted to refine exposure estimates by categorizing the exposure based on the number of years employed in a specific occupation as a surrogate for exposure duration, obtaining supplier records on the amount of herbicides purchased to estimate the level of exposure, or estimating acres sprayed to quantify the amount used (Wigle et al., 1990; Morrison et al., 1992). In some cases, self-reported information on exposure was obtained, including direct handling of the herbicide, whether it was applied by tractor or hand-held spray, and what type of protective equipment was worn or what safety precautions were exercised, if any (Hoar et al., 1986; Zahm et al., 1990). Some studies attempted to validate self-reported information, based on verification using written records, signed statements, or telephone contacts with coworkers or former employers (Carmelli et al., 1981; Woods and Polissar, 1989).

Forestry workers and other outdoor workers, such as highway maintenance workers, are likely to have been exposed to herbicides and other chemicals to varying degrees. Exposure has been classified in a manner similar to other studies, for example, by number of years employed, job category, and occupational title.

Herbicide/Pesticide Sprayers

Studies of herbicide sprayers are relevant because it can be presumed that applicators had more sustained exposure to herbicides; however, applicators were also likely to be exposed to a multiplicity of chemicals, complicating the assessment of any individual or group exposure to specifically phenoxy herbicides or TCDD. Some studies have attempted to quantify exposure of applicators based on information from work records on the number of acres sprayed or the number of days of herbicide spraying. Employment records can also be used to extract information on the type of chemicals sprayed.

One surrogate indicator of herbicide exposure is receipt of a license to perform spraying. Several studies have specifically identified licensed or registered pesticide and herbicide applicators (Smith et al., 1981, 1982; Blair et al., 1983; Wiklund et al., 1988b, 1989; Swaen et al., 1992). Individual estimates of the intensity and frequency of exposure were rarely quantified in the studies the committee examined, however, and often applicators were known to have applied many different kinds of herbicides, pesticides, and other chemicals. In addition, herbicide spraying is generally a seasonal occupation, and information may not be available on possible exposure-related activities during the rest of the year.

One study provided information on serum TCDD concentrations in herbicide sprayers, that of Smith et al. (1992). Blood from nine professional spray applicators in New Zealand, who first sprayed before 1960 and were also spraying in 1984, was analyzed. The duration of actual spray work varied from 80 to 370 months. The serum levels ranged from 3 to 131 ppt TCDD on a lipid basis, with a mean of 53 ppt. The corresponding values for age-matched controls ranged from 2 to 11 ppt; the mean was 6 ppt. Serum TCDD levels were positively correlated with the number of months of professional spray application.

Several studies have evaluated various herbicide exposures during spraying in terms of type of exposure, routes of entry, and routes of excretion: Kolmodin-Hedman and Erne (1980); Kolmodin-Hedman et al. (1983), Lavy et al. (1980a,b), Ferry et al. (1982), Libich et al. (1984), Frank et al. (1985). Based on these studies, it would appear that the major route of exposure is through dermal absorption, with 2 to 4 percent of that on the skin being absorbed into the body during a normal work day. Air concentrations were usually less than 0.2 mg/m^3. The absorbed phenoxy acid herbicides are virtually cleared within one day, primarily through urinary excretion. Typical measured excretion levels for ground crews ranged from 0.1 to 5 mg/day and less for air crews.

Paper and Pulp Mill Workers

Another occupational group likely to be exposed to TCDD and chlorinated phenols consists of paper and pulp mill workers. These workers are likely to have received varying degrees of exposure as part of the bleaching process in the production of paper and paper products. Pulp and paper production workers are also likely to be exposed to other chemicals in the workplace, which vary, for example, according to the type of paper mill or pulping operation, and the final product manufactured (Robinson et al., 1986; Henneberger et al., 1989; Solet et al., 1989; Jappinen and Pukkala, 1991) In a study of a cohort of Danish paper mill workers, Rix et al. (1998), there were no direct measures of exposure for these workers, and a qualitative assessment of chemicals used in paper manufacture by department does not include chlorinated organic compounds although chlorine, chlorine dioxide, and hypochlorite were used.

Sawmill Workers

Workers in sawmills may be exposed to pentachlorophenates, which are contaminated with higher chlorinated PCDDs (Cl_6–Cl_8) or tetrachlorophenates, which are less contaminated with higher chlorinated PCDDs. The wood is dipped in these chemicals and then cut and planed in the mills. Most exposure is dermal, although some exposure can occur via inhalation (Teschke et al., 1994; Hertzman et al., 1997).

Environmental Studies

Studies of environmental exposures related primarily to unintentional releases of TCDD into the environment at Seveso, Italy, and Times Beach, Missouri. In these cases, the simplest measure of exposure was classification according to place of residence. Intensity of exposure has been estimated by years of residence in a contaminated area; this measure does not take into account the concentration of TCDD or herbicide, or the frequency of individual contact with contaminated soil or water.

One of the largest industrial accidents involving environmental exposures to TCDD occurred in Seveso, in July 1976, as a result of an uncontrolled reaction during trichlorophenol production. A variety of indicators were used to estimate individual exposure; soil contamination by TCDD has been the most extensively used. On the basis of soil sampling, three areas were defined about the release point. They were zone A, the most heavily contaminated, from which all residents were evacuated within 20 days; zone B, an area of lesser contamination that children and pregnant women in their first trimester were urged to avoid during daytime; and zone R, a region with some contamination, in which consumption of local crops was prohibited (Bertazzi et al., 1989). The samples so obtained are virtually unique in that they were numerous and were obtained prior to elimination and degradation of TCDD in the sample media.

Data on serum concentrations of zone A residents have been presented by Mocarelli et al. (1990, 1991) and earlier by the CDC (1988a). For those with severe chloracne ($N = 10$) the TCDD levels ranged from 828 to 56,000 ppt lipid weight. Those without chloracne ($N = 10$) had levels from 1,770 to 10,400 ppt. The levels in all controls but one were not detectable. The highest of these levels exceeded any that had been estimated at the time for TCDD-exposed workers, based on backward extrapolation with a half-life of seven years. Data on nearby soil levels, number of days an individual stayed in zone A, and whether local food was consumed were considered in evaluating TCDD levels. None of these data correlated with serum TCDD levels, strongly suggesting that the exposure of importance was fallout on the day of the accident. The presence and degree of chloracne did correlate with TCDD levels; however, it appears that adults are much less likely to develop chloracne than children following an acute exposure, but surveillance bias may have played some role in this finding. Recent updates (Bertazzi et al., 1998, 2001) have not changed the exposure assessment approach in any way.

A number of reports have provided information on exposure to TCDD from environmental contamination in Missouri (Patterson et al., 1986; Andrews et al., 1989). In 1971, TCDD-contaminated sludge from a hexachlorophene production facility was mixed with waste oil and sprayed in various community areas for dust control. Soil contamination in some samples exceeded 100 parts per billion (ppb). One of the Missouri sites with the highest TCDD soil concentrations was the Quail Run mobile home park. Residents were considered exposed if they had lived in the park for at least six months during the time the contamination occurred (Hoffman et al., 1986). Other investigations of Times Beach have estimated exposure risk based on residents' reported occupational and recreational activities in the sprayed area. Levels of exposure have been estimated from duration of residence and TCDD soil concentrations.

Andrews et al. (1989) provided the most extensive data on human adipose tissue levels for 51 persons who had ridden or cared for horses at arenas sprayed with TCDD-contaminated oil; persons exposed in residential areas where such oil had been sprayed; individuals involved in TCP production; persons exposed in TCP nonproduction activities, such as lab and maintenance workers; and 128 controls. Persons were considered exposed if they lived, worked, or had other contact for two years or more with TCDD-contaminated soil at levels of 20–100 ppb or for six months or more with soil contaminated with TCDD at levels greater than 100 ppb. Of the exposed population samples, 87 percent of adipose tissue TCDD levels were less than 200 ppt; however TCDD concentrations in 7 of the 51 exposed ranged from 250 to 750 ppt. For nonexposed persons, adipose tissue TCDD concentrations ranged from nondetectable to 20 ppt, with a median of 6 ppt. Based on a seven-year half-life it is calculated that two of the study participants would have had adipose tissue TCDD levels near 3,000 ppt at the time of the last date of exposure.

Viel et al. (2000) reported on an investigation of apparent clusters of soft-tissue sarcoma and non-Hodgkin's lymphoma cases in the vicinity of a municipal solid waste incinerator in Doubs, France. The presumptive source of dioxin in this region is a municipal solid waste incinerator in the Besançon electoral ward in the west of Doubs. A measurement of dioxin emissions from the incinerator showed a level of 16.3 ng I-TEQ/m^3, far in excess of the EU standard of 0.1 ng I-TEQ/m^3. In addition, measurements of dioxin in cow's milk from three farms near the incinerators suggested that dioxin content of the milk was highest at the farm closest to the incinerator. These measurements were all well below the guideline of 6 ng I-TEQ/kg of fat, however.

Vietnamese Studies

Several studies have investigated exposure to herbicides among the residents of southern Vietnam (Constable and Hatch, 1985), comparing unexposed residents of the South to residents of the North. Other studies have attempted to identify veterans of northern Vietnam who served in the South during the Vietnam era. Records of herbicide sprays have been used to refine exposure measurements, comparing individuals who lived in sprayed villages in the South with those living in unsprayed villages. In some studies, residents of villages were considered exposed if a recorded herbicide mission passed within 10 km of the village center (Dai et al., 1990). Other criteria for classifying exposure included length of residence in a sprayed area and number of times the area had reportedly been sprayed.

A small number of studies provide information on TCDD concentrations in Vietnamese civilians exposed during the war. Schecter et al. (1986) detected

TCDD in 12 of 15 samples of adipose tissue taken at surgery or autopsy in southern Vietnam during 1984. The concentrations in the positive samples were from 3 to 103 ppt. No detectable levels of TCDD were found in nine samples from residents of northern Vietnam who had never been in the South. The detection sensitivity was 2–3 ppt. Analysis of three breast milk samples collected in 1973 from Vietnamese women thought to have been exposed to Agent Orange varied from 77 to 230 ppt on a lipid basis.

MILITARY USE OF HERBICIDES IN VIETNAM

Background

The military use of herbicides in Vietnam began in 1962, was expanded during 1965 and 1966, and reached a peak from 1967 to 1969. Herbicides were used extensively in Vietnam by the U.S. Air Force's Operation Ranch Hand to defoliate inland hardwood forests, coastal mangrove forests, and to a lesser extent, cultivated land, by aerial spraying from C-123 aircraft and helicopters. According to military records of Operation Ranch Hand, from August 1965 to February 1971 a total of 17.6 million gallons of herbicide was sprayed over approximately 3.6 million acres in Vietnam (NAS, 1974). Soldiers also sprayed herbicides on the ground to defoliate the perimeters of base camps and fire bases; this spraying was executed from the rear of trucks and from spray units mounted on the backs of soldiers on foot. Navy river boats also sprayed herbicides along riverbanks. The purpose of spraying herbicides was to improve the ability to detect enemy base camps and enemy forces along lines of communication and infiltration routes and around U.S. base camps and fire bases. Spraying was also used to destroy the crops of the Vietcong and North Vietnamese (Dux and Young, 1980).

Four major compounds were used in the Ranch Hand herbicide formulations—2,4-dichlorophenoxyacetic acid (2,4-D), 2,4,5-trichlorophenoxyacetic acid (2,4,5-T), picloram, and cacodylic acid. These compounds have been used worldwide for the control of weeds and unwanted vegetation, although the application of 2,4,5-T is no longer permitted in the United States following a series of Environmental Protection Agency directives in the 1970s.

Which of these four major chemicals (2,4-D, 2,4,5-T, picloram, or cacodylic acid) was chosen for a specific application depended on the desired effects. 2,4-D and 2,4,5-T are chlorinated phenoxy acids, and each is effective against a wide array of broadleaf plant species (Irish et al., 1969). They persist in soil only a few weeks (Buckingham, 1982). Picloram, like 2,4-D and 2,4,5-T, regulates plant growth. Compared to 2,4-D, picloram is more mobile and therefore better able to penetrate the plant's roots and be transported throughout plant tissues. Unlike the phenoxy herbicides, picloram is extremely persistent in soils. The fourth compound, cacodylic acid, contains an organic form of arsenic. Cacodylic acid is a desiccant, causing a plant's tissues to lose their moisture and eventually killing the plant.

The different types of herbicide used by U.S. forces in Vietnam were identified by a code name referring to the color of the band around the 55-gallon drum that contained the chemical. These included Agents Orange, White, Blue, Purple, Pink, and Green (see Table 5-1). From 1962 to 1965, small quantities of Agents Purple, Blue, Pink, and Green were used. From 1965 to 1970, Agents Orange, White, and Blue were employed; from 1970 to 1971, only Agents White and Blue were used in the defoliation program (Young and Reggiani, 1988).

Agent Purple was a 5:3:2 mixture of the n-butyl ester of 2,4-D and the n-butyl and isobutyl esters of 2,4,5-T that was used on broadleaf plants. Because of its volatility, Agent Purple was replaced by Agent Orange in 1965. Blue was the code designation for a liquid formulation of cacodylic acid and its sodium salt. The term Blue was first applied to cacodylic acid in a powder form that was mixed in the field with water. It was later replaced by the liquid formulation Phytar 560-G. Cacodylic acid is a highly soluble organic arsenic compound that is readily broken down in soil. Approximately one-half of all Agent Blue was used for crop destruction missions; it was the agent of choice for destruction of rice crops. The remainder was used in defoliation or sprayed around base perimeters, being delivered by helicopters or ground vehicles with sprayers attached to them (Young et al., 1978).

Agents Pink and Green were used in small quantities; however, official records of herbicide sprays during the early years of the program (1962–1964), when these two herbicides were used, are incomplete. Agent Green was a single-component formulation of the n-butyl ester of 2,4,5-T, used primarily in defoliation missions (Young et al., 1978).

In January 1965, two additional herbicides, code named Orange and White,

TABLE 5-1 Major Herbicides Used in Operation Ranch Hand: 1962–1971

Code Name	Formulation	Purpose	No. of Gallons Sprayed	Period of Use
Purple	2,4-D; 2,4,5-T	General defoliation	145,000	1962–1964
Blue (Phytar 560-G)	Cacodylic acid	Rapid defoliation, grassy plant control, rice destruction	1,124,307	1962–1971
Pink	2,4,5-T	Defoliation	122,792	1962–1964
Green	2,4,5-T	Crop destruction	8,208	1962–1964
Orange, Orange II	2,4-D; 2,4,5-T	General defoliation	11,261,429	1965–1970
White (Tordon 101)	2,4-D; picloram	Forest defoliation, long-term control	5,246,502	1965–1971

SOURCES: MRI, 1967; NAS, 1974; Young and Reggiani, 1988.

were introduced into the herbicide program. Agent Orange, a 1:1 mixture of 2,4-D and the *n*-butyl ester of 2,4,5-T, accounted for approximately 61 percent of the recorded herbicide use. Orange was the general-purpose herbicide for defoliation and crop destruction. According to military estimates of herbicide use, 90 percent of Agent Orange was used in Ranch Hand forest defoliation missions; 8 percent was used in Ranch Hand crop destruction missions; and 2 percent was sprayed from the ground around base perimeters and cache sites, waterways, and communication lines (NAS, 1974).

Orange II was introduced later in the program. It differed from the original Agent Orange in that the *n*-butyl ester of 2,4,5-T was replaced by the isooctyl ester; however, their herbicidal effects were similar. According to procurement records, less than 10 percent of the total Agent Orange used was Orange II (Craig, 1975).

White was the code name for Tordon 101, a liquid mixture of 2,4-D and picloram. More than 95 percent of Agent White was applied in defoliation missions (NAS, 1974; Young and Reggiani, 1988). Because of the persistence of Agent White in soil, it was not recommended for use on crops but was most often used in areas where longer persistence rather than immediate defoliation was desired, such as inland forests.

In addition to these four major compounds, Dinoxol, Trinoxol, and diquat were applied on native grasses and bamboo (Brown, 1962). Soil-applied herbicides were also reportedly used around base camp perimeters, minefields, ammunition storage areas, and other specialized sites requiring control of grasses and woody vegetation (Darrow et al., 1969). Additional accounts include the use of fungicides, insecticides, wetting agents, wood preservatives, insect repellents, and other herbicides (Gonzales, 1992). The number of military personnel potentially exposed to these chemicals is not available.

An undetermined amount of herbicides and insecticides was procured and distributed by Australian forces in Vietnam during 1966–1971. The use of these chemicals was confined largely to defoliation around base camps, improving security, and controlling mosquito-borne diseases. It appears that the chemicals were largely dispersed by use of ground delivery techniques, although low-volume aerial applications of insecticides, usually by helicopter, have been reported. The chemicals tested and used included 2,4-D, chlordane, DDT, diazinon, lindane, malathion, and picloram (Australian Senate Standing Committee, 1982).

The military use of 2,4,5-T, and thus Agent Orange, was suspended by the U.S. Department of Defense in April 1970 (Young and Reggiani, 1988). On February 12, 1971, U.S. Military Assistance Command, Vietnam, announced that herbicides would no longer be used for crop destruction in Vietnam, and the last Ranch Hand fixed-wing aircraft (C-123) was flown. Subsequent spraying of herbicides was limited to controlled use around U.S. fire bases by helicopter or ground troops (MACV, 1972). On October 31, 1971, nearly 10 years after the herbicide program began in Vietnam, the last U.S. helicopter herbicide operation was flown (NAS, 1974).

Ground Spraying of Herbicides

Although the number of U.S. military personnel exposed to herbicides is impossible to determine precisely, the majority of those assigned to Operation Ranch Hand can be presumed to have been exposed to Agent Orange and other herbicides. During the entire operation, approximately 1,250 military personnel served in Ranch Hand units. Although the Air Force maintained complete records of its Operation Ranch Hand fixed-wing herbicide missions, documentation of spraying conducted on the ground by boat, truck, or backpack and authorized at the unit level was less systematic. Authorization for herbicide missions by helicopter or surface spraying from river boats, trucks, and hand-operated backpacks was delegated to the Republic of Vietnam and U.S. authorities at the Corps level; these operations required only the approval of the unit commanders or senior advisors. "Free-spraying" areas, including the Demilitarized Zone (DMZ) at the seventeenth parallel and the first 100 meters outside base camps, were also exempt from Ranch Hand regulations (NAS, 1974). This delegation of authority for spraying to the Corps level reduced the lag time that existed from proposal to completion of small defoliation projects, for example, around depots, airfields, and outposts (Collins, 1967). However, because these helicopter and ground sprays were less rigidly controlled than fixed-wing aerial spraying, the recording of such sprays was not as systematic as those of Operation Ranch Hand.

The U.S. Army Chemical Corps, using hand equipment and H-34-type helicopters, conducted smaller spray operations, such as defoliation around Special Forces camps; clearance of perimeters surrounding airfields, depots, and other bases; and small-scale crop destruction (Warren, 1968; Thomas and Kang, 1990). Twenty-two Army Chemical Corps units were assigned to South Vietnam between 1966 and 1971. Approximately 950 veterans who served in the Army Chemical Corps in Vietnam between 1966 and 1971 have been identified from unit morning reports. Men serving in these units were trained in the preparation and application of chemicals, as well as in the cleaning and maintenance of spray equipment (Thomas and Kang, 1990).

Units and individuals other than members of the Air Force Ranch Hand and Army Chemical Corps were also likely to have handled or sprayed herbicides around bases or lines of communication. For example, Navy river patrols were reported to have used herbicides for clearance of inland waterways. Engineering personnel required the use of herbicides for removal of underbrush and dense growth in constructing fire support bases. It is estimated that 10 to 12 percent of the total volume of herbicides was dispensed from the ground by spraying from backpacks, boats, trucks, and buffalo turbines (NAS, 1974). The buffalo turbine was a trailer-mounted spray system used for roadside spraying and perimeter applications, which essentially "shot" the herbicide with a velocity up to 240 km/hour and a volume of 280 m^3/min (Young and Reggiani, 1988). Hand spray units consisted of a backpack type of dispenser with a capacity of 3 gallons (Collins, 1967).

Although some information is documented in military records, it is impossible to determine accurately from military records alone the extent of spraying conducted on the ground or the number of personnel involved in these operations with potential herbicide exposure. An unknown number of non-Ranch Hand personnel likely received various degrees of exposure to herbicides. Young and Reggiani (1988) report that the actual number "may be in the thousands since at least 100 helicopter spray equipment units were used in South Vietnam, and most military bases had vehicle-mounted and backpack spray units available for use in routine vegetation control programs." According to official documents, the "small-scale use of herbicides, for example around friendly base perimeters, were at the discretion of area commanders. Such uses seemed so obvious and so uncontroversial at the time that little thought was given to any detailed or permanent record of the uses or results" (U.S. Army, 1972).

The Department of Defense (DoD) took few precautions to prevent troop exposure to herbicides since they were considered to be a low health hazard. Precautions prescribed were consistent with those applied in the domestic use of herbicides existing before the Vietnam conflict (U.S. GAO, 1979). The Army added that exposure of ground troops was very unlikely since DoD personnel did not enter a Ranch Hand-sprayed area until approximately 4 to 6 weeks after the mission, when defoliation was complete and the herbicide had been biodegraded or photodegraded (U.S. Army, 1972). The restriction placed on troops entering a previously sprayed area was primarily for operational reasons, to prevent troops from being injured by the fighter aircraft that often accompanied the herbicide spraying aircraft (U.S. GAO, 1979).

A very different picture arose when the U.S. General Accounting Office (U.S. GAO, 1979) examined the military defoliation operation in the Con Thieu province of I Corps between January 1966 and December 1969. During this period, more than 2 million gallons of herbicides were sprayed in I Corps. By using average troop strength and turnover figures, an estimated 218,000 Marine infantry personnel were determined to have been assigned to I Corps during this period. By randomly selecting 276 of 976 Marine monthly battalion reports, the GAO tracked troop movement and compared troop locations to herbicide mission data. Nearly 26,000 U.S. Marines and Navy medical personnel were identified who entered within a radius of 2.5 km of the defoliated target areas within 1 day of spraying; 4,300 troops were identified as being within 0.5 km of the flight path; 11,700 were within 2.5 km within 4 weeks. In the Khe Sanh–Thon Son Lam area, an estimated 4,300–8,000 troops were within 0.5 km of the sprayed area within 1 day of spraying; within 28 days, 33,600–45,300 troops were determined to have been within 2.5 km of the defoliation target. Army records were found to lack sufficient information, so that the number of Army personnel close to sprayed areas could not be estimated. The GAO report concluded that "the chances that ground troops were exposed to herbicide Orange are higher than the DoD previously acknowledged . . . the group of personnel most likely to have been exposed could include ground troops as well as herbicide handlers and aircraft crew members" (U.S. GAO, 1979).

Level of Dioxin (TCDD) in Herbicides Used in Vietnam

2,3,7,8-Tetrachlorodibenzo-p-dioxin (2,3,7,8-TCDD, TCDD, or dioxin) is a contaminant of 2,4,5-T. Small quantities of other dioxins are present in 2,4-D. The levels of TCDD found in any given lot of 2,4,5-T depend on the manufacturing process (Young et al., 1976), and different manufacturers produced 2,4,5-T with various concentrations of TCDD. The primary source of 2,4,5-T in the herbicides used in Vietnam was Agent Orange.

Of all the herbicides used in South Vietnam, only Agent Orange was formulated differently from the materials for commercial application that were readily available in the United States (Young et al., 1978). TCDD concentrations in individual shipments were not recorded, and levels of TCDD varied in sampled inventories of herbicides containing 2,4,5-T. Analysis of the TCDD concentration in stocks of Agent Orange remaining after the conflict, which either had been returned from South Vietnam or had been procured but not shipped, ranged from less than 0.05 to almost 50 parts per million (ppm), averaging 1.98 and 2.99 ppm in two sets of samples (NAS, 1974; Young et al., 1978). Comparable manufacturing standards for the domestic use of 2,4,5-T in 1974 required that TCDD levels be less than 0.05 ppm (NAS, 1974). Therefore, depending on which stocks were sampled, the level of dioxin contamination in Agent Orange could have been up to 1,000 times higher than the level of dioxin found in phenoxy herbicides domestically available at the time.

Agents Green, Pink, and Purple, also contained 2,4,5-T and were used from 1962 through mid-1965. These 2,4,5-T formulations used early in the program (prior to 1965) contained 16 times the mean dioxin content of formulations used during 1965–1970 (Young et al., 1978). Analysis of archive samples of Agent Purple reported levels of TCDD as high as 45 ppm (Young, 1992). The mean concentration of TCDD in Agent Purple was estimated to be 32.8 ppm; the estimate for Agents Pink and Green was 65.6 ppm (Young et al., 1978). As a result of TCDD contamination in the herbicides, it has been estimated that about 368 pounds of dioxin was sprayed in Vietnam over a 6-year period (Gough, 1986).

EXPOSURE ASSESSMENT IN STUDIES OF VIETNAM VETERANS

Different approaches have been used to estimate the exposure of Vietnam veterans, including self-reported exposures, records-based exposure estimates, or biomarkers of TCDD exposure. Each approach is limited in its ability to determine precisely the degree of individual exposure. Some studies rely on gross markers such as service in Vietnam—perhaps enhanced by branch of service, military region, military specialty, or combat experience—as proxies for exposure to herbicides. Studies of this type include the Centers for Disease Control and Prevention's (CDC's) Vietnam Experience Study and Selected Cancers Study, the Department of Veterans Affairs' (DVA's) mortality studies, and most studies of veterans conducted by states. This approach almost surely dilutes whatever health effects of herbicides exist, because many members of the cohort presumed to be exposed to herbicides may, in reality, not have been.

Ranch Hands and Army Chemical Corps

Military occupation has been shown to be a valid exposure classification for two specific occupations that involved the direct handling and distribution of herbicides: the Air Force Ranch Hands, who were responsible for aerial spraying of herbicides, and the Army Chemical Corps, which performed ground and helicopter chemical operations. Biomarker studies of the Ranch Hands are consistent with their exposure to TCDD as a group. When the Ranch Hand cohort was further classified by military occupation, a general increase in serum TCDD levels was detected for jobs that involved more frequent handling of herbicides. The median TCDD level for enlisted ground crew (24 parts per trillion [ppt], range 0–618 ppt) was higher than the median level for enlisted flyers (18 ppt, range 0–196 ppt), and three times greater than the median level for officers (8 ppt, range 0–43 ppt) (AFHS, 1991).

The exposure index initially proposed in the Air Force Ranch Hand study relied upon military records of TCDD-containing herbicides (Agents Orange, Purple, Pink, and Green) sprayed as reported in the HERBS tapes for the period after July 1965 and on military procurement records and dissemination information for the period prior to July 1965. A TCDD weighting factor (based on the concentration of TCDD in the herbicide and the duration of spraying) was applied to the number of gallons of herbicides sprayed during each subject's tour of duty in Vietnam. The dates of each subject's tour(s) in Vietnam were determined by a manual review of military records. The HERBS tapes were used with quarterly operations reports to construct a table of gallons of TCDD-containing herbicides sprayed for each month during the Ranch Hand operation.

The exposure index for a Ranch Hand was defined as the product of the TCDD weighting factor and the number of gallons of TCDD herbicides sprayed during an individual's tour of duty, divided by the number of Ranch Hands sharing such duties during this individual's tour. Each Ranch Hand was placed in an exposure category (high, medium, or low) based on the value of the individual's exposure index. The index included exposure from recorded Ranch Hand sprays only—the measure did not allow for other unrecorded herbicide exposures, such as chemical dumps or perimeter sprays, or other non-Ranch Hand herbicide applications. In 1991, the exposure index was compared to the results of the Ranch Hand serum TCDD analysis. The exposure index and the TCDD body burden were weakly correlated.

Michalek et al. (1995) developed several indices of herbicide exposure for members of the Ranch Hand cohort and tried to relate these to the levels of serum TCDD measured between 1987 and 1992. Self-administered questionnaires completed by veterans of Operation Ranch Hand were used to develop three indices for herbicide or TCDD exposure: (1) the number of days of skin exposure; (2) the percentage of skin area exposed; and (3) the number of days of skin exposure, times the percentage of skin exposed, times a factor for the concentration of TCDD in the herbicide. A fourth index used no information gathered from individual subjects. It was calculated as the volume of herbicide sprayed during a specific individual's tour of duty, times the concentration of TCDD in herbicides sprayed in that period, divided by the number of crew members at that time in each job specialty.

Each of the four models tested was significantly related to the serum TCDD level, although each explained only between 19 and 27 percent of the variability in serum TCDD. Days of skin exposure had the highest correlation. Military job classification (non-Ranch Hand combat troops, Ranch Hand administrators, Ranch Hand flight engineers, and Ranch Hand ground crew), which is separate from the four indices, explained 60 percent of the variance in serum TCDD concentrations. When the questionnaire-derived indices were applied within each job classification, days of skin exposure added significantly, but not substantially, to the variability explained by job alone.

Other Vietnam Veterans

Surveys of Vietnam veterans who were not part of the Ranch Hands or Chemical Corps groups indicate that 25 to 55 percent believe they were exposed to herbicides (Erickson et al., 1984a,b; Stellman and Stellman, 1986; CDC, 1989). A few attempts have been made to estimate exposures of the Vietnam veterans who were not part of the Ranch Hand or Chemical Corps groups. The CDC was involved in two such studies: the CDC Agent Orange Study (CDC, 1985) and the CDC Birth Defects Study which developed an exposure opportunity index (EOI) to score Agent Orange exposures (Erickson et al., 1984a,b).

As part of a case-control study to determine if there was an increased risk of birth defects among the offspring of Vietnam veterans, an Agent Orange exposure assessment was done (Erickson et al., 1984a,b). The potential for an individual Vietnam veteran's exposure to Agent Orange ("exposure opportunity") was estimated by military records specialists of the Army Agent Orange Task Force without knowledge of case or control status. The EOI scores ranged from a value of 1 (minimum opportunities for exposure) to a value of 5 (most numerous opportunities for exposure). Higher values signify a greater likelihood of exposure but do not necessarily indicate a higher degree (duration or intensity) of exposure.

All individual veterans were given two index scores: one was derived from self-reported information on dates and location of service, and military duties, obtained during the interview; the second was developed based on a review of military records. The records-based EOI used unit location data determined from the Operational Report Lessons Learned. The proximity of these general unit locations was compared to Agent Orange and other herbicide spray data by using the HERBS tapes and other data available on base perimeter sprays to construct the index scores.

Approximately 25 percent of interviewed Vietnam veterans reported that they had been exposed to Agent Orange. Fifty-two percent received the same score in both the index score and the self-reported Agent Orange exposure. A higher proportion of subjects who thought they had been exposed received 4 or 5 on the military records index score than did subjects who thought they had not been exposed.

In 1983, the CDC was assigned by the U.S. government to conduct a study of the possible long-term health effects of Vietnam veterans' exposures to Agent Orange. The Agent Orange Study attempted to classify veterans' exposure to herbicides that occurred during military service. This was to be accomplished by determining the proximity of troops to Agent Orange spraying using military records to track troop movement and the HERBS tapes to locate herbicide spraying patterns. The original study was to involve three cohorts, each containing approximately 8,500 men.

The DoD Environmental Services Group assisted CDC in the abstraction of military records on troop locations. According to the CDC protocol, 65 battalions were to be selected from III Corps. Herbicide exposure "scores" were calculated at the company level (about 250 men), based on a reported unit location occurring within a specified time and distance from a known herbicide application. Three exposure scores were proposed—short, intermediate, and chronic—to estimate an individual's likelihood of exposure. These scores attempted to account for variations in TCDD half-life, dispersion of herbicides, error in the calculated distances from spray lines, and uncertainties regarding the time between spraying and possible exposure, as well as whether the exposure could be viewed as acute, chronic, or intermediate. The CDC initially concluded that "many veterans were in close enough proximity to applications of Agent Orange to be classified as highly likely to have been exposed to the herbicide" and that there was substantial variability in exposure scores among units and among individual veterans (CDC, 1985).

To test the validity of several indirect methods for estimating exposure of ground troops to Agent Orange in Vietnam, in 1987 the CDC Agent Orange Validation Study measured serum TCDD levels in a nonrandom sample of Vietnam veterans and Vietnam era veterans who did not serve in Vietnam (CDC,

1988b). Vietnam veterans were selected for further study based on their estimated number of Agent Orange hits, derived from the number of days for which at least one company location was within 2 km and 6 days of a recorded Agent Orange spray: the "low-" exposure group included 298 veterans, the "medium-" exposure group included 157 veterans, and the "high-" exposure group included 191 veterans. Blood samples were obtained from 66 percent of Vietnam veterans ($N = 646$) and 49 percent of the eligible comparison group of veterans ($N = 97$). More than 94 percent of those whose serum was obtained had served in one of five battalions.

Five indirect exposure scores based on military records and two scores based on self-reports were used to rank veterans according to their likelihood of exposure to Agent Orange. The five indirect scores incorporated a variety of assumptions concerning possible sources of TCDD exposure, the estimated half-life of TCDD in the environment, and the completeness of data on troop and spray location. Two Agent Orange exposure scores were calculated based on proximity to recorded Agent Orange sprays. Two similar scores were computed for recorded sprays of "unknown" agents. The fifth score, an area score, depended less on precise military unit location data than the other four scores. It was computed based on the number of days a company was in one of five heavily sprayed areas in III Corps during 1967 and 1968. Two self-assessed exposure scores were determined based on the number of days an individual reported direct and indirect exposure to herbicides during military service (CDC, 1988b).

The median TCDD level in Vietnam veterans was 4 ppt, with a range of less than 1 to 45 ppt and two veterans having levels greater than 20 ppt; the distributions of these measurements were nearly identical to those for the control group of 97 non-Vietnam veterans. In other words, the CDC's Validation Study found that study subjects could not be distinguished from controls based on serum TCDD levels. In addition, none of the records-derived estimates of exposure and neither type of self-reported exposure to herbicides identified Vietnam veterans who were likely to have currently elevated serum TCDD levels (CDC, 1988b). The study concluded it is unlikely that military records can be used to identify a large number of U.S. Army veterans who might have been heavily exposed to TCDD in Vietnam.

In addition, these serum TCDD levels in Vietnam veterans suggest that the exposure to TCDD in Vietnam was substantially less, *on average*, than that of occupationally exposed workers; of persons exposed as a result of the industrial explosion in Seveso, Italy; or of the heavily exposed occupational workers that are the focus of many of the studies evaluated by the committee. As noted above, this estimation of *average* exposure does not preclude the existence of a heavily exposed subgroup of Vietnam veterans.

In 1997, a committee convened by the Institute of Medicine developed a Request for Proposals (RFP) seeking individuals and organizations capable of conducting research to develop one or more historic exposure reconstruction approaches suitable for epidemiologic studies of herbicide exposure among U.S. veterans during the Vietnam war (IOM, 1997). These approaches were to incorporate information from, for example, existing data bases, biomarker data, and supplemental material gathered from surveys of military personnel, governmental and nongovernmental organizations, and other sources. Work funded under this RFP began in 1998 and was still under way at the end of 2000.

REFERENCES

AFHS (Air Force Health Study). 1991. An Epidemiologic Investigation of Health Effects in Air Force Personnel Following Exposure to Herbicides. Serum Dioxin Analysis of 1987 Examination Results. Brooks AFB, TX: USAF School of Aerospace Medicine. 9 vols.

Andrews JS Jr, Garrett WA Jr, Patterson DG Jr, Needham LL, Roberts DW, Bagby JR, Anderson JE, Hoffman RE, Schramm W. 1989. 2,3,7,8-Tetrachlorodibenzo-*p*-dioxin levels in adipose tissue of persons with no known exposure and in exposure persons. Chemosphere 18:499–506.

Australian Senate Standing Committee on Science and the Environment. 1982. Pesticides and the Health of Australian Vietnam Veterans. First report. 240 pp.

Becher H, Flesch-Janys D, Kauppinen T, Kogevinas M, Steindorf K, Manz A, Wahrendorf J. 1996. Cancer mortality in German male workers exposed to phenoxy herbicides and dioxins. Cancer Causes and Control 7(3):312–321.

Bertazzi PA, Zocchetti C, Pesatori AC, Guercilena S, Sanarico M, Radice L. 1989. Ten-year mortality study of the population involved in the Seveso incident in 1976. American Journal of Epidemiology 129:1187–1200.

Bertazzi PA, Bernucci I, Brambilla G, Consonni D, Pesatori AC. 1998. The Seveso studies on early and long-term effects of dioxin exposure: a review. Environmental Health Perspectives 106(Suppl 2): 625–633.

Bertazzi PA, Consonni D, Bachetti S, Rubagotti M, Baccarelli A, Zocchetti C, Pesatori AC. 2001. Health effects of dioxin exposure: a 20-year mortality study. American Journal of Epidemiology 153(11):1031-1044.

Blair A, White DW. 1985. Leukemia cell types and agricultural practices in Nebraska. Archives of Environmental Health 40:211–214.

Blair A, Grauman DJ, Lubin JH, Fraumeni JF Jr. 1983. Lung cancer and other causes of death among licensed pesticide applicators. Journal of the National Cancer Institute 71:31–37.

Brown JW. 1962. Vegetational Spray Test in South Vietnam. Fort Detrick, MD: U.S. Army Chemical Corps Biological Laboratories. DDC Number AD 476961. 119 pp.

Buckingham WA. 1982. Operation Ranch Hand: The Air Force and Herbicides in Southeast Asia 1961–1971. Washington, DC: U.S. Air Force Office of Air Force History.

Bueno de Mesquita HB, Doornbos G, van der Kuip DA, Kogevinas M, Winkelmann R. 1993. Occupational exposure to phenoxy herbicides and chlorophenols and cancer mortality in the Netherlands. American Journal of Industrial Medicine 23:289–300.

Burmeister LF. 1981. Cancer mortality in Iowa farmers: 1971–1978. Journal of the National Cancer Institute 66:461–464.

Cantor KP. 1982. Farming and mortality from non-Hodgkin's lymphoma: a case-control study. International Journal of Cancer 29:239–247.

Carmelli D, Hofherr L, Tomsic J, Morgan RW. 1981. A Case-Control Study of the Relationship Between Exposure to 2,4-D and Spontaneous Abortions in Humans. SRI International. Prepared for the National Forest Products Association and the U.S. Department of Agriculture, Forest Service.

CDC (Centers for Disease Control). 1985. Agent Orange Projects Interim Report Number 2: Exposure Assessment for the Agent Orange Study. Atlanta: CDC, Center for Environmental Health, Division of Chronic Disease Control, Agent Orange Projects.

CDC. 1988a. Preliminary report: 2,3,7,8-tetrachlorodibenzo-p-dioxin exposure in humans-Seveso, Italy. Morbidity and Mortality Weekly Report 37:733–736.

CDC. 1988b. Serum 2,3,7,8-tetrachlorodibenzo-p-dioxin levels in U.S. Army Vietnam era veterans. Journal of the American Medical Association 260:1249–1254.

CDC. 1989. Health Status of Vietnam Veterans. Vietnam Experience Study. Atlanta: U.S. Department of Health and Human Services. Vols. I–V, Supplements A–C.

Coggon D, Pannett B, Winter PD, Acheson ED, Bonsall J. 1986. Mortality of workers exposed to 2 methyl-4 chlorophenoxyacetic acid. Scandinavian Journal of Work, Environment, and Health 12:448–454.

Coggon D, Pannett B, Winter P. 1991. Mortality and incidence of cancer at four factories making phenoxy herbicides. British Journal of Industrial Medicine 48:173–178.

Collins CV. 1967. Herbicide Operations in Southeast Asia, July 1961–June 1967. San Francisco: Headquarters, Pacific Air Forces. NTIS AD-779-796.

Constable JD, Hatch MC. 1985. Reproductive effects of herbicide exposure in Vietnam: recent studies by the Vietnamese and others. Teratogenesis, Carcinogenesis, and Mutagenesis 5:231–250.

Cook RR, Bond GG, Olson RA. 1986. Evaluation of the mortality experience of workers exposed to the chlorinated dioxins. Chemosphere 15:1769–1776.

Craig DA. 1975. Use of Herbicides in Southeast Asia. Historical Report. Kelly AFB, TX: San Antonio Logistics Center, Directorate of Energy Management. 58 pp.

Dai LC, Phuong NTN, Thom LH, Thuy TT, Van NTT, Cam LH, Chi HTK, Thuy LB. 1990. A comparison of infant mortality rates between two Vietnamese villages sprayed by defoliants in wartime and one unsprayed village. Chemosphere 20:1005–1012.

Darrow RA, Irish KR, Minarik CD. 1969. Herbicides Used in Southeast Asia. Kelly AFB, TX. Technical Report SAOQ-TR-69-11078. 60 pp.

Dux J, Young PJ. 1980. Agent Orange: The Bitter Harvest. Sydney: Hodder and Stoughton.

Erickson JD, Mulinare J, Mcclain PW. 1984a. Vietnam veterans' risks for fathering babies with birth defects. Journal of the American Medical Association 252:903–912.

Erickson JD, Mulinare J, Mcclain PW, Fitch TG, James LM, McClearn AB, Adams MJ. 1984b. Vietnam Veterans' Risks for Fathering Babies with Birth Defects. Atlanta: U.S. Department of Health and Human Services, Centers for Disease Control.

Ferry DG, Gazeley LR, Edwards IR. 1982. 2,4,5-T absorption in chemical applicators. Proceedings of the University Otago Medical School 60:31–34.

Fingerhut MA, Halperin WE, Marlow DA, Piacitelli LA, Honchar PA, Sweeney MH, Greife AL, Dill PA, Steenland K, Suruda AJ. 1991. Cancer mortality in workers exposed to 2,3,7,8-tetrachlorodibenzo-p-dioxin. New England Journal of Medicine 324:212–218.

Flesch-Janys D, Berger J, Gurn P, Manz A, Nagel S, Waltsgott H, Dwyer. 1995. Exposure to polychlorinated dioxins and furans (PCDD/F) and mortality in a cohort of workers from a herbicide-producing plant in Hamburg, Federal Republic of Germany. American Journal of Epidemiology 142:1165–1175.

Frank R, Campbell RA, Sirons GJ. 1985. Forestry workers involved in aerial application of 2,4-dichlorophenoxyacetic acid (2,4-D): exposure and urinary excretion. Archives of Environmental Contamination and Toxicology 14:427–435.

Gonzales J. 1992. List of Chemicals Used in Vietnam. Presented to the Institute of Medicine Committee to Review the Health Effects in Vietnam Veterans of Exposure to Herbicides. Illinois Agent Orange Committee, Vietnam Veterans of America.

Gordon JE, Shy CM. 1981. Agricultural chemical use and congenital cleft lip and/or palate. Archives of Environmental Health 36:213–221.

Gough M. 1986. Dioxin, Agent Orange: The Facts. New York: Plenum Press.

Hansen ES, Hasle H, Lander F. 1992. A cohort study on cancer incidence among Danish gardeners. American Journal of Industrial Medicine 21:651–660.

Henneberger PK, Ferris BG Jr, Monson RR. 1989. Mortality among pulp and paper workers in Berlin, New Hampshire. British Journal of Industrial Medicine 46:658–664.

Hertzman C, Teschke K, Ostry A, Hershler R, Dimich-Ward H, Kelly S, Spinelli JJ, Gallagher RP, McBride M, Marion SA. 1997. Mortality and cancer incidence among sawmill workers exposed to chlorophenate wood preservatives. American Journal of Public Health 87(1):71–79.

Hoar SK, Blair A, Holmes FF, Boysen CD, Robel RJ, Hoover R, Fraumeni JF. 1986. Agricultural herbicide use and risk of lymphoma and soft-tissue sarcoma. Journal of the American Medical Association 256:1141–1147.

Hoffman RE, Stehr-Green PA, Webb KB, Evans RG, Knutsen AP, Schramm WF, Staake JL, Gibson BB, Steinberg KK. 1986. Health effects of long-term exposure to 2,3,7,8-tetrachlorodibenzo-p-dioxin. Journal of the American Medical Association 255:2031–2038.

Hooiveld M, Heederik DJ, Kogevinas M, Boffetta P, Needham LL, Patterson DG Jr, Bueno de Mesquita HB. 1998. Second follow-up of a Dutch cohort occupationally exposed to phenoxy herbicides, chlorophenols, and contaminants. American Journal of Epidemiology 147(9):891–901.

IOM (Institute of Medicine). 1994. Veterans and Agent Orange Health Effects of Herbicides Used in Vietnam. Washington, DC: National Academy Press.

IOM. 1996. Veterans and Agent Orange: Update 1996. Washington, DC: National Academy Press.

IOM. 1997. Characterizing Exposure of Veterans to Agent Orange and Other Herbicides Used in Vietnam: Scientific Considerations Regarding a Request for Proposals for Research. Washington, DC: National Academy Press.

IOM. 1999. Veterans and Agent Orange: Update 1998. Washington, DC: National Academy Press.

Irish KR, Darrow RA, Minarik CE. 1969. Information Manual for Vegetation Control in Southeast Asia. Misc. Publication 33. Fort Detrick, MD: Department of the Army, Plant Sciences Laboratories, Plant Physiology Division. NTIS AD-864-443.

Jappinen P, Pukkala E. 1991. Cancer incidence among pulp and paper workers exposed to organic chlorinated compounds formed during chlorine pulp bleaching. Scandinavian Journal of Work, Environment, and Health 17:356–359.

Kolmodin-Hedman B, Erne K. 1980. Estimation of occupational exposure to phenoxy acids (2,4-D and 2,4,5-T). Archives of Toxicology Supplement 4:318–321.

Kolmodin-Hedman B, Hoglund S, Akerblom M. 1983. Studies on phenoxy acid herbicides. I. Field study. Occupational exposure to phenoxy acid herbicides (MCPA, dichlorprop, mecoprop and 2,4-D) in agriculture. Archives of Toxicology 54:257–265.

Lavy TL, Shepard JS, Mattice JD. 1980a. Exposure measurements of applicators spraying (2,4,5-trichlorophenoxy)acetic acid in the forest. Journal of Agricultural and Food Chemistry 28:626–630.

Lavy TL, Shepard JS, Bouchard DC. 1980b. Field worker exposure and helicopter spray pattern of 2,4,5-T. Bulletin of Environmental Contamination and Toxicology 24:90–96.

Libich S, To JC, Frank R, Sirons GJ. 1984. Occupational exposure of herbicide applicators to herbicides used along electric power transmission line right-of-way. American Industrial Hygiene Association Journal 45:56–62.

MACV (Military Assistance Command, Vietnam), Military History Branch. 1972. Chronology of Events Pertaining to U.S. Involvement in the War in Vietnam and Southeast Asia.

Manz A, Berger J, Dwyer JH, Flesch-Janys D, Nagel S, Waltsgott H. 1991. Cancer mortality among workers in chemical plant contaminated with dioxin. Lancet 338:959–964.

Michalek JE, Wolfe WH, Miner JC, Papa TM, Pirkle JL. 1995. Indices of TCDD exposure and TCDD body burden in veterans of Operation Ranch Hand. Journal of Exposure Analysis and Environmental Epidemiology 5(2):209–223.

MRI (Midwest Research Institute). 1967. Assessment of Ecological Effects of Extensive or Repeated Use of Herbicides. MRI Project No. 3103-B. Kansas City, MO: MRI. NTIS AD-824–314.

Mocarelli P, Patterson DG Jr, Marocchi A, Needham LL. 1990. Pilot study (phase II) for determining polychlorinated dibenzo-p-dioxin (PCDD) and polychlorinated dibenzofuran (PCDF) levels in serum of Seveso, Italy residents collected at the time of exposure: future plans. Chemosphere 20:967–974.

Mocarelli P, Needham LL, Marocchi A, Patterson DG Jr, Brambilla P, Gerthoux PM, Meazza L, Carreri V. 1991. Serum concentrations of 2,3,7,8-tetrachlorobdibenzo-p-dioxin and test results from selected residents of Seveso, Italy. Journal of Toxicology and Environmental Health 32:357–366.

Morrison HI, Semenci RM, Morison D, Magwood S, Mao Y. 1992. Brain cancer and farming in western Canada. Neuroepidemiology 11: 267–276.

Musicco M, Sant M, Molinari S, Filippini G, Gatta G, Berrino F. 1988. A case-control study of brain gliomas and occupational exposure to chemical carcinogens: the risks to farmers. American Journal of Epidemiology 128:778–785.

NAS (National Academy of Sciences), National Research Council, Assembly of Life Sciences. 1974. The Effects of Herbicides in South Vietnam. Washington, DC: National Academy Press.

Ott MG, Holder BB, Olson RD. 1980. A mortality analysis of employees engaged in the manufacture of 2,4,5-trichlorophenoxyacetic acid. Journal of Occupational Medicine 22:47–50.

Patterson DG Jr, Hoffman RE, Needham LL, Roberts DW, Bagby JR, Pirkle JL, Falk H, Sampson EJ, Houk VN. 1986. 2,3,7,8-tetrachlorodibenzo-p-dioxin levels in adipose tissue of exposed and control persons in Missouri. An interim report. Journal of the American Medical Association 256:2683–2686.

Rix BA, Villadsen E, Engholm G, Lynge E. 1998. Hodgkin's disease, pharyngeal cancer, and soft tissue sarcomas in Danish paper mill workers. Journal of Occupational and Environmental Medicine 40(1):55–62.

Robinson CF, Waxweiler RJ, Fowler DP. 1986. Mortality among production workers in pulp and paper mills. Scandinavian Journal of Work, Environment, and Health 12:552–560.

Ronco G, Costa G, Lynge E. 1992. Cancer risk among Danish and Italian farmers. British Journal of Industrial Medicine 49:220–225.

Saracci R, Kogevinas M, Bertazzi PA, Bueno De Mesquita BH, Coggon D, Green LM, Kauppinen T, L'Abbe KA, Littorin M, Lynge E, Mathews JD, Neuberger M, Osman J, Pearce N, Winkelmann R. 1991. Cancer mortality in workers exposed to chlorophenoxy herbicides and chlorophenols. Lancet 338:1027–1032.

Schecter A, Ryan JJ, Constable JD. 1986. Chlorinated dibenzo-p-dioxin and dibenzofuran levels in human adipose tissue and milk samples from the north and south of Vietnam. Chemosphere 15:1613–1620.

Smith AH, Matheson DP, Fisher DO, Chapman CJ. 1981. Preliminary report of reproductive outcomes among pesticide applicators using 2,4,5-T. New Zealand Medical Journal 93:177–179.

Smith AH, Fisher DO, Pearce N, Chapman CJ. 1982. Congenital defects and miscarriages among New Zealand 2,4,5-T sprayers. Archives of Environmental Health 37:197–200.

Smith AH, Patterson DG Jr, Warner ML, Mackenzie R, Needham LL. 1992. Serum 2,3,7,8-tetrachlorodibenzo-p-dioxin levels of New Zealand pesticide applicators and their implication for cancer hypotheses. Journal of the National Cancer Institute 84:104–108.

Solet D, Zoloth SR, Sullivan C, Jewett J, Michaels DM. 1989. Patterns of mortality in pulp and paper workers. Journal of Occupational Medicine 31:627–630.

Steenland K, Piacitelli L, Deddens J, Fingerhut M, Chang LI. 1999. Cancer, heart disease, and diabetes in workers exposed to 2,3,7,8-tetrachlorodibenzo-p-dioxin. Journal of the National Cancer Institute 91(9):779–786.

Stellman SD, Stellman JM. 1986. Estimation of exposure to Agent Orange and other defoliants among American troops in Vietnam: a methodological approach. American Journal of Industrial Medicine 9:305–321.

Swaen GMH, van Vliet C, Slangen JJM, Sturmans F. 1992. Cancer mortality among licensed herbicide applicators. Scandinavian Journal of Work, Environment, and Health 18:201–204.

Teschke K, Hertzman C, Morrison B. 1994. Level and distribution of employee exposures to total and respirable wood dust in two Canadian sawmills. American Industrial Hygiene Association Journal 55(3):245–250.

Thomas TL, Kang HK. 1990. Mortality and morbidity among Army Chemical Corps Vietnam veterans: a preliminary report. American Journal of Industrial Medicine 18:665–673.

U.S. Army. 1972. Herbicides and Military Operations. Vols. I and II. Washington, DC: Department of the Army, Engineer Strategic Studies Group, Office, Chief of Engineers.

U.S. GAO (U.S. General Accounting Office). 1979. U.S. Ground Troops in South Vietnam Were in Areas Sprayed with Herbicide Orange. Report by the Comptroller General of the United States, FPCD 80 23. Washington, DC: GAO.

Viel JF, Arveux P, Baverel J, Cahn JY. 2000. Soft-tissue sarcoma and non-Hodgkin's lymphoma clusters around a municipal solid waste incinerator with high dioxin emission levels. American Journal of Epidemiology 152(1):13–19.

Vineis P, Terracini B, Ciccone G, Cignetti A, Colombo E, Donna A, Maffi L, Pisa R, Ricci P, Zanini E, Comba P. 1986. Phenoxy herbicides and soft-tissue sarcomas in female rice weeders. A population-based case-referent study. Scandinavian Journal of Work, Environment, and Health 13:9–17.

Warren WF. 1968. A Review of the Herbicide Program in South Vietnam. San Francisco: Scientific Advisory Group. Working Paper No. 10-68. NTIS AD-779–797.

Wigle DT, Semenciw RB, Wilkins K, Riedel D, Ritter L, Morrison HI, Mao Y. 1990. Mortality study of Canadian male farm operators: non-Hodgkin's lymphoma mortality and agricultural practices in Saskatchewan. Journal of the National Cancer Institute 82:575–582.

Wiklund K, Holm LE. 1986. Soft tissue sarcoma risk in Swedish agricultural and forestry workers. Journal of the National Cancer Institute 76:229–234.

Wiklund K, Lindefors BM, Holm LE. 1988a. Risk of malignant lymphoma in Swedish agricultural and forestry workers. British Journal of Industrial Medicine 45:19–24.

Wiklund K, Dich J, Holm LE. 1988b. Soft tissue sarcoma risk in Swedish licensed pesticide applicators. Journal of Occupational Medicine 30:801–804.

Wiklund K, Dich J, Holm LE. 1989. Risk of soft tissue sarcoma, Hodgkin's disease and non-Hodgkin lymphoma among Swedish licensed pesticide applicators. Chemosphere 18:395–400.

Woods JS, Polissar L. 1989. Non-Hodgkin's lymphoma among phenoxy herbicide-exposed farm workers in western Washington State. Chemosphere 18:401–406.

Young AL. 1992. The Military Use of Herbicides in Vietnam. Presentation to the Institute of Medicine Committee to Review the Health Effects in Vietnam Veterans of Exposure to Herbicides. December 8, 1992. Washington, DC.

Young AL, Reggiani GM, eds. 1988. Agent Orange and Its Associated Dioxin: Assessment of a Controversy. Amsterdam: Elsevier.

Young AL, Thalken CE, Arnold EL, Cupello JM, Cockerham LG. 1976. Fate of 2,3,7,8-Tetrachlorodibenzo-p-dioxin (TCDD) in the Environment: Summary and Decontamination Recommendations. Colorado Springs: U.S. Air Force Academy. USAFA TR 76 18.

Young AL, Calcagni JA, Thalken CE, Tremblay JW. 1978. The Toxicology, Environmental Fate, and Human Risk of Herbicide Orange and Its Associated Dioxin. Brooks AFB, TX: Air Force Occupational and Environmental Health Lab. USAF OEHL TR 78 92.

Zack JA, Gaffey WR. 1983. A mortality study of workers employed at the Monsanto company plant in Nitro, West Virginia. Environmental Science Research 26:575–591.

Zahm SH, Weisenburger DD, Babbitt PA, Saal RC, Vaught JB, Cantor KP, Blair A. 1990. A case-control study of non-Hodgkin's lymphoma and the herbicide 2,4-dichlorophenoxyacetic acid (2,4-D) in eastern Nebraska. Epidemiology 1:349–356.

Zober A, Messerer P, Huber P. 1990. Thirty-four-year mortality follow up of BASF employees exposed to 2,3,7,8-TCDD after the 1953 accident. International Archives of Occupational and Environmental Health 62:139–157.

6

Epidemiologic Studies

In seeking evidence for associations between health outcomes and exposure to herbicides and TCDD (2,3,7,8-tetrachlorodibenzo-p-dioxin), many different kinds of epidemiologic studies must be considered. Each study type has varying degrees of strengths and weaknesses and contributes evidence to an association with the health outcomes considered in Chapters 7–10. The three main groups of individuals studied with respect to herbicide exposure are those with occupational, environmental, and military exposures. The committee highly values studies of Vietnam veterans, but does not consider either the presence or absence of a particular health effect in a study of veterans to be definitive. The committee believes that a broad based evaluation meets its charge under P.L.102–4 to "determine, to the extent that available data permitted meaningful determinations … whether a statistical association with herbicide exposure exists."

A detailed description of the groups studied was examined in Chapter 2 of *Veterans and Agent Orange* (hereafter referred to as *VAO)* (IOM, 1994). A discussion of the criteria for inclusion in the review is detailed in Appendix A of *VAO.*

This chapter summarizes the epidemiologic studies and reports reviewed by the committee. Included are new studies published after *Veterans and Agent Orange: Update 1998* (hereafter, *Update 1998*) (IOM, 1999), studies that were not reviewed by the committees that wrote the prior reports, and studies that have been updated since publication of *Update 1998*. Tables 6-1, 6-2, and 6-3 (which begin on page 182) provide a brief overview of the epidemiologic studies reviewed in both the prior reports and this document. The summaries include the study method used and, if available, how the study subjects were selected; how the data were collected; the inclusion criteria; and how exposure was determined. The tables also list the numbers of subjects in the study and comparison populations, and provide a brief description of the study. No studies are evaluated in this chapter; rather, a methodologic framework is provided for the health outcome chapters that follow. Qualitative critique of the study design, population size, methods of data collection, case and control ascertainment, or quality of exposure assessment has been reserved for the individual health outcome chapters in which the results of these studies are discussed.

The text and tables in this chapter are organized into three basic sections—occupational studies, environmental studies, and studies of Vietnam veterans—with subsections included under each heading. The studies address exposures to 2,4-D (2,4-dichlorophenoxyacetic acid); 2,4,5-T (2,4,5-trichlorophenoxyacetic acid) and its contaminant TCDD; cacodylic acid; and picloram. In some cases, the committee examined studies addressing compounds chemically related to the herbicides used in Vietnam, such as 2-methyl-4-chlorophenoxyacetic acid (MCPA), hexachlorophene, and chlorophenols, including trichlorophenol. In other instances, investigators did not indicate specific herbicides to which study participants were exposed or the level of exposure. These complicating factors were considered when the committee weighed the relevance of a study to its findings. Where available, details are given with regard to exposure assessment and how exposure was subsequently used in the analysis.

The occupational section includes studies of production workers, agricultural and forestry workers (including herbicide and pesticide appliers), and paper and pulp workers, as well as case-control studies of specific cancers and the association with exposures to herbicides or related compounds. The environmental section includes studies of populations accidentally exposed to unusual levels of herbicides or dioxins as a result of the location in which they live, for example, the residents of Seveso, Italy; Times Beach, Missouri; and the southern portion of Vietnam. The section on Vietnam veterans includes studies conducted in the United States by the Air Force; the Centers for Disease Control and Prevention (CDC), the Department of Veterans Affairs (DVA, formerly the Veterans Administration [VA]); the American Legion; and the State of Michigan, as well as other groups. Studies of Australian Vietnam veterans are also presented there.

Many cohorts potentially exposed to dioxin and the herbicides used in Vietnam are monitored on an ongoing basis. Studies of the groups that are assessed regularly include the National Institute for Occupational Safety and Health (NIOSH), International Agency for Research on Cancer (IARC), National Cancer Institute (NCI), Seveso, and Ranch Hand cohorts. Typically, the risks between exposure to herbicides and specific health outcomes are updated every 3 to 5 years. For example, the health of the Ranch Hand cohort was assessed in 1982, 1987, 1992, and 1997. *For such studies, the committee has chosen to focus on the most recent update, when multiple reports on the same cohort are available.* For the sake of thoroughness, the discussion of specific health outcomes in Chapters 7–10 includes reference to all studies, including those subsumed by the most recent update.

Similarly, researchers investigating the constituent cohorts used in some large multicenter studies may publish reports based solely on the individuals they monitor. Examples include the IARC and NCI cohort studies. *The committee has chosen to focus on the studies of the larger multicenter cohorts.* However, for the sake of thoroughness, Chapters 7–10 reference all of these studies, including those subsumed by the larger multicenter cohorts.

OCCUPATIONAL STUDIES

Several occupational groups in the United States and elsewhere have been exposed to the types of herbicides used in Vietnam and, more specifically, to TCDD, a contaminant of some herbicides and other products. Occupational groups exposed to these chemicals include farmers, agricultural and forestry workers, herbicide sprayers, workers in chemical production plants, and workers involved in paper and pulp manufacturing. In addition, studies that use job titles as broad surrogates of exposure and studies that rely on disease registry data have been conducted. Exposure characterization varies widely in these studies in terms of measurement, quantification, level of detail, confounding by other exposures, and individual versus surrogate or group (ecological) measures.

Production Workers

National Institute for Occupational Safety and Health

In 1978, NIOSH began a study to identify all U.S. workers potentially exposed to TCDD between 1942 and 1984 (Fingerhut et al., 1991). In a total of 12 chemical companies, 5,132 workers were identified from personnel and payroll records as having been involved in production or maintenance processes associated with TCDD contamination. Their possible exposure resulted from working with certain chemicals in which TCDD was a contaminant, including 2,4,5-trichlorophenol (TCP) and 2,4,5-T, Silvex, Erbon, Ronnel, and hexachlorophene. An additional 172 workers identified previously by their employers as being exposed to TCDD were also included in the study cohort. The 12 plants involved were large manufacturing sites of major chemical companies. Thus, many of the study subjects were potentially exposed to many other chemicals, some of which could be carcinogenic.

Prior to the publication of the cohort study, NIOSH conducted a cross-sectional study that included a comprehensive medical history, medical examination, and measurement of pulmonary function of workers employed in the manufacture of chemicals with TCDD contamination at two of the plants in the full cohort. These included workers at two chemical plants in Newark, New Jersey, from 1951 to 1969, and in Verona, Missouri, from 1968 to 1969 and from 1970 to 1972 (Sweeney et al., 1989, 1993; Calvert et al., 1991, 1992; Alderfer et al., 1992). The plant in New Jersey manufactured TCP and 2,4,5-T; the Missouri plant manufactured TCP, 2,4,5-T, and hexachlorophene. A number of studies were later conducted that looked at specific health outcomes among the cohort, including pulmonary function (Calvert et al., 1991), liver and gastrointestinal function (Calvert et al., 1992), mood (Alderfer et al., 1992), the peripheral nervous system (Sweeney et al., 1993), porphyria cutanea tarda (Calvert et al., 1994), and reproductive hormones (Egeland et al., 1994). Sweeney et al. (1996, 1997/1998) also evaluated noncancer end points including liver function, gastrointestinal disorders, chloracne, serum glucose, hormone and lipid levels, and diabetes in a subgroup of the original Calvert et al. (1991) cohort. A cross-sectional medical survey reported blood serum TCDD concentrations and surrogates of cytochrome P450 induction in that cohort (Halperin et al., 1995). *VAO, Veterans and Agent Orange: Update 1996* (hereafter, *Update 1996*) and *Update 1998* describe the details of each of those studies.

Since *Update 1998*, Calvert et al. (1998, 1999) and Halperin et al. (1998) have published follow-up results on the cohort of workers employed more than 15 years earlier at the chemical plants in New Jersey and Missouri. Occupationally exposed individuals were compared to a referent group composed of age-, neighborhood-, race-, and sex-matched individuals with no self-reported occupational exposure to TCDD. The relationship between serum TCDD concentrations (measured as picograms per gram of lipid) and various end points were assessed in those follow-up reports. In Calvert et al. (1998) the association between exposure to TCDD and cardiovascular effects (increased risk of myocardial infarction, angina, cardiac arrhythmias, hypertension, and abnormal peripheral arterial flow) was examined in the cohort. Blood samples were analyzed for total cholesterol, triglyceride, high-density lipoprotein (HDL) cholesterol, and glucose. A general physical examination was conducted, which included measurement of blood pressure, as well as a Doppler examination of the peripheral pulses, a chest X-ray, and electrocardiograms (ECG). Calvert et al. (1999) examined the relationship among TCDD exposure and diabetes mellitus, thyroid function, and indicators of endocrine function in the same cohort. Serum glucose, thyroid-stimulating hormone, total thyroxine (T_4), and thyroid hormone binding resin levels were measured. Halperin et al. (1998) evaluated immune parameters in this cohort; lymphocyte subsets, natural killer cell cytotoxic activity, and lymphocyte proliferative responses to stimulation were studied.

Steenland et al. (1999) studied the association between TCDD exposure and cause of death in the cohort from the 12 U.S. chemical plants described by Fingerhut et al. (1991). Those researchers investigated any association between exposure and cancer (all and site specific), respiratory disease, cardiovascular disease, and diabetes. In addition, a similar analysis was conducted in a subgroup of workers who had previously been diagnosed with chloracne, indicating a higher exposure to TCDD on average.

Monsanto

Included in the NIOSH study cohort (Fingerhut et al., 1991) are a number of individual cohort members from Monsanto's production facilities on whom studies have been conducted. One set of Monsanto studies is based on an accidental exposure that occurred on March 8, 1949, in the trichlorophenol production process at the Nitro, West Virginia, plant of Monsanto (Zack and Suskind, 1980; Moses et al., 1984; Collins et al., 1993). Other studies focused on exposure of Monsanto workers involved in numerous aspects of 2,4,5-T production (Zack and Gaffey, 1983; Moses et al., 1984; Suskind and Hertzberg, 1984). These studies are discussed in more detail in *VAO*. No new studies have been published on these cohorts.

Dow

Several studies have been conducted on Dow Chemical Company production workers and are summarized in *VAO, Update 1996*, and *Update 1998*. The populations in these studies, except for one report by Bond et al. (1988), are included in the NIOSH cohort (Fingerhut et al., 1991). Originally, Dow Chemical Company conducted a study on the work force engaged in the production of 2,4,5-T (Ott et al., 1980) and a study on TCP manufacturing workers exhibiting chloracne (Cook et al., 1980). Extension and follow-up studies compared potential exposure to TCDD and medical examination frequency and morbidity (Bond et al., 1983), as well as reproductive outcomes after potential paternal TCDD exposure (Townsend et al., 1982). A prospective mortality study was also conducted of Dow employees diagnosed with chloracne or classified as having chloracne on the basis of clinical description (Bond et al., 1987).

In addition, Dow Chemical Company assembled a large cohort at the Midland, Michigan, plant (Cook et al., 1986, 1997; Bond et al., 1989b). Exposure to TCDD was characterized in this cohort based on chloracne diagnosis (Bond et al., 1989a). Within this large Midland cohort, a cohort study of women (Ott et al., 1987) and a case-control study of soft-tissue sarcoma (STS) (Sobel et al., 1987) were conducted. Dow Chemical Company has also undertaken a large-scale cohort mortality study of workers exposed to herbicides in several Dow plants (Bond et al., 1988; Bloemen et al., 1993; Ramlow et al., 1996). No new studies have been published on the Dow cohort since *Update 1998*.

BASF

In Germany, an accident on November 17, 1953, during the manufacture of trichlorophenol at BASF Aktiengesellschaft, resulted in the exposure of some workers in the plant to predominantly TCDD. *VAO, Update 1996*, and *Update 1998* summarize studies of these workers. The studies include a mortality study of persons initially exposed or later involved in cleanup operations (Thiess et al., 1982), an update and expansion of that study (Zober et al., 1990), and a morbidity follow-up (Zober et al., 1994). In addition, Ott and Zober (1996) examined cancer incidence and mortality in another cohort of workers exposed to TCDD after the accident during reactor cleanup, maintenance, or demolition.

Since *Update 1998*, Zober et al. (1997) have summarized their studies on the BASF cohort, but no new analyses of the cohort have been reported.

IARC

To avoid problems of small studies with insufficient power to detect increased cancer risks, IARC created a multinational registry of workers exposed to phenoxy herbicides, chlorophenols, and their contaminants (Saracci et al., 1991). The IARC registry includes information on mortality and exposures of 18,390 workers—16,863 men and 1,527 women. *Update 1996* describes the individual national cohorts included in this multinational registry.

In a study including cohorts from 10 countries, cancer mortality from soft-tissue sarcoma (STS) and malignant lymphoma was evaluated (Kogevinas et al., 1992). Two nested case-control studies were also undertaken within this cohort to evaluate the relationship between STS and non-Hodgkin's lymphoma (Kogevinas et al., 1995). In an update and expansion, Kogevinas et al. (1997) assembled national studies from 12 countries that used the same protocol, jointly developed by study participants and coordinated by IARC, and studied cancer mortality. A cohort study of cancer incidence and mortality was conducted among 701 women occupationally exposed to chlorophenoxy herbicides, chlorophenols, and dioxins from seven countries (Kogevinas et al., 1993). *VAO, Update 1996,* and *Update 1998* highlight these studies.

In addition, a number of the individual cohorts have been evaluated apart from the IARC-coordinated efforts. These cohorts include Danish production workers studied by Lynge (1985, 1993); British production workers studied by Coggon et al. (1986, 1991); Dutch production workers studied by Bueno de Mesquita et al. (1993); and German production workers studied by Manz et al. (1991), Becher et al. (1996), and Flesch-Janys et al. (1995). *VAO, Update 1996,* and *Update 1998* discuss these studies in more detail.

Since *Update 1998*, Vena et al. (1998) published a study on nonneoplastic mortality in the cohort in which Kogevinas et al. (1997) studied cancer mortality. The cohort is composed of 21,863 workers who were employed in the production or spraying of phenoxyacetic herbicides. In the study by Vena et al. (1998), data on workers from all 36 cohorts from 12 countries were studied; data for workers from cohorts for which minimum employment periods were specified were not included. Exposures were estimated by job records, company exposure questionnaires, and in some cohorts, serum, adipose, or workplace TCDD measurements. Workers were divided into three exposure categories: exposed to TCDD or higher-chlorinated dioxins, not exposed, and unknown exposure status. Standard mortality ratios (SMRs) were calculated for all major noncancer causes of death.

Hooiveld et al. (1998) analyzed data from one study at a factory in the Netherlands that followed the protocol of, and was included in, the IARC study. Exposure status was based on departmental occupational history, as well as exposure to the accident. Serum concentrations of polychlorinated dibenzodioxins (PCDDs), polychlorinated dibenzofurans (PCDFs), and polychlorinated biphenyls (PCBs) were measured in a subset of survivors who were employed prior to the end of the last TCDD-contaminated process. Maximum TCDD concentrations were estimated from the measured TCDD concentrations using a one-compartment, first-order kinetic model and a half-life of 7.1 years. SMRs and relative risks were calculated by cause of death in two cohorts: 549 male workers exposed to phenoxy herbicides, chlorophenols, and contaminants; and 140 male workers exposed as a result of an accident at the plant.

Flesch-Janys (1997) summarized exposure and mortality data on employees of the Hamburg Boehringer Company plant that produced 2,4,5-T, 2,4,5-TCP, and hexachlorocyclohexane (HCH) until 1984. The cohort, which had been studied previously by Flesch-Janys et al. (1995), consisted of all regular employees of a chemical plant ($N = 1,189$ males). Flesch-Janys (1997) used half-life data previously determined in a subgroup of the cohort (Flesch-Janys et al., 1996) to estimate blood TCDD levels in 190 workers. From that they determined department-specific exposures and, from that, estimated exposures (TCDD and toxic equivalents) for the entire cohort (Flesch-Janys et al., 1995). Using these estimates, dose–response analyses were conducted for SMRs from different causes of death.

Neuberger et al. (1999) studied the health effects of TCDD in an Austrian cohort that is part of the IARC study. Preliminary results are presented in Neuberger et al. (1998) and in an article with an English abstract (Jäger et al., 1998). Individuals in the Austrian cohort had been diagnosed with chloracne and were exposed to polychlorinated dibenzodioxin or dibenzofuran (PCDD/F) (mainly TCDD) in a 2,4,5-T production facility in Linz, Austria. At the time of the study, of 159 individuals identified as having chloracne, 124 remained in Austria and were invited to participate in a health examination survey: 56 individuals participated in the survey and 50 individuals donated blood and urine and answered all questions. Age- and sex-matched controls who had recently participated in health checkups similar to those of the cases were employed. Two such control groups were used, one drawn from the same occupational health center in Linz and one from another prospective study on workers from a chemical plant located 66 km from the 2,4,5-T plant. Occupational and medical histories, including smoking and alcohol consumption, were obtained from cases and controls. PCDF, PCDD, and PCB concentrations were measured in plasma. Chloracne, general health status (e.g., neurological symptoms, liver disease, stomach problems, arthritis), and clinical chemistry parameters (e.g., blood sugar, cholesterol, enzyme levels, leukocyte levels) were assessed in the three groups.

Other Chemical Plants

Previous studies have reviewed health outcomes among chemical workers in the United Kingdom exposed to TCDD as a result of an industrial accident in 1968 (May, 1982, 1983; Jennings et al., 1988); production workers in the former USSR involved in the production of 2,4-D (Bashirov, 1969); factory workers in Prague, Czechoslovakia, who exhibited symptoms of TCDD toxicity 10 years after occupational exposure to 2,4,5-T (Pazderova-Vejlupkova et al., 1981); 2,4-D and 2,4,5-T production workers in the United States (Poland et al., 1971); white male workers employed at a chemical plant in the United States manufacturing flavors and fragrances (Thomas, 1987); and the long-term immune system effects of TCDD in 11 industrial workers involved in production and maintenance operations at a German chemical factory producing 2,4,5-T (Tonn et al., 1996). *VAO* and *Update 1998* detail these studies.

Since *Update 1998*, Hryhorczuk et al. (1998) has examined employees in a chemical plant in southwestern Illinois who were engaged in the production of PCP, lower-chlorinated phenols, and esters of chlorophenoxy acids. The study population was defined based on company personnel records. The unexposed comparison population consisted of workers from the same plant who, according to company records, had never worked in areas where they would have been exposed to PCP. Of the 743 eligible exposed workers, 473 participated in the medical examination, of whom 366 were engaged in the production of PCP. Of the 559 eligible unexposed workers, 303 participated in the medical examination. The exposed and unexposed groups were examined for general health status, chloracne, and porphyria.

Jung et al. (1998) evaluated immune effects in a cohort of workers formerly employed at a German pesticide-producing plant. Of 450 former workers, 192 (8 women) chose to participate in comprehensive health status checks that were offered following the closing of the plant and were used in the study. PCDD/F concentrations were measured in blood lipids and expressed as toxicity equivalents (TEQs). Study participants were observed clinically and were asked about medical and work history. Measurements of immunological parameters, including erythrocyte sedimentation rate, full blood count, serum electrophoresis, presence of specific antibodies, immunoglobulin (Ig) levels, and lymphocyte surface marker measurements, were conducted. The results of specific tests, however, were not presented for the full cohort (e.g., tetanus antibodies before and 3 weeks after vaccination, $N = 53$; IgA, IgG, and IgM levels, $N = 53$). No explanation is provided for the variable number of participants in the different immunological assays. In addition, a subgroup of the 29 most highly exposed individuals was compared to 28 unexposed individuals for proliferation of lymphocytes and chromate resistance.

Agricultural and Forest Products Workers

Cohort Studies

Agricultural Workers *VAO*, *Update 1996*, and *Update 1998* detail a number of cohort studies examining health effects in individuals involved in agricultural activity. These include studies of proportionate mortality among Iowa farmers (Burmeister, 1981) and among male and female farmers from 23 states (Blair et al., 1993); cancer mortality among Danish and Italian farmers (Ronco et al., 1992) and among a cohort of rice growers in the Novara Province of northern Italy (Gambini et al., 1997); cancer incidence among farmers licensed to spray pesticides in the southern Piedmont area of Italy (Corrao et al., 1989) and among female Danish gardeners (Hansen et al., 1992); sperm abnormalities among Argentinean farmers (Lerda and Rizzi, 1991); cancer birth defects among the offspring of Norwegian farmers (Kristensen et al., 1997); and immunological changes in 10 farmers who mixed and applied commercial formulations containing the chlorophenoxy herbicides (Faustini et al., 1996). In addition, a set of Canadian studies, called the Mortality Study of Canadian Male Farm Operators, evaluated the risk to farmers of general mortality and specific health outcomes including non-Hodgkin's lymphoma (NHL) (Wigle et al., 1990; Morrison et al., 1994), prostate cancer (Morrison et al., 1992), brain cancer (Morrison et al., 1993), multiple myeloma (Semenciw et al., 1993), leukemia (Semenciw et al., 1994), and asthma (Senthilselvan et al., 1992). Based on data from the Swedish Cancer Environment Register (which links population census data, including occupation, with the Swedish Cancer Registry), cohort studies evaluated cancer mortality and farm work (Wiklund, 1983); STS and malignant lymphoma among agricultural and forestry workers (Wiklund and Holm, 1986; Wiklund et al., 1988a); and the risk of NHL, Hodgkin's disease (HD), and multiple myeloma in relation to numerous occupational activities (Eriksson et al., 1992). Brain, lymphatic, and hematopoietic cancers in Irish agricultural workers have also been studied (Dean, 1994).

Since *Update 1998*, Arbuckle et al. (1999) examined the incidence of spontaneous abortion in couples living on family farms in Ontario, Canada, selected from the 1986 Canadian Census of Agriculture. Farming families were contacted by telephone and were considered eligible if they were married or "living as married," if they lived year-round on the farm, and if the wife was not older than

44. Eligible families were sent three questionnaires. One questionnaire, addressed to the farm operator, collected data on pesticide use (current and historical use). Another questionnaire, addressed to the husband, collected demographic, socioeconomic, and life-style information, medical history, and information on his activities on the farm, date of moving to the farm, and pesticide exposures both at home and on the farm. Another questionnaire, addressed to the wife, collected information similar to that of the husbands, but also collected a complete reproductive history. Pesticide use was recorded by specific pesticide by month and year. Spontaneous abortion occurrence was self-reported at <20 weeks of gestation and was categorized by occurrence at <12 weeks and occurrence between 12 and 19 weeks of gestation. This subgrouping provided an indirect estimate of the frequency of chromosomal anomalies because these anomalies are a much more common cause of early abortions than later abortions. Pregnancy outcome data were merged with pesticide use at the corresponding time. Potential confounders were also recorded (e.g., parental age, smoking, alcohol consumption), along with the time period during which they were present. Telephone screening identified 2,946 eligible couples (36.5 percent of all operating farms). Pregnancies were excluded if there was missing information (e.g., outcome, delivery date, gestational age at delivery), if it occurred when the woman was not living on the farm, if the study husband might not have been the father, or in the case of multiple gestations, ectopic pregnancies, or hydatidiform mole pregnancies. A total of 2,110 women were enrolled in the study with a total of 5,853 pregnancies, of which 3,396 were included in the analysis.

Forestry Workers Studies have been conducted among forestry workers potentially exposed to the types of herbicides used in Vietnam. These studies include a cohort mortality study among men employed at a Canadian public utility (Green, 1987, 1991) and a briefly outlined Dutch study of forestry workers exposed to 2,4,5-T that investigated the prevalence of acne and liver dysfunction (van Houdt et al., 1983). *VAO* describes these studies in greater detail.

Since *Update 1998*, Thörn et al. (2000) have reported on mortality and cancer incidence in a cohort of Swedish lumberjacks. The cohort analyzed consisted of males and females who were Swedish residents and employed by one Swedish forestry company at some time between 1954 and 1967. Approximate volume and concentration of phenoxy acids used daily in a particular work task or job category were obtained from former employees. Pay slips were used to determine time spent at particular work tasks, and exposure to phenoxy acids was estimated by the time spent at particular job categories. Employees who were exposed to phenoxy acids for more than 5 working days were considered to have been exposed; employees not exposed to any types of pesticides were used as the unexposed or control group; individuals who were exposed to other pesticides (including DDT) were excluded from the study. Mortality was determined from the National Register of Causes of Death, new cancer cases were determined from the Swedish Cancer Register, and death certificates with underlying cause of death were provided by Statistics Sweden. Data were available for 261 exposed and 243 unexposed members of the cohort. SMRs and cancer incidence (all and site specific) ratios were calculated for each group using ratios expected from the death and cancer registries.

Herbicide and Pesticide Sprayers A number of cohort studies have assessed health outcomes among herbicide and pesticide appliers including cancer mortality among Swedish railroad workers (Axelson and Sundell, 1974; Axelson et al., 1980), mortality among pesticide appliers in Florida (Blair et al., 1983), general and cancer mortality and morbidity measured prospectively among Finnish male 2,4-D and 2,4,5-T appliers (Riihimaki et al., 1982, 1983; Asp et al., 1994), and reproductive outcomes among male chemical appliers in New Zealand (Smith et al., 1981, 1982). Other studies examined the risk of cancer including STS, HD, and NHL among pesticide and herbicide appliers in Sweden (Wiklund et al., 1987, 1988b, 1989a,b), general and cancer mortality among Dutch male herbicide appliers (Swaen et al., 1992), cancer mortality among Minnesota highway maintenance workers (Bender et al., 1989) and Minnesota pesticide appliers (Garry et al., 1994, 1996a,b), lung cancer morbidity in male agricultural plant protection workers in the former German Democratic Republic (Barthel, 1981), British Columbia sawmill workers potentially exposed to chlorophenate wood preservatives (Dimich-Ward et al., 1996; Hertzman et al., 1997; Heacock et al. 1998), and cancer risk among pesticide users in Iceland (Zhong and Rafnsson, 1996). Some of these studies include agricultural and forestry worker cohorts; the details are included in *VAO*, *Update 1996*, and *Update 1998*.

More recently, data from the first 2 years of a 10-year Agricultural Health Study in Iowa and North Carolina have been published (Alavanja et al., 1998). In that study, pesticide appliers completed a self-administered questionnaire that asked about hospital or doctor visits resulting from pesticide exposures. Questionnaires were administered at testing and training sessions, which are required every 3 years for certification or recertification of pesticide appliers in these states. Out of 51,256 appliers who attended the sessions, 35,879 (3 percent of those enrolled in the study were women and 3.1 percent were minorities) completed the questionnaire, which asked about general information on pesticide use, as well as specific information on the use of 50 individual pesticides. In addition, for 22 pesticides, information on the number of years and the average number of days of application per year was gathered. Questions on the use of protective clothing, application procedures, crops and livestock raised in the past year, farm size, smoking and alcohol consumption history, diet, and basic demographics were included. Cumulative lifetime application days for herbicides, insecticides, fumigants, and fungicides were calculated based on the responses, and relative risks for health care visits were determined.

Dich and Wiklund (1998) studied a cohort of 20,025 males who were licensed for pesticide application in Sweden between 1965 and 1976. This cohort had been studied previously by Wiklund et al. (1987, 1988b, 1989a,b). The use of pesticides in a random sample of 268 of these applicators has been described (Wiklund et al., 1989a). Information gathered included types of pesticides used, frequency of application, years used, application methods, use of protective clothing, smoking, and occupational history. Prostate cancer occurrence in the cohort was determined from the Swedish Cancer Registry, with all registered cases of malignant prostatic tumors included. The expected rate of tumors was based on the annual incidence of prostate tumors in the male Swedish population in 5-year age groups.

Case-Control Studies

In 1977, case series reports in Sweden (Hardell, 1977, 1979) of a potential connection between soft-tissue sarcoma and exposure to phenoxyacetic acids prompted several case-control studies in Sweden to further investigate the possible association (Hardell and Sandstrom, 1979; Eriksson et al., 1979, 1981, 1990; Hardell and Eriksson, 1988; Wingren et al., 1990). Following the initial reports on STS (Hardell, 1977, 1979), case-control studies of other cancer outcomes were also conducted in Sweden, including studies of HD, NHL, and other lymphomas (Hardell et al., 1980, 1981; Hardell and Bengtsson, 1983); HD and NHL (Persson et al., 1989, 1993); NHL (Olsson and Brandt, 1988); nasal and nasopharyngeal carcinomas (Hardell et al., 1982); and primary or unspecified liver cancer (Hardell et al., 1984). To address criticism regarding potential observer bias in some of these case-control series, Hardell (1981) conducted another case-control study on colon cancer. Hardell et al. (1994) also examined the relationship between occupational exposure to phenoxyacetic acids and chlorophenols, and various parameters related to NHL, including histopathology, stage, and anatomical location, on the basis of the NHL cases from a previous study (Hardell et al., 1981).

Prompted by the Swedish studies (Hardell, 1977, 1979), a set of case-control studies was undertaken in New Zealand to evaluate the risks of phenoxy herbicide and chlorophenol exposure and STS incidence and mortality (Smith et al., 1983, 1984; Smith and Pearce, 1986). Additional case-control studies and an expanded case series were conducted on phenoxy herbicide and chlorophenol exposure and the risks of malignant lymphoma, NHL, and multiple myeloma (Pearce et al., 1985, 1986a,b, 1987).

Elevated leukemia mortality in geographic patterns for white males in the central part of the United States prompted a study of the leukemia mortality of Nebraska farmers (Blair and Thomas, 1979). Additional case-control studies were later conducted on leukemia in Nebraska (Blair and White, 1985); in Iowa (Burmeister et al., 1982) based on the cohort study of Burmeister (1981); and in

Iowa and Minnesota (Brown et al., 1990); as well as on leukemia associated with NHL in eastern Nebraska (Zahm et al., 1990).

Case-control studies have been conducted on other cancers in various U.S. populations, including NHL (Cantor, 1982; Cantor et al., 1992; Zahm et al., 1993; Tatham et al., 1997); multiple myeloma (Morris et al., 1986; Boffetta et al., 1989; Brown et al., 1993); cancers of the stomach, prostate, NHL, and multiple myeloma (Burmeister et al., 1983); STS, HD, and NHL (Hoar et al., 1986); NHL and HD (Dubrow et al., 1988); and STS and NHL (Woods et al., 1987; Woods and Polissar, 1989).

Other studies have been conducted outside the United States looking at cancer end points: ovarian cancer in the Piedmont region of Italy (Donna et al., 1984); brain gliomas in two hospitals in Milan, Italy (Musicco et al., 1988); STS and other cancers from the 15 regional cancer registries that constitute the National Cancer Register in England (Balarajan and Acheson, 1984); STS and malignant lymphomas in the Victorian Cancer Registry of Australia (Smith and Christophers, 1992); lymphoid cancer in Milan, Italy (LaVecchia et al., 1989); STS among rice weeders in northern Italy (Vineis et al., 1986); primary lung cancer among pesticide users in Saskatchewan (McDuffie et al., 1990); and renal cell carcinoma from the Denmark Cancer Registry (Mellemgaard et al., 1994). In addition, Nanni et al. (1996) conducted a population-based case-control study, based on the work of Amadori et al. (1995), of occupational and chemical risk factors for lymphocytic leukemia and NHL in northeastern Italy.

Noncancer end points have also been investigated in case-control studies. End points studied include spontaneous abortions (Carmelli et al., 1981); immunosuppression and subsequently decreased host resistance to infection among AIDS patients with Kaposi's sarcoma (Hardell et al., 1987); mortality of U.S. Department of Agriculture (USDA) extension agents (Alavanja et al., 1988, 1989); risk of spina bifida in offspring by investigating paternal occupation (Blatter et al., 1997); mortality from neurodegenerative diseases by looking at occupational risk factors (Schulte et al., 1996); Parkinson's disease (PD) in terms of occupational and environmental risk factors (Liou et al., 1997); PD by looking at various rural factors, including exposure to herbicides and wood preservatives (Seidler et al., 1996); PD by examining occupational risk factors (Semchuk et al., 1993); and birth defects among agricultural workers (Nurminen et al., 1994). Those earlier studies are discussed in detail in *VAO, Update 1996,* or *Update 1998.*

More recently, García et al. (1998) conducted a case-control study in an agricultural region of Spain assessing the association between paternal occupational exposure to pesticides and congenital malformations. The base population for the study was selected from couples who gave birth at selected hospitals in the study area in 1993 and 1994. From this base, study cases were chosen when they exhibited the presence of malformations or groups of defects with a relatively high prevalence at birth which were also conditions identified in earlier epidemiologic research as being related to pesticide exposure. One matched control was included for each case. From a total of 336 cases and 355 controls originally identified, 261 cases and 261 controls participated in the study. Interviews were conducted by telephone when possible and in person otherwise. A questionnaire asked about possible exposures to pesticides (e.g., involvement in agricultural work and pesticide application) for 3 months preceding conception and during the first trimester for the father, and for 1 month prior to conception and during the first trimester for the mother. Individuals involved in pesticide application were then interviewed in person to collect detailed information on the characteristics of the agricultural work; exposure to pesticides, including details of the crops sprayed, duration, and types of pesticide treatments; and other sources of pesticide exposure. One individual involved in training pesticide appliers and one individual working at the local agricultural department independently assessed the exposure of individuals based on the questionnaires; a consensus rating of exposure was obtained from the two assessments. Risk estimates were calculated jointly for all congenital malformations in association with exposure to major classes of pesticides and specific active ingredients.

Ekstrom et al. (1999) published a case-control study on different geographic regions of Sweden that have different rates of gastric cancer. Three counties have gastric cancer incidences close to the national average; two other counties have Sweden's highest incidences of gastric cancer. Individuals born in Sweden who were between 40 and 79 years of age and lived in one of five counties in Sweden during the study period were eligible for the study. New cases of histologically confirmed gastric adenocarcinoma were identified by clinicians working in hospitals in the study area, by surveillance of definite or suspected cases evaluated at county pathology departments, by checking regional cancer registries, and by a final check with the national Cancer Register 20 months after the end of the study period. Identified cases were asked by their clinicians to participate in an interview for the study, with a total of 567 cases interviewed (out of 908 identified individuals). Two age- and gender-matched controls were randomly identified and interviewed for each case. A total of 1,165 individuals were interviewed out of 1,534 control subjects who were contacted. Interviews were conducted in person by professional interviewers at Statistics Sweden. Occupation was coded by title for any position held for at least 1 year and was stratified both as "ever" and also by duration (1–10 years, >10 years). Inquiries were also made as to exposure to particular occupations and chemicals, including mining and paper mills, and asbestos, organic solvents, and specific pesticide groups. Based on job histories and the interview data, individuals were assigned an exposure status, and cumulative duration of exposure was estimated. Socioeconomic status, education level, area of residence, smoking habits, and diets were assessed as covariates. Because gastric cancer is the end point of interest, a subset of the cases and controls was assessed for antibodies to *Helicobacter pylori* as a potential confounder.

Hardell and Eriksson (1999) investigated the relationship between exposure to pesticides and NHL in Sweden. Males greater than 25 years of age diagnosed with NHL between 1987 and 1990 in five counties of Sweden were identified through regional cancer registries. Cases had to have been diagnosed histopathologically and the pathological diagnosis was confirmed for the study. A total of 442 cases were included. Two male controls were matched to each case. Controls for deceased cases were matched for age and year of death. A questionnaire was mailed to subjects or next of kin to collect information on work history and exposure to different chemicals, including information on years of exposure and cumulative exposure in days. Information on smoking, dietary habits, and previous diseases was also collected. Most individuals were also interviewed over the phone to clarify confusing answers or complete unanswered questions; 404 cases and 741 controls answered the questionnaire.

Paper and Pulp Workers

Workers in the paper and pulp industry may be exposed to TCDD and other dioxins that are generated during the bleaching process used in the production and treatment of some paper and paper products. *VAO* describes studies of workers potentially exposed to TCDD at paper and pulp mills and various health outcomes, including general mortality of workers at five mills in Washington, Oregon, and California (Robinson et al., 1986); cancer incidence among male Finnish paper mill workers (Jappinen and Pukkala, 1991); respiratory health in a New Hampshire mill (Henneberger et al., 1989); and cause-specific mortality among white males employed in plants identified by the United Paperworkers International Union (Solet et al., 1989).

More recently, Rix et al. (1998) investigated the relationship between working in the paper industry and cancer risk. A historical cohort was made up of workers in three paper mills in Denmark owned by the same company, with 1890 as the earliest year of employment. None of the mills ever produced pulp. Work history was determined from company records, and individuals were located by either personal identification numbers or the National Mortality Register. A total of 14,362 people were identified out of 14,789 in the overall cohort. Cancer cases occurring from 1943 to 1993 were identified from the Danish Cancer Register, which started in 1943. Expected cancer incidences were calculated from Danish population incidences. Overall cancer risk and site-specific cancer risks were calculated.

Schildt et al. (1999) conducted a case-control study in Sweden investigating the risk of oral cancer from occupational exposures and particular occupations. The cases consisted of all histopathologically verified squamous cell oral cancer cases in the Cancer Register for four counties in Sweden. A total of 410 cases out of 419 identified individuals were used. One control was matched for each case on the basis of age, sex, county of residence, and age at death if the case was deceased. Questionnaires were sent to all living subjects and next of kin for deceased subjects to assess exposure. Information on lifetime occupational history, smoking, other exposure factors of interest, and socioeconomic status was collected. Follow-up telephone interviews were used to clarify answers or complete unanswered questions and with any individuals who were employed in farming or forestry to ensure uniform assessment of exposures of these individuals to pesticides. A total of 354 matched pairs participated in the study (354 cases and 354 controls).

ENVIRONMENTAL STUDIES

The occurrence of accidents and industrial disasters has offered opportunities to evaluate the long-term health effects of exposure to dioxin and other potentially hazardous chemicals.

Seveso, Italy

One of the largest industrial accidents involving environmental exposures to TCDD occurred in Seveso, Italy, in July 1976 as a result of an uncontrolled reaction during trichlorophenol production. A variety of indicators were used to estimate individual exposure; soil contamination by TCDD has been the most extensively used. On the basis of soil sampling, three areas were defined about the release point: zone A, the most heavily contaminated, from which all residents were evacuated within 20 days; zone B, an area of lesser contamination that children and pregnant women in their first trimester were urged to avoid during daytime; and zone R, a region with some contamination, in which consumption of local crops was prohibited (Bertazzi et al., 1989a,b).

Several cohort studies based on these exposure categories have been conducted. These studies are reviewed extensively in *VAO*, *Update 1996,* and *Update 1998* and are summarized here. Caramaschi et al. (1981) presented the distribution of chloracne among Seveso children, while Mocarelli et al. (1986) tested the children for laboratory levels of several chemicals in blood and urine based on previous chloracne. In a follow-up to these studies, dermatologic findings and laboratory tests were conducted among a group of the children with chloracne compared to controls (Assennato et al., 1989a).

Other studies looked at specific health effects associated with TCDD exposure among Seveso residents, including chloracne, birth defects, spontaneous abortions, crude birth and death rates (Bisanti et al., 1980); chloracne and peripheral nervous system conditions (Barbieri et al., 1988); hepatic enzyme-associated conditions (Ideo et al., 1982, 1985); abnormal birth outcomes (Mastroiacovo et al., 1988); cytogenetic abnormalities in maternal and fetal tissues (Tenchini et al., 1983); neurological disorders (Boeri et al., 1978; Filippini et al., 1981); cancer incidence (Pesatori et al., 1992, 1993; Bertazzi et al., 1993); and the sex ratio among offspring who were born in zone A (Mocarelli et al., 1996). A 2-year prospective controlled study was conducted of workers potentially exposed to TCDD during cleanup of the most highly contaminated areas following the accident (Assennato et al., 1989b).

Seveso residents have had long-term follow-up of their health outcomes, especially cancer. Bertazzi and colleagues conducted 10-year mortality follow-up studies among adults and children age 1 to 19 at the time of the accident (Bertazzi et al., 1989a,b, 1992) and 15-year follow-up studies (Bertazzi et al., 1997, 1998).

Since *Update 1998*, Pesatori et al. (1998) have updated the noncancer mortality causes for the 15 years from July 1976 to June 1991 for individuals living in zone A, B, or R at the time of the accident. Data were obtained from vital statistics registries. Vital status was obtained for more than 99 percent of the cohort, with information on 805 individuals from zone A; 5,943 individuals from zone B; 38,625 individuals from zone R; and 232,747 reference individuals.

Bertazzi et al. (2001) conducted a 20.5-year mortality study (1976–1996) of individuals living in zone A, B, or R at the time of the accident or who moved to the area in the 10 years after the accident. Vital statistics and cause of death for deceased subjects were determined through local vital statistics offices. Tracing was high with only 2.3 percent of the original cohort not traced; information was obtained on 804 individuals from zone A; 5,941 individuals from zone B; 38,624 individuals from zone R; and 232,745 reference individuals. In addition to analysis of the full cohort, data for zones A and B were analyzed by years since first exposure to assess latency effects and by gender, age category, calendar time, duration of residence, and residence at the time of exposure.

Times Beach and Quail Run

During early 1971, by-products of a hexachlorophene and 2,4,5-T production facility in Verona, Missouri, were mixed with waste oils and sprayed on various sites around the state for dust control. TCDD was a contaminant of the mixtures sprayed, and the contamination was reported by the Environmental Protection Agency (EPA). A number of studies were conducted to evaluate health effects from the potential exposure (Evans et al., 1988; Hoffman et al., 1986; Stehr et al., 1986; Stehr-Green et al., 1987; Stockbauer et al., 1988; Webb et al., 1987). *VAO* discusses these studies in greater detail, and no more recent studies have been published.

Vietnam

Vietnamese researchers have conducted studies of the native population exposed to the spraying that occurred during the Vietnam conflict. In a review paper, Constable and Hatch (1985) summarized the unpublished results of these studies. The review article included nine reports that focus primarily on reproductive outcomes (Can et al., 1983a,b; Huong and Phuong, 1983; Khoa, 1983; Lang et al., 1983a,b; Nguyen, 1983; Phuong and Huong, 1983; Trung and Chien, 1983). Vietnamese researchers later published results of four additional studies conducted in Vietnam—two focusing on reproductive abnormalities (Phuong et al., 1989a,b), one on mortality (Dai et al., 1990), and one on hepatocellular carcinoma (Cordier et al., 1993). *VAO* and *Update 1996* discuss these studies in more detail. No studies have been published since *Update 1996*.

Other Environmental Studies

VAO, Update 1996, and *Update 1998* reported on numerous studies focusing on reproductive outcomes of potential environmental exposure in Oregon (U.S. EPA, 1979); Arkansas (Nelson et al., 1979); Iowa and Michigan (Gordon and Shy, 1981); New Brunswick, Canada (White et al., 1988); Skaraborg, Sweden (Jansson and Voog, 1989); and Northland, New Zealand (Hanify et al., 1981).

Numerous other studies have focused on different outcomes resulting from environmental exposure. These studies include examinations of STS and connective tissue cancers in Midland County, Michigan (Michigan Department of Public Health, 1983); NHL in Yorkshire, England (Cartwright et al., 1988); cancer in Finland (Lampi et al., 1992); lymphomas and STS in Italy (Vineis et al., 1991); neuropsychological effects in Germany (Peper et al., 1993); young-onset Parkinson's disease in Oregon and Washington (Butterfield et al., 1993); adverse health effects following an electrical transformer fire in Binghamton, New York (Fitzgerald et al., 1989); skin cancer in Alberta, Canada (Gallagher et al., 1996); NHL, HD, and chronic lymphocytic leukemia (CLL) in a rural Michigan community (Waterhouse et al., 1996); HD, NHL, multiple myelomas, and acute myeloid leukemias in various regions of Italy (Masala et al., 1996); inhalation exposure to TCDD and the effects of related compounds in wood preservatives on cell-mediated immunity in German day care center employees (Wolf and Karmaus, 1995); mortality and cancer incidence in two cohorts of Swedish fishermen for whom it is assumed that diet constitutes the primary exposure route (Svensson et al., 1995); immune effects in hobby fishermen in the Frierfjord in southeastern Norway (Lovik et al., 1996); and immunological effects of pre- and postnatal PCB or TCDD exposure in Dutch infants from birth to 18 months of age (Weisglas-Kuperus et al., 1995).

Since *Update 1998*, Schreinemachers (2000) has examined cancer mortality from 1980–1989 in four northern wheat-producing states. Information on total land area, total crop land, and individual harvested crop acreage by county was obtained for Minnesota, North Dakota, South Dakota, and Montana from the 1982 USDA Agricultural Census data base. Wheat acreage per county was used as a surrogate for exposure to chlorophenoxy herbicides (including 2,4-D). Counties with less than 20 percent crop land or more than 50 percent urban population were excluded. Remaining counties were divided into tertiles based on wheat acreage. Cancer mortality data for 1980–1989, collected by the National Center for Health Statistics, were summarized for 34 cancers. Data were grouped by 5-year age intervals, sex, race, and county and state of residence. Age-standardized mortality rate ratios (SRRs) were calculated by comparing the top two tertiles to the first tertile for white subjects. SRRs for rare cancers were calculated by dividing counties into two groups based on the median of wheat per county. Frequently occurring cancers were investigated using individual counties as the unit of observation; analysis focussed on counties that reported five or more cancers.

VIETNAM VETERAN STUDIES

Studies of Vietnam veterans who were potentially exposed to herbicides, including Agent Orange, have been conducted in the United States at the national and state levels, as well as in Australia and Vietnam. Exposure measures in these studies have been done on a variety of levels, and evaluations of health outcomes have been made using a variety of different comparison or control groups. This section is organized primarily by the sponsors of the research, because this format is more conducive to methodologic presentation of the articles. In these studies, exposure measures fall along a crude scale from individual levels for Ranch Hands, as reflected in serum dioxin measurements, to use of service in Vietnam as a surrogate for TCDD exposure in some state studies.

It should also be noted that a variety of comparison groups have been used for the veteran cohort studies: (a) Vietnam veterans who were stationed in areas essentially not exposed to active herbicide missions and were unlikely to have been in areas sprayed with herbicides; (b) Vietnam era veterans who were in the military at the time of the conflict but did not serve in Vietnam; (c) non-Vietnam veterans who served in other wars or conflicts such as the Korean War or World War II; and (d) various U.S. male populations (either state or national). This is also discussed in Chapter 5 of this report.

United States

Ranch Hands

The men responsible for the majority of aerial spraying of herbicides in Vietnam were volunteers from the Air Force who participated in Operation Ranch Hand. To determine whether there are adverse health effects associated with exposure to herbicides, including Agent Orange, the Air Force made a commitment to Congress and the White House in 1979 to conduct an epidemiologic study of Ranch Hands (AFHS, 1982). *VAO, Update 1996, Update 1998,* and *Veterans and Agent Orange: Herbicide/Dioxin Exposure and Type 2 Diabetes* (hereafter referred to as *Type 2 Diabetes*) (IOM, 2000) discuss reports and papers addressing this cohort in more detail.

A retrospective matched cohort study design was implemented to examine morbidity and mortality, with follow-up scheduled to continue until 2002. National Personnel Records Center and U.S. Air Force Human Resources Laboratory records were searched and cross-referenced to ascertain completely all Ranch Hand personnel (AFHS, 1982; Michalek et al., 1990). A total of 1,269 participants were originally identified (AFHS, 1983). A control population of 24,971 C-130 crew members and support personnel assigned to duty in Southeast Asia but not occupationally exposed to herbicides (AFHS, 1983) was selected from the same data sources used to identify the Ranch Hand population. Controls were individually matched on age, type of job (using Air Force specialty code), and race (white or not white). The rationale for matching on these variables was to control for age-related effects, educational and socioeconomic status, and potential differences by race in development of chronic disease. Since Ranch Hands and controls performed similar combat or combat-related jobs, many potential confounders related to the physical and psychophysiologic effects of combat stress and the Southeast Asia environment were potentially controlled (AFHS, 1982). Rank was also used as a surrogate of exposure. Alcohol and smoking were controlled for when they are known risk factors for the endpoint of interest.

Ten matches for each exposed subject formed a control set. For the mortality study, each subject classified as exposed and a random sample of half of each subject's control set are being followed for 20 years, in a 1:5 matched design. The morbidity component of follow-up consists of a 1:1 matched design, using the first control randomized to the mortality ascertainment component of the study. If a control is noncompliant, another control from the matched "pool" is selected; controls who die are not replaced.

The baseline exam occurred in 1982, and future exams are scheduled until 2002. Morbidity is ascertained through questionnaire and physical examination, which emphasize dermatologic, neuropsychiatric, hepatic, immunologic, reproductive, and neoplastic conditions. There were 1,208 Ranch Hands and 1,668 comparison subjects eligible for baseline examination. Initial questionnaire response rates were 97 percent for the exposed cohort and 93 percent for the unexposed; baseline physical exam responses were 87 and 76 percent, respectively (Wolfe et al., 1990). For the 1987 examination and questionnaire (Wolfe et al., 1990), 84 percent of Ranch Hands ($N = 955$) and 75 percent of comparison subjects ($N = 1,299$) were fully compliant. Mortality outcome was obtained and reviewed by using U.S. Air Force Military Personnel Center records, the DVA's Death Beneficiary Identification and Record Location System (BIRLS), and the Internal Revenue Service's data base of active social security numbers. Death certificates were obtained from the appropriate health departments (Michalek et al., 1990). For this study, 84 percent of the 1,148 eligible Ranch Hands ($N = 952$), 76 percent of the original comparison group ($N = 912$), and 65 percent of the 567 replacement comparisons ($N = 369$) invited to the 1992 follow-up chose to participate in the examination and questionnaire (AFHS, 1995). The methods used to assess mortality and morbidity were identical to the methods described previously for the 1982 and 1987 examinations.

Ranch Hands were divided into three categories on the basis of their potential exposures:

1. *Low potential*: This group included pilots, copilots, and navigators. Exposure was primarily through preflight checks and during actual spraying.

2. *Moderate potential*: This group included crew chiefs, aircraft mechanics, and support personnel. Exposure could occur by contact during dedrumming and aircraft loading operations, on-site repair of aircraft, and repair of spray equipment.

3. *High potential*: This group included spray console operators and flight engineers.

Results have been published for the baseline morbidity (AFHS, 1984a) and baseline mortality studies (AFHS, 1983); the first (1984b), second (1987), and third (1992) follow-up examinations (AFHS, 1987, 1990, 1995); and the reproductive outcomes study (AFHS, 1992; Wolfe et al., 1995). Mortality updates have been published for 1984–1986, 1989, and 1991 (AFHS, 1984b, 1985, 1986, 1989, 1991a). An interim technical report updated the cause-specific mortality among Ranch Hands through the end of 1993 (AFHS, 1996; Michalek et al., 1998b). Serum dioxin levels were measured in 1982 (36 Ranch Hands; Pirkle et al., 1989); 1987 (866 Ranch Hands; AFHS, 1991b); and 1992 (455 Ranch Hands; AFHS, 1995). Serum dioxin analysis of the 1987 follow-up examinations was published in 1991 (AFHS, 1991b).

Other Ranch Hand publications have addressed the relationship between serum dioxin and reproductive hormones (Henriksen et al., 1996); TCDD and diabetes mellitus, glucose, and insulin levels (Henriksen et al., 1997); and dioxin levels and infant death (Michalek et al., 1998a).

Since *Update 1998*, Burton et al. (1998) have investigated the incidence of skin disorders in veterans of Operation Ranch Hand, updating the previous study by Wolfe et al. (1990). Dermatological examinations were conducted in 1982, 1985, 1987, and 1992 by dermatologists who had undertaken a review program to become familiar with the clinical features of chloracne. Statistical analyses were adjusted for age, race, and military occupation. Veterans were excluded from the statistical analyses of acne located in the eyelids, ears, or temples if they had a history of acne prior to service in Southeast Asia or if they had no history of acne. Veterans were excluded if their dioxin concentration was missing. Data from 930 Ranch Hand and 1,200 comparison veterans were analyzed in the study. The association between categorized serum dioxin levels and chloracne, the occurrence of acne relative to the tour of duty in Southeast Asia, and the anatomical location of acne after service in Southeast Asia were investigated.

Michalek et al. (1998b) reported on a 15-year follow-up of postservice mortality in veterans of Operation Ranch Hand. The report updates cause-specific mortality in the population studied by Michalek et al. (1990) and described above. Cumulative mortality through December 31, 1993, for Ranch Hand veterans and comparison veterans was analyzed. There were 31 veterans whose service dates could not be located; these veterans were excluded from the analysis. A total of 1,261 Ranch Hands and 19,080 comparison veterans were included in the analysis. Exposure was based on military occupation. SMRs were calculated for major causes of death.

Michalek et al. (1998c) report the sex ratio in offspring of veterans of Operation Ranch Hand studied previously (Wolfe et al., 1990, 1995; Henriksen et al., 1996; Michalek et al., 1990). Sex ratios in offspring born after a father's service in Southeast Asia were evaluated in 1,208 Ranch Hand veterans and 1,549 comparison Vietnam veterans. Pregnancies were categorized as being conceived less than 1 month, 1 year, or 5 years after service or at any time during the postservice period. The percentage of female children was compared among dioxin exposure categories.

Michalek et al. (1998d) report on reproductive outcomes in the Vietnam veterans cohort of Wolfe et al. (1990). Reproductive outcomes were assessed in the health evaluations, including the 1992 health evaluation, by questions regarding the health of children. Participants were also asked to provide access to medical records documenting each pregnancy and the health of each child through 18 years of age. Histories of smoking and alcohol consumption during each pregnancy were obtained during interviews with wives and partners. Blood dioxin levels were estimated as described previously for this cohort. Attempts were made to verify pregnancies through retrieval of medical documents, birth certificates, death certificates, and autopsy reports. Attempts were made to verify the existence, lineage, birthweight, gestation, and vital status of all live births. Reproductive outcomes were assessed in singleton live births fathered by study participants with a quantifiable dioxin level, conceived during or after paternal service in Southeast Asia. Any unverifiable children, children of comparison veterans who had dioxin levels greater than 10 parts per trillion (ppt), and children without a recorded birthweight were excluded. The total number of children assessed in this study was 2,082 (1,223 children of comparison veterans, 859 children of veterans of Operation Ranch Hand). Relative risks were calculated for preterm birth, intrauterine growth retardation, and infant and neonatal death.

Ketchum et al. (1999) studied cancer and exposure to dioxin in Ranch Hand veterans, in the cohort previously described by Wolfe et al. (1990). Participants were examined, and medical records were retrieved in 1982, 1985, 1987, and 1992. Cancer was defined as a malignant neoplasm and was considered if it occurred in the postservice period. Veterans with cancer prior to service, with a missing dioxin measurement, with a dioxin measurement that could not be quantified, or with a cancer that could not be verified were excluded. All cancers and site-specific cancers were analyzed. The cancer analyses (except for skin cancer) were adjusted for birth year, military occupation, race, percentage of body fat at time of dioxin blood draw, smoking, alcohol consumption, and exposure to asbestos, ionizing radiation, industrial chemicals, herbicides, insecticides, and degreasing chemicals. Only nonblack veterans were included in the analysis of skin cancer; the analyses were not adjusted for race, smoking, alcohol consumption, and exposure to asbestos but were adjusted for skin coloring (dark, medium, pale, dark peach, pale peach), hair color, eye color, reaction of skin to 2 hours of sun, and average lifetime residential latitude.

Immunological responses in the cohort described by Wolfe et al. (1990) were examined (Michalek et al., 1999b). Veterans who had no dioxin measurement, or a nonquantifiable dioxin measurement, and comparison veterans with a dioxin measurement greater than 10 ppt, were excluded from the analyses. Veterans taking non-aspirin anti-inflammatory or immunosuppressant medication at the time of the 1992 exam, veterans who had recently received radiation or chemotherapy treatment for cancer, and veterans who tested positive for human immunodeficiency virus were also excluded. Exposure dioxin levels were estimated using serum levels and back-calculating with a constant half-life of 8.7 years. Exposures were categorized as background, low, or high as described above. Skin tests, immunoglobulin studies, and autoantibody panel tests were conducted on all subjects in the study; lymphocyte counts (total and subsets) were conducted on a random sample of the veterans (approximately 40 percent). Analyses were adjusted for percentage of body fat, age, race, military occupation, alcohol use, and smoking. Odds ratios were calculated for the various immunological end points.

Michalek et al. (1999a) studied insulin, fasting glucose, and sex hormone-binding globulin (SHBG) in the Ranch Hand cohort previously described by Wolfe et al. (1990). Medical records and laboratory results were reviewed to determine diabetic status. Veterans with a verified history of diabetes or with a postchallenge glucose of ≥200 mg/dl before July 1995 were classified as diabetic. Veterans taking hormone medications; individuals with cancer of the prostate, testes, or other genital organ; and individuals with a history of diabetes prior to service in Southeast Asia were excluded from the study because these cancers could confound examination of the outcomes of interest. Individuals without a dioxin measurement and comparison veterans with dioxin measurements greater than 10 ppt were also excluded. After exclusions, 871 exposed and 1,121 comparison veterans were included in correlation analyses for the end points of interest.

Longnecker and Michalek (2000) studied the relationship between serum dioxin levels and diabetes mellitus in Vietnam veterans who had never had contact with dioxin-contaminated herbicides (i.e., among the comparison veterans) because they were interested in health effects from background levels of dioxin. Diagnosis of diabetes (all were Type 2) was based on self-reported physician diagnosis and subsequent verification of medical records by June 1995 or a postchallenge glucose of ≥200 mg/dl in 1992. Any individuals with serum dioxin levels greater than 10 ng/kg lipid or with missing dioxin data, waist size, postchallenge glucose levels, or triglyceride levels were excluded. A total of 1,197 individuals were included in the cohort. Logistic regression was conducted to examine the relationship between diabetes and serum dioxin levels. Results were adjusted for race, military occupation, family history of diabetes, age, body mass index, waist size, and serum triglycerides (for odds ratios).

In February 2000, the Air Force Heath Study (AFHS) released a report based on data from the 1997 physical examination of Ranch Hand veterans and their comparison cohort (AFHS, 2000). The cohort is described above and by Wolfe et al. (1990). In this study, four different models were used to determine if there were any effects in veterans of Operation Ranch Hand.

Model 1 uses group (Ranch Hands, comparisons) and military occupation (officer, enlisted flycr, and enlisted ground crew) as proxies for exposure. As indicated above, prior AFHS analyses report that on average, enlisted ground crew had the highest dioxin exposure, followed by enlisted flyers, and then officers. This model does not include any direct dioxin measure.

Model 2 is applied only to Ranch Hands. The exposure estimate is an individual's serum dioxin level extrapolated to a time-of-exposure value (initial) adjusted for a 1987 body fat measure. Extrapolations were calculated based on a first-order elimination assumption of an exponential decrease in dioxin body burden with time; the half-life of 8.7 years is based on a sample of Ranch Hand participants with repeat dioxin measures over time. It is further limited to Ranch Hands with serum dioxin levels greater than 10 ppt measured at the 1987, 1992, or 1997 physical exam.

Model 3 divides the Ranch Hand veterans in Model 2 into two discrete dioxin categories—"low" and "high"—based on current serum dioxin levels extrapolated to initial values. This model also includes as a third category "background" Ranch Hand veterans who had been excluded from Model 2 because current serum dioxin measures were less than 10 ppt and as a fourth category all comparison subjects with serum levels less than 10 ppt. All exposure values are adjusted for 1987 body fat. The specific category definitions follow:

- *Comparisons*: comparison subjects with up to 10 ppt lipid-adjusted serum dioxin level
- *Background:* Ranch Hand veterans with up to 10 ppt lipid-adjusted serum dioxin level
- *Low:* Ranch Hand veterans with more than 10 ppt lipid-adjusted serum dioxin *but at most* 94 ppt estimated initial serum dioxin level
- *High:* Ranch Hand veterans with more than 10 ppt lipid-adjusted serum dioxin *and more than* 94 ppt estimated initial serum dioxin level

Model 4, restricted to the Ranch Hand cohort only, uses the serum dioxin level measured in 1987 (the year in which most Ranch Hand veterans were initially assayed) or a later measurement extrapolated to a 1987 value. All Ranch Hand veterans with available dioxin measurements were considered in Model 4 analyses, including those with levels less than 10 ppt who were excluded from Model 2 and treated as a separate category in Model 3.

Models 2, 3, and 4 all use the same 1987 serum dioxin measures (or later where a 1987 value was not available), and the authors note that the extrapolations in Models 2 and 3 assume that the dioxin elimination rate is constant across individuals. Models 2 and 3 use serum dioxin values adjusted for body fat at the time of dioxin measure. All four models were run both "unadjusted" and "adjusted" for a set of potential confounders: age, race, military occupation, personality type, body fat, and family history of diabetes.

The authors evaluated 266 health-related end points, including 10 clinical areas: general health, neoplasia, neurological, psychological, gastrointestinal, cardiovascular, hematologic, endocrine, immunologic, and pulmonary.

Centers for Disease Control and Prevention

The CDC has undertaken a series of studies to examine various health outcomes of Vietnam veterans, as directed by Congress (Veterans Health Programs Extension and Improvement Act of 1979, Public Law 96-151; and Veterans' Health Care, Training, and Small Business Loan Act of 1981, Public Law 97-72). *VAO* and *Update 1996* describe these studies in more detail. The first of these was a case-control interview study of birth defects among offspring of fathers serving in Vietnam (Erickson et al., 1984a,b).

To examine concerns about Agent Orange more directly, the CDC conducted the Agent Orange Validation Study to evaluate TCDD levels in U.S. Army veterans, compared to exposure estimates based on military records and TCDD levels of veterans who did not serve in Vietnam (CDC, 1989a). Using the exposure estimates from this study, the CDC subsequently conducted the Vietnam Experience Study (VES), a historical cohort study of the health experience of Vietnam veterans (CDC, 1989b). The study was divided into three parts: (1) physical health; (2) reproductive outcomes and child health; and (3) psychosocial characteristics (CDC, 1987, 1988a,b,c, 1989b).

Using data from the VES, the CDC also examined the postservice mortality (through 1983) of a cohort of 9,324 U.S. Army veterans who served in Vietnam, compared to 8,989 Vietnam era Army veterans who served in Korea, Germany, or the United States (Boyle et al., 1987; CDC, 1987). An additional study (O'Brien et al., 1991) combined the mortality and interview data to identify all veterans with NHL. To evaluate whether self-reported assessment of exposure to herbicides influences the reporting of adverse health outcomes, the CDC designed a study using VES subjects (Decoufle et al., 1992).

Finally, the CDC undertook the Selected Cancers Study (CDC, 1990a) to investigate the effects of military service in Vietnam and exposure to herbicides on the health of American veterans. Outcomes studied were NHL (CDC, 1990b); STS and other sarcomas (CDC, 1990c); and HD, nasal, nasopharyngeal, and primary liver cancers (CDC, 1990d).

No new CDC studies have been published.

Department of Veterans Affairs

The DVA has conducted numerous cohort and case-control studies, which *VAO*, *Update 1996*, and *Update 1998* discuss in greater detail. One of the first of these was a proportionate mortality study conducted by Breslin et al. (1988). Study subjects were ground troops who served in the U.S. Army or Marine Corps at any time from July 4, 1965, through March 1, 1973. A list of 186,000 Vietnam era veterans who served in the Army or Marine Corps and were reported deceased as of July 1, 1982, was assembled from DVA's BIRLS. A random sample of 75,617 names was selected from this group. Cause of death was ascertained for 51,421 men, including 24,235 who served in Vietnam. Based on this proportionate mortality study (Breslin et al., 1988), Burt et al. (1987) conducted a nested case-control study of NHL with controls selected from among the cardiovascular disease mortality deaths. Later, Bullman et al. (1990) examined whether Army I Corps Vietnam veterans had cancer mortality experiences similar to other Army Vietnam era veterans, based on the study design of Breslin et al. (1988). Watanabe et al. (1991) conducted an additional study comparing the Vietnam veteran mortality experience of Breslin et al. (1988) with three different referent groups and with additional follow-up through 1984. A third follow-up proportionate mortality study using the veterans from Breslin et al. (1988) and Watanabe et al. (1991) was also conducted (Watanabe and Kang, 1996).

The DVA also examined the morbidity and mortality experience of a subgroup of Vietnam veterans potentially exposed to high levels of herbicides from certain U.S. Army Chemical Corps units (Thomas and Kang, 1990). In an extension of Thomas and Kang (1990), Dalager and Kang (1997) compared mortality among veterans of the Chemical Corps specialties, including Vietnam veterans and non-Vietnam veterans. Watanabe and Kang (1995) also examined postservice mortality among Marine Vietnam veterans compared to Vietnam era Marines who did not actually serve in Vietnam. Mortality among women Vietnam veterans was assessed by Thomas et al. (1991) and updated in Dalager et al. (1995a).

The DVA has evaluated specific disease and health outcomes, including case-control studies of STS (Kang et al., 1986, 1987), NHL (Dalager et al., 1991), testicular cancer (Bullman et al., 1994), Hodgkin's disease (Dalager et al., 1995b), and lung cancer (Mahan et al., 1997), as well as conducting a co-twin study of self-reported physical health in a series of Vietnam era monozygotic twins (Eisen et al., 1991).

Other outcomes including posttraumatic stress disorder (PTSD) (True et al.,

1988; Bullman et al., 1991), suicide, motor vehicle accidents (Farberow et al., 1990), and smoking behavior (McKinney et al., 1997) among Vietnam veterans, as well as cause-specific mortality among veterans with nonlethal (combat and noncombat) wounds sustained during the Vietnam War (Bullman and Kang, 1996), have also been examined by the DVA. *VAO* and *Update 1998* discuss these studies in greater detail. In many of the studies, exposure to Agent Orange is not discussed; exposure to "combat" is evaluated as the risk factor of interest.

Since *Update 1998*, the DVA has published a study on pregnancy outcomes among U.S. women Vietnam veterans (Kang et al., 2000). Of a total of 5,230 women, 4,390 women whose permanent tour of duty included service in Vietnam were found alive as of January 1, 1992. From a pool of 6,657 potential control subjects whose military unit did not include service in Vietnam, 4,390 women who were alive as of January 1, 1992, were randomly selected as controls. A questionnaire was administered on demographic background; general health; lifestyle; menstrual history; pregnancy history; pregnancy outcomes; and military experience, including nursing occupation and combat exposure. Information on pregnancy complications, including smoking, infections, medications, exposure to X-rays, occupational history, exposure to anesthetic gases, ethylene oxide, herbicides, and pesticides was also collected for each pregnancy. The first pregnancy after the beginning of Vietnam service was designated as the index pregnancy for each woman. For the comparison group, the first pregnancy after July 4, 1965, was used as the index pregnancy. Odds ratios were calculated for reproductive history and pregnancy outcomes. A total of 3,392 Vietnam and 3,038 non-Vietnam veterans and a total of 1,665 Vietnam and 1,912 non-Vietnam veterans indexed pregnancies were analyzed in the study.

American Legion

The American Legion conducted a cohort study of the health and well-being of Vietnam veterans who belonged to the American Legion, a voluntary veterans service organization. A series of studies examining physical health and reproductive outcomes, social–behavioral consequences, and PTSD were conducted on veterans who had served in Southeast Asia compared with veterans who served elsewhere (Snow et al., 1988; Stellman et al., 1988a,b,c). No new studies have been published on this cohort.

State Studies

Several states have conducted studies of Vietnam veterans. Most of these studies remain unpublished in the scientific literature. *VAO* and *Update 1996* review studies from Hawaii (Rellahan, 1985); Iowa (Wendt, 1985); Maine (Deprez et al., 1991); Massachusetts (Kogan and Clapp, 1985, 1988; Levy, 1988; Clapp et al., 1991; Clapp, 1997); Michigan (Visintainer et al., 1995); New Jersey

(Kahn et al., 1988; Fielder and Gochfeld, 1992; Kahn et al., 1992a,b,c); New Mexico (Pollei et al., 1986); New York (Greenwald et al., 1984; Lawrence et al., 1985); Pennsylvania (Goun and Kuller, 1986); Texas (Newell, 1984); West Virginia (Holmes et al., 1986); and Wisconsin (Anderson et al., 1986a,b).

Other U.S. Vietnam Veteran Studies

Additional studies have been conducted to examine a number of health outcomes including spontaneous abortion (Aschengrau and Monson, 1989) and late adverse pregnancy outcomes in spouses of veterans (Aschengrau and Monson, 1990), and PTSD among monozygotic twins who served during the Vietnam era (Goldberg et al., 1990). After a published study indicating a potential association with testicular cancer in dogs that served in Vietnam (Hayes et al., 1990), Tarone et al. (1991) conducted a case-control study of testicular cancer in male veterans. *VAO* summarizes these studies, and no new studies have been published.

Australia

The Australian government has also commissioned studies to investigate the health risks of Australian veterans. Studies of birth anomalies (Donovan et al., 1983, 1984; Evatt, 1985); mortality (Commonwealth Institute of Health, 1984a,b,c; Evatt, 1985; Fett et al., 1987a,b; Forcier et al., 1987; Crane et al., 1997a,b); deaths from all causes (Fett et al., 1987b); and cause-specific mortality (Fett et al., 1987a) have been conducted. An independent study in Tasmania evaluated numerous reproductive and childhood health problems for association with paternal Vietnam service (Field and Kerr, 1988). In addition, O'Toole et al. (1996a,b,c) described self-reported health status in a random sample of Australian Army Vietnam veterans. *VAO* and *Update 1998* describe the studies.

Since *Update 1998*, the government of Australia has published three studies of Australian Vietnam veterans to assess the health and well-being of Vietnam veterans, their spouses, and their children (CDVA, 1998a,b; AIHW, 1999). Data on male veterans (CDVA, 1998a), data on female veterans (CDVA, 1998b), and a validation of the male veterans study (AIHW, 1999) have been published. All members of the Australian Defence Force and the Citizen Military Force who landed in Vietnam or entered Vietnamese water between May 1962 and July 1973 were considered Vietnam veterans. Besides those involved in combat, this included entertainers, medical teams, war correspondents, and philanthropy workers. All of these individuals who could be located were surveyed by mail. The self-report data gathered were compared with age-matched Australian national data. Three distinct questionnaires were mailed to male veterans (49,944 mailed, 80 percent response rate); female veterans (278 mailed, 81 percent response rate); and widow(er), separated, or divorced partners (691 mailed, 45.1 percent response rate). A comparable control group was not used; comparison was drawn by reference to community data for individuals of comparable age where data were available. The self-reported survey sent to male veterans inquired about their own health, both physical and mental; the physical and mental health of their partner(s) and children; and their reproductive history (CDVA, 1998a). A similar questionnaire was sent to female veterans (CDVA, 1998b). The study of female veterans, however, was limited by the small sample cohort—only 57 percent (278 of 484) of eligible veterans were located, and the authors speculated that married veterans were underrepresented in this sample since married women were more likely to have changed their name and thus less likely to have been found. The objective of the validation study was to medically confirm selected conditions, including a number of specific cancers and degenerative diseases of the nervous system in male Vietnam veterans and congenital abnormalities, cancers, and deaths in their children. The validation study population consisted of 6,842 male veterans and their children. Validation was done using medical documents (e.g., pathology results), doctor's certification (e.g., a response to a validation study questionnaire or a standard doctor's certificate), and records on a disease or death registry.

Other Vietnam Veteran Studies

A team of Vietnamese scientists examined Vietnamese veterans who served in a "dioxin-sprayed zone" looking at antinuclear and sperm autoantibodies (Chinh et al., 1996). Available details of this study are presented in *Update 1998*. No other studies in similar cohorts have been published.

OBSERVATIONS AND RESEARCH RECOMMENDATIONS

As noted above, the Air Force Health Study (AFHS) is an epidemiologic study whose purpose is to determine whether exposure to the herbicides used in Vietnam may be responsible for any adverse health conditions observed in a cohort of Air Force personnel responsible for conducting aerial spray missions (the Ranch Hands). A baseline morbidity study of the Ranch Hands and a matched comparison cohort (comprising over 2,000 individuals total) was conducted in 1982, with follow-up assessments in 1985, 1987, 1992, and 1997. In accordance with the study protocol, one additional assessment is planned for 2002, after which a final report will be issued.

Because the study represents one of the few primary sources of information on the health of Vietnam veterans and is coming close to its scheduled end, the committee believes it is timely to offer some observations and recommendations concerning it.

The AFHS cohorts represent an unusually thoroughly studied population. Some of the data generated in the course of the study are already or will soon be available to the public. However, there are also medical records and biological specimens that are not amenable to such public disclosure. The committee believes that there is scientific merit in retaining and maintaining these medical records and samples, so that—with proper respect for the privacy of the study participants—they could be available for future research. It therefore recommends that the federal government examine whether and how the various forms of data and specimens collected in the course of the Air Force Health Study could be retained and maintained, and what form of oversight should be established for their future use. The committee further recommends that consideration be given to whether it is appropriate to continue the study past its planned completion date. It notes that the AFHS cohorts are only now reaching the age where several health outcomes of interest may be expected to manifest. The committee cannot draw a conclusion on whether or not a continuation of research on the AFHS cohorts will inform specific questions regarding the health effects of exposure to the herbicides used in Vietnam. However, the committee's judgment is that continued research on the health of the Ranch Hand and Comparison veterans is likely to yield important information on the determinants of health and disease in males who served in the military during the Vietnam era and perhaps their offspring. If the records were to be retained and maintained and/or the research continued, this would have to be done with the full knowledge and consent of the AFHS population, and to be subject to controls that would respect the privacy of the participants.

REFERENCES

AFHS (Air Force Health Study). 1982. An Epidemiologic Investigation of Health Effects in Air Force Personnel Following Exposure to Herbicides: Study Protocol, Initial Report. Brooks AFB, TX: USAF School of Aerospace Medicine. SAM-TR-82-44. 189 pp.

AFHS. 1983. An Epidemiologic Investigation of Health Effects in Air Force Personnel Following Exposure to Herbicides. Baseline Mortality Study Results. Brooks AFB, TX: USAF School of Aerospace Medicine. NTIS AD-A130 793.

AFHS. 1984a. An Epidemiologic Investigation of Health Effects in Air Force Personnel Following Exposure to Herbicides. Baseline Morbidity Study Results. Brooks AFB, TX: USAF School of Aerospace Medicine. NTIS AD-A138 340. 362 pp.

AFHS. 1984b. An Epidemiologic Investigation of Health Effects in Air Force Personnel Following Exposure to Herbicides. Mortality Update: 1984. Brooks AFB, TX: USAF School of Aerospace Medicine.

AFHS. 1985. An Epidemiologic Investigation of Health Effects in Air Force Personnel Following Exposure to Herbicides. Mortality Update: 1985. Brooks AFB, TX: USAF School of Aerospace Medicine.

AFHS. 1986. An Epidemiologic Investigation of Health Effects in Air Force Personnel Following Exposure to Herbicides. Mortality Update: 1986. Brooks AFB, TX: USAF School of Aerospace Medicine. USAFSAM-TR-86-43. 12 pp.

AFHS. 1987. An Epidemiologic Investigation of Health Effects in Air Force Personnel Following Exposure to Herbicides. First Follow-up Examination Results. 2 vols. Brooks AFB, TX: USAF School of Aerospace Medicine. USAFSAM-TR-87-27. 629 pp.

AFHS. 1989. An Epidemiologic Investigation of Health Effects in Air Force Personnel Following Exposure to Herbicides. Mortality Update: 1989. Brooks AFB, TX: USAF School of Aerospace Medicine. USAFSAM-TR-89-9. 35 pp.

AFHS. 1990. An Epidemiologic Investigation of Health Effects in Air Force Personnel Following Exposure to Herbicides. 2 vols. Brooks AFB, TX: USAF School of Aerospace Medicine. USAFSAM-TR-90-2.

AFHS. 1991a. An Epidemiologic Investigation of Health Effects in Air Force Personnel Following Exposure to Herbicides. Mortality Update: 1991. Brooks AFB, TX: Armstrong Laboratory. AL-TR-1991-0132. 33 pp.

AFHS. 1991b. An Epidemiologic Investigation of Health Effects in Air Force Personnel Following Exposure to Herbicides. Serum Dioxin Analysis of 1987 Examination Results. Brooks AFB, TX: USAF School of Aerospace Medicine. 9 vols.

AHFS. 1992. An Epidemiologic Investigation of Health Effects in Air Force Personnel Following Exposure to Herbicides. Reproductive Outcomes. Brooks AFB, TX: Armstrong Laboratory. AL-TR-1992-0090. 602 pp.

AFHS. 1995. An Epidemiologic Investigation of Health Effects in Air Force Personnel Following Exposure to Herbicides. 1992 Follow-up Examination Results. 10 vols. Brooks AFB, TX: Epidemiologic Research Division; Armstrong Laboratory.

AFHS. 1996. An Epidemiologic Investigation of Health Effects in Air Force Personnel Following Exposure to Herbicides. Mortality Update 1996. Brooks AFB, TX: Epidemiologic Research Division; Armstrong Laboratory. AL/AO-TR-1996-0068. 31 pp.

AFHS. 2000. An Epidemiologic Investigation of Health Effects in Air Force Personnel Following Exposure to Herbicides. 1997 Follow-up Examination and Results. Reston, VA: Science Application International Corporation. F41624–96–C1012.

AIHW (Australian Institute of Health and Welfare). 1999. Morbidity of Vietnam Veterans: A Study of the Health of Australia's Vietnam Veteran Community: Volume 3: Validation Study. Canberra.

Alavanja MC, Blair A, Merkle S, Teske J, Eaton B. 1988. Mortality among agricultural extension agents. American Journal of Industrial Medicine 14:167–176.

Alavanja MC, Merkle S, Teske J, Eaton B, Reed B. 1989. Mortality among forest and soil conservationists. Archives of Environmental Health 44:94–101.

Alavanja MC, Sandler DP, Mcdonnell CJ, Lynch CF, Pennybacker M, Zahm SH, Lubin J, Mage D, Steen WC, Wintersteen W, Blair, A. 1998. Factors associated with self-reported, pesticide-related visits to health care providers in the agricultural health study. Environmental Health Perspectives 106(7):415–420.

Alderfer R, Sweeney M, Fingerhut M, Hornung R, Wille K, Fidler A. 1992. Measures of depressed mood in workers exposed to 2,3,7,8-tetrachlorodibenzo-p-dioxin (TCDD). Chemosphere 25: 247–250.

Amadori D, Nanni O, Falcini F, Saragoni A, Tison V, Callea A, Scarpi E, Ricci M, Riva N, Buiatti E. 1995. Chronic lymphocytic leukemias and non-Hodgkin's lymphomas by histological type in farming-animal breeding workers: a population case-control study based on job titles. Occupational and Environmental Medicine 52(6):374–379.

Anderson HA, Hanrahan LP, Jensen M, Laurin D, Yick WY, Wiegman P. 1986a. Wisconsin Vietnam Veteran Mortality Study: Proportionate Mortality Ratio Study Results. Madison: Wisconsin Division of Health.

Anderson HA, Hanrahan LP, Jensen M, Laurin D, Yick WY, Wiegman P. 1986b. Wisconsin Vietnam Veteran Mortality Study: Final Report. Madison: Wisconsin Division of Health.

Arbuckle TE, Schrader SM, Cole D, Hall JC, Bancej CM, Turner LA, Claman P. 1999. 2,4-Dichlorophenoxyacetic acid residues in semen of Ontario farmers. Reproductive Toxicology 13(6): 421–429.

Aschengrau A, Monson RR. 1989. Paternal military service in Vietnam and risk of spontaneous abortion. Journal of Occupational Medicine 31:618–623.
Aschengrau A, Monson RR. 1990. Paternal military service in Vietnam and the risk of late adverse pregnancy outcomes. American Journal of Public Health 80:1218–1224.
Asp S, Riihimaki V, Hernberg S, Pukkala E. 1994. Mortality and cancer morbidity of Finnish chlorophenoxy herbicide applicators: an 18-year prospective follow-up. American Journal of Industrial Medicine 26:243–253.
Assennato G, Cervino D, Emmett E, Longo G, Merlo F. 1989a. Follow-up of subjects who developed chloracne following TCDD exposure at Seveso. American Journal of Industrial Medicine 16:119–125.
Assennato G, Cannatelli P, Emmett E, Ghezzi I, Merlo F. 1989b. Medical monitoring of dioxin clean-up workers. American Industrial Hygiene Association Journal 50:586–592.
Axelson O, Sundell L. 1974. Herbicide exposure, mortality and tumor incidence. An epidemiological investigation on Swedish railroad workers. Scandinavian Journal of Work, Environment, and Health 11:21–28.
Axelson O, Sundell L, Andersson K, Edling C, Hogstedt C, Kling H. 1980. Herbicide exposure and tumor mortality: an updated epidemiologic investigation on Swedish railroad workers. Scandinavian Journal of Work, Environment, and Health 6:73–79.
Balarajan R, Acheson ED. 1984. Soft tissue sarcomas in agriculture and forestry workers. Journal of Epidemiology and Community Health 38:113–116.
Barbieri S, Pirovano C, Scarlato G, Tarchini P, Zappa A, Maranzana M. 1988. Long-term effects of 2,3,7,8-tetrachlorodibenzo-*p*-dioxin on the peripheral nervous system. Clinical and neurophysiological controlled study on subjects with chloracne from the Seveso area. Neuroepidemiology 7:29–37.
Barthel E. 1981. Increased risk of lung cancer in pesticide-exposed male agricultural workers. Journal of Toxicology and Environmental Health 8:1027–1040.
Bashirov AA. 1969. The health of workers involved in the production of amine and butyl 2,4-D herbicides. Vrachebnoye Delo 10:92–95.
Becher H, Flesch-Janys D, Kauppinen T, Kogevinas M, Steindorf K, Manz A, Wahrendorf J. 1996. Cancer mortality in German male workers exposed to phenoxy herbicides and dioxins. Cancer Causes and Control 7(3):312–321.
Bender AP, Parker DL, Johnson RA, Scharber WK, Williams AN, Marbury MC, Mandel JS. 1989. Minnesota highway maintenance worker study: cancer mortality. American Journal of Industrial Medicine 15:545–556.
Bertazzi PA, Zocchetti C, Pesatori AC, Guercilena S, Sanarico M, Radice L. 1989a. Mortality in an area contaminated by TCDD following an industrial incident. Medicina Del Lavoro 80:316–329.
Bertazzi PA, Zocchetti C, Pesatori AC, Guercilena S, Sanarico M, Radice L. 1989b. Ten-year mortality study of the population involved in the Seveso incident in 1976. American Journal of Epidemiology 129:1187–1200.
Bertazzi PA, Zocchetti C, Pesatori AC, Guercilena S, Consonni D, Tironi A, Landi MT. 1992. Mortality of a young population after accidental exposure to 2,3,7,8-tetrachlorodibenzodioxin. International Journal of Epidemiology 21:118–123.
Bertazzi A, Pesatori AC, Consonni D, Tironi A, Landi MT, Zocchetti C. 1993. Cancer incidence in a population accidentally exposed to 2,3,7,8-tetrachlorodibenzo-*para*-dioxin [see comments]. Epidemiology 4:398–406.
Bertazzi PA, Zochetti C, Guercilena S, Consonni D, Tironi A, Landi MT, Pesatori AC. 1997. Dioxin exposure and cancer risk: a 15-year mortality study after the "Seveso accident." Epidemiology 8(6):646–652.

Bertazzi PA, Bernucci I, Brambilla G, Consonni D, Pesatori AC. 1998. The Seveso studies on early and long-term effects of dioxin exposure: a review. Environmental Health Perspectives 106 (Suppl 2):625–633.

Bertazzi PA, Consonni D, Bachetti S, Rubagotti M, Baccarelli A, Zocchetti C, Pesatori AC. 2001. Health effects of dioxin exposure: a 20-year mortality study. American Journal of Epidemiology 153911):1031–1044.

Bisanti L, Bonetti F, Caramaschi F, Del Corno G, Favaretti C, Giambelluca SE, Marni E, Montesarchio E, Puccinelli V, Remotti G, Volpato C, Zambrelli E, Fara GM. 1980. Experiences from the accident of Seveso. Acta Morphologica Academiae Scientarum Hungaricae 28:139–157.

Blair A, Thomas TL. 1979. Leukemia among Nebraska farmers: a death certificate study. American Journal of Epidemiology 110:264–273.

Blair A, White DW. 1985. Leukemia cell types and agricultural practices in Nebraska. Archives of Environmental Health 40:211–214.

Blair A, Grauman DJ, Lubin JH, Fraumeni JF Jr. 1983. Lung cancer and other causes of death among licensed pesticide applicators. Journal of the National Cancer Institute 71:31–37.

Blair A, Mustafa D, Heineman EF. 1993. Cancer and other causes of death among male and female farmers from twenty-three states. American Journal of Industrial Medicine 23:729–742.

Blatter BM, Hermens R, Bakker M, Roeleveld N, Verbeek AL, Zielhuis GA. 1997. Paternal occupational exposure around conception and spina bifida in offspring. American Journal of Industrial Medicine 32(3):283–291.

Bloemen LJ, Mandel JS, Bond GG, Pollock AF, Vitek RP, Cook RR. 1993. An update of mortality among chemical workers potentially exposed to the herbicide 2,4-dichlorophenoxyacetic acid and its derivatives. Journal of Occupational Medicine 35:1208–1212.

Boeri R, Bordo B, Crenna P, Filippini G, Massetto M, Zecchini A. 1978. Preliminary results of a neurological investigation of the population exposed to TCDD in the Seveso region. Rivista di Patologia Nervosa e Mentale 99:111–128.

Boffetta P, Stellman SD, Garfinkel L. 1989. A case-control study of multiple myeloma nested in the American Cancer Society prospective study. International Journal of Cancer 43:554–559.

Bond GG, Ott MG, Brenner FE, Cook RR. 1983. Medical and morbidity surveillance findings among employees potentially exposed to TCDD. British Journal of Industrial Medicine 40:318–324.

Bond GG, Cook RR, Brenner FE, McLaren EA. 1987. Evaluation of mortality patterns among chemical workers with chloracne. Chemosphere 16:2117–2121.

Bond GG, Wetterstroem NH, Roush GJ, McLaren EA, Lipps TE, Cook RR. 1988. Cause specific mortality among employees engaged in the manufacture, formulation, or packaging of 2,4-dichlorophenoxyacetic acid and related salts. British Journal of Industrial Medicine 45:98–105.

Bond GG, McLaren EA, Brenner FE, Cook RR. 1989a. Incidence of chloracne among chemical workers potentially exposed to chlorinated dioxins. Journal of Occupational Medicine 31:771–774.

Bond GG, McLaren EA, Lipps TE, Cook RR. 1989b. Update of mortality among chemical workers with potential exposure to the higher chlorinated dioxins. Journal of Occupational Medicine 31:121–123.

Boyle C, Decoufle P, Delaney RJ, DeStefano F, Flock ML, Hunter MI, Joesoef MR, Karon JM, Kirk ML, Layde PM, McGee DL, Moyer LA, Pollock DA, Rhodes P, Scally MJ, Worth RM. 1987. Postservice Mortality Among Vietnam Veterans. Atlanta: Centers for Disease Control. CEH 86-0076. 143 pp.

Breslin P, Kang H, Lee Y, Burt V, Shepard BM. 1988. Proportionate mortality study of U.S. Army and U.S. Marine Corps veterans of the Vietnam War. Journal of Occupational Medicine 30:412–419.

Brown LM, Blair A, Gibson R, Everett GD, Cantor KP, Schuman LM, Burmeister LF, Van Lier SF, Dick F. 1990. Pesticide exposures and other agricultural risk factors for leukemia among men in Iowa and Minnesota. Cancer Research 50:6585–6591.

Brown LM, Burmeister LF, Everett GD, Blair A. 1993. Pesticide exposures and multiple myeloma in Iowa men. Cancer Causes and Control 4:153–156.

Bueno de Mesquita HB, Doornbos G, van der Kuip DA, Kogevinas M, Winkelmann R. 1993. Occupational exposure to phenoxy herbicides and chlorophenols and cancer mortality in the Netherlands. American Journal of Industrial Medicine 23:289–300.

Bullman TA, Kang HK. 1996. The risk of suicide among wounded Vietnam veterans. American Journal of Public Health 86(5):662–667.

Bullman TA, Kang HK, Watanabe KK. 1990. Proportionate mortality among U.S. Army Vietnam veterans who served in Military Region I. American Journal of Epidemiology 132:670–674.

Bullman TA, Kang H, Thomas TL. 1991. Posttraumatic stress disorder among Vietnam veterans on the Agent Orange Registry: a case-control analysis. Annals of Epidemiology 1:505–512.

Bullman TA, Watanabe KK, Kang HK. 1994. Risk of testicular cancer associated with surrogate measures of Agent Orange exposure among Vietnam veterans on the Agent Orange Registry. Annals of Epidemiology 4:11–16.

Burmeister LF. 1981. Cancer mortality in Iowa farmers: 1971–1978. Journal of the National Cancer Institute 66:461–464.

Burmeister LF, Van Lier SF, Isacson P. 1982. Leukemia and farm practices in Iowa. American Journal of Epidemiology 115:720–728.

Burmeister LF, Everett GD, Van Lier SF, Isacson P. 1983. Selected cancer mortality and farm practices in Iowa. American Journal of Epidemiology 118:72–77.

Burt VL, Breslin PP, Kang HK, Lee Y. 1987. Non-Hodgkin's lymphoma in Vietnam veterans. Washington, DC: Department of Medicine and Surgery, Veterans Administration.

Burton JE, Michalek JE, Rahe AJ. 1998. Serum dioxin, chloracne, and acne in veterans of Operation Ranch Hand. Archives of Environmental Health 53(3):199–204.

Butterfield PG, Valanis BG, Spencer PS, Lindeman CA, Nutt JG. 1993. Environmental antecedents of young-onset Parkinson's disease. Neurology 43:1150–1158.

Calvert GM, Sweeney MH, Morris JA, Fingerhut MA, Hornung RW, Halperin WE. 1991. Evaluation of chronic bronchitis, chronic obstructive pulmonary disease, and ventilatory function among workers exposed to 2,3,7,8-tetrachlorodibenzo-p-dioxin. American Review of Respiratory Disease 144:1302–1306.

Calvert GM, Hornung RW, Sweeney MH, Fingerhut MA, Halperin WE. 1992. Hepatic and gastrointestinal effects in an occupational cohort exposed to 2,3,7,8-tetrachlorodibenzo-*para*-dioxin. Journal of the American Medical Association 267:2209–2214.

Calvert GM, Sweeney MH, Fingerhut MA, Hornung RW, Halperin WE. 1994. Evaluation of porphyria cutanea tarda in U.S. workers exposed to 2,3,7,8-tetrachlorodibenzo-p-dioxin. American Journal of Industrial Medicine 25:559–571.

Calvert GM, Wall DK, Sweeney MH, Fingerhut MA. 1998. Evaluation of cardiovascular outcomes among U.S. workers exposed to 2,3,7,8-tetrachlorodibenzo-p-dioxin. Environmental Health Perspectives 106(Suppl 2):635–643.

Calvert GM, Sweeney MH, Deddens J, Wall DK. 1999. Evaluation of diabetes mellitus, serum glucose, and thyroid function among United States workers exposed to 2,3,7,8-tetrachlorodibenzo-p-dioxin. Occupational and Environmental Medicine 56(4):270–276.

Can N, Xiem NT, Tong NK, Duong DB. 1983a. A case-control survey of congenital defects in My Van District, Hai Hung Province. Summarized in: Constable JD, Hatch MC. Reproductive effects of herbicide exposure in Vietnam: recent studies by the Vietnamese and others. Teratogenesis, Carcinogenesis, and Mutagenesis 5:231–250, 1985.

Can N, Xiem NT, Tong NK, Duong DB. 1983b. An epidemiologic survey of pregnancies in Viet Nam. Summarized in: Constable JD, Hatch MC. Reproductive effects of herbicide exposure in Vietnam: recent studies by the Vietnamese and others. Teratogenesis, Carcinogenesis, and Mutagenesis 5:231–250, 1985.

Cantor KP. 1982. Farming and mortality from non-Hodgkin's lymphoma: a case-control study. International Journal of Cancer 29:239–247.

Cantor KP, Blair A, Everett G, Gibson R, Burmeister LF, Brown LM, Schuman L, Dick FR. 1992. Pesticides and other agricultural risk factors for non-Hodgkin's lymphoma among men in Iowa and Minnesota. Cancer Research 52:2447–2455.

Caramaschi F, Del Corno G, Favaretti C, Giambelluca SE, Montesarchio E, Fara GM. 1981. Chloracne following environmental contamination by TCDD in Seveso, Italy. International Journal of Epidemiology 10:135–143.

Carmelli D, Hofherr L, Tomsic J, Morgan RW. 1981. A Case-Control Study of the Relationship Between Exposure to 2,4-D and Spontaneous Abortions in Humans. SRI International. Prepared for the National Forest Products Association and the U.S. Department of Agriculture, Forest Service.

Cartwright RA, McKinney PA, O'Brien C, Richards IDG, Roberts B, Lauder I, Darwin CM, Bernard SM, Bird CC. 1988. Non-Hodgkin's lymphoma: case-control epidemiological study in Yorkshire. Leukemia Research 12:81–88.

CDC (Centers for Disease Control). 1987. Postservice mortality among Vietnam veterans. Journal of the American Medical Association 257:790–795.

CDC. 1988a. Health status of Vietnam veterans. I. Psychosocial characteristics. Journal of the American Medical Association 259:2701–2707.

CDC. 1988b. Health status of Vietnam veterans. II. Physical health. Journal of the American Medical Association 259:2708–2714.

CDC. 1988c. Health status of Vietnam veterans. III. Reproductive outcomes and child health. Journal of the American Medical Association 259:2715–2717.

CDC. 1989a. Comparison of Serum Levels of 2,3,7,8-Tetrachlorodibenzo-p-Dioxin with Indirect Estimates of Agent Orange Exposure Among Vietnam Veterans: Final Report. Atlanta: U.S. Department of Health and Human Services.

CDC. 1989b. Health Status of Vietnam Veterans: Vietnam Experience Study. Vols. I–V, Supplements A–C. Atlanta: U.S. Department of Health and Human Services.

CDC. 1990a. The Association of Selected Cancers with Service in the U.S. Military in Vietnam: Final Report. Atlanta: U.S. Department of Health and Human Services.

CDC. 1990b. The association of selected cancers with service in the U.S. military in Vietnam. I. Non-Hodgkin's lymphoma. Archives of Internal Medicine 150:2473–2483.

CDC. 1990c. The association of selected cancers with service in the U.S. military in Vietnam. II. Soft-tissue and other sarcomas. Archives of Internal Medicine 150:2485–2492.

CDC. 1990d. The association of selected cancers with service in the U.S. military in Vietnam. III. Hodgkin's disease, nasal cancer, nasopharyngeal cancer, and primary liver cancer. Archives of Internal Medicine 150:2495–2505.

CDVA (Commonwealth Department of Veterans' Affairs). 1998a. Morbidity of Vietnam Veterans: A Study of the Health of Australia's Vietnam Veteran Community. Volume 1: Male Vietnam Veterans Survey and Community Comparison Outcomes. Canberra: Department of Veterans' Affairs.

CDVA. 1998b. Morbidity of Vietnam Veterans: A Study of the Health of Australia's Vietnam Veteran Community. Volume 2: Female Vietnam Veterans Survey and Community Comparison Outcomes. Canberra: Department of Veterans' Affairs.

Chinh TT, Phi PT, Thuy NT. 1996. Sperm auto-antibodies and anti-nuclear antigen antibodies in chronic dioxin-exposed veterans. Chemosphere 32(3):525–530.

Clapp RW. 1997. Update of cancer surveillance of veterans in Massachusetts, USA. International Journal of Epidemiology 26(3):679–681.

Clapp RW, Cupples LA, Colton T, Ozonoff DM. 1991. Cancer surveillance of veterans in Massachusetts, 1982–1988. International Journal of Epidemiology 20:7–12.

Coggon D, Pannett B, Winter PD, Acheson ED, Bonsall J. 1986. Mortality of workers exposed to 2-methyl-4-chlorophenoxyacetic acid. Scandinavian Journal of Work, Environment, and Health 12:448–454.

Coggon D, Pannett B, Winter P. 1991. Mortality and incidence of cancer at four factories making phenoxy herbicides. British Journal of Industrial Medicine 48:173–178.

Collins JJ, Strauss ME, Levinskas GJ, Conner PR. 1993. The mortality experience of workers exposed to 2,3,7,8-tetrachlorodibenzo-p-dioxin in a trichlorophenol process accident. Epidemiology 4:7–13.

Commonwealth Institute of Health. 1984a. Australian Veterans Health Studies. Mortality Report. Part I. A Retrospective Cohort Study of Mortality Among Australian National Servicemen of the Vietnam Conflict Era, and Executive Summary of the Mortality Report. Canberra: Australian Government Publishing Service.

Commonwealth Institute of Health. 1984b. Australian Veterans Health Studies. The Mortality Report. Part II. Factors Influencing Mortality Rates of Australian National Servicemen of the Vietnam Conflict Era. Canberra: Australian Government Publishing Service.

Commonwealth Institute of Health. 1984c. Australian Veterans Health Studies. The Mortality Report. Part III. The Relationship Between Aspects of Vietnam Service and Subsequent Mortality Among Australian National Servicemen of the Vietnam Conflict Era. Canberra: Australian Government Publishing Service.

Constable JD, Hatch MC. 1985. Reproductive effects of herbicide exposure in Vietnam: recent studies by the Vietnamese and others. Teratogenesis, Carcinogenesis, and Mutagenesis 5:231–250.

Cook RR, Townsend JC, Ott MG, Silverstein LG. 1980. Mortality experience of employees exposed to 2,3,7,8-tetrachlorodibenzo-p-dioxin (TCDD). Journal of Occupational Medicine 22:530–532.

Cook RR, Bond GG, Olson RA. 1986. Evaluation of the mortality experience of workers exposed to the chlorinated dioxins. Chemosphere 15:1769–1776.

Cook RR, Bond GG, Olson RA, Ott MG. 1987. Update of the mortality experience of workers exposed to chlorinated dioxins. Chemosphere 16:2111–2116.

Cordier S, Le TB, Verger P, Bard D, Le CD, Larouze B, Dazza MC, Hoang TQ, Abenhaim L. 1993. Viral infections and chemical exposures as risk factors for hepatocellular carcinoma in Vietnam. International Journal of Cancer 55:196–201.

Corrao G, Caller M, Carle F, Russo R, Bosia S, Piccioni P. 1989. Cancer risk in a cohort of licensed pesticide users. Scandinavian Journal of Work, Environment, and Health 15:203–209.

Crane PJ, Barnard DL, Horsley KW, Adena MA. 1997a. Mortality of Vietnam veterans: the veteran cohort study. A report of the 1996 retrospective cohort study of Australian Vietnam veterans. Canberra: Department of Veterans' Affairs.

Crane PJ, Barnard DL, Horsley KW, Adena MA. 1997b. Mortality of National Service Vietnam veterans: A report of the 1996 retrospective cohort study of Australian Vietnam veterans. Canberra: Department of Veterans' Affairs.

Dai LC, Phuong NTN, Thom LH, Thuy TT, Van NTT, Cam LH, Chi HTK, Thuy LB. 1990. A comparison of infant mortality rates between two Vietnamese villages sprayed by defoliants in wartime and one unsprayed village. Chemosphere 20:1005–1012.

Dalager NA, Kang HK. 1997. Mortality among Army Chemical Corps Vietnam veterans. American Journal of Industrial Medicine 31(6):719–726.

Dalager NA, Kang HK, Burt VL, Weatherbee L. 1991. Non-Hodgkin's lymphoma among Vietnam veterans. Journal of Occupational Medicine 33:774–779.

Dalager NA, Kang HK, Thomas TL. 1995a. Cancer mortality patterns among women who served in the military: the Vietnam experience. Journal of Occupational and Environmental Medicine 37:298–305.

Dalager NA, Kang HK, Burt VL, Weatherbee L. 1995b. Hodgkin's disease and Vietnam service. Annals of Epidemiology 5(5):400–406.

Dean G. 1994. Deaths from primary brain cancers, lymphatic and haematopoietic cancers in agricultural workers in the Republic of Ireland. Journal of Epidemiology and Community Health 48:364–368.

Decoufle P, Holmgreen P, Boyle CA, Stroup NE. 1992. Self-reported health status of Vietnam veterans in relation to perceived exposure to herbicides and combat. American Journal of Epidemiology 135:312–323.

Deprez RD, Carvette ME, Agger MS. 1991. The Health and Medical Status of Maine Veterans: A Report to the Bureau of Veterans Services, Commission of Vietnam and Atomic Veterans. Portland, ME: Public Health Resource Group.

Dich J, Wiklund K. 1998. Prostate cancer in pesticide applicators in Swedish agriculture. Prostate 34(2):100–112.

Dimich-Ward H, Hertzman C, Teschke K, Hershler R, Marion SA, Ostry A, Kelly S. 1996. Reproductive effects of paternal exposure to chlorophenate wood preservatives in the sawmill industry. Scandinavian Journal of Work, Environment, and Health 22(4):267–273.

Donna A, Betta PG, Robutti F, Crosignani P, Berrino F, Bellingeri D. 1984. Ovarian mesothelial tumors and herbicides: a case-control study. Carcinogenesis 5:941–942.

Donovan JW, Adena MA, Rose G, Battistutta D. 1983. Case-Control Study of Congenital Anomalies and Vietnam Service: Birth Defects Study. Report to the Minister for Veterans' Affairs. Canberra: Australian Government Publishing Service.

Donovan JW, MacLennan R, Adena M. 1984. Vietnam service and the risk of congenital anomalies: a case-control study. Medical Journal of Australia 140:394–397.

Dubrow R, Paulson JO, Indian RW. 1988. Farming and malignant lymphoma in Hancock County, Ohio. British Journal of Industrial Medicine 45:25–28.

Egeland GM, Sweeney MH, Fingerhut MA, Wille KK, Schnorr TM, Halperin WE. 1994. Total serum testosterone and gonadotropins in workers exposed to dioxin. American Journal of Epidemiology 139:272–281.

Eisen S, Goldberg J, True WR, Henderson WG. 1991. A co-twin control study of the effects of the Vietnam War on the self-reported physical health of veterans. American Journal of Epidemiology 134:49–58.

Ekstrom AM, Eriksson M, Hansson LE, Lindgren A, Signorello LB, Nyren O, Hardell L. 1999. Occupational exposures and risk of gastric cancer in a population-based case-control study. Cancer Research 59(23):5932–5937.

Erickson JD, Mulinare J, McClain PW, Fitch TG, James LM, McClearn AB, Adams MJ Jr. 1984a. Vietnam Veterans' Risks for Fathering Babies with Birth Defects. Atlanta: U.S. Department of Health and Human Services, Centers for Disease Control.

Erickson JD, Mulinare J, McClain PW, Fitch TG, James LM, McClearn AB, Adams MJ Jr. 1984b. Vietnam veterans' risks for fathering babies with birth defects. Journal of the American Medical Association 252:903–912.

Eriksson M, Hardell L, Berg NO, Moller T, Axelson O. 1979. Case-control study on malignant mesenchymal tumor of the soft tissue and exposure to chemical substances. Lakartidningen 76:3872–3875 [in Swedish].

Eriksson M, Hardell L, Berg NO, Moller T, Axelson O. 1981. Soft-tissue sarcomas and exposure to chemical substances: a case-referent study. British Journal of Industrial Medicine 38:27–33.

Eriksson M, Hardell L, Adami HO. 1990. Exposure to dioxins as a risk factor for soft tissue sarcoma: a population-based case-control study. Journal of the National Cancer Institute 82:486–490.

Eriksson M, Hardell L, Malker H, Weiner J. 1992. Malignant lymphoproliferative diseases in occupations with potential exposure to phenoxyacetic acids or dioxins: a register-based study. American Journal of Industrial Medicine 22:305–312.

Evans RG, Webb KB, Knutsen AP, Roodman ST, Roberts DW, Bagby JR, Garrett WA Jr, Andrews JS Jr. 1988. A medical follow-up of the health effects of long-term exposure to 2,3,7,8-tetrachlorodibenzo-p-dioxin. Archives of Environmental Health 43:273–278.

Evatt P. 1985. Royal Commission on the Use and Effect of Chemical Agents on Australian Personnel in Vietnam, Final Report. Canberra: Australian Government Publishing Service. 9 vols.

Farberow NL, Kang H, Bullman T. 1990. Combat experience and postservice psychosocial status as predictors of suicide in Vietnam veterans. Journal of Nervous and Mental Disease 178:32–37.

Faustini A. Settimi L, Pacifici R, Fano V, Zuccaro P, Forastiere F. 1996. Immunological changes among farmers exposed to phenoxy herbicides: preliminary observations. Occupational and Environmental Medicine 53(9):583–585.

Fett MJ, Adena MA, Cobbin DM, Dunn M. 1987a. Mortality among Australian conscripts of the Vietnam conflict era. I. Death from all causes. American Journal of Epidemiology 126:869–877.

Fett MJ, Nairn JR, Cobbin DM, Adena MA. 1987b. Mortality among Australian conscripts of the Vietnam conflict era. II. Causes of death. American Journal of Epidemiology 125:878–884.

Field B, Kerr C. 1988. Reproductive behaviour and consistent patterns of abnormality in offspring of Vietnam veterans. Journal of Medical Genetics 25:819–826.

Fielder N, Gochfeld M. 1992. Neurobehavioral Correlates of Herbicide Exposure in Vietnam Veterans. New Jersey Agent Orange Commission.

Filippini G, Bordo B, Crenna P, Massetto N, Musicco M, Boeri R. 1981. Relationship between clinical and electrophysiological findings and indicators of heavy exposure to 2,3,7,8-tetrachlorodibenzodioxin. Scandinavian Journal of Work, Environment, and Health 7:257–262.

Fingerhut MA, Halperin WE, Marlow DA, Piacitelli LA, Honchar PA, Sweeney MH, Greife AL, Dill PA, Steenland K, Suruda AJ. 1991. Cancer mortality in workers exposed to 2,3,7,8-tetrachlorodibenzo-p-dioxin. New England Journal of Medicine 324:212–218.

Fitzgerald EF, Weinstein AL, Youngblood LG, Standfast SJ, Melius JM. 1989. Health effects three years after potential exposure to the toxic contaminants of an electrical transformer fire. Archives of Environmental Health 44:214–221.

Flesch-Janys D. 1997. Analyses of exposure to polychlorinated dibenzo-p-dioxins, furans, and hexachlorocyclohexane and different health outcomes in a cohort of former herbicide-producing workers in Hamburg, Germany. Teratogenesis, Carcinogenesis and Mutagenesis 17(4-5):257–264.

Flesch-Janys D, Berger J, Gurn P, Manz A, Nagel S, Waltsgott H, Dwyer. 1995. Exposure to polychlorinated dioxins and furans (PCDD/F) and mortality in a cohort of workers from a herbicide-producing plant in Hamburg, Federal Republic of Germany. American Journal of Epidemiology 142(11):1165–1175.

Flesch-Janys D, Becher H, Gurn P, et al. 1996. Elimination of polychlorinated dibenzo-p-dioxins and dibenzofurans in occupationally exposed persons. Journal of Toxicology and Environmental Health 47(4):363–378.

Forcier L, Hudson HM, Cobbin DM, Jones MP, Adena MA, Fett MJ. 1987. Mortality of Australian veterans of the Vietnam conflict and the period and location of their Vietnam service. Military Medicine 152:9–15.

Gallagher RP, Bajdik CD, Fincham S, Hill GB, Keefe AR, Coldman A, McLean DI. 1996. Chemical exposures, medical history, and risk of squamous and basal cell carcinoma of the skin. Cancer Epidemiology, Biomarkers and Prevention 5(6):419–424.

Gambini GF, Mantovani C, Pira E, Piolatto PG, Negri E. 1997. Cancer mortality among rice growers in Novara Province, northern Italy. American Journal of Industrial Medicine 31(4):435–441.

Garcia AM, Benavides FG, Fletcher T, Orts E. 1998. Paternal exposure to pesticides and congenital malformations. Scandinavian Journal of Work, Environment and Health 24(6):473–480.

Garry VF, Kelly JT, Sprafka JM, Edwards S, Griffith J. 1994. Survey of health and use characterization of pesticide appliers in Minnesota. Archives of Environmental Health 49:337–343.

Garry VF, Tarone RE, Long L, Griffith J, Kelly JT, Burroughs B. 1996a. Pesticide appliers with mixed pesticide exposure: G-banded analysis and possible relationship to non-Hodgkin's lymphoma. Cancer Epidemiology, Biomarkers and Prevention 5(1):11–16.

Garry VF, Schreinemachers D, Harkins ME, Griffith J. 1996b. Pesticide appliers, biocides, and birth defects in rural Minnesota. Environmental Health Perspectives 104(4):394–399.

Goldberg J, True WR, Eisen SA, Henderson WG. 1990. A twin study of the effects of the Vietnam war on posttraumatic stress disorder. Journal of the American Medical Association 263:1227–1232.

Gordon JE, Shy CM. 1981. Agricultural chemical use and congenital cleft lip and/or palate. Archives of Environmental Health 36:213–221.

Goun BD, Kuller LH. 1986. Final Report: A Case-Control Mortality Study on the Association of Soft Tissue Sarcomas, Non-Hodgkin's Lymphomas, and Other Selected Cancers and Vietnam Military Service in Pennsylvania Males. Pittsburgh, PA: University of Pittsburgh.

Green LM. 1987. Suicide and exposure to phenoxy acid herbicides. Scandinavian Journal of Work, Environment, and Health 13:460.

Green LM. 1991. A cohort mortality study of forestry workers exposed to phenoxy acid herbicides. British Journal of Industrial Medicine 48:234–238.

Greenwald P, Kovasznay B, Collins DN, Therriault G. 1984. Sarcomas of soft tissues after Vietnam service. Journal of the National Cancer Institute 73:1107–1109.

Halperin W, Kalow W, Sweeney MH, Tang BK, Fingerhut M, Timpkins B, Wille K. 1995. Induction of P-450 in workers exposed to dioxin. Occupational and Environmental Medicine 52(2):86–91.

Halperin W, Vogt R, Sweeney MH, Shopp G, Fingerhut M, Petersen M. 1998. Immunological markers among workers exposed to 2,3,7,8-tetrachlorodibenzo-*p*-dioxin. Occupational and Environmental Medicine 55(11):742–749.

Hanify JA, Metcalf P, Nobbs CL, Worsley KJ. 1981. Aerial spraying of 2,4,5-T and human birth malformations: an epidemiological investigation. Science 212:349–351.

Hansen ES, Hasle H, Lander F. 1992. A cohort study on cancer incidence among Danish gardeners. American Journal of Industrial Medicine 21:651–660.

Hardell L. 1977. Malignant mesenchymal tumors and exposure to phenoxy acids: a clinical observation. Lakartidningen 74:2753–2754 [in Swedish].

Hardell L. 1979. Malignant lymphoma of histiocytic type and exposure to phenoxyacetic acids or chlorophenols. Lancet 1(8106):55–56.

Hardell L. 1981. Relation of soft-tissue sarcoma, malignant lymphoma and colon cancer to phenoxy acids, chlorophenols and other agents. Scandinavian Journal of Work, Environment, and Health 7:119–130.

Hardell L, Eriksson M. 1988. The association between soft tissue sarcomas and exposure to phenoxyacetic acids: a new case-referent study. Cancer 62:652–656.

Hardell L, Eriksson M. 1999. A case-control study of non-Hodgkin lymphoma and exposure to pesticides. Cancer 85(6):1353–1360.

Hardell L, Sandstrom A. 1979. Case-control study: soft-tissue sarcomas and exposure to phenoxyacetic acids or chlorophenols. British Journal of Cancer 39:711–717.

Hardell L, Bengtsson NO. 1983. Epidemiological study of socioeconomic factors and clinical findings in Hodgkin's disease, and reanalysis of previous data regarding chemical exposure. British Journal of Cancer 48:217–225.

Hardell L, Eriksson M, Lenner P. 1980. Malignant lymphoma and exposure to chemical substances, especially organic solvents, chlorophenols and phenoxy acids. Lakartidningen 77:208–210.

Hardell L, Eriksson M, Lenner P, Lundgren E. 1981. Malignant lymphoma and exposure to chemicals, especially organic solvents, chlorophenols and phenoxy acids: a case-control study. British Journal of Cancer 43:169–176.

Hardell L, Johansson B, Axelson O. 1982. Epidemiological study of nasal and nasopharyngeal cancer and their relation to phenoxy acid or chlorophenol exposure. American Journal of Industrial Medicine 3:247–257.

Hardell L, Bengtsson NO, Jonsson U, Eriksson S, Larsson LG. 1984. Aetiological aspects on primary liver cancer with special regard to alcohol, organic solvents and acute intermittent porphyria: an epidemiological investigation. British Journal of Cancer 50:389–397.

Hardell L, Moss A, Osmond D, Volberding P. 1987. Exposure to hair dyes and polychlorinated dibenzo-p-dioxins in AIDS patients with Kaposi sarcoma: an epidemiological investigation. Cancer Detection and Prevention Supplement 1:567–570.

Hardell L, Eriksson M, Degerman A. 1994. Exposure to phenoxyacetic acids, chlorophenols, or organic solvents in relation to histopathology, stage, and anatomical localization of non-Hodgkin's lymphoma. Cancer Research 54:2386–2389.

Hayes HM, Tarone RE, Casey HW, Huxsoll DL. 1990. Excess of seminomas observed in Vietnam service U.S. military working dogs. Journal of the National Cancer Institute 82:1042–1046.

Heacock H, Hogg R, Marion SA, Hershler R, Teschke K, Dimich-Ward H, Demers P, Kelly S, Ostry A, Hertzman C. 1998. Fertility among a cohort of male sawmill workers exposed to chlorophenate fungicides. Epidemiology 9(1):56–60.

Henneberger PK, Ferris BG Jr, Monson RR. 1989. Mortality among pulp and paper workers in Berlin, New Hampshire. British Journal of Industrial Medicine 46:658–664.

Henriksen GL, Michalek JE, Swaby JA, Rahe AJ. 1996. Serum dioxin, testosterone, and gonadotropins in veterans of Operation Ranch Hand. Epidemiology 7(4):352–357.

Henriksen GL, Ketchum NS, Michalek JE, Swaby JA. 1997. Serum dioxin and diabetes mellitus in veterans of Operation Ranch Hand. Epidemiology 8(3):252–258.

Hertzman C, Teschke K, Ostry A, Hershler R, Dimich-Ward H, Kelly S, Spinelli JJ, Gallagher RP, McBride M, Marion SA. 1997. Mortality and cancer incidence among sawmill workers exposed to chlorophenate wood preservatives. American Journal of Public Health 87(1):71–79.

Hoar SK, Blair A, Holmes FF, Boysen CD, Robel RJ, Hoover R, Fraumeni JF. 1986. Agricultural herbicide use and risk of lymphoma and soft-tissue sarcoma. Journal of the American Medical Association 256:1141–1147.

Hoffman RE, Stehr-Green PA, Webb KB, Evans RG, Knutsen AP, Schramm WF, Staake JL, Gibson BB, Steinberg KK. 1986. Health effects of long-term exposure to 2,3,7,8-tetrachlorodibenzo-p-dioxin. Journal of the American Medical Association 255:2031–2038.

Holmes AP, Bailey C, Baron RC, Bosanac E, Brough J, Conroy C, Haddy L. 1986. West Virginia Department of Health Vietnam-Era Veterans Mortality Study, Preliminary Report. Charleston: West Virginia Health Department.

Hooiveld M, Heederik DJ, Kogevinas M, Boffetta P, Needham LL, Patterson DG Jr, Bueno de Mesquita HB. 1998. Second follow-up of a Dutch cohort occupationally exposed to phenoxy herbicides, chlorophenols, and contaminants. American Journal of Epidemiology 147(9):891–901.

Hryhorczuk DO, Wallace WH, Persky V, Furner S, Webster JR Jr, Oleske D, Haselhorst B, Ellefson R, Zugerman C. 1998. A morbidity study of former pentachlorophenol-production workers. Environmental Health Perspectives 106(7):401–408.

Huong LD, Phuong NTN. 1983. The state of abnormal pregnancies and congenital malformations at the Gyneco-Obstetrical Hospital of Ho Chi Minh City (formerly Tu Du Hospital). Summarized in: Constable JD, Hatch MC. Reproductive effects of herbicide exposure in Vietnam: recent studies by the Vietnamese and others. Teratogenesis, Carcinogenesis, and Mutagenesis 5:231–250, 1985.

Ideo G, Bellati G, Bellobuono A, Mocarelli P, Marocchi A, Brambilla P. 1982. Increased urinary d-glucaric acid excretion by children living in an area polluted with tetrachlorodibenzo-*para*-dioxin (TCDD). Clinica Chimica Acta 120:273–283.

Ideo G, Bellati G, Bellobuono A, Bissanti L. 1985. Urinary d-glucaric acid excretion in the Seveso area, polluted by tetrachlorodibenzo-p-dioxin (TCDD): five years of experience. Environmental Health Perspectives 60:151–157.

IOM (Institute of Medicine). 1994. Veterans and Agent Orange Health Effects of Herbicides Used in Vietnam. Washington, DC: National Academy Press.
IOM. 1996. Veterans and Agent Orange: Update 1996. Washington, DC: National Academy Press.
IOM. 1999. Veterans and Agent Orange: Update 1998. Washington, DC: National Academy Press.
IOM. 2000. Veterans and Agent Orange: Herbicide/Dioxin Exposure and Type 2 Diabetes. Washington, DC: National Academy Press.
Jäger R, Neuberger M, Rappe C, Kundi M, Pigler B, Smith AG. 1998. Chloracne and other symptoms 23 years after dioxin-exposure. Atemwegs- Und Lungenkrankheiten 24 (SUPPL. 1):S101–S104.
Jansson B, Voog L. 1989. Dioxin from Swedish municipal incinerators and the occurrence of cleft lip and palate malformations. International Journal of Environmental Studies 34:99–104.
Jappinen P, Pukkala E. 1991. Cancer incidence among pulp and paper workers exposed to organic chlorinated compounds formed during chlorine pulp bleaching. Scandinavian Journal of Work, Environment, and Health 17:356–359.
Jennings AM, Wild G, Ward JD, Ward AM. 1988. Immunological abnormalities 17 years after accidental exposure to 2,3,7,8-tetrachlorodibenzo-p-dioxin. British Journal of Industrial Medicine 45:701–704.
Jung D, Berg PA, Edler L, Ehrenthal W, Fenner D, Flesch-Janys D, Huber C, Klein R, Koitka C, Lucier G, Manz A, Muttray A, Needham L, Päpke O, Pietsch M, Portier C, Patterson D, Prellwitz W, Rose DM, Thews A, Konietzko J. 1998. Immunological findings in formerly exposed workers to 2,3,7,8-tetrachlorodibenzo-p-dioxin (TCDD) and related compounds in pesticide production. Arbeitsmedizin Sozialmedizin Umweltmedizin, Supplement 24:38–43.
Kahn PC, Gochfeld M, Nygren M, Hansson M, Rappe C, Velez H, Ghent-Guenther T, Wilson WP. 1988. Dioxins and dibenzofurans in blood and adipose tissue of Agent Orange-exposed Vietnam veterans and matched controls. Journal of the American Medical Association 259:1661–1667.
Kahn PC, Gochfeld M, Lewis WW. 1992a. Dibenzodioxin and Dibenzofuran Congener Levels in Four Groups of Vietnam Veterans Who Did Not Handle Agent Orange. New Jersey Agent Orange Commission.
Kahn PC, Gochfeld M, Lewis WW. 1992b. Immune Status and Herbicide Exposure in the New Jersey Pointman I Project. New Jersey Agent Orange Commission.
Kahn PC, Gochfeld M, Lewis WW. 1992c. Semen Analysis in Vietnam Veterans with Respect to Presumed Herbicide Exposure. New Jersey Agent Orange Commission.
Kang HK, Weatherbee L, Breslin PP, Lee Y, Shepard BM. 1986. Soft tissue sarcomas and military service in Vietnam: a case comparison group analysis of hospital patients. Journal of Occupational Medicine 28:1215–1218.
Kang HK, Enzinger FM, Breslin P, Feil M, Lee Y, Shepard B. 1987. Soft tissue sarcoma and military service in Vietnam: a case-control study. Journal of the National Cancer Institute 79:693–699 [published erratum appears in Journal of the National Cancer Institute 79:1173].
Kang HK, Mahan CM, Lee KY, Magee CA, Mather SH, Matanoski G. 2000. Pregnancy outcomes among U.S. women Vietnam veterans. American Journal Industrial Medicine 38(4):447–454.
Ketchum NS, Michalek JE, Burton JE. 1999. Serum dioxin and cancer in veterans of Operation Ranch Hand. American Journal of Epidemiology 149(7):630–639.
Khoa ND. 1983. Some biologic parameters collected on the groups of people in an area affected by chemicals. Summarized in: Constable JD, Hatch MC. Reproductive effects of herbicide exposure in Vietnam: recent studies by the Vietnamese and others. Teratogenesis, Carcinogenesis, and Mutagenesis 5:231–250, 1985.
Kogan MD, Clapp RW. 1985. Mortality Among Vietnam Veterans in Massachusetts, 1972–1983. Boston: MA. Massachusetts Office of the Commissioner of Veterans Services, Agent Orange Program.

Kogan MD, Clapp RW. 1988. Soft tissue sarcoma mortality among Vietnam veterans in Massachusetts, 1972 to 1983. International Journal of Epidemiology 17:39–43.

Kogevinas M, Saracci R, Bertazzi PA, Bueno De Mesquita BH, Coggon D, Green LM, Kauppinen T, Littorin M, Lynge E, Mathews JD, Neuberger M, Osman J, Pearce N, Winkelmann R. 1992. Cancer mortality from soft-tissue sarcoma and malignant lymphomas in an international cohort of workers exposed to chlorophenoxy herbicides and chlorophenols. Chemosphere 25:1071–1076.

Kogevinas M, Saracci R, Winkelmann R, Johnson ES, Bertazzi PA, Bueno de Mesquita BH, Kauppinen T, Littorin M, Lynge E, Neuberger M. 1993. Cancer incidence and mortality in women occupationally exposed to chlorophenoxy herbicides, chlorophenols, and dioxins. Cancer Causes and Control 4:547–553.

Kogevinas M, Kauppinen T, Winkelmann R, Becher H, Bertazzi PA, Bas B, Coggon D, Green L, Johnson E, Littorin M, Lynge E, Marlow DA, Mathews JD, Neuberger M, Benn T, Pannett B, Pearce N, Saracci R. 1995. Soft tissue sarcoma and non-Hodgkin's lymphoma in workers exposed to phenoxy herbicides, chlorophenols and dioxins: two nested case-control studies. Epidemiology 6:396–402.

Kogevinas M, Becher H, Benn T, Bertazzi PA, Boffetta P, Bueno de Mesquita HB, Coggon D, Colin D, Flesch-Janys D, Fingerhut M, Green L, Kauppinen T, Littorin M, Lynge E, Mathews JD, Neuberger M, Pearce N, Saracci R. 1997. Cancer mortality in workers exposed to phenoxy herbicides, chlorophenols, and dioxins. An expanded and updated international cohort study. American Journal of Epidemiology 145(12):1061–1075.

Kristensen P, Irgens LM, Andersen A, Bye AS, Sundheim L. 1997. Birth defects among offspring of Norwegian farmers, 1967–1991. Epidemiology 8(5):537–544.

Lampi P, Hakulinen T, Luostarinen T, Pukkala E, Teppo L. 1992. Cancer incidence following chlorophenol exposure in a community in southern Finland. Archives of Environmental Health 47:167–175.

Lang TD, Tung TT, Van DD. 1983a. Mutagenic effects on the first generation after exposure to "Orange Agent." Summarized in: Constable JD, Hatch MC. Reproductive effects of herbicide exposure in Vietnam: recent studies by the Vietnamese and others. Teratogenesis, Carcinogenesis, and Mutagenesis 5:231–250, 1985.

Lang TD, Van DD, Dwyer JH, Flamenbuam C, Dwyer KM, Fantini D. 1983b. Self-reports of exposure to herbicides and health problems: a preliminary analysis of survey data from the families of 432 veterans in northern Vietnam. Summarized in: Constable JD, Hatch MC. Reproductive effects of herbicide exposure in Vietnam: recent studies by the Vietnamese and others. Teratogenesis, Carcinogenesis, and Mutagenesis 5:231–250, 1985.

LaVecchia C, Negri E, D'Avanzo B, Franceschi S. 1989. Occupation and lymphoid neoplasms. British Journal of Cancer 60:385–388.

Lawrence CE, Reilly AA, Quickenton P, Greenwald P, Page WF, Kuntz AJ. 1985. Mortality patterns of New York State Vietnam veterans. American Journal of Public Health 75:277–279.

Lerda D, Rizzi R. 1991. Study of reproductive function in persons occupationally exposed to 2,4-dichlorophenoxyacetic acid (2,4-D). Mutation Research 262:47–50.

Levy CJ. 1988. Agent Orange exposure and posttraumatic stress disorder. Journal of Nervous and Mental Disorders 176:242–245.

Liou HH, Tsai MC, Chen CJ, Jeng JS, Chang YC, Chen SY, Chen RC. 1997. Environmental risk factors and Parkinson's disease: a case-control study in Taiwan. Neurology 48(6):1583–1588.

Longnecker MP, Michalek JE. 2000. Serum dioxin level in relation to diabetes mellitus among Air Force veterans with background levels of exposure. Epidemiology 11(1):44–48.

Lovik M, Johansen HR, Gaarder PI, Becher G, Aaberge IS, Gdynia W, Alexander J. 1996. Halogenated organic compounds and the human immune system: preliminary report on a study in hobby fishermen. Archives of Toxicology Supplement 18:15–20.

Lynge E. 1985. A follow-up study of cancer incidence among workers in manufacture of phenoxy herbicides in Denmark. British Journal of Cancer 52:259–270.

Lynge E. 1993. Cancer in phenoxy herbicide manufacturing workers in Denmark, 1947–87—an update. Cancer Causes and Control 4:261–272.

Mahan CM, Bullman TA, Kang HK, Selvin S. 1997. A case-control study of lung cancer among Vietnam veterans. Journal of Occupational and Environmental Medicine 39(8):740–747.

Manz A, Berger J, Dwyer JH, Flesch-Janys D, Nagel S, Waltsgott H. 1991. Cancer mortality among workers in chemical plant contaminated with dioxin. Lancet 338:959–964.

Masala G, Di Lollo S, Picoco C, Crosignani P, Demicheli V, Fontana A, Funto I, Miligi L, Nanni O, Papucci A, Ramazzotti V, Rodella S, Stagnaro E, Tumino R, Vigano C, Vindigni C, Seniori Costantini A, Vineis P. 1996. Incidence rates of leukemias, lymphomas and myelomas in Italy: geographic distribution and NHL histotypes. International Journal of Cancer 68(2):156–159.

Mastroiacovo P, Spagnolo A, Marni E, Meazza L, Bertollini R, Segni G, Borgna-Pignatti C. 1988. Birth defects in the Seveso area after TCDD contamination. Journal of the American Medical Association 259:1668–1672 [published erratum appears in the Journal of the American Medical Association 1988, 260:792].

May G. 1982. Tetrachlorodibenzodioxin: a survey of subjects ten years after exposure. British Journal of Industrial Medicine 39:128–135.

May G. 1983. TCDD: a study of subjects 10 and 14 years after exposure. Chemosphere 12:771–778.

McDuffie HH, Klaassen DJ, Dosman JA. 1990. Is pesticide use related to the risk of primary lung cancer in Saskatchewan? Journal of Occupational Medicine 32:996–1002.

McKinney WP, McIntire DD, Carmody TJ, Joseph A. 1997. Comparing the smoking behavior of veterans and nonveterans. Public Health Reports 112(3):212–217.

Mellemgaard A, Engholm G, McLaughlin JK, Olsen JH. 1994. Occupational risk factors for renal-cell carcinoma in Denmark. Scandinavian Journal of Work, Environment, and Health 20:160–165.

Michalek JE, Rahe AJ, Boyle CA. 1998a. Paternal dioxin, preterm birth, intrauterine growth retardation, and infant death. Epidemiology 9(2):161–167.

Michalek JE, Ketchum NS, Akhtar FZ. 1998b. Postservice mortality of U.S. Air Force veterans occupationally exposed to herbicides in Vietnam: 15-year follow-up. American Journal of Epidemiology 148(8):786–792.

Michalek JE, Rahe AJ, Boyle CA. 1998c. Paternal dioxin and the sex of children fathered by veterans of Operation Ranch Hand (2). Epidemiology 9(4):474–475.

Michalek JE, Albanese RA, Wolfe WH. 1998d. Project Ranch Hand II: an epidemiologic investigation of health effects in Air Force personnel following exposure to herbicides—reproductive outcome update. Government Reports Announcements and Index.

Michalek JE, Wolfe WH, Miner JC. 1990. Health status of Air Force veterans occupationally exposed to herbicides in Vietnam. II. Mortality. Journal of the American Medical Association 264:1832–1836.

Michalek JE, Akhtar FZ, Kiel JL. 1999a. Serum dioxin, insulin, fasting glucose, and sex hormone-binding globulin in veterans of Operation Ranch Hand. Journal of Clinical Endocrinology and Metabolism 84(5):1540–1543.

Michalek JE, Ketchum NS, Check IJ. 1999b. Serum dioxin and immunologic response in veterans of Operation Ranch Hand. American Journal of Epidemiology 149(11):1038–1046.

Michigan Department of Public Health. 1983. Evaluation of Soft and Connective Tissue Cancer Mortality Rates for Midland and Other Selected Michigan Counties. Michigan Department of Public Health.

Mocarelli P, Marocchi A, Brambilla P, Gerthoux P, Young DS, Mantel N. 1986. Clinical laboratory manifestations of exposure to dioxin in children. A six-year study of the effects of an environmental disaster near Seveso, Italy. Journal of the American Medical Association 256:2687–2695.

Mocarelli P, Brambilla P, Gerthoux PM, Patterson DG Jr, Needham LL. 1996. Change in sex ratio with exposure to dioxin. Lancet 348(9024):409.

Morris PD, Koepsell TD, Daling JR, Taylor JW, Lyon JL, Swanson GM, Child M, Weiss NS. 1986. Toxic substance exposure and multiple myeloma: a case-control study. Journal of the National Cancer Institute 76:987–994.

Morrison H, Semenciw RM, Morison D, Magwood S, Mao Y. 1992. Brain cancer and farming in western Canada. Neuroepidemiology 11:267–276.

Morrison H, Savitz D, Semenciw RM, Hulka B, Mao Y, Morison D, Wigle D. 1993. Farming and prostate cancer mortality. American Journal of Epidemiology 137:270–280.

Morrison HI, Semenciw RM, Wilkins K, Mao Y, Wigle DT. 1994. Non-Hodgkin's lymphoma and agricultural practices in the prairie provinces of Canada. Scandinavian Journal of Work, Environment, and Health 20:42–47.

Moses M, Lilis R, Crow KD, Thornton J, Fischbein A, Anderson HA, Selikoff IJ. 1984. Health status of workers with past exposure to 2,3,7,8-tetrachlorodibenzo-p-dioxin in the manufacture of 2,4,5-trichlorophenoxyacetic acid: comparison of findings with and without chloracne. American Journal of Industrial Medicine 5:161–182.

Musicco M, Sant M, Molinari S, Filippini G, Gatta G, Berrino F. 1988. A case-control study of brain gliomas and occupational exposure to chemical carcinogens: the risks to farmers. American Journal of Epidemiology 128:778–785.

Nanni O, Amadori D, Lugaresi C, Falcini F, Scarpi E, Saragoni A, Buiatti E. 1996. Chronic lymphocytic leukaemias and non-Hodgkin's lymphomas by histological type in farming-animal breeding workers: a population case-control study based on a priori exposure matrices. Occupational and Environmental Medicine 53(10):652–657.

Nelson CJ, Holson JF, Green HG, Gaylor DW. 1979. Retrospective study of the relationship between agricultural use of 2,4,5-T and cleft palate occurrence in Arkansas. Teratology 19:377–383.

Neuberger M, Kundi M, Jäger R. 1998. Chloracne and morbidity after dioxin exposure (preliminary results). Toxicology Letters 96,97:347–350.

Neuberger M, Rappe C, Bergek S, Cai H, Hansson M, Jäger R, Kundi M, Lim CK, Wingfors H, Smith AG. 1999. Persistent health effects of dioxin contamination in herbicide production. Environmental Research 81(3):206–214.

Newell GR. 1984. Development and Preliminary Results of Pilot Clinical Studies. Report of the Agent Orange Advisory Committee to the Texas Department of Health. University of Texas System Cancer Center.

Nguyen HD. 1983. Pregnancies at the Polyclinic of Tay Ninh Province. Summarized in: Constable JD, Hatch MC. Reproductive effects of herbicide exposure in Vietnam: recent studies by the Vietnamese and others. Teratogenesis, Carcinogenesis, and Mutagenesis 5:231–250, 1985.

Nurminen T, Rantala K, Kurppa K, Holmberg PC. 1994. Agricultural work during pregnancy and selected structural malformations in Finland. Epidemiology 1:23–30.

O'Brien TR, Decoufle P, Boyle CA. 1991. Non-Hodgkin's lymphoma in a cohort of Vietnam veterans. American Journal of Public Health 81:758–760.

Olsson H, Brandt L. 1988. Risk of non-Hodgkin's lymphoma among men occupationally exposed to organic solvents. Scandinavian Journal of Work, Environment, and Health 14:246–251.

O'Toole BI, Marshall RP, Grayson DA, Schureck RJ, Dobson M, Ffrench M, Pulvertaft B, Meldrum L, Bolton J, Vennard J. 1996a. The Australian Vietnam Veterans Health Study: I. Study design and response bias. International Journal of Epidemiology 25(2):307–318.

O'Toole BI, Marshall RP, Grayson DA, Schureck RJ, Dobson M, Ffrench M, Pulvertaft B, Meldrum L, Bolton J, Vennard J. 1996b. The Australian Vietnam Veterans Health Study: II. Self-reported health of veterans compared with the Australian population. International Journal of Epidemiology 25(2):319–330.

O'Toole BI, Marshall RP, Grayson DA, Schureck RJ, Dobson M, Ffrench M, Pulvertaft B, Meldrum L, Bolton J, Vennard J. 1996c. The Australian Vietnam Veterans Health Study: III. Psychological health of Australian Vietnam veterans and its relationship to combat. International Journal of Epidemiology 25(2):331–340.

Ott MG, Zober A. 1996. Cause specific mortality and cancer incidence among employees exposed to 2,3,7,8-TCDD after a 1953 reactor accident. Occupational and Environmental Medicine 53(9): 606–612.

Ott MG, Holder BB, Olson RD. 1980. A mortality analysis of employees engaged in the manufacture of 2,4,5-trichlorophenoxyacetic acid. Journal of Occupational Medicine 22:47–50.

Ott MG, Olson RA, Cook RR, Bond GG. 1987. Cohort mortality study of chemical workers with potential exposure to the higher chlorinated dioxins. Journal of Occupational Medicine 29:422–429.

Pazderova-Vejlupkova J, Lukas E, Nemcova M, Pickova J, Jirasek L. 1981. The development and prognosis of chronic intoxication by tetrachlorodibenzo-*p*-dioxin in men. Archives of Environmental Health 36:5–11.

Pearce NE, Smith AH, Fisher DO. 1985. Malignant lymphoma and multiple myeloma linked with agricultural occupations in a New Zealand cancer registry-based study. American Journal of Epidemiology 121:225–237.

Pearce NE, Smith AH, Howard JK, Sheppard RA, Giles HJ, Teague CA. 1986a. Case-control study of multiple myeloma and farming. British Journal of Cancer 54:493–500.

Pearce NE, Smith AH, Howard JK, Sheppard RA, Giles HJ, Teague CA. 1986b. Non-Hodgkin's lymphoma and exposure to phenoxyherbicides, chlorophenols, fencing work, and meat works employment: a case-control study. British Journal of Industrial Medicine 43:75–83.

Pearce NE, Sheppard RA, Smith AH, Teague CA. 1987. Non-Hodgkin's lymphoma and farming: an expanded case-control study. International Journal of Cancer 39:155–161.

Peper M, Klett M, Frentzel-Beyme R, Heller WD. 1993. Neuropsychological effects of chronic exposure to environmental dioxins and furans. Environmental Research 60:124–135.

Persson B, Dahlander AM, Fredriksson M, Brage HN, Ohlson C-G, Axelson O. 1989. Malignant lymphomas and occupational exposures. British Journal of Industrial Medicine 46:516–520.

Persson B, Fredriksson M, Olsen K, Boeryd B, Axelson O. 1993. Some occupational exposures as risk factors for malignant lymphomas. Cancer 72:1773–1778.

Pesatori AC, Consonni D, Tironi A, Landi MT, Zocchetti C, Bertazzi PA. 1992. Cancer morbidity in the Seveso area, 1976–1986. Chemosphere 25:209–212.

Pesatori AC, Consonni D, Tironi A, Zocchetti C, Fini A, Bertazzi PA. 1993. Cancer in a young population in a dioxin-contaminated area. International Journal of Epidemiology 22:1010–1013.

Pesatori AC, Zocchetti C, Guercilena S, Consonni D, Turrini D, Bertazzi PA. 1998. Dioxin exposure and nonmalignant health effects: a mortality study. Occupational and Environmental Medicine 55(2):126–131.

Peters JM, Narotsky MG, Elizondo G, Fernandez-Salguero PM, Gonzalez FJ, Abbott BD. 1999. Amelioration of TCDD-induced eratogenesis in aryl hydrocarbon receptor (AhR)-null mice. Toxicological Sciences 47(1):86–92.

Phuong NTN, Huong LTD. 1983. The effects of toxic chemicals on the pregnancy of the women living at two localities in the South of Vietnam. Summarized in: Constable JD, Hatch MC. Reproductive effects of herbicide exposure in Vietnam: recent studies by the Vietnamese and others. Teratogenesis, Carcinogenesis, and Mutagenesis 5:231–250, 1985.

Phuong NTN, Thuy TT, Phuong PK. 1989a. An estimate of differences among women giving birth to deformed babies and among those with hydatidiform mole seen at the Ob-Gyn hospital of Ho Chi Minh City in the south of Vietnam. Chemosphere 18:801–803.

Phuong NTN, Thuy TT, Phuong PK. 1989b. An estimate of reproductive abnormalities in women inhabiting herbicide sprayed and non-herbicide sprayed areas in the south of Vietnam, 1952–1981. Chemosphere 18:843–846.

Pirkle JL, Wolfe WH, Patterson DG, Needham LL, Michalek JE, Miner JC, Peterson MR, Phillips DL. 1989. Estimates of the half-life of 2,3,7,8-tetrachlorodibenzo-p-dioxin in Vietnam veterans of Operation Ranch Hand. Journal of Toxicology and Environmental Health 27:165–171.

Poland AP, Smith D, Metter G, Possick P. 1971. A health survey of workers in a 2,4-D and 2,4,5-T plant with special attention to chloracne, porphyria cutanea tarda, and psychologic parameters. Archives of Environmental Health 22:316–327.

Pollei S, Mettler FA Jr, Kelsey CA, Walters MR, White RE. 1986. Follow-up chest radiographs in Vietnam veterans: are they useful? Radiology 161:101–102.

Ramlow JM, Spadacene NW, Hoag SR, Stafford BA, Cartmill JB, Lerner PJ. 1996. Mortality in a cohort of pentachlorophenol manufacturing workers, 1940–1989. American Journal of Industrial Medicine 30(2):180–194.

Rellahan WL. 1985. Aspects of the Health of Hawaii's Vietnam-Era Veterans. Honolulu: Hawaii State Department of Health, Research, and Statistics Office.

Riihimaki V, Asp S, Hernberg S. 1982. Mortality of 2,4-dichlorophenoxyacetic acid and 2,4,5-trichlorophenoxyacetic acid herbicide applicators in Finland: first report of an ongoing prospective cohort study. Scandinavian Journal of Work, Environment, and Health 8:37–42.

Riihimaki V, Asp S, Pukkala E, Hernberg S. 1983. Mortality and cancer morbidity among chlorinated phenoxyacid applicators in Finland. Chemosphere 12:779–784.

Rix BA, Villadsen E, Engholm G, Lynge E. 1998. Hodgkin's disease, pharyngeal cancer, and soft tissue sarcomas in Danish paper mill workers. Journal of Occupational and Environmental Medicine 40(1):55–62.

Robinson CF, Waxweiler RJ, Fowler DP. 1986. Mortality among production workers in pulp and paper mills. Scandinavian Journal of Work, Environment, and Health 12:552–560.

Ronco G, Costa G, Lynge E. 1992. Cancer risk among Danish and Italian farmers. British Journal of Industrial Medicine 49:220–225.

Saracci R, Kogevinas M, Bertazzi PA, Bueno De Mesquita BH, Coggon D, Green LM, Kauppinen T, L'Abbe KA, Littorin M, Lynge E, Mathews JD, Neuberger M, Osman J, Pearce N, Winkelmann R. 1991. Cancer mortality in workers exposed to chlorophenoxy herbicides and chlorophenols. Lancet 338:1027–1032.

Schildt EB, Eriksson M, Hardell L, Magnuson A. 1999. Occupational exposures as risk factors for oral cancer evaluated in a Swedish case-control study. Oncology Reports 6 (2):317–320.

Schreinemachers DM. 2000. Cancer mortality in four northern wheat-producing states. Environmental Health Perspectives 108(9):873–881.

Schulte PA, Burnett CA, Boeniger MF, Johnson J. 1996. Neurodegenerative diseases: occupational occurrence and potential risk factors, 1982 through 1991. American Journal of Public Health 86(9):1281–1288.

Seidler A, Hellenbrand W, Robra BP, Vieregge P, Nischan P, Joerg J, Oertel WH, Ulm G, Schneider E. 1996. Possible environmental, occupational, and other etiologic factors for Parkinson's disease: a case-control study in Germany. Neurology 46(5):1275–1284.

Semchuk KM, Love EJ, Lee RG. 1993. Parkinson's disease: a test of the multifactorial etiologic hypothesis. Neurology 43:1173–1180.

Semenciw RM, Morrison HI, Riedel D, Wilkins K, Ritter L, Mao Y. 1993. Multiple myeloma mortality and agricultural practices in the prairie provinces of Canada. Journal of Occupational Medicine 35:557–561.

Semenciw RM, Morrison HI, Morison D, Mao Y. 1994. Leukemia mortality and farming in the prairie provinces of Canada. Canadian Journal of Public Health 85:208–211.

Senthilselvan A, Mcduffie HH, Dosman JA. 1992. Association of asthma with use of pesticides: results of a cross-sectional survey of farmers. American Review of Respiratory Disease 146: 884–887.
Smith AH, Pearce NE. 1986. Update on soft tissue sarcoma and phenoxyherbicides in New Zealand. Chemosphere 15:1795–1798.
Smith AH, Matheson DP, Fisher DO, Chapman CJ. 1981. Preliminary report of reproductive outcomes among pesticide applicators using 2,4,5-T. New Zealand Medical Journal 93:177–179.
Smith AH, Fisher DO, Pearce N, Chapman CJ. 1982. Congenital defects and miscarriages among New Zealand 2,4,5-T sprayers. Archives of Environmental Health 37:197–200.
Smith AH, Fisher DO, Giles HJ, Pearce N. 1983. The New Zealand soft tissue sarcoma case-control study: interview findings concerning phenoxyacetic acid exposure. Chemosphere 12:565–571.
Smith AH, Pearce NE, Fisher DO, Giles HJ, Teague CA, Howard JK. 1984. Soft tissue sarcoma and exposure to phenoxyherbicides and chlorophenols in New Zealand. Journal of the National Cancer Institute 73:1111–1117.
Smith JG, Christophers AJ. 1992. Phenoxy herbicides and chlorophenols: a case-control study on soft tissue sarcoma and malignant lymphoma. British Journal of Cancer 65:442–448.
Snow BR, Stellman JM, Stellman SD, Sommer, JF. 1988. Post-traumatic stress disorder among American Legionnaires in relation to combat experience in Vietnam: associated and contributing factors. Environmental Research 47:175–192.
Sobel W, Bond GG, Skowronski BJ, Brownson PJ, Cook RR. 1987. A soft tissue sarcoma case-control study in a large multi-chemical manufacturing facility. Chemosphere 16:2095–2099.
Solet D, Zoloth SR, Sullivan C, Jewett J, Michaels DM. 1989. Patterns of mortality in pulp and paper workers. Journal of Occupational Medicine 31:627–630.
Steenland K, Piacitelli L, Deddens J, Fingerhut M, Chang LI. 1999. Cancer, heart disease, and diabetes in workers exposed to 2,3,7,8-tetrachlorodibenzo-p-dioxin. Journal of the National Cancer Institute 91(9):779–786.
Stehr PA, Stein G, Webb K, Schramm W, Gedney WB, Donnell HD, Ayres S, Falk H, Sampson E, Smith SJ. 1986. A pilot epidemiologic study of possible health effects associated with 2,3,7,8-tetrachlorodibenzo-p-dioxin contaminations in Missouri. Archives of Environmental Health 41:16–22.
Stehr-Green P, Hoffman R, Webb K, Evans RG, Knusten A, Schramm W, Staake J, Gibson B, Steinberg K. 1987. Health effects of long-term exposure to 2,3,7,8-tetrachlorodibenzo-p-dioxin. Chemosphere 16:2089–2094.
Stellman SD, Stellman JM, Sommer JF Jr. 1988a. Combat and herbicide exposures in Vietnam among a sample of American Legionnaires. Environmental Research 47:112–128.
Stellman SD, Stellman JM, Sommer JF Jr. 1988b. Health and reproductive outcomes among American Legionnaires in relation to combat and herbicide exposure in Vietnam. Environmental Research 47:150–174.
Stellman JM, Stellman SD, Sommer JF. 1988c. Social and behavioral consequences of the Vietnam experience among American Legionnaires. Environmental Research 47:129–149.
Stockbauer JW, Hoffman RE, Schramm WF, Edmonds LD. 1988. Reproductive outcomes of mothers with potential exposure to 2,3,7,8-tetrachlorodibenzo-p-dioxin. American Journal of Epidemiology 128:410–419.
Suskind RR, Hertzberg VS. 1984. Human health effects of 2,4,5-T and its toxic contaminants. Journal of the American Medical Association 251:2372–2380.
Svensson BG, Mikoczy Z, Stromberg U, Hagmar L. 1995. Mortality and cancer incidence among Swedish fishermen with a high dietary intake of persistent organochlorine compounds. Scandinavian Journal of Work, Environment, and Health 21(2):106–115.
Swaen GMH, van Vliet C, Slangen JJM, Sturmans F. 1992. Cancer mortality among licensed herbicide applicators. Scandinavian Journal of Work, Environment, and Health 18:201–204.

Sweeney MH, Fingerhut MA, Connally LB, Halperin WE, Moody PL, Marlow DA. 1989. Progress of the NIOSH cross-sectional study of workers occupationally exposed to chemicals contaminated with 2,3,7,8-TCDD. Chemosphere 19:973–977.

Sweeney MH, Fingerhut MA, Arezzo JC, Hornung RW, Connally LB. 1993. Peripheral neuropathy after occupational exposure to 2,3,7,8-tetrachlorodibenzo-*p*-dioxin (TCDD). American Journal of Industrial Medicine 23:845–858.

Sweeney MH, Calvert G, Egeland GA, Fingerhut MA, Halperin WE, Piacitelli. 1996. Review and update of the results of the NIOSH medical study of workers exposed to chemicals contaminated with 2,3,7,8-tetrachlorodibenzodioxin. Presented at the symposium Dioxin Exposure and Human Health—An Update, Berlin June 17.

Sweeney MH, Calvert GM, Egeland GA, Fingerhut MA, Halperin WE, Piacitelli LA. 1997/98. Review and update of the results of the NIOSH medical study of workers exposed to chemicals contaminated with 2,3,7,8-tetrachlorodibenzodioxin. Teratogenesis, Carcinogenesis, and Mutagenesis 17(4–5):241–247.

Tarone RE, Hayes HM, Hoover RN, Rosenthal JF, Brown LM, Pottern LM, Javadpour N, O'Connell KJ, Stutzman RE. 1991. Service in Vietnam and risk of testicular cancer. Journal of the National Cancer Institute 83:1497–1499.

Tatham L, Tolbert P, Kjeldsberg C. 1997. Occupational risk factors for subgroups of non-Hodgkin's lymphoma. Epidemiology 8(5):551–558.

Tenchini ML, Crimaudo C, Pacchetti G, Mottura A, Agosti S, De Carli L. 1983. A comparative cytogenetic study on cases of induced abortions in TCDD-exposed and nonexposed women. Environmental Mutagenesis 5:73–85.

Thiess AM, Frentzel-Beyme R, Link R. 1982. Mortality study of persons exposed to dioxin in a trichlorophenol-process accident that occurred in the BASF AG on November 17, 1953. American Journal of Industrial Medicine 3:179–189.

Thomas TL. 1987. Mortality among flavour and fragrance chemical plant workers in the United States. British Journal of Industrial Medicine 44:733–737.

Thomas TL, Kang HK. 1990. Mortality and morbidity among Army Chemical Corps Vietnam veterans: a preliminary report. American Journal of Industrial Medicine 18:665–673.

Thomas TL, Kang H, Dalager N. 1991. Mortality among women Vietnam veterans, 1973–1987. American Journal of Epidemiology 134:973–980.

Thorn A, Gustavsson P, Sadigh J, Westerlund-Hannestrand B, Hogstedt C. 2000. Mortality and cancer incidence among Swedish lumberjacks exposed to phenoxy herbicides. Occupational and Environmental Medicine 57(10):718–720.

Tonn T, Esser C, Schneider EM, Steinmann-Steiner-Haldenstatt W, Gleichmann E. 1996. Persistence of decreased T-helper cell function in industrial workers 20 years after exposure to 2,3,7,8-tetrachlorodibenzo-*p*-dioxin. Environmental Health Perspectives 104(4):422–426.

Townsend JC, Bodner KM, Van Peenen PFD, Olson RD, Cook RR. 1982. Survey of reproductive events of wives of employees exposed to chlorinated dioxins. American Journal of Epidemiology 115:695–713.

True WR, Goldberg J, Eisen SA. 1988. Stress symptomatology among Vietnam veterans. Analysis of the Veterans Administration Survey of Veterans II. American Journal of Epidemiology 128:85–92.

Trung CB, Chien NT. 1983. Spontaneous abortions and birth defects in area exposed to toxic chemical sprays in Giong Trom District. Summarized in: Constable JD, Hatch MC. Reproductive effects of herbicide exposure in Vietnam: recent studies by the Vietnamese and others. Teratogenesis, Carcinogenesis, and Mutagenesis 5:231–250, 1985.

U.S. EPA (Environmental Protection Agency). 1979. Report of Assessment of a Field Investigation of Six-Year Spontaneous Abortion Rates in Three Oregon Areas in Relation to Forest 2,4,5-T Spray Practices. Washington: DC. Epidemiologic Studies Program, Human Effects Monitoring Branch.

van Houdt JJ, Fransman LG, Strik JJ. 1983. Epidemiological case-control study in personnel exposed to 2,4,5-T. Chemosphere 12:575.
Vena J, Boffetta P, Becher H, Benn T, Bueno de Mesquita HB, Coggon D, Colin D, Flesch-Janys D, Green L, Kauppinen T, Littorin M, Lynge E, Mathews JD, Neuberger M, Pearce N, Pesatori AC, Saracci R, Steenland K, Kogevinas M. 1998. Exposure to dioxin and nonneoplastic mortality in the expanded IARC international cohort study of phenoxy herbicide and chlorophenol production workers and sprayers. Environmental Health Perspectives 106 (Suppl 2):645–653.
Vineis P, Terracini B, Ciccone G, Cignetti A, Colombo E, Donna A, Maffi L, Pisa R, Ricci P, Zanini E, Comba P. 1986. Phenoxy herbicides and soft-tissue sarcomas in female rice weeders. A population-based case-referent study. Scandinavian Journal of Work, Environment, and Health 13:9–17.
Vineis P, Faggiano F, Tedeschi M, Ciccone G. 1991. Incidence rates of lymphomas and soft-tissue sarcomas and environmental measurements of phenoxy herbicides. Journal of the National Cancer Institute 83:362–363.
Visintainer PF, Barone M, McGee H, Peterson EL. 1995. Proportionate mortality study of Vietnam-era veterans of Michigan. Journal of Occupational and Environmental Medicine 37(4):423–428.
Watanabe KK, Kang HK. 1995. Military service in Vietnam and the risk of death from trauma and selected cancers. Annals of Epidemiology 5(5):407–412.
Watanabe KK, Kang HK. 1996. Mortality patterns among Vietnam veterans: a 24-year retrospective analysis. Journal of Occupational and Environmental Medicine 38(3):272–278.
Watanabe KK, Kang HK, Thomas TL. 1991. Mortality among Vietnam veterans: with methodological considerations. Journal of Occupational Medicine 33:780–785.
Waterhouse D, Carman WJ, Schottenfeld D, Gridley G, McLean S. 1996. Cancer incidence in the rural community of Tecumseh, Michigan: a pattern of increased lymphopoietic neoplasms. Cancer 77(4):763–770.
Webb K, Evans RG, Stehr P, Ayres SM. 1987. Pilot study on health effects of environmental 2,3,7,8-TCDD in Missouri. American Journal of Industrial Medicine 11:685–691.
Weisglas-Kuperus N, Sas TC, Koopman-Esseboom C, van der Zwan CW, De Ridder MA, Beishuizen A, Hooijkaas H, Sauer PJ. 1995. Immunologic effects of background prenatal and postnatal exposure to dioxins and polychlorinated biphenyls in Dutch infants. Pediatric Research 38(3):404–410.
Wendt AS. 1985. Iowa Agent Orange Survey of Vietnam Veterans. Iowa State Department of Health.
White FMM, Cohen FG, Sherman G, McCurdy R. 1988. Chemicals, birth defects and stillbirths in New Brunswick: associations with agricultural activity. Canadian Medical Association Journal 138:117–124.
Wigle DT, Semenciw RB, Wilkins K, Riedel D, Ritter L, Morrison HI, Mao Y. 1990. Mortality study of Canadian male farm operators: non-Hodgkin's lymphoma mortality and agricultural practices in Saskatchewan. Journal of the National Cancer Institute 82:575–582.
Wiklund K. 1983. Swedish agricultural workers: a group with a decreased risk of cancer. Cancer 51:566–568.
Wiklund K, Holm LE. 1986. Soft tissue sarcoma risk in Swedish agricultural and forestry workers. Journal of the National Cancer Institute 76:229–234.
Wiklund K, Dich J, Holm LE. 1987. Risk of malignant lymphoma in Swedish pesticide appliers. British Journal of Cancer 56:505–508.
Wiklund K, Lindefors BM, Holm LE. 1988a. Risk of malignant lymphoma in Swedish agricultural and forestry workers. British Journal of Industrial Medicine 45:19–24.
Wiklund K, Dich J, Holm LE. 1988b. Soft tissue sarcoma risk in Swedish licensed pesticide applicators. Journal of Occupational Medicine 30:801–804.

Wiklund K, Dich J, Holm LE, Eklund G. 1989a. Risk of cancer in pesticide applicators in Swedish agriculture. British Journal of Industrial Medicine 46:809–814.

Wiklund K, Dich J, Holm LE. 1989b. Risk of soft tissue sarcoma, Hodgkin's disease and non-Hodgkin lymphoma among Swedish licensed pesticide applicators. Chemosphere 18:395–400.

Wingren G, Fredrikson M, Brage HN, Nordenskjold B, Axelson O. 1990. Soft tissue sarcoma and occupational exposures. Cancer 66:806–811.

Wolf N, Karmaus W. 1995. Effects of inhalative exposure to dioxins in wood preservatives on cell-mediated immunity in day-care center teachers. Environmental Research 68(2):96–105.

Wolfe WH, Michalek JE, Miner JC, Rahe A, Silva J, Thomas WF, Grubbs WD, Lustik MB, Karrison TG, Roegner RH, Williams DE. 1990. Health status of Air Force veterans occupationally exposed to herbicides in Vietnam. I. Physical health. Journal of the American Medical Association 264:1824–1831.

Wolfe WH, Michalek JE, Miner JC, Rahe AJ, Moore CA, Needham LL, Patterson D.G. 1995. Paternal serum dioxin and reproductive outcomes among veterans of Operation Ranch Hand. Epidemiology 6(1):17–22.

Woods JS, Polissar L. 1989. Non-Hodgkin's lymphoma among phenoxy herbicide-exposed farm workers in western Washington State. Chemosphere 18:401–406.

Woods JS, Polissar L, Severson RK, Heuser LS, Kulander BG. 1987. Soft tissue sarcoma and non-Hodgkin's lymphoma in relation to phenoxy herbicide and chlorinated phenol exposure in western Washington. Journal of the National Cancer Institute 78:899–910.

Zack JA, Gaffey WR. 1983. A mortality study of workers employed at the Monsanto company plant in Nitro, West Virginia. Environmental Science Research 26:575–591.

Zack JA, Suskind RR. 1980. The mortality experience of workers exposed to tetrachlorodibenzodioxin in a trichlorophenol process accident. Journal of Occupational Medicine 22:11–14.

Zahm SH, Weisenburger DD, Babbitt PA, Saal RC, Vaught JB, Cantor KP, Blair A. 1990. A case-control study of non-Hodgkin's lymphoma and the herbicide 2,4-dichlorophenoxyacetic acid (2,4-D) in eastern Nebraska. Epidemiology 1:349–356.

Zahm SH, Weisenburger DD, Saal RC, Vaught JB, Babbitt PA, Blair A. 1993. The role of agricultural pesticide use in the development of non-Hodgkin's lymphoma in women. Archives of Environmental Health 48:353–358.

Zhong Y, Rafnsson V. 1996. Cancer incidence among Icelandic pesticide users. International Journal of Epidemiology 25(6):1117–1124.

Zober A, Messerer P, Huber P. 1990. Thirty-four-year mortality follow-up of BASF employees exposed to 2,3,7,8-TCDD after the 1953 accident. International Archives of Occupational and Environmental Health 62:139–157.

Zober A, Ott MG, Messerer P. 1994. Morbidity follow-up study of BASF employees exposed to 2,3,7,8-tetrachlorodibenzo-p-dioxin (TCDD) after a 1953 chemical reactor incident. Occupational and Environmental Medicine 51:479–486.

Zober A, Messerer P, Ott MG. 1997. BASF studies: epidemiological and clinical investigations on dioxin-exposed chemical workers. Teratogenesis, Carcinogenesis, and Mutagenesis 17(4–5): 249–256.

TABLE 6-1 Epidemiologic Studies—Occupational Exposure

Reference	Study	Design Description	Study Group (N)	Comparison Group (N)[a]
Production Workers				
New NIOSH Studies				
Calvert et al., 1999	Cohort	Continuing follow-up of workers employed more than 15 years ago at two plants that manufactured substances contaminated with TCDD to evaluate associations between serum TCDD and serum glucose (diabetes), TSH, total T_4, and T_3	281	260
Steenland et al., 1999	Cohort	Mortality study of workers at 12 industrial plants that produced chemicals contaminated with TCDD, using a job-exposure matrix to estimate TCDD exposure categories. End points reported are all cancers, ischemic heart disease, and diabetes	5,132 (3,538 with exposure data divided into septiles of cumulative exposure; 608 who had chloracne)	—
Calvert et al., 1998	Cohort	Continuing follow-up of workers employed more than 15 years ago at two plants that manufactured substances contaminated with TCDD to evaluate the association between TCDD exposure and cardiovascular outcomes	281	260

Halperin et al., 1998	Cohort	Continuing study of a cohort of TCDD-exposed workers at two plants that manufactured substances contaminated with TCDD to assess the association between serum TCDD and immunological outcome variables for eligible workers and matched neighborhood controls	259	243
NIOSH Studies Reviewed in Update 1998				
Sweeney et al., 1996, 1997/1998	Cross-sectional	Study of numerous noncancer end points for liver function, gastrointestinal disorders, chloracne, serum glucose, hormone and lipid levels, and diabetes in same group as Calvert et al. (1991)	281	260
Halperin et al., 1995	Cross-sectional	Study of surrogates for cytochrome P450 induction in same group as Calvert et al. (1991)	281	260
NIOSH Studies Reviewed in Update 1996				
Calvert et al., 1994	Cross-sectional	Study of porphyria cutanea tarda in same group as Calvert et al. (1991)	281	260
Egeland et al., 1994	Cohort	Study of total serum testosterone and gondadotropin levels in chemical production workers exposed to dioxin, in same group as Calvert et al. (1991)	248	231

continued

TABLE 6-1 Continued

Reference	Study	Design Description	Study Group (N)	Comparison Group (N)[a]
NIOSH Studies Reviewed in VAO				
Sweeney et al., 1993	Cohort	Peripheral neuropathy in same group as Calvert et al. (1991)	281	260
Alderfer et al., 1992	Cohort	Assessment of psychological variables to determine depression in same group as Calvert et al. (1991)	281	260
Calvert et al., 1992	Cohort	Assessment of liver and gastrointestinal systems in same group as Calvert et al. (1991)	281	260
Calvert et al., 1991	Cohort	Study of workers employed at one of two plants manufacturing substances contaminated with TCDD at least 15 years prior to assessment of chronic bronchitis, COPD, ventilatory function, thorax, and lung abnormalities, compared to matched neighborhood controls	281	260
Fingerhut et al., 1991	Cohort	Cancer mortality in male workers from 12 plants producing TCDD contaminated chemicals (1942–1984), compared to U.S. population	5,172	—

Monsanto Studies Reviewed in VAO

Reference	Type	Description	N	
Collins et al., 1993	Cohort	Mortality of workers (through 1987) exposed and unexposed to dioxin between March 8, 1949, and November 22, 1949, as indicated by presence of chloracne, compared to local population mortality rates	122 with chloracne; 632 without chloracne	—
Moses et al., 1984	Cohort	Study of health outcomes in Monsanto workers (1948–1969) with chloracne reported as a surrogate to 2,4,5-T exposure compared to health outcomes in workers without chloracne as surrogate for no exposure	117	109
Suskind and Hertzberg, 1984	Cohort	Evaluation of health outcomes (1979) at clinical examination among workers exposed to 2,4,5-T (1948–1969) compared to nonexposed workers at same Monsanto plant	204	163
Zack and Gaffey, 1983	Cohort	Study of mortality experience of all white male workers (1955–1977) employed at a Monsanto plant through Dec. 31 1977, compared to mortality rates of standardized U.S. population	884	—

continued

TABLE 6-1 Continued

Reference	Study	Design Description	Study Group (N)	Comparison Group (N)[a]
Zack and Suskind, 1980	Cohort	Evaluation of mortality experience among employees with chloracne exposed to TCP process accident in 1949 at Monsanto, compared to U.S. male population standard	121	—
Dow Studies Reviewed in Update 1998				
Ramlow et al., 1996	Cohort	Study of mortality in a cohort of workers exposed to pentachlorophenol (PCP)	770	36,804 unexposed workers; U.S. population
Dow Studies Reviewed in Update 1996				
Bloemen et al., 1993	Cohort	Additional years of follow-up of Bond et al. (1988) study cohort through 1986	878	U.S. population; 36,804 unexposed workers
Dow Studies Reviewed in VAO				
Bond et al., 1989a	Cohort	Study of incidence of chloracne among a cohort of workers potentially exposed to TCDD, and association with other risk factors	2,072	Internal comparison
Bond et al., 1989b	Cohort	Extension of Ott et al. (1987) study through 1984	2,187	—

Bond et al., 1988	Cohort	Study of mortality (through 1982) among workers potentially exposed to 2,4-D (1945–1983) compared to U.S. white males and all other male employees not exposed	878	U.S. white male population; 36,804 employees not exposed
Bond et al., 1987	Cohort	Extension of Cook et al. (1980) study, mortality through 1982	322	U.S. white male population; 2,026 employees without chloracne
Cook et al., 1987; Ott et al., 1987	Cohort	Expanded Cook et al. (1986) study an additional three years, through 1982	2,187	—
Sobel et al., 1987	Case-control	Study of STS among Dow chemical employees (1940–1979) compared to employees without STS for possible association with several chemical exposures	14	126
Cook et al., 1986	Cohort	Mortality experience (1940–1979) of men manufacturing chlorinated phenols compared to U.S. white men	2,189	—
Bond et al., 1983	Cross-sectional	Study of differences in workers potentially exposed and unexposed to TCDD during chemical production for (1) morbidity and (2) medical examination frequency between 1976 and 1978	(1) 183 (2) 114	(1) 732 (2) 456

continued

TABLE 6-1 Continued

Reference	Study	Design Description	Study Group (N)	Comparison Group (N)[a]
Townsend et al., 1982	Cohort	Study of adverse reproductive outcomes among wives of Dow chemical employees potentially exposed to TCDD (1939–1975) compared to reproductive outcomes among wives whose husbands were not exposed	370	345
Cook et al., 1980	Cohort	Mortality experience (through 1978) of male workers involved in a chloracne incident (1964) from TCDD exposure, compared to mortality experience of U.S. white men	61	—
Ott et al., 1980	Cohort	Mortality experience among workers exposed to 2,4,5-T in manufacturing (1950–1971) compared to mortality experience of U.S. white men	204	—
New BASF Studies				
Zober et al., 1997	Cohort (1953 accident) Cross-sectional (1988 cohort)	Review and summary of previous BASF studies of morbidity and mortality in workers exposed to TCDD after BASF accidents in 1953 and 1988	154 surviving (as of 1989) members of 1953 accident cohort 42 exposed (1988) extruder personnel	No comparison group

BASF Studies Reviewed in Update 1998			
Ott and Zober, 1996	Cohort	Cancer incidence and mortality experience (through 1992) of workers exposed to TCDD after the BASF accident, during reactor cleanup, maintenance, or demolition (based on the cohort of Zober et al. 1990)	243	—
BASF Studies Reviewed in Update 1996			
Zober et al., 1994	Cohort	Morbidity experience in the same group as Zober et al. (1990)	158	161
BASF Studies Reviewed in VAO			
Zober et al., 1990	Cohort	Mortality experience of workers exposed to TCDD (1954–1987) at BASF plant compared to population of Federal Republic of Germany (FRG)	247	—
Thiess et al., 1982	Cohort	Study of mortality experience among BASF employees potentially exposed to TCDD during Nov. 17, 1953, accident compared to population and other workers not exposed	74	180,000 (town); 1.8 million (district); 60.5 million (FRG); two groups of 74 each from other cohort studies
New IARC Studies			
Neuberger et al., 1999	Austrian chloracne cohort	Morbidity up to 1993 of exposed chemical workers assessed by health insurance data and health examination, laboratory measures, and interviews with participating survivors and controls	159, including 50 who participated in examination	Two control groups comparable to the 50 participants—numbers not given

continued

TABLE 6-1 Continued

Reference	Study	Design Description	Study Group (N)	Comparison Group (N)[a]
Hooiveld et al., 1998	Cohort	Mortality (through 1991), using SMRs, of workers at one Dutch factory assessed in relation to work and exposure history. SMR and relative risk analyses	562 (serum samples for 50); 140 males at accident	567
Jager et al., 1998	Cohort	Preliminary data from Neuberger et al. (1999; English abstract only)	159 in original cohort; 56 screened; 49 full data	Matched nonexposed controls
Neuberger et al., 1998	Cohort of exposed cases	Preliminary data from Neuberger et al. (1999)	50	Age- and sex-matched controls; number not given
Vena et al., 1998	Cohort	International study (36 cohorts from 12 countries) of workers producing or spraying phenoxy acid herbicides and chlorophenols, categorized into one of three TCDD or higher chlorinated dioxin categories. Noncancer mortality (from 1939 to 1992) was analyzed by standardized mortality rate comparisons and by Poisson multiple regression	21,863	No comparison group

Flesch-Janys, 1997	Cohort	Mortality (from 1952 to 1984) study of German workers exposed to TCDD and other contaminants in the production of herbicides and insecticides. SMRs and Cox regression models were calculated	1,189	—
IARC Studies Reviewed in Update 1998				
Kogevinas et al., 1997	Cohort	Mortality study (through 1992) of workers engaged in the production or application of phenoxy herbicides and composed of (1) the Saracci et al. (1991) cohorts, (2) the German cohorts of Becher et al. (1996), and (3) the NIOSH cohorts of Fingerhut et al. (1991)	26,615 total (21,863 exposed; 4,160 probably exposed; 592 unknown exposure)	—
Becher et al., 1996	Cohort	Cancer mortality (through 1989) among German workers in four chemical factories exposed to 2,4,5-T and/or trichlorophenol (subcohorts I and II) and phenoxy herbicides and chlorophenols (subcohorts III and IV)	2,479	—
Flesch-Janys et al., 1995	Cohort	Cancer and circulatory system mortality among workers in a chemical plant in Hamburg, Germany exposed in varying degrees to herbicides contaminated with PCDD/F	1,189	(1) population (2) 2,528 gas workers

continued

TABLE 6-1 Continued

Reference	Study	Design Description	Study Group (N)	Comparison Group (N)[a]
IARC Studies Reviewed in Update 1996				
Kogevinas et al., 1995	Case-control	Two nested case-control studies of the relationship between STS and NHL and occupational exposures in members of the IARC cohort	STS: 11 cases NHL: 32 cases	5 controls per case
Kogevinas et al., 1993	Cohort	Cancer incidence and mortality experience of female workers in seven countries, potentially exposed to chlorophenoxy herbicides, chlorophenols, and dioxin compared to national death rates and cancer incidence rates	701	—
Lynge, 1993	Cohort	Cancer incidence in the same group as Lynge (1985), with follow-up extended through 1987	3,390 men 1,071 women	—
Kogevinas et al., 1992	Cohort	Study of mortality from STS and malignant lymphomas in an international cohort of production workers and herbicide sprayers (same group as Saracci et al., 1991)	14,439 (13,482 exposed; 416 probably exposed; 541 unknown exposure)	3,951 nonexposed employees

IARC Studies Reviewed in VAO				
Bueno de Mesquita et al., 1993	Cohort	Mortality experience of production workers exposed to phenoxy herbicides and chlorophenols in the Netherlands compared to national rates	2,310	—
Coggon et al., 1991	Cohort	Mortality experience among four cohorts of workers potentially exposed (1963–1985) to phenoxy herbicides and chlorophenols compared to national (England and Wales) expected numbers and to the local population where factory is located	1,104 Factory A 271 Factory B 345 Factory C 519 Factory D	—
Manz et al., 1991	Cohort	Mortality experience of workers (1952–1984) at Hamburg plant of Boehringer exposed to TCDD compared to national mortality and workers from another company	1,184 men 399 women	(a) population (b) 3,120 gas workers
Saracci et al., 1991	Cohort	Study of mortality experience of 20 international cohorts of herbicide sprayers and production workers compared to mortality experience expected for the nation	16,863 men 1,527 women	—

continued

TABLE 6-1 Continued

Reference	Study	Design Description	Study Group (N)	Comparison Group (N)[a]
Coggon et al., 1986	Cohort	Study of mortality experience (through 1983) among workers manufacturing and spraying MCPA (1947–1975) compared to expected numbers of deaths among men of England and Wales and for rural areas	5,754	—
Lynge, 1985	Cohort	Study of cancer incidence among Danish workers exposed to phenoxyherbicides compared to expected results from the general population	3,390 men 1,069 women	—
New Studies from Other Chemical Plants				
Hryhorczuk et al., 1998	Cohort	Morbidity study of workers involved in pentachlorophenol production at one factory between 1938 and 1978 and unexposed workers at the same factory. Assesses chloracne, prophyria, and general health status	366	303

Jung et al., 1998	Cohort	Self-selected group of former workers at pesticide-producing factory participated in physical examination, laboratory measures, and questionnaires. Associations between serum PCDD/F, infectious disease, and immunologic measures were assessed	192
		Lymphocyte proliferation and chromate resistance tests were compared between a subgroup of the mostly highly exposed workers at the study factory and an unexposed group of workers in another industry	29 (highly exposed subgroup) 28 (external unexposed group)

Studies from Other Chemical Plants Reviewed in Update 1998

Tonn et al., 1996	Cohort	Study of the long-term immune system effects of TCDD in industrial workers involved in production and maintenance operations at a German chemical factory producing 2,4,5-T between 1966 and 1976	11 10

Studies from Other Chemical Plants Reviewed in VAO

Jennings et al., 1988	Cohort	Assessment of immunological abnormalities among workers exposed to TCDD during accident manufacturing 2,4,5-T compared to matched controls	18 15

continued

TABLE 6-1 Continued

Reference	Study	Design Description	Study Group (N)	Comparison Group (N)[a]
Thomas, 1987	Cohort	Assessment of mortality experience as of Jan. 1, 1981, for white men employed in fragrance and flavors plant with possible exposure to TCDD, compared to U.S. white men and for cancers compared to local men	1,412	—
May, 1982, 1983	Cohort	Health outcomes among workers exposed and probably exposed to TCDD following a 1968 accidents, compared to unexposed workers	41 exposed 54 possibly exposed	31
Pazderova-Vejlupkova et al., 1981	Descriptive	Study of development of TCDD intoxication among men in Prague (1965–1968)	55	No comparison group
Poland et al., 1971	Cross-sectional	Assessment of porphyria cutanea tarda (PCT), chloracne, hepatotoxicity, and neuropsychiatric symptoms among 2,4-D and 2,4,5-T workers compared to other plant workers	73 total (20 administrators; 11 production supervisors; 28 production workers; 14 maintenance workers)	Internal comparison

196

Bashirov, 1969	Cross-sectional	Descriptive results of examination of workers involved in production of herbicides and study of workers at examination of cardiovascular and digestive systems compared to unexposed controls	292 (descriptive) 50 (examined)	20 (examined)

Agricultural and Forest Products
New Cohort Studies of Agricultural Workers Studies

Arbuckle et al., 1999	Cohort	Spontaneous abortions in couples living on full-time family-run farms in Ontario, Canada	2,110 women (3,936 pregnancies)	None

Cohort Studies of Agricultural Workers Reviewed in Update 1998

Gambini et al., 1997	Cohort	Cancer mortality (1957–1992) among a cohort of rice growers in the Novara Province of northern Italy	958	—
Kristensen et al., 1997	Cohort	Birth defects among the offspring of Norwegian farmers born after 1924	192,417 births	61,351 births
Faustini et al., 1996	Cohort	Study of immune system components and functions among farmers who mixed and applied commercial formulations containing the chlorophenoxy herbicides 2,4-D and MCPA	10	Internal comparison

continued

TABLE 6-1 Continued

Reference	Study	Design Description	Study Group (N)	Comparison Group (N)[a]
Cohort Studies of Agricultural Workers Reviewed in Update 1996				
Dean, 1994	Cohort	Study of mortality from brain and hematopoietic cancers of agricultural workers compared to nonagricultural workers in Ireland (1971–1987)	(population size unclear)	—
Morrison et al., 1994	Cohort	Update of mortality experience in Wigle et al. (1990) cohort through 1987, with addition of farmers from Alberta and Manitoba	155,547	—
Semenciw et al., 1994	Cohort	Study of leukemia mortality in same group as Morrison et al. (1993)	155,547	—
Blair et al., 1993	Cohort	Study of causes of death, including cancer, among farmers in 23 states (1984–1988)	119,648 white men; 2,400 white women; 11,446 nonwhite men; 2,066 nonwhite women	—
Semenciw et al., 1993	Cohort	Study of multiple myeloma mortality of male farmers compared to male population of the three prairie provinces of Canada (1971–1987)	155,547	—

Senthilselvan et al., 1992	Cross-sectional	Study of the association between pesticide exposure and asthma in male farmers	1,939	No comparison group

Cohort Studies of Agricultural Workers Reviewed in VAO

Morrison et al., 1993	Cohort	Mortality experience of male Canadian farmers 45 years or older in Manitoba, Saskatchewan, and Alberta, Canada, (1971–1987) compared to Canadian prairie province mortality rates	145,383	—
Eriksson et al., 1992	Cohort	Study of incidence of NHL, HD, and multiple myeloma (1971–1984) among selected occupational groups in Swedish men and women, compared to expected rates of disease in general population	Number in occupational group unknown	—
Hansen et al., 1992	Cohort	Study of cancer incidence among male and female Danish gardeners compared to incidence expected among the general population	4,015 (859 women; 3,156 men)	—
Morrison et al., 1992	Cohort	Mortality experience of male farmers 35 or older (1971–1987) compared to Canadian prairie province rates	155,547	—

continued

TABLE 6-1 *Continued*

Reference	Study	Design Description	Study Group (N)	Comparison Group (N)[a]
Ronco et al., 1992	Cohort	Study of cancer incidence (1970–1980) among male and female Danish farm workers 15 to 74 years old, compared to expected numbers of cancers among persons economically active, and study of cancer mortality (November 1981–April 1982) among male and female Italian farmers 18 to 74 years old compared to persons in other occupational groups	No N given	No N given
Lerda and Rizzi, 1991	Cohort	Study of farmers exposed to 2,4-D, as measured in urine, compared to unexposed men for differences in sperm volume death, count, motility, and abnormalities between March and June 1989	32	25
Wigle et al., 1990	Cohort	Mortality experience from NHL of male farmers 35 years or older (1971–1985) in Saskatchewan, Canada, compared to age- and period-specific mortality rates expected for Saskatchewan males	69,513	—

Corrao et al., 1989	Cohort	Study of cancer incidence among male farmers licensed (1970–1974) to use pesticides, compared to number of cancers expected among licensed nonusers	642	18,839
Wiklund et al., 1988a	Cohort	Malignant lymphoma incidence among agricultural and forestry workers in Sweden compared to the general population of men; 1960 census	354,620	1,725,845
Wiklund and Holm, 1986	Cohort	STS incidence among agricultural and forestry workers in Sweden compared to the general population of men; 1960 census	354,620	1,725,845
Wiklund, 1983	Cohort	Study of cancer incidence (diagnosed 1961–1973) among agricultural workers in Sweden compared to rates expected from the 1960 population census	19,490	—
Burmeister, 1981	Cohort	Study of mortality of farmers compared to nonfarmers in Iowa (1971–1978)	6,402	13,809
New Cohort Studies of Forestry Workers				
Thorn et al., 2000	Cohort	Study of mortality and cancer incidence in a cohort of Swedish lumberjacks exposed to phenoxy herbicides	261	243

continued

TABLE 6-1 Continued

Reference	Study	Design Description	Study Group (N)	Comparison Group (N)[a]
Cohort Studies of Forestry Workers Reviewed in VAO				
Green, 1991	Cohort	Mortality experience of male forestry workers (1950–1982) in Ontario, compared to expected mortality of the male Ontario population	1,222	—
Green, 1987	Cohort	Suicide experience in a cohort of Canadian forestry workers by number of years in forestry trade as a surrogate for exposure to phenoxy herbicides compared to population	1,222	—
Van Houdt et al., 1983	Cross-sectional	Study of acne and liver dysfunction in a select group of Dutch forestry workers exposed to 2,4,5-T and unexposed	54	54
New Cohort Studies of Herbicide and Pesticide Sprayers				
Alavanja et al., 1998	Cohort	Analysis of self-reported health care visits having resulted from pesticide use by Iowa and North Carolina pesticide appliers	35,879	None
Dich et al., 1998	Cohort	Study of men licensed for pesticide application in Sweden. Cancer cases ascertained from cancer registry and standardized incidence ratio reported for prostate cancer	20,025	—

Cohort Studies of Herbicide and Pesticide Sprayers Reviewed in Update 1998

Reference	Study Design	Description	Exposed	Controls
Heacock et al., 1998	Cohort	Fertility study among British Columbia workers potentially exposed to chlorophenate wood preservatives in 14 sawmills between 1955 and 1988; includes the cohort of Hertzman et al. (1997)	18,016 births	1,668 births
Hertzman et al., 1997	Cohort	Mortality study among British Columbia workers potentially exposed to chlorophenate wood preservatives in 11 sawmills between 1950 and 1985	23,829	2,658
Dimich-Ward et al., 1996	Cohort; Nested case-control	Analysis of birth defects among offspring born between 1952 and 1988 of the Hertzman et al. (1997) cohort	19,675 births among 9,512 fathers	5 nondefect births as controls per case
Garry et al., 1996a	Cohort	Study of chromosome abnormalities based on the cohort of Garry et al. (1994)	23 fumigant appliers; 18 insecticide appliers; 20 herbicide appliers	33
Garry et al., 1996b	Cohort	Birth defects among the offspring of male pesticide appliers in Minnesota born between 1989 and 1992	4,935 births among 34,772 pesticide appliers (125 with birth anomalies)	3,666 births with anomalies in the general population
Zhong and Rafnsson, 1996	Cohort	Cancer mortality among various subgroups of pesticide users in Iceland	2,449 (1,860 males and 589 females)	—

continued

203

TABLE 6-1 Continued

Reference	Study	Design Description	Study Group (N)	Comparison Group (N)[a]
Cohort Studies of Herbicide and Pesticide Sprayers Reviewed in Update 1996				
Asp et al., 1994	Cohort	Mortality and cancer morbidity experience of male chlorophenoxy herbicide appliers (same cohort as Riihimaki et al., 1982, 1983) in Finland (1955–1971), through 1989, compared to general population rates for morbidity and mortality	1,909	—
Garry et al., 1994	Cross-sectional	Evaluation of health outcomes resulting from exposure to pesticides by male pesticide appliers in Minnesota	719	No comparison group
Cohort Studies of Herbicide and Pesticide Sprayers Reviewed in VAO				
Swaen et al., 1992	Cohort	Cancer mortality experience (through 1987) among Dutch male herbicide appliers licensed before 1980, compared to total male Dutch population	1,341	—
Bender et al., 1989	Cohort	Cancer mortality of Minnesota highway maintenance workers compared to expected numbers based on white Minnesota men	4,849	—
Wiklund et al., 1989a	Cohort	Risk of cancer in Wiklund et al. (1987) cohort through 1982	20,245	—

Reference	Study Design	Description	Sample Size	Exposed
Wiklund et al., 1989b	Cohort	Risk of STS, HD, and NHL in Wiklund et al. (1987) cohort through 1984	20,245	—
Wiklund et al., 1988b	Cohort	Risk of STS in Wiklund et al. (1987) cohort through 1984	20,245	—
Wiklund et al., 1987	Cohort	Risk of HD and NHL among Swedish pesticide appliers from date of license through 1982, compared to expected number of cases in the total population	20,245	—
Blair et al., 1983	Cohort	Mortality experience of white male Florida pesticide appliers compared to U.S. and Florida men	3,827	—
Riihimaki et al., 1983	Cohort	Cancer morbidity and mortality in cohort of Riihimaki et al. (1982), through 1980	1,926	—
Riihimaki et al., 1982	Cohort	Study of mortality among herbicide appliers exposed to 2,4-D and 2,4,5-T in Finland compared to mortality expected in the population	1,926	—
Smith et al., 1982	Cohort	Study of adverse reproductive outcomes among chemical appliers and agricultural contractors by category of exposure: none; chemicals not 2,4,5-T; 2,4,5-T	113 pregnancies (chemicals not 2,4,5-T); 486 pregnancies (2,4,5-T)	401 pregnancies (not exposed)

continued

TABLE 6-1 Continued

Reference	Study	Design Description	Study Group (N)	Comparison Group (N)[a]
Barthel, 1981	Cohort	Study of male agricultural production workers (1948–1972) for incidence of cancer, compared to incidence rates expected in the population	1,658	
Smith et al., 1981	Cohort	Study of chemical appliers (1973–1979) in New Zealand compared to agricultural contractors for differences in adverse reproductive outcomes	459	422
Axelson et al., 1980	Cohort	Additional years of follow-up to cohort established in Axelson and Sundell (1974)	348	—
Axelson and Sundell, 1974	Cohort	Study of mortality and cancer incidence among cohorts of Swedish railroad workers spraying herbicides (>45 days) compared to the expected number of deaths (1957–1972) from Swedish age- and sex-specific rates	348 total herbicide exposure; 207 phenoxy acids and combinations; 152 amitrole and combinations; 28 other herbicides and combinations	—

Case-Control Studies
New Case-Control Studies

Study	Type	Description	N1	N2
Ekstrom et al., 1999	Case-control	All new cases of histologically confirmed gastric adenocarcinoma in two geographic areas in Sweden; age- and gender-matched control group randomly selected using computerized population register	565	1,164
Hardell and Eriksson, 1999	Case-control	Male cases 25 or older with histopathologically confirmed NHL during 1987–1990 in northern and mid-Sweden; age matched controls from National Population Registry	404	741
Garcia et al., 1998	Case-control	Matched-paired study of congenital malformations or defects in an agricultural region of Spain	261	261

Case-Control Studies Reviewed in Update 1998

Study	Type	Description	N1	N2
Blatter et al., 1997	Case-control	Multicenter Dutch study of paternal occupation and risk of spina bifida in offspring (1980–1992)	222	764
Liou et al., 1997	Case-control	Study of occupational and environmental risk factors and Parkinson's disease (PD) in Taiwan (1993–1995)	120	240

continued

TABLE 6-1 Continued

Reference	Study	Design Description	Study Group (N)	Comparison Group (N)[a]
Tatham et al., 1997	Nested case-control	Population-based study of occupational risk factors for subgroups of NHL patients based on the CDC's Selected Cancers Study (CDC, 1990a,b,c,d)	1,048	1,659
Nanni et al., 1996	Case-control	Population-based study in northeastern Italy of occupational and chemical risk factors for chronic lymphocytic leukemia (CLL) and NHL (1987–1990)	187	977
Schulte et al., 1996	PMR analysis with nested case-control	Study of neurodegenerative diseases and occupational risk factors from 27 states	Based on 130,420 death certificates	
Seidler et al., 1996	Case-control	Study of PD and various rural factors, including exposure to herbicides and wood preservatives in Germany	380	379 neighborhood controls; 376 regional controls
Case-Control Studies Reviewed in Update 1996				
Hardell et al., 1994	Case-control	Study of the association between occupational exposures and parameters related to NHL in white males in Sweden	105	335

208

Reference	Study Type	Description		
Mellemgaard et al., 1994	Case-control	Study of cases of renal cell carcinoma (20–79 years) in Denmark, compared to population-based sample without cancer for identification of occupational risk factors	365	396
Nurminen et al., 1994	Case-control	Study of structural defects in infants born to mothers engaged in agricultural work during the first trimester of pregnancy, compared to infants with structural defects born to mothers who did not engage in agricultural work during the first trimester	1,306	1,306
Brown et al., 1993	Case-control	Population-based case-control study of multiple myeloma in Iowa men for association with pesticide exposures	173	650
Persson et al., 1993	Case-control	Study of risk factors potentially associated with HD and NHL in males identified from the Regional Cancer Registry in Sweden	NHL: 93 HD: 31	204
Semchuk et al., 1993	Case-control	Study of cases of PD (36–90 years) in Canada, compared to population-based sample for association with occupational exposure to herbicides and other exposures	75 men 55 women	150 men 110 women

continued

TABLE 6-1 Continued

Reference	Study	Design Description	Study Group (N)	Comparison Group (N)[a]
Zahm et al., 1993	Case-control	Study of NHL and exposure to pesticides in white women diagnosed with NHL between July 1, 1983, and June 30, 1986	206	824
McDuffie et al., 1990	Case-control	Study of pesticide exposure in male cases of primary lung cancer in Saskatchewan, compared to control subjects matched by age, sex, and location of residence	273	187
Case-Control Studies Reviewed in VAO				
Cantor et al., 1992	Case-control	Population-based case-control study of NHL in Iowa and Minnesota men for association with farming exposures	622	1,245
Smith and Christophers, 1992	Case-control	Study of STS and malignant lymphomas in men diagnosed 1982–1988 in Australia, compared to other cancers for association with exposure to phenoxy herbicides and chlorophenols	82	82 other cancers; 82 population controls
Brown et al., 1990	Case-control	Population-based case-control study of leukemia in Iowa and Minnesota men for association with farming exposures	578	1,245

Eriksson et al., 1990	Case-control	Study of male cases of STS (25–80 years) diagnosed 1978–1986 in central Sweden compared to population-based sample without cancer for association with occupational exposure to phenoxyacetic acids and chlorophenols	218	212
Wingren et al., 1990	Case-control	Study of male cases of STS (25–80 years) diagnosed 1975–1982 in southeast Sweden, compared to two referent groups: (1) population-based sample, (2) with other cancers, for association with phenoxyacetic acids and chlorophenols	71	315 population based; 164 other cancers
Zahm et al., 1990	Case-control	Study of white men 21 years or older diagnosed with NHL (1983–1986) in Nebraska, compared to residents of the same area without NHL, HD, multiple myeloma (MM), chronic lymphocytic leukemia for association with herbicides (2,4-D) on farms	201	725

continued

211

TABLE 6-1 Continued

Reference	Study	Design Description	Study Group (N)	Comparison Group (N)[a]
Alavanja et al., 1989	PMR analysis with nested case-control	Mortality experience of United States Department of Agriculture (USDA) forest or soil conservationists (1970–1979) evaluated for specific cancer excess; case-control study of specific cancers identified from PMR analysis	1,411	—
Boffetta et al., 1989	Nested case-control	National study of MM compared to other cancer controls for association with exposures including pesticides and herbicides	282	1,128
LaVecchia et al., 1989	Case-control	Study of Italian men and women with HD, NHL, and MM (1983–1988), compared to population of Italy for association with occupations and herbicide use	69 HD 153 NHL 110 MM	396
Persson et al., 1989	Case-control	Study of HD and NHL among living men and women in Sweden, compared to those without these cancers for association with occupational exposures, including phenoxy herbicides	54 HD 106 NHL	275

Woods and Polissar, 1989	Case-control	Study of NHL from the Woods et al. (1987) cohort for association with phenoxy herbicides in farm workers	576	694
Alavanja et al., 1988	PMR analysis with nested case-control	Mortality experience of USDA extension agents (1970–1979) evaluated for specific cancer excess; case-control study of specific cancers identified from PMR analysis	1,495	—
Dubrow et al., 1988	Case-control	Death certificate study (1958–1983) of NHL and HD among white male residents of Hancock County, Ohio, compared to a random sample of those dying from other causes for association with farming	61 NHL 15 HD	304
Hardell and Eriksson, 1988	Case-control	Study of male cases of STS (25–80 years) diagnosed between 1978 and 1983 in northern Sweden compared to two referent groups: (1) population based, (2) with other cancers, for association with occupational exposure to phenoxyacetic acids and chlorophenols	55	330 population based; 190 other cancers

continued

TABLE 6-1 Continued

Reference	Study	Design Description	Study Group (N)	Comparison Group (N)[a]
Musicco et al., 1988	Case-control	Study of brain gliomas diagnosed 1983–1984 in men and women in Italy, compared to (1) patients with nonglioma nervous system tumors and (2) patients with other neurologic diseases, for association with chemical exposures in farming	240	(1) 465 (2) 277
Olsson and Brandt, 1988	Case-control	Study of NHL (1978–1981) in Swedish men, compared to two groups of men without NHL for association with occupational exposures including phenoxy acids	167	50 same area; 80 other parts of Sweden
Hardell et al., 1987	Case-control	Study of Kaposi's sarcoma in AIDS patients (23–53 years of age) compared to controls for association with TCDD and pesticide exposure in Sweden	50	50
Pearce et al., 1987	Case-control	Expanded study (Pearce et al., 1986b) of NHL to include ICD•9 200-diagnosed cases and additional controls for association with farming exposures	183	338

Woods et al., 1987	Case-control	Study of STS or NHL in men 20–79 years old (1983–1985) in western Washington State compared to a population sample without these cancers for association with occupational exposure to phenoxy herbicides and chlorinated phenols	128 STS 576 NHL	694
Hoar et al., 1986	Case-control	Study of STS, NHL, and HD in Kansas (1976–1982), compared to controls without cancer for association with 2,4-D, 2,4,5-T, and other herbicides in white men 21 years or older	133 STS 121 HD 170 NHL	948
Morris et al., 1986	Case-control	Study of multiple myeloma (1977–1981) in four SEER areas compared to population controls for risk factors associated with MM, including farm use of herbicides	698	1,683
Pearce et al., 1986a	Case-control	Study of male MM cases diagnosed 1971–1981 in New Zealand, compared to controls for other cancers for potential association with phenoxy herbicides and chlorophenols	76	315

continued

TABLE 6-1 *Continued*

Reference	Study	Design Description	Study Group (N)	Comparison Group (N)[a]
Pearce et al., 1986b	Case-control	Study of NHL cases (ICD-9 202) in men diagnosed between 1977 and 1981 in New Zealand, compared to sample with other cancers and population sample, for association with occupational exposure to phenoxy herbicides and chlorophenols	83	168 other cancers; 228 general population
Smith and Pearce, 1986	Case-control	Update of Smith et al. (1983) with diagnoses through 1982	51 in update (133 when combined with Smith et al., 1983)	315 (407)
Vineis et al., 1986	Case-control	Study of cases of STS in men and women diagnosed 1981–1983 in northern Italy, compared to population sample of controls for association with phenoxy herbicide exposure	37 men 31 women	85 men 73 women
Blair and White, 1985	Case-control	Study of leukemia cases by cell type in Nebraska (1957–1974) compared to nonleukemia deaths for association with agricultural practices	1,084	2,168

216

Pearce et al., 1985	Case-control	Study of malignant lymphoma and multiple myeloma in men diagnosed 1977–1981 in New Zealand, compared to men with other cancers for association with agricultural occupations	734	2,936
Balarajan and Acheson, 1984	Case-control	Study of STS (1968–1976) diagnosed in men in England and Wales compared to men with other cancers for association with farming, agriculture, and forestry occupations	1,961	1,961
Donna et al., 1984	Case-control	Study of ovarian cancer in women (1974–1980) for association with herbicide use, compared to women without ovarian cancer	60	127
Hardell et al., 1984	Case-control	Study of primary liver cancer diagnosed 1974–1981 in men 25–80 years residing in northern Sweden compared to population based controls for association with occupational exposure to phenoxyacetic acids and chlorophenols	98	200

continued

TABLE 6-1 Continued

Reference	Study	Design Description	Study Group (N)	Comparison Group (N)[a]
Smith et al., 1984	Case-control	Study of STS among New Zealand residents (1976–1980) compared to those without these cancers for association with occupational exposures, including phenoxy herbicides	82	92
Burmeister et al., 1983	Case-control	Study of multiple myeloma, NHL, prostate, and stomach cancer mortality (1964–1978) in white men 30 years or older compared to mortality from other causes for association with farming practices including herbicide use in Iowa	550 MM 1,101 NHL 4,827 prostate 1,812 stomach	1,100 2,202 9,654 3,624
Hardell and Bengtsson, 1983	Case-control	Study of HD diagnosed in men 25–85, between 1974 and 1978 in northern Sweden, compared to population-based sample without cancer for association with occupational exposure to phenoxyacetic acid and chlorophenols	60	335

Smith et al., 1983	Case-control	Preliminary report of men with STS reported 1976–1980 in New Zealand, compared to controls with other cancers for association with phenoxyacetic acid exposure	80	92
Burmeister et al., 1982	Case-control	Study of leukemia deaths (1964–1978) in white men 30 years or older in Iowa, compared to nonleukemia deaths for association with farming	1,675	3,350
Cantor, 1982	Case-control	Study of NHL in Wisconsin among males (1968–1976) compared to men dying from other causes for association with farming exposures	774	1,651
Hardell et al. 1982	Case-control	Study of nasal and nasopharyngeal cancers diagnosed 1970–1979 in men 25–85 years residing in northern Sweden, compared to controls selected from previous studies (Hardell and Sandstrom, 1979; Hardell et al., 1981) for association with occupational exposure to phenoxyacetic acids and chlorophenols	44 nasal; 27 nasopharyngeal	541

continued

TABLE 6-1 *Continued*

Reference	Study	Design Description	Study Group (N)	Comparison Group (N)[a]
Carmelli et al., 1981	Case-control	Cases of spontaneous abortions occurring to women (1978–1980) compared to live births for association with paternal exposure to 2,4-D	134	311
Eriksson et al., 1979, 1981	Case-control	Cases of STS diagnosed between 1974 and 1978 in southern Sweden compared to population based sample without cancer for association with occupational exposure to phenoxyacetic acids and chlorophenols	110	219
Hardell, 1981	Case-control	(1) Cases of STS (Hardell and Sandstrom, 1979) and malignant lymphomas (Hardell et al., 1981) compared to colon cancer cases (2) Colon-cancer cases compared to population-based controls for association with occupational exposure to phenoxyacetic acids and chlorophenols	(1) 221 (2) 154	154 541

Reference	Study Type	Description	Cases	Total
Hardell et al., 1980; Hardell et al., 1981	Case-control	Cases of malignant lymphomas (HD, NHL, unknown) diagnosed in men age 25–85, between 1974 and 1978 in northern Sweden, compared to population-based controls for association with occupational exposure to phenoxyacetic acids and chlorophenols	60 HD 109 NHL	338
Blair and Thomas, 1979	Case-control	Cases in Nebraska (1957–1974) compared to deaths from other causes for association with agricultural practices	1,084	2,168
Hardell and Sandstrom, 1979	Case-control	Cases of STS (26–80 years) diagnosed between 1970 and 1977 in northern Sweden, compared to population-based controls for association with occupational exposure to phenoxyacetic acids and chlorophenols	52	206
Paper and Pulp Workers				
New Paper and Pulp Worker Studies				
Schildt et al., 1999	Case-control	Matched study of histo-pathologically verified oral cancer cases. Mailed exposure questionnaire on lifetime occupational history, oral cancer risk factors, pesticide use, smoking, SES, and place of residence	410	410

continued

TABLE 6-1 Continued

Reference	Study	Design Description	Study Group (N)	Comparison Group (N)[a]
Rix et al., 1998	Cohort	Cancer incidence rates of blue-collar workers at three Danish paper mills were compared to population rates from national population and mortality registers	14,788 (14,362 were identified for follow-up)	—
Paper and Pulp Worker Studies Reviewed in VAO				
Jappinen and Pukkala, 1991	Cohort	Cancer incidence (through 1987) among male Finnish pulp and paper workers (1945–1961), compared to rates in the local central hospital district	152	Approximately 135,000
Henneberger et al., 1989	Cohort	Mortality experience through August 1985 of white men employed in Berlin, N.H., paper and pulp industry, compared to expected mortality in U.S. white men	883	—

| Solet et al., 1989 | Cohort | Mortality (1970–1984) among white male United Paperworkers International union members, compared to expected number of deaths in U.S. men | 201 | — |
| Robinson et al., 1986 | Cohort | Mortality experience through March 1977 of white male workers employed in five paper or pulp mills compared to expected number of deaths among U.S. population | 3,572 | — |

NOTE: CDC = Centers for Disease Control and Prevention; COPD = chronic obstructive pulmonary disease; HD = Hodgkin's disease; IARC = International Agency for Research on Cancer; ICD = International Classification of Diseases; NHL = non-Hodgkin's lymphoma; NIOSH = National Institute for Occupational Safety and Health; PCDD/F = polychlorinated dibenzodioxin or dibenzofuran; PMR = proportionate mortality ratio; SEER = surveillance, epidemiology, and end results; SES = socio-economic status; STS = soft-tissue sarcoma; T_3 = Triiodothyronine; T_4 = thyroxine; TSH = Thyroid-stimulating hormone; *Update 1998* = *Veterans and Agent Orange: Update 1998* (IOM, 1999); *Update 1996* = *Veterans and Agent Orange: Update 1996* (IOM, 1996); and *VAO* = *Veterans and Agent Orange: Health Effects of Herbicides Used in Vietnam* (IOM, 1994). [a]The dash (—) indicates the comparison group is based on a population (e.g., U.S. white males, country rates), and details are given in the text for specifics of the actual population.

TABLE 6-2 Epidemiologic Studies—Environmental Exposure

Reference	Study Design	Description	Study Group (N)	Comparison Group (N)[a]
New Studies from Seveso				
Bertazzi et al., 2001	Cohort	Mortality (through 1996) study of residents in industrial accident exposure-related geographic regions	804 zone A 5,941 zone B 38,624 zone R	232,745
Bertazzi et al., 1998; Pesatori et al., 1998	Cohort	Mortality (through 1991) study of residents in industrial accident exposure-related geographic regions	805 zone A 51,943 zone B 38,625 zone R	232,747
Seveso Studies Reviewed in Update 1998				
Bertazzi et al., 1997	Cohort	Study of cancer incidence among Seveso residents in contaminated zones (A, B, R) after 15 years of follow-up through 1991	45,373 total 805 zone A 5,943 zone B 38,625 zone R	232,747
Mocarelli et al., 1996	Cohort	Study of sex ratio among the offspring of Seveso residents born in zone A from (1) 1977 to 1984 and (2) 1985 to 1994	(1) 74 births (28 male, 48 female) (2) 124 births (60 male, 48 female)	
Seveso Studies Reviewed in Update 1996				
Bertazzi et al., 1993	Cohort	Study of cancer incidence in Seveso residents (aged 20 to 74 years) in contaminated zones (A, B, R) exposed to TCDD on July 10, 1976, compared to neighboring residents in unexposed areas	724 zone A 4,824 zone B 31,647 zone R	181,579

Reference	Study Type	Description	Exposed	Controls
Pesatori et al., 1993	Cohort	Evaluation of cancer incidence in Seveso residents aged 1–19 years in the first postaccident decade compared to age-matched residents of neighboring unexposed areas	Approximately 20,000	167,391
Seveso Studies Reviewed in VAO				
Bertazzi et al., 1992	Cohort	Comparison of mortality of children (1976–1986) exposed during Seveso accident compared to children in uncontaminated areas	306 zone A 2,727 zone B 16,604 zone R	95,339
Pesatori et al., 1992	Cohort	Cancer incidence (1976–1986) among those in zones A, B, R around Seveso compared to residents of uncontaminated surrounding areas	Data given in person-years	Data given in person-years
Assennato et al., 1989a	Cohort	Comparison of dermatologic and laboratory findings in children during periodic exams following accident in Seveso	193 with chloracne	123
Assennato et al., 1989b	Cohort	Study of health outcomes in workers assigned to cleanup or referent group following Seveso accident	36	36
Bertazzi et al., 1989a,b	Cohort	Comparison of mortality experience (1976–1986) of residents of contaminated zones (A, B, R) around Seveso to mortality experience of unexposed residents in neighboring towns	556 zone A 3,920 zone B 26,227 zone R	167,391
Barbieri et al., 1988	Cohort	Comparison of prevalence of peripheral nervous system involvement among Seveso residents with chloracne, compared to residents of unexposed areas	152	123

continued

TABLE 6-2 *Continued*

Reference	Study Design	Description	Study Group (N)	Comparison Group (N)[a]
Mastroiacovo et al., 1988	Cohort	Comparison of birth defects occurring among zone A, B, and R mothers with live and stillbirths to birth mothers who were non-A, B, or R residents	26 zone A 435 zone B 2,439 zone R	12,391 (non-A, B, or R)
Mocarelli et al., 1986	Cross-sectional	Study of laboratory measures of serum and urine in Seveso zone A and B children measured over 6 years (1977–1982), compared to zone R children	69 zone A 528 zone B 874 zone R	241, subset of zone R
Ideo et al., 1985	Cross-sectional	Evaluation of levels of enzyme activity among residents of Seveso zone B and an uncontaminated community	117 adults	127 adults
Tenchini et al., 1983	Cross-sectional	Cytogenetic analysis of maternal and fetal tissue among Seveso exposed, compared to control sample	19	16
Ideo et al., 1982	Cross-sectional	Evaluation of hepatic enzymes in children exposed in Seveso compared to normal values	16 zone A 51 zone B	60 Bristo Assizio 26 Cannero
Caramaschi et al., 1981	Cohort	Evaluation of chloracne among children in Seveso, compared to children with no chloracne, and association with other health outcomes between chloracne and no-chloracne groups	146	182
Filippini et al., 1981	Cohort	Comparison of prevalence of peripheral neuropathy on two screening examinations among Seveso residents, compared to residents in unexposed areas	308	305

Study	Design	Description	Exposed	Comparison
Bisanti et al., 1980	Descriptive	Descriptive report of selected health outcomes among residents of Seveso located in zones A, B, R	730 zone A 4,737 zone B 31,800 zone R	No comparison group
Boeri et al., 1978	Cohort	Evaluation of neurological disorders among Seveso residents exposed to TCDD on July 10, 1976, compared to residents in unexposed areas	470 zone A	152 zone R
Times Beach/Quail Run Studies Reviewed in VAO				
Evans et al., 1988	Cross-sectional	Comparison of retesting for skin delayed-type hypersensitivity among nonresponders in earlier test (Stehr et al., 1986)	28	15
Stockbauer et al., 1988	Cohort	Study of adverse reproductive outcomes (1972–1982) among mothers potentially exposed to TCDD-contaminated areas of Missouri (1971) compared to births among unexposed mothers	402 births	804 births
Webb et al., 1987	Cross-sectional	Pilot study of Missouri residents exposed to TCDD in the environment (1971) for health effects, comparing potentially high-exposed to low-exposed residents	68 (high exposure)	36 (low exposure)
Stehr et al., 1986	Cross-sectional	Pilot study of Missouri residents exposed to TCDD in the environment (1971) for health effects, comparing potentially high-exposed to low-exposed residents	68 (high exposure)	36 (low exposure)
Studies of Vietnamese Reviewed in Update 1996				
Cordier et al., 1993	Case-control	Study of cases of hepatocellular carcinoma (1989–1992) in males living in Vietnam, compared to other hospitalized patients for association with a range of exposures including herbicides	152	241

continued

TABLE 6-2 Continued

Reference	Study Design	Description	Study Group (N)	Comparison Group (N)[a]
Studies of Vietnamese Reviewed in VAO				
Dai et al., 1990	Cohort	Study of infant mortality (1966–1986) in two South Vietnam villages exposed to Agent Orange spraying compared to infant mortality in unsprayed area	5,609	3,306
Phuong et al., 1989a	Case-control	Study of deformed babies and hydatidiform mole compared to normal births (1982) in Ho Chi Minh City for association with mother's exposure to Agent Orange and TCDD in Vietnam conflict	15 birth defects 50 hydatidiform moles	104 134
Phuong et al., 1989b	Cohort	Comparison of reproductive anomalies among births to women (May 1982–June 1982) living in areas heavily sprayed with herbicides in southern Vietnam, to women from Ho Chi Minh City	7,327 births	6,690 births
Constable and Hatch, 1985	Review	Summaries of reproductive outcomes among Vietnamese populations, includes nine unpublished studies		
Other New Environmental Studies				
Schreinemachers, 2000	Cross-sectional	Study of cancer mortality rates in four northern wheat-producing states using wheat acreage per county as surrogate for exposure	—	—

228

Other Environmental Studies Reviewed in Update 1998

Reference	Study Design	Study Description	Exposed	Controls
Gallagher et al., 1996	Case-control	Community-based study of primary basal cell carcinoma (BCC) and patients with primary squamous cell carcinoma (SCC) in Alberta, Canada	BCC: 226 SCC: 180	406
Lovik et al., 1996	Cohort	Study of immune system parameters in hobby fishermen in the Frierfjord in southeastern Norway	24	10
Masala et al., 1996	Case-control	Multicenter study of NHL, HD, multiple myeloma (MM), and acute myeloid leukemia (AML) in Italy by region	HD: 421 NHL: 1,822 MM: 325 AML: 263	Internal comparison by region
Svensson et al., 1995	Cohort	Mortality and cancer incidence experience in two cohorts of Swedish fishermen	East coast: 2,896	West coast: 8,477
Weisglas-Kuperus et al., 1995	Cohort	Study of the immunological effects of pre- and postnatal PCB or TCDD exposure in 207 Dutch infants from birth to 18 months	105 breast-fed	102 bottle-fed
Wolf and Karmaus, 1995	Cross-sectional	Study of the effects of inhalative exposure to TCDD and related compounds in wood preservatives on cell-mediated immunity in German day care center employees	221	189

Other Environmental Studies Reviewed in Update 1996

Reference	Study Design	Study Description	Exposed	Controls
Butterfield et al., 1993	Case-control	Study of possible environmental risk factors associated with young-onset Parkinson's disease	63	68
Peper et al., 1993	Descriptive	Study of environmental exposure to dioxins and furans and potential association with adverse neuropsychological effects in Germany	19	None

continued

TABLE 6-2 *Continued*

Reference	Study Design	Description	Study Group (N)	Comparison Group (N)[a]
Other Environmental Studies Reviewed in VAO				
Lampi et al., 1992	Nested case-control/cohort	Study of cancer incidence among a community in Finland exposed to water and food contaminated with chlorophenols (1987), compared to other communities; study of several cancers compared to population controls for association with potential risk factors including food and water consumption	56 colon cancer; 40 bladder cancer; 8 STS; 7 HD; 23 NHL; 43 leukemia	688
Vineis et al., 1991	Ecological	Presentation of rates (1985–1988) of NHL, HD, and STS in men and women 15–74 years living in provinces in Italy where phenoxy herbicides are used in rice weeding and defined in two categories	63 HD 253 NHL 49 STS	No unexposed control
Fitzgerald et al., 1989	Cohort	Health outcomes in group exposed to electrical transformer fire in 1981 compared to standardized rates among upstate New York residents	377	—
Jansson and Voog, 1989	Cohort/case study	Case study of facial cleft (April–August 1987) and study of facial clefts (1975–1987) compared to the rates expected in Swedish county with incinerators	20,595 births after incineration 6 case studies	71,665 births before incineration
Cartwright et al., 1988	Case-control	Study of living cases of NHL (1979–1984) in Yorkshire, England, compared to other hospitalized patients for association with a range of exposures including fertilizers or herbicides	437	724

Study	Design	Description	County rates	State and national rates
Michigan Department of Public Health, 1983	Descriptive	Comparison of Michigan county rates of mortality for STS and connective tissue cancer (1960–1981), compared to state and national rates for potential excess in areas where dioxin may be in the environment		
Gordon and Shy, 1981	Case-control	Study of agricultural chemical exposures and potential association with cleft palate or lip in Iowa and Michigan, compared to other live births	187	985
Hanify et al., 1981	Ecological design	Study of adverse birth outcomes occurring 1960–1966, compared to 1972–1977 for association with 2,4,5-T spraying in the later period	9,614 births	15,000 births
Nelson et al., 1979	Ecological design	Study of prevalence of oval cleft palates in high, medium, and low 2,4,5-T sprayed areas in Arkansas (1948–1974)	—	—
U.S. EPA, 1979	Ecological design	Study of spontaneous abortions occurring during 1972–1977 in herbicide-sprayed areas around Alsea, Oregon, compared to spontaneous abortions occurring in unsprayed areas	2,344 births	1,666 births—unsprayed area; 4,120 births—urban area

NOTE: HD = Hodgkin's disease; NHL = non-Hodgkin's lymphoma; STS = soft-tissue sarcoma; *Update 1998* = *Veterans and Agent Orange: Update 1998* (IOM, 1999); *Update 1996* = *Veterans and Agent Orange: Update 1996* (IOM, 1996); *VAO* = *Veterans and Agent Orange: Health Effects of Herbicides Used in Vietnam* (IOM, 1994). [a]The dash (—) indicates the comparison group is based on a population (e.g., U.S. white males, country rates), with details given in the text for specifics of the actual population.

TABLE 6-3 Epidemiologic Studies—Veterans' Exposure

Reference	Study Design	Description	Study Group (N)	Comparison Group (N)[a]
United States Studies				
New Ranch Hand Studies				
AFHS, 2000	Cohort	Evaluation of 266 health-related end points, including assessments of 10 clinical areas: general health, neoplasia, neurological, psychological, gastrointestinal, cardiovascular, hematologic, endocrine, immunologic, and pulmonary	995	1,299
Longnecker and Michalek, 2000	Cohort	Based on physical examination and medical record review through 1992, analyzed association between serum dioxin levels and diabetes mellitus among the comparison group (no Ranch Hands)	—	1,281 1,197
Ketchum et al., 1999	Cohort	Based on physical examination and medical record review through 1992, analyzed association between serum dioxin levels and cancer, skin cancer, and other than skin cancer	1,109 980 922 980	1,493 1,275 1,202 1,275
Michalek et al., 1999a	Cohort	To further elucidate the relationship between dioxin and diabetes mellitus, this analysis studies the effect of dioxin body burden on the relationship between sex hormone-binding globulin and insulin and fasting glucose	952 871	1,281 1,121
Michalek et al., 1999b	Cohort	Based on physical examinations in 1982, 1985, 1987, and 1992, examination of immunologic response and exposure to dioxin among Ranch Hand and comparison cohorts	952 914 372 358	1,281 1,186 491 456

Burton et al., 1998	Cohort	Based on physical examination and medical record review through 1992, analyzed association between serum dioxin levels and occurrence and timing (relative to Southeast Asia service) of chloracne and acne	952 930 476	1,281 1,200 598
Michalek et al., 1998b	Cohort	Updates all-cause and cause-specific postservice mortality (through 1993) among veterans of Operation Ranch Hand, using standardized mortality ratios	1,261	19,080
Michalek et al., 1998c	Cohort	Prospective study of exposure and long-term health, survival, or reproductive outcome	1,208 veterans 903 offspring	1,549 veterans 1,254 offspring
Michalek et al., 1998d	Cohort	Third report in a series investigating dioxin body burden and preterm birth, intrauterine growth retardation, and infant death among offspring of Ranch Hand veterans	995 932 859	1,299 1,202 1,223

Ranch Hand Studies Reviewed in Update 1998

Michalek et al., 1998a	Cohort	Paternal serum dioxin levels and infant death among offspring of Ranch Hands	859 children: 323 background exposure, 267 low exposure, 269 high exposure	1,223 children
Henriksen et al., 1997	Cohort	Study of the relationship between serum dioxin and glucose levels, insulin levels, and diabetes mellitus in Ranch Hands through 1992	989	1,276

continued

TABLE 6-3 Continued

Reference	Study Design	Description	Study Group (N)	Comparison Group (N)[a]
AFHS, 1996; Michalek et al., 1998b	Cohort	Mortality update of Ranch Hands through the end of 1993 in the same cohort as AFHS (1983, 1984b, 1985, 1986, 1989, 1991a, 1995)	1,261	19,080
Henriksen et al., 1996	Cohort	Study of serum dioxin and reproductive hormones in Ranch Hands in 1982, 1985, 1987, and 1992	1,045 (participants, 1982) 474 (provided semen)	1,224 (participants, 1982) 532 (provided semen)
Ranch Hand Studies Reviewed in Update 1996				
AFHS, 1995	Cohort	Mortality updates of Ranch Hands tasked with herbicide spraying operations during the Vietnam conflict, compared with Air Force C-130 air and ground crew veterans in Southeast Asia who did not participate in herbicide spraying missions	1,261 (original cohort)	19,101 (original cohort)
Wolfe et al., 1995	Cohort	Paternal serum dioxin levels and reproductive outcomes of Ranch Hand veterans compared with Air Force veterans from Southeast Asia who did not participate in herbicide spraying missions	932	1,202
Ranch Hand Studies Reviewed in VAO				
AFHS, 1992	Cohort	Reproductive outcomes of participants in the Air Force Health Study (AFHS)	791	942

AFHS, 1984a, 1987, 1990, 1991b, 1995	Cohort	Baseline morbidity and follow-up exam results of the AFHS	1,208 (baseline)	1,668 (baseline)
AFHS, 1983, 1984b, 1985, 1986, 1989, 1991a	Cohort	Mortality updates of Ranch Hands tasked with herbicide spraying operations during the Vietnam conflict, compared with Air Force C-130 air and ground crew veterans in Southeast Asia who did not participate in herbicide spraying missions	1,261 (original cohort)	19,101 (original cohort)
Michalek et al., 1990	Cohort	Mortality of Ranch Hands compared with Air Force C-130 air and ground crew veterans in Southeast Asia	1,261	19,101
Wolfe et al., 1990	Cohort	Health status of Ranch Hands at second follow-up, compared with Air Force C-130 air and ground crew veterans in Southeast Asia	995	1,299

Centers for Disease Control (CDC) Studies Reviewed in VAO

Decoufle et al., 1992	Cohort	Association between self-reported health outcomes and perception of exposure to herbicides based on Vietnam Experience Study (VES)	7,924	7,364
O'Brien et al., 1991	Cohort	Interview report and mortality for NHL based on VES	8,170	7,564

continued

TABLE 6-3 *Continued*

Reference	Study Design	Description	Study Group (N)	Comparison Group (N)[a]
CDC, 1990a	Case-control	Selected Cancers Study—population-based case-control study of all men born between 1921 and 1953; cases diagnosed area covered by eight cancer registries and controls selected by random-digit dialing	1,157 NHL; 342 STS; 310 HD; 48 nasal carcinoma; 80 nasopharyngeal carcinoma; 130 primary liver cancer	1,776
CDC, 1990b	Case-control	Selected Cancers Study—population-based case-control study of all men born between 1921 and 1953; cases diagnosed area covered by eight cancer registries and controls selected by random-digit dialing: NHL	1,157	1,776
CDC, 1990c	Case-control	Selected Cancers Study: soft-tissue sarcoma	342	1,776
CDC, 1990d	Case-control	Selected Cancers Study: HD, nasal cancer, nasopharyngeal cancer, and primary liver cancer	310 HD; 48 nasal carcinoma; 80 nasopharyngeal carcinoma; 130 primary liver cancer	1,776
CDC, 1989b	Cohort	Vietnam Experience Study—random sample of U.S. Army enlisted men 1965–1971	2,490	1,972

CDC, 1988a	Cohort	VES—random sample of U.S. Army enlisted men 1965–1971: psychosocial outcomes	2,490	1,972	
CDC, 1988b	Cohort	VES: physical health outcomes	2,490	1,972	
CDC, 1988c	Cohort	VES: reproductive outcomes	12,788 children	11,910 children	
CDC, 1987; Boyle et al., 1987	Cohort	VES: mortality	9,324	8,989	
Erickson et al., 1984 a,b	Case-control	CDC birth defects study of children born in the Atlanta area between 1968 and 1980, comparing fathers' Vietnam experience and potential Agent Orange exposure between birth defects cases and normal controls	7,133	4,246	

New Department of Veterans Affairs (DVA) Studies

Kang et al., 2000	Cohort	Self-reported pregnancy outcomes for female Vietnam veterans compared to contemporary Vietnam veterans not deployed to Vietnam. Odds ratios were calculated for reproductive history and various birth defects	3,392 women; 1,665 women with an indexed pregnancy	3,038 women; 1,912 women with an indexed pregnancy	

DVA Studies Reviewed in Update 1998

Dalager and Kang,1997	Cohort	Morbidity and mortality experience (1968–1987) of Army Chemical Corps Vietnam veterans compared to U.S. men; extension of Thomas and Kang (1990)	2,872	2,737	
Mahan et al., 1997	Case-control	Study of lung cancer among Vietnam veterans (1983–1990)	329	269 men hospitalized without cancer; 111 patients with colon cancer	

continued

TABLE 6-3 Continued

Reference	Study Design	Description	Study Group (N)	Comparison Group (N)[a]
McKinney et al., 1997	Cross-sectional	Study of the smoking behavior of veterans and nonveterans using the 1987 National Medical Expenditure Survey (NMES)	15,000	—
Bullman and Kang, 1996	Cohort	Mortality study of veterans with nonlethal (combat and noncombat) wounds sustained during the Vietnam war	34,534	—
Watanabe and Kang, 1996	Cohort	Mortality experience (1965–1988) of Army and Marine Corps Vietnam veterans; extension of Breslin et al. (1988) and Watanabe et al. (1991)	33,833	36,797
Dalager et al., 1995b	Case-control	Cases of HD diagnosed 1969–1985 among Vietnam era veterans	283	404
Watanabe and Kang, 1995	Cohort	Postservice mortality among Marine Vietnam veterans	10,716	9,346
DVA Studies Reviewed in Update 1996				
Dalager et al., 1995a	Cohort	Update of Thomas et al. (1991) through December 31, 1995	4,586	5,325
Bullman et al., 1994	Case-control	Study of the association between testicular cancer and surrogate measures of exposure to Agent Orange in male Vietnam veterans	97	311

DVA Studies Reviewed in VAO

Bullman et al., 1991	Case-control	PTSD cases in Vietnam veterans compared to Vietnam veterans without PTSD for association with traumatic combat experience	374	373
Dalager et al., 1991	Case-control	Cases of NHL diagnosed 1969–1985 among Vietnam era veterans compared to cases of other malignancies among Vietnam era veterans for association with Vietnam service	201	358
Eisen et al., 1991	Cohort	Health effects of male monozygotic twins serving in the armed forces during Vietnam era (1965–1975)	2,260	2,260
Thomas et al., 1991	Cohort	Mortality experience (1973–1987) among women Vietnam veterans compared to women non-Vietnam veterans and for each cohort compared to U.S. women	4,582	5,324
Watanabe et al., 1991	Cohort	Mortality experience (1965–1984) of Army and Marine Corps Vietnam veterans compared to: (1) branch-specific (Army and Marine) Vietnam era veterans; (2) all Vietnam era veterans combined; (3) the U.S. male population	24,145 Army, 5,501 Marines	(1) 27,145 Army, 4,505 Marines (2) 32,422 combined Vietnam era (3) U.S. male population
Bullman et al., 1990	Cohort	Mortality experience of Army I Corps Vietnam veterans compared to Army Vietnam era veterans	6,668 deaths	27,917 deaths

continued

TABLE 6-3 Continued

Reference	Study Design	Description	Study Group (N)	Comparison Group (N)[a]
Farberow et al., 1990	Case-control	Psychological profiles and military factors associated with suicide and motor vehicle accident (MVA) fatalities in Los Angeles County Vietnam era veterans (1977–1982)	22 Vietnam suicides; 19 Vietnam era suicides	21 Vietnam MVA; 20 Vietnam era MVA
Thomas and Kang, 1990	Cohort	Morbidity and mortality experience (1968–1987) of Army Chemical Corps Vietnam veterans compared to U.S. men	894	—
True et al., 1988	Cross-sectional	PTSD and Vietnam combat experience evaluated among Vietnam era veterans	775	1,012
Breslin et al., 1988 Burt et al., 1987	Cohort	Mortality experience (1965–1982) of Army and Marine Corps Vietnam veterans, compared to Vietnam era veterans who did not serve in Southeast Asia standardized by age and race; nested case-control study of NHL	24,235	26,685
Kang et al., 1987	Case-control	STS cases (1975–1980) diagnosed at the Armed Forces Institute of Pathology, compared to controls identified from patient logs of referring pathologists or their departments for association with Vietnam service and likelihood of Agent Orange exposure	217	599
Kang et al., 1986	Case-control	STS cases (1969–1983) in Vietnam era veterans for association with branch of Vietnam service as a surrogate for Agent Orange exposure	234	13,496

American Legion Studies Reviewed in VAO

Reference	Design	Description		
Snow et al., 1988	Cohort	Assessment of PTSD in association with traumatic combat experience among American Legionnaires serving in Southeast Asia (1961–1975)	2,858	Study group subdivided for internal comparison
Stellman et al., 1988b	Cohort	Assessment of physical health and reproductive outcomes among American Legionnaires who served in Southeast Asia (1961–1975) for association with combat and herbicide exposure	2,858	3,933
Stellman et al., 1988c	Cohort	Assessment of social and behavioral outcomes among American Legionnaires who served in Southeast Asia (1961–1975) for association with combat and herbicide exposure	2,858	3,933

State Studies Reviewed in Update 1998

Reference	Design	Description		
Clapp, 1997	Case-control	Selected cancers identified (1988–1993) among Massachusetts Vietnam veterans, compared to Massachusetts Vietnam era veterans with cancers of other sites; update of Clapp et al. (1991)	245	999

State Studies Reviewed in Update 1996

Reference	Design	Description		
Visintainer et al., 1995	Cohort	Mortality experience (1965–1971) among male Michigan Vietnam veterans, compared to non-Vietnam veterans from Michigan	3,364 deaths	5,229 deaths

State Studies Reviewed in VAO

Reference	Design	Description		
Fiedler and Gochfeld, 1992; Kahn et al., 1992a,b,c	Cohort	New Jersey study of outcomes in select group of herbicide-exposed Army, Marine, and Navy Vietnam veterans, compared to veterans self-reported as unexposed	10 Pointman I 55 Pointman II	17 Pointman I 15 Pointman II

continued

241

TABLE 6-3 Continued

Reference	Study Design	Description	Study Group (N)	Comparison Group (N)[a]
Clapp et al., 1991	Case-control	Selected cancers identified (1982–1988) among Massachusetts Vietnam veterans, compared to Massachusetts Vietnam era veterans with cancers of other sites	214	727
Deprez et al., 1991	Descriptive	Study of Maine Vietnam veterans compared to atomic test veterans and general population for health status and reproductive outcomes	249	113 atomic test veterans
Levy, 1988	Cross-sectional	Study of PTSD in chloracne as indicator of TCDD-exposed and control Vietnam veterans in Massachusetts	6	25
Anderson et al., 1986a	Cohort	Mortality experience of Wisconsin veterans compared to nonveterans (Phase 1); mortality experience of Wisconsin Vietnam veterans and Vietnam era veterans compared to nonveterans and other veterans (Phase 2)	110,815 white male veteran deaths; 2,494 white male Vietnam era veteran deaths; 923 white male Vietnam veteran deaths	342,654 white male nonveteran deaths 109,225 white male other veteran deaths
Anderson et al., 1986b	Cohort	Mortality experience of Wisconsin Vietnam era veterans and Vietnam veterans compared to U.S. men, Wisconsin men, Wisconsin nonveterans, and Wisconsin other veterans	122,238 Vietnam era veterans 43,398 Vietnam veterans	—

Goun and Kuller, 1986	Case-control	Cases of STS, NHL, and selected rare cancers compared to controls without cancer for Vietnam experience in Pennsylvania men (1968–1983)	349	349 deceased
Holmes et al., 1986	Cohort	Mortality experience (1968–1983) of West Virginia veterans, Vietnam veterans, and Vietnam era veterans compared to nonveterans; Vietnam veterans compared to Vietnam era veterans	615 Vietnam veterans 610 Vietnam era veterans	—
Pollei et al., 1986	Cohort	Study of chest radiographs of New Mexico Agent Orange Registry Vietnam veterans compared to radiographs of control Air Force servicemen for pulmonary and cardiovascular pathology	422	105
Kogan and Clapp, 1985, 1988	Cohort	Mortality experience (1972–1983) among white male Massachusetts Vietnam veterans, compared to non-Vietnam veterans and to all other nonveteran white males in Massachusetts	840 deaths	2,515 deaths of Vietnam era veterans
Lawrence et al., 1985	Cohort	Mortality experience of New York State (1) Vietnam era veterans compared to nonveterans and (2) Vietnam veterans compared to Vietnam era veterans	(1) 4,558 (2) 555	17,936 941
Rellahan, 1985	Cohort	Study of health outcomes in Vietnam era (1962–1972) veterans residing in Hawaii associated with Vietnam experience	232	186

continued

TABLE 6-3 *Continued*

Reference	Study Design	Description	Study Group (N)	Comparison Group (N)[a]
Wendt, 1985	Descriptive	Descriptive findings of health effects and potential exposure to Agent Orange among Iowa veterans who served in Southeast Asia	10,846	None
Greenwald et al., 1984	Case-control	Cases of STS in New York State compared to controls without cancer for Vietnam service and herbicide exposure including Agent Orange, dioxin, or 2,4,5-T	281	281 live controls 130 deceased controls
Newell, 1984	Cross-sectional	Preliminary (1) cytogenetic, (2) sperm, and (3) immune response tests in Texas Vietnam veterans compared to controls	(1) 30 (2) 32 (3) 66	30 32 66
Other U.S. Veteran Studies Reviewed in VAO				
Tarone et al., 1991	Case-control	Study of cases between January 1976 and June 1981 with testicular cancer (18–42 years old) compared to hospital controls for association with Vietnam service	137	130
Aschengrau and Monson, 1990	Case-control	Study of cases with late adverse pregnancy outcomes compared to normal control births for association with paternal Vietnam service (1977–1980)	857 congenital anomalies 61 stillbirths 48 neonatal deaths	998
Goldberg et al., 1990	Cohort	Study of male twin pairs who served in Vietnam era (1965–1975) for association between Vietnam service and PTSD	2,092	2,092

Aschengrau and Monson, 1989	Case-control	Association between husband's military service and women having spontaneous abortion at or by 27 weeks compared to women delivering at 37 weeks	201 1,119
Australian Studies			
New Australian Studies			
AIHW, 1999	Cohort	Validation of the male veterans study (CDVA, 1998a) using medical documents, doctors' certification and records on a disease or death registry	6,842 —
CDVA, 1998a	Cohort	Self-reported data on male members of the Australian Defence Force and the Citizen Military Force who landed in Vietnam or entered Vietnamese water. Questions on physical (including reproductive history) and mental health, and that of their partner(s) and children	49,944 mailed; 39,955 responded —
CDVA, 1998b	Cohort	Self-reported data on female members of the Australian Defence Force and the Citizen Military Force who landed in Vietnam or entered Vietnamese water. Questions on physical (including reproductive history) and mental health, and that of their partner(s) and children	278 mailed 225 responded —
Australian Studies Reviewed in Update 1998			
Crane et al., 1997a	Cohort	Mortality experience (through 1994) of Australian veterans who served in Vietnam	59,036 males 484 females —

continued

245

TABLE 6-3 Continued

Reference	Study Design	Description	Study Group (N)	Comparison Group (N)[a]
Crane et al., 1997b	Cohort	Mortality experience (through 1994) of Australian national servicemen who served in Vietnam	18,949	24,646
O'Toole et al., 1996a,b,c	Cross-sectional	Survey of self-reported health status (1989–1990) of Australian Army Vietnam veterans	641	—
Australian Studies Reviewed in VAO				
Field and Kerr, 1988	Cohort	Study of Tasmanian Vietnam veterans compared to neighborhood controls for adverse reproductive and childhood health outcomes	357	281
Fett et al., 1987a	Cohort	Australian study of mortality experience of Vietnam veterans compared to Vietnam era veterans through 1981	19,205	25,677
Fett et al., 1987b	Cohort	Australian study of cause-specific mortality experience of Vietnam veterans compared to Vietnam era veterans through 1981	19,205	25,677
Forcier et al., 1987	Cohort	Australian study of mortality in Vietnam veterans by job classification, location, and time of service	19,205	Internal comparison

| Donovan et al., 1983, 1984 | Case-control | Australian study of cases of congenital anomalies in children born (1969–1979), compared to infants born without anomalies for association with paternal Vietnam service | 8,517 | 8,517 |

Other Vietnam Veterans Studies Reviewed in Update 1998

| Chinh et al., 1996 | Cohort | Study of antinuclear antibodies and sperm autoantibodies among Vietnamese veterans who served 5–10 years in a "dioxin-sprayed zone" | 25 | 63 age-matched controls; 36 additional male controls |

NOTE: CDVA = Commonwealth Department of Veterans' Affairs; HD = Hodgkin's disease; NHL = non-Hodgkin's lymphoma; PTSD = posttraumatic stress disorder; STS = soft-tissue sarcoma; *Update 1998* = *Veterans and Agent Orange: Update 1998* (IOM, 1999); *Update 1996* = *Veterans and Agent Orange: Update 1996* (IOM, 1996); VAO = *Veterans and Agent Orange: Health Effects of Herbicides Used in Vietnam* (IOM, 1994). ªThe dash (—) indicates the comparison group is based on a population (e.g., U.S. white males, country rates), with details given in the text for specifics of the actual population.

7

Cancer

Cancer is the second leading cause of death in the United States. Among males aged 45–64, the group that describes most Vietnam veterans, the risk of dying from cancer nearly equals the risk from heart disease, the overall leading cause of death in the United States (U.S. Census, 1999). This year about 552,200 Americans are expected to die of cancer—more than 1,500 people a day. In the United States, one of every four deaths is from cancer (ACS, 2000b).

In this chapter, the committee summarizes and reaches conclusions about the strength of the evidence in epidemiologic studies regarding associations between exposure to herbicides and 2,3,7,8-tetrachlorodibenzo-*p*-dioxin (TCDD) and each type of cancer under consideration in this report. The cancer types are, with minor exceptions, discussed in the order in which they are listed in the *International Classification of Diseases*, Ninth Edition (ICD·9). ICD·9 is a standardized means of classifying medical conditions used by physicians and researchers around the world. Appendix B lists ICD·9 codes for the major forms of cancer.

In assessing a possible relation between herbicide exposure and risk of cancer, one key issue is the level of exposure of those included in a study. As noted in Chapter 5, the detail and accuracy of exposure assessment vary widely among the studies reviewed by the committee. A small number of studies use a biomarker of exposure, for example, the presence of dioxin in serum or tissues; some develop an index of exposure from employment or activity records; and others use a surrogate measure of exposure, such as being present when herbicides were used. Inaccurate assessment of exposure can obscure the presence or absence of exposure–disease associations and thus make it less likely that a true risk will be identified.

The outcomes reviewed in this chapter follow a common format. Each section begins by providing some background information about the cancer under discussion, including data concerning its incidence in the general U.S. population. A brief summary of the findings described in the first three Agent Orange reports—*Veterans and Agent Orange: Health Effects of Herbicides Used in Vietnam* (hereafter referred to as *VAO;* IOM, 1994), *Veterans and Agent Orange: Update 1996* (hereafter, *Update 1996*; IOM, 1996), and *Veterans and Agent Orange: Update 1998* (hereafter, *Update 1998*; IOM, 1999)—is then presented, followed by a discussion of the most recent scientific literature and a synthesis of the material reviewed. Where appropriate, reviews are separated by the type of exposure (occupational, environmental, Vietnam veteran) being addressed. Each section concludes with the committee's finding regarding the strength of the evidence in epidemiologic studies, biologic plausibility, and evidence regarding Vietnam veterans.

Expected Number of Cancer Cases Among Vietnam Veterans in the Absence of Any Increase in Risk Due to Herbicide Exposure

To provide some background for the consideration of cancer risks in Vietnam veterans, this chapter also reports information on cancer incidence in the general U.S. population. Incidence rates are reported for individuals between the ages of 45 and 59 because most Vietnam era veterans are in this age group. The data, which were collected as part of the Surveillance, Epidemiology, and End Results (SEER) Program of the National Center for Health Statistics (NCHS), are categorized by sex, age, and race because these factors can have a profound effect on the estimated level of risk. Prostate cancer incidence, for example, is nearly 11 times higher in men age 55–59 than in 45–49-year-olds and more than twice as high in African Americans age 45–59 as in whites of this age group (NCI, 2000). The figures presented for each cancer are estimates for the entire U.S. population, not precise predictions for the Vietnam veteran cohort. It should be remembered that numerous factors may influence the incidence reported here—including personal behavior (e.g., smoking and diet), genetic predisposition, and other risk factors such as medical history. These factors may make a particular individual more or less likely than average to contract a given cancer. Incidence data are reported for all races and also separately for African Americans and whites. The data reported are for 1993–1997, the most recent data available at the time this report was written.

As detailed in Chapter 6, here, and in the following chapters, great uncertainties remain about the magnitude of potential risk from exposure to herbicides and dioxin in the occupational, environmental, and veteran studies reviewed by the committee. Many have inadequate controls for important confounders, and the information needed to extrapolate from the level of exposure in the studies to that of individual Vietnam veterans is lacking. The committee therefore cannot quantify the degree of risk likely to have been experienced by Vietnam veterans due to exposure to herbicides in Vietnam. It offers qualitative observations where data permit.

GASTROINTESTINAL TRACT TUMORS

Background

As a group, this category includes some of the major cancers in the United States and the world. The committee reviewed the data on colon cancer (ICD·9 153.0–153.9), rectal cancer (ICD·9 154.0–154.1), stomach cancer (ICD·9 151.0–151.9), and pancreatic cancer (ICD·9 157.0–157.9). According to American Cancer Society estimates, approximately 180,000 individuals will be diagnosed with these cancers in the United States in 2000 and some 97,500 individuals will die from them (ACS, 2000a). Colon cancer accounts for about half of these diagnoses and deaths. Collectively, gastrointestinal (GI) tract tumors are expected to account for 15 percent of new diagnoses and 18 percent of cancer deaths in 2000.

Average Annual Cancer Incidence (per 100,000 individuals) in the United States[a]
Selected Gastrointestinal Cancers

	45–49 Years of Age			50–54 Years of Age			55–59 Years of Age		
	All Races	White	Black	All Races	White	Black	All Races	White	Black
Stomach									
Males	6.0	4.9	11.1	10.9	9.8	20.9	20.0	16.7	35.2
Females	2.6	2.0	4.7	4.4	3.5	7.3	7.8	6.6	14.1
Colon									
Males	15.6	14.6	23.7	34.2	31.4	59.8	62.9	61.7	81.4
Females	14.8	13.0	24.1	27.1	23.9	49.0	49.9	48.3	72.7
Rectal									
Males	7.7	6.9	10.1	14.8	13.6	17.9	24.8	24.6	27.1
Females	4.9	4.6	5.4	9.4	8.8	12.7	13.7	12.8	16.6
Pancreatic									
Males	5.4	4.9	10.6	12.5	11.7	24.7	21.6	19.6	46.7
Females	3.9	3.5	6.7	8.1	7.5	13.7	13.8	13.4	22.6

[a] SEER nine standard registries, crude age-specific rate, 1993–1997.

The incidence of stomach, colon, rectal, and pancreatic cancers increases with age for individuals between 45 and 59. In general, incidence in males is higher than in females, and incidence in African Americans exceeds that in whites. Risk factors besides age and race vary for these cancers but always include family history of the same form of cancer, certain diseases of the affected organ, and dietary factors. Cigarette smoking is a risk factor for pancreatic cancer and may also increase the risk of stomach cancer (Miller et al., 1996).

Infection with the bacterium *Helicobacter pylori* also increases the risk of stomach cancer.

Summary of *VAO*, *Update 1996*, and *Update 1998*

The committee responsible for *VAO* found there to be limited or suggestive evidence of *no* association between exposure to herbicides used in Vietnam or the contaminant dioxin and gastrointestinal tumors. Additional information available to the committees responsible for *Update 1996* and *Update 1998* did not change this finding. Tables 7-1, 7-2, 7-3, and 7-4 provide summaries of the results of studies underlying these findings and a list of reports that contain details of the research.

Update of the Scientific Literature

Occupational Studies

The largest industrial cohort exposed to dioxins is the group of 5,132 U.S. workers known as the NIOSH (National Institute of Occupational Safety and Health) cohort. This group was assembled from employees of 12 major chemical manufacturers that produced 2,4,5-trichlorophenol, 2,4,5-trichlorophenoxyacetic acid (2,4,5-T), Silvex, Erbon, Ronnel, and hexachlorophene. Workers engaged in production and maintenance were exposed to TCDD as a contaminant of these chemicals. The first study of mortality through 1987 among these workers (Fingerhut, 1991) found a slight excess cancer mortality for all cancers combined (standardized mortality ratio [SMR] = 1.2, 95 percent confidence interval [95% CI] 1.0–1.3); however, no elevated risk was observed for cancers of the stomach, colon, rectum, or pancreas. This cohort has been updated through 1993, and an exposure–response analysis on a subcohort (approximately 69 percent of the population) has been conducted (Steenland et al., 1999).

In that study, mortality from cancer of the small intestine and colon (1.2, 0.8–1.6), rectum (0.9, 0.3–1.9), stomach (1.0, 0.6–1.8), and pancreas (1.0, 0.6–1.6) is not different from expected. Similar results are reported for a subcohort of 608 workers whose medical records stated that they had chloracne, indicating higher TCDD exposures during their working years.

A quantitative exposure assessment was conducted on workers employed in 8 (of a total of 12) plants that had sufficient information on the level of TCDD contamination in their products and detailed work histories. For this subcohort, a job–exposure matrix was constructed, and exposure scores were calculated using three factors: (1) the concentration of TCDD in the process materials, (2) the fraction of the day each worker spent in the specific process that resulted in contact with these materials, and (3) a weighting factor for the level of contact by skin contamination or inhalation of TCDD-containing material. In the analysis of this subcohort, several exposure metrics were calculated including a cumulative exposure score, the log of this score, the average exposure score (cumulative divided by duration), and cumulative exposure categorized into septiles.

Excess cancer risk was confined largely to the highest two exposure class septiles, with an all-cancer SMR of 1.5 (1.2–1.8). Site-specific GI cancers are not reported, and for all digestive cancers (ICD·9 150–159), this highest-exposure class (the two highest septiles) had a nonsignificantly elevated excess risk (1.4, 0.9–2.2).

In a study of a cohort of Danish paper mill workers, Rix et al. (1998) examined mortality from a wide range of causes. Substantial dioxin exposure among these workers is unlikely, since paper pulp was never produced at the three mills studied. Rather, they manufactured paper from imported bleached and unbleached pulp. There are no direct measures of exposure for these workers, and a qualitative assessment of chemicals used in paper manufacture by department does not include chlorinated organic compounds, although chlorine, chlorine dioxide, and hypochlorite were used. For two of the mills, the period of follow-up was January 1, 1943, to December 31, 1993, while for the third mill, follow-up started at January 1, 1965. Incident cancer cases were identified from the Danish Cancer Register, and expected numbers of cases were calculated using the rates for the total Danish population by gender, 5-year age group, and calendar time. For cancer sites of specific interest, Poisson regression models were used to analyze by duration and years since first employment and by department of employment.

For GI cancers, no statistically significant excesses were observed in men or women (standardized incidence ratios [SIRs] reported separately for esophagus, stomach, colon, rectum, and pancreas). When analyzed by department of work, men employed in maintenance and repair had a nonsignificantly elevated risk of stomach cancer (SIR = 1.5, CI not reported, 15 cases), while men employed in the power station had an SIR of 1.7 (4 cases). For pancreatic cancer, men in the paper machine department had an SIR of 1.6 (6 cases), while men in the storage and transport departments had an SIR of 1.6 (8 cases).

Hooiveld et al. (1998) reported on an update of a mortality study of workers at two chemical factories in the Netherlands. This group is included in the multinational International Agency for Research on Cancer (IARC) study of cancer and exposure to organochlorine compounds. This update of the Dutch cohort added 6.5 years of follow-up to a previous study of these workers (Bueno de Mesquita et al., 1993) and included analysis by estimated maximum TCDD serum level. This value was estimated for each member of the cohort by measuring serum TCDD levels for 144 subjects, including production workers known to be exposed to dioxins, workers in herbicide production, nonexposed production workers, and workers known to be exposed as a result of an accident that occurred in 1963. By assuming first-order TCDD elimination with an estimated half-life of 7.1 years, $TCDD_{max}$ was extrapolated for 47 of these workers, and a regression model was constructed to estimate the effect of exposure as a result of the accident, duration of employment in the main production department, and time of first exposure before (or after) 1970 on the estimated $TCDD_{max}$ for each cohort member.

For gastrointestinal cancers (esophagus, 1 case; stomach, 3 cases; intestine, 3 cases; rectum, 1 case; pancreas, 4 cases; other sites, 1 case), no excess mortality was observed among 549 exposed male workers by comparison to national (Dutch) death rates. For workers known to be exposed as a result of the 1963 accident, a nonsignificant elevation of cancer of the esophagus was reported (SMR = 4.3, 0.1–24.0, 1 case); the other GI sites were not reported. Gastrointestinal cancer was not reported in the results of the comparison between exposed and unexposed male workers in the cohort or by comparison of workers with low, medium, and high levels of predicted $TCDD_{max}$.

In a meta-analysis of occupational exposures and pancreatic cancer, Ojajärvi et al. (2000) surveyed publications for the period 1969–1998, searching Medline, Toxline, and Cancerlit for studies addressing occupational exposure and pancreatic cancer. They reduced the number of studies from 1,902 to 92 studies of 161 populations after excluding studies that did not report on pancreatic cancer, did not include sufficient information for meta-analysis, were not the most recent update, or did not include verifiable information on exposure to one or more of 23 specific chemical and physical agents. This information on exposure may have been direct estimates of risk for one or more of the 23 agents or information on job title that verified exposure to one or more of these agents. Herbicides were among the 23 specific agents included; however this broad class of chemical agents was not stratified by type of herbicide. Other agents of interest included chlorinated hydrocarbon solvents, fungicides, insecticides, and polycyclic aromatic hydrocarbons, as well as several heavy metals (cadmium, chromium, iron, lead, and nickel). The set of studies included in the meta-analysis consisted of 23 studies described as administrative (linkage of administrative records or proportional mortality ratio [PMR], proportionate cancer mortality ratio, or mortality odds ratio studies); 88 studies of industrial cohorts; 7 industry-based nested case-control studies; and 43 population- or hospital-based case-control studies. Most studies included were mortality studies. Studies were analyzed using simple random effects models to calculate meta-risk ratios (MRRs). In cases where excesses were observed, population etiological fractions and etiological fractions among the exposed groups were calculated. Data were reported based on exposed populations rather than by study. For the 10 studies in which herbicide exposure was reported, the MRR was 1.0 (0.8–1.3), and the range of point estimates in these studies was 0.6–5.9. The p-value for heterogeneity by agent (herbicides) was .3. These results were virtually unchanged when stratified for gender and quality of diagnosis (MRR = 1.2, 0.8–2.0 for men, not reported for women; 0.9, 0.7–1.2 when gender was unspecified or both). None of the studies included information on the histological verification of the pancreatic cancer diagnosis. When examined by study type, the MRRs for the nine SMR or SIR studies (1.1,

0.8–1.5) were virtually identical to the one case-control study (0.9, 0.7–1.8). Population etiological fraction and etiological fraction among the exposed groups were not calculated for herbicides. The authors concluded that the meta-analysis suggested increased risk of pancreatic cancer with exposure to chlorinated hydrocarbon solvents, nickel and its compounds, and chromium and its compounds. There was more limited evidence of increased risk for organochlorine pesticides, silica, and aliphatic and alicyclic hydrocarbon solvents. There was no evidence of increased risk with herbicide exposure.

Environmental Studies

In a review of early, mid-term, and long-term health effects, Bertazzi et al. (1998) continued the follow-up of people environmentally exposed to TCDD in the Seveso accident. The events that led to the exposure and the methods used to study this population have been fully described previously. Their 1998 report reviews the full range of indicators of exposure and effects on animal and human health. At least in the case of GI cancer mortality, the report does not appear to add any new information to Bertazzi et al. (1997), which was reviewed in *Update 1998*. After 15 years' follow-up (1976–1991), death from cancer of the rectum was significantly elevated for men in zone B (relative risk [RR] = 2.9, 1.3–6.2, 7 observed deaths). A statistically significant increase in stomach cancer in women in Zone B observed after 10 years (RR = 2.4, 1.0–6.0, 5 deaths) was not seen in the 15-year follow-up (RR = 1.0, 0.5–2.2, 7 observed deaths). Excess mortality from esophageal cancer (RR = 1.6, 1.1–2.4, 30 deaths) was reported among men in zone R (considered to be the low-exposure region). No other significant elevation of death from digestive cancer overall or at any of the GI sites was observed in men or women in any exposure zone.

In another report, Bertazzi et al. (2001) extended the mortality analysis through the end of 1996. They examined mortality from GI cancer and found a pattern of mixed results, similar to those seen in their earlier studies of the Seveso population. In this study, digestive cancer overall (ICD·9 150–159) was not elevated in either zone A or zone B. When examined on a site-specific basis, cancer of the rectum (ICD·9 154) was elevated in zone B (RR = 1.9, 1.1–3.5, 11 cases) but not in zone A (1.2, 0.2–8.6, 1 case). Digestive cancers classified as "other" (ICD·9 159) were nonsignificantly elevated in zones A and B, while all other digestive cancer sites had RRs of 1.0 or less. More detailed examination including stratification of the zone A and zone B populations (done both separately and combined) by 5-year intervals of latency did not reveal any significant excess risk estimates, except for an excess in stomach cancer for zone B women in the 10–14-year latency group (2.5, 1.1–5.7, 6 cases). Cancer of the rectum was also elevated among all zone B men (2.4, 1.2–4.9, 8 cases).

Vietnam Veteran Studies

In the Air Force Health Study final report (AFHS, 2000), gastrointestinal cancers as a group are not addressed; however, results for esophageal cancer and cancer of the colon and rectum are reported. Because of the absence of cases of malignant neoplasms of the esophagus in Ranch Hands, statistical analysis was not performed. A malignant neoplasm of the esophagus was observed in two members of the comparison group. For malignant neoplasms of the colon and rectum, no excess risk was seen for the Ranch Hand veterans after analyses were adjusted for covariates.

Approximately 50,000 members of the Australian Defence Force and Citizen Military Forces served in the Vietnam theater over the war years. The government of Australia conducted mail surveys of all individuals with Vietnam service, which included those involved in combat, medical teams, war correspondents, entertainers, and philanthropy workers (CDVA, 1998a,b). Questionnaires were mailed to 49,944 male veterans (80 percent response rate) and 278 female veterans (81 percent response rate). The self-reported data gathered were compared with age-matched Australian national data.

The study found that 405 male veterans and 1 female veteran indicated a doctor had told them they had colorectal cancer since their first day of service in Vietnam. For male veterans, this was higher than the expected number of 117 (96–138), while for female veterans, it corresponded to expected community rates. The authors cited possible reporting errors such as misclassification of intestinal and rectal cancers as colon cancers and reporting pre- or nonmalignant polyps as possible explanations for the high number of cases reported by male veterans.

A follow-up to the Commonwealth Department of Veterans' Affairs (CDVA) study of male Vietnam veterans was conducted to medically confirm selected conditions reported in the survey study described above (AIHW, 1999). Sources used to validate reported conditions included clinicians, several Australian morbidity and mortality data bases, CDVA data, and documentation provided by veterans. Results from this study showed there was no significant difference in prevalence of colorectal cancer between the veterans and an Australian community standard.

Synthesis

With only rare exceptions, studies on gastrointestinal cancers and exposure to herbicide in production, from agricultural use, from environmental sources, and among veteran populations found RRs close to 1.0, providing no evidence of any increase in risk. Most of the recent studies were occupational.

The updated analysis of mortality among U.S. chemical workers did not report site-specific GI cancers, and there was a nonsignificantly elevated excess risk for all GI cancers in the highest-exposed subgroups. A study of Danish paper mill workers found some nonsignificant elevations of GI cancers, but the possible link with dioxin exposure was not well established. An update of a cohort of Dutch chemical workers found no significant excess of GI cancer among the workers exposed to phenoxy herbicides or chlorophenols. A meta-analysis of studies of pancreatic cancer and occupational exposures found no evidence of associations with herbicide exposures. Updates of the Seveso cohort found some statistically significant excess risks, but these were based on relatively small numbers of cases and do not seem to occur with any consistency over the range of latency periods and exposure zones for the cohort. Among studies of Vietnam veterans, there is no significant evidence of an association between exposure and any gastrointestinal cancer.

Conclusions

Strength of Evidence in Epidemiologic Studies

VAO and the previous updates concluded that there is limited/suggestive evidence of *no* association between exposure to herbicides (2,4-dichlorophenoxyacetic acid [2,4-D], 2,4,5-T and its contaminant TCDD, cacodylic acid, and picloram) and gastrointestinal cancers (stomach, pancreatic, rectal, and colon cancers). The evidence regarding association was drawn from occupational and other studies in which subjects were exposed to a variety of herbicides and herbicide components. There is no evidence found by this committee to suggest that the conclusion of limited/suggestive evidence of *no* association should be changed.

Biologic Plausibility

No animal studies have found an increased incidence of gastrointestinal cancer. A summary of the biologic plausibility for the carcinogenicity of TCDD and the herbicides in general is presented in the conclusion to this chapter. A discussion of toxicological studies that concern biologic plausibility is contained in Chapter 3.

Increased Risk of Disease Among Vietnam Veterans

The available data on Vietnam veterans do not suggest there is an association between TCDD or herbicide exposure and any gastrointestinal cancers.

(text continues on page 267)

TABLE 7-1 Selected Epidemiologic Studies—Stomach Cancer

Reference	Study Population	Exposed Cases[a]	Estimated Risk (95% CI)[a]
OCCUPATIONAL			
New Studies			
Steenland et al., 1999	U.S. chemical production workers	13	1.0 (0.6–1.8)
Hooiveld et al., 1998	Dutch chemical production workers	3	1.0 (0.2–2.9)
Rix et al., 1998	Danish paper mill workers		
	Male	48	1.1 (0.8–1.4)
	Female	7	1.0 (0.4–2.1)
Studies Reviewed in *Update 1998*			
Gambini et al., 1997	Italian rice growers	39	0.9 (0.7–1.3)
Kogevinas et al., 1997	IARC cohort		
	Workers exposed to TCDD (or higher-chlorinated dioxins)	42	0.9 (0.6–1.2)
	Workers not exposed to TCDD (or higher-chlorinated dioxins)	30	0.9 (0.6–1.3)
	Workers exposed to any phenoxy herbicide or chlorophenol	72	0.9 (0.7–1.1)
Becher et al., 1996	German chemical production workers		
	Plant I	12	1.3 (0.7–2.2)
	Plant II	0	
	Plant III	0	
	Plant IV	2	0.6 (0.1–2.3)
Ott and Zober, 1996	BASF cleanup workers	3	1.0 (0.2–2.9)
	TCDD <0.1 µg/kg body wt	0	
	TCDD 0.1–0.99 µg/kg body wt	1	1.3 (0.0–7.0)
	TCDD >1 µg/kg body wt	2	1.7 (0.2–6.2)
Ramlow et al., 1996	Pentachlorophenol production workers		
	0-year latency	4	1.7 (0.4–4.3)
	15-year latency	3	1.8 (0.4–5.2)
Studies Reviewed in *Update 1996*			
Blair et al., 1993	U.S. farmers in 23 states		
	White males	657	1.0 (1.0–1.1)
	Nonwhite females	23	1.9 (1.2–2.8)
Bueno de Mesquita et al., 1993	Phenoxy herbicide workers		NS
Collins et al., 1993	Monsanto 2,4-D production workers		NS
Kogevinas et al., 1993	IARC cohort—female		NS
Studies Reviewed in *VAO*			
Ronco et al., 1992	Danish male self-employed farm workers	286	0.9
Swaen et al., 1992	Dutch herbicide appliers	1	0.5 (0.0–2.7)[b]
Fingerhut et al., 1991	NIOSH cohort	10	1.0 (0.5–1.9)
Manz et al., 1991	German production workers	12	1.2 (0.6–2.1)
Saracci et al., 1991	IARC cohort	40	0.9 (0.6–1.2)
Wigle et al., 1990	Canadian farmers	246	0.9 (0.8–1.0)
Zober et al., 1990	BASF production workers—basic cohort	3	3.0 (0.8–11.8)
Alavanja et al., 1989	USDA forest or soil conservationists	9	0.7 (0.3–1.3)
Henneberger et al., 1989	Paper and pulp workers	5	1.2 (0.4–2.8)

TABLE 7-1 *Continued*

Reference	Study Population	Exposed Cases[a]	Estimated Risk (95% CI)[a]
Solet et al., 1989	Paper and pulp workers	1	0.5 (0.1–3.0)
Alavanja et al., 1988	USDA agricultural extension agents	10	0.7 (0.4–1.4)
Bond et al., 1988	Dow 2,4-D production workers	0	— (0.0–3.7)
Thomas, 1987	Flavor and fragrance chemical production workers		1.4
Coggon et al., 1986	British MCPA production workers	26	0.9 (0.6–1.3)
Robinson et al., 1986	Paper and pulp workers	17	1.2 (0.7–2.1)
Lynge, 1985	Danish male production workers	12	1.3
Blair et al., 1983	Florida pesticide appliers	4	1.2
Burmeister et al., 1983	Iowa residents		
	Farming exposures		1.3 ($p < .05$)
Wiklund, 1983	Swedish agricultural workers	2,599	1.1 (1.0–1.2)[c]
Burmeister, 1981	Farmers in Iowa	338	1.1 ($p < .01$)
Axelson et al., 1980	Swedish railroad workers—total exposure	3	2.2
ENVIRONMENTAL			
New Studies			
Bertazzi et al., 2001	Seveso residents—20-year follow-up		
	Zone A males	1	0.5 (0.1–3.2)
	Zone A females	2	1.4 (0.3–5.5)
	Zone B males	15	1.0 (0.6–1.6)
	Zone B females	9	1.0 (0.5–1.9)
Bertazzi et al., 1998	Seveso residents—15-year follow-up		
	Zone A females	1	0.9 (0.1–6.7)
	Zone B males	10	0.8 (0.4–1.5)
	Zone B females	7	1.0 (0.5–2.2)
Studies Reviewed in *Update 1998*			
Bertazzi et al., 1997	Seveso residents—15-year follow-up		
	Zone A females	1	0.9 (0.0–5.3)
	Zone B males	10	0.8 (0.4–1.5)
	Zone B females	7	1.0 (0.4–2.1)
	Zone R males	76	0.9 (0.7–1.1)
	Zone R females	58	1.0 (0.8–1.3)
Svensson et al., 1995	Swedish fishermen, mortality		
	East coast	17	1.4 (0.8–2.2)
	West coast	63	0.9 (0.7–1.2)
	Swedish fishermen, incidence		
	East coast	24	1.6 (1.0–2.4)
	West coast	71	0.9 (0.7–1.2)
Studies Reviewed in *Update 1996*			
Bertazzi et al., 1993	Seveso residents—10-year follow-up, morbidity		
	Zone B males	7	1.0 (0.5–2.1)
	Zone B females	2	0.6 (0.2–2.5)
	Zone R males	45	0.9 (0.7–1.2)
	Zone R females	25	1.0 (0.6–1.5)

TABLE 7-1 Continued

Reference	Study Population	Exposed Cases[a]	Estimated Risk (95% CI)[a]
Studies Reviewed in *VAO*			
Pesatori et al., 1992	Seveso residents		
	Zones A, B males	7	0.9 (0.4–1.8)
	Zones A, B females	3	0.8 (0.3–2.5)
Bertazzi et al., 1989a	Seveso residents—10-year follow-up		
	Zones A, B, R males	40	0.8 (0.6–1.2)
	Zones A, B, R females	22	1.0 (0.6–1.5)
Bertazzi et al., 1989b	Seveso residents—10-year follow-up		
	Zone B males	7	1.2 (0.6–2.6)
VIETNAM VETERANS			
Studies Reviewed in *Update 1998*			
Crane et al., 1997a	Australian military Vietnam veterans	32	1.1 (0.7–1.5)
Crane et al., 1997b	Australian national service Vietnam veterans	4	1.7 (0.3–>10)
Studies Reviewed in VAO			
Breslin et al., 1988	Army Vietnam veterans	88	1.1 (0.9–1.5)
	Marine Vietnam veterans	17	0.8 (0.4–1.6)
Anderson et al., 1986a	Wisconsin Vietnam veterans	3	—
Anderson et al., 1986b	Wisconsin Vietnam veterans	1	—

NOTE: MCPA = methyl-4-chlorophenoxyacetic acid; NS = not significant; USDA = United States Department of Agriculture.
[a] Given when available.
[b] Risk estimate is for stomach and small intestine.
[c] 99% CI.

TABLE 7-2 Selected Epidemiologic Studies—Colon Cancer

Reference	Study Population	Exposed Cases[a]	Estimated Risk (95% CI)[a]
OCCUPATIONAL			
New Studies			
Steenland et al., 1999	U.S. chemical production workers	34	1.2 (0.8–1.6)
Hooiveld et al., 1998	Dutch chemical production workers	3	1.4 (0.3–4.0)
Rix et al., 1998	Danish paper mill workers		
	Males	58	1.0 (0.7–1.2)
	Females	23	1.1 (0.7–1.7)
Studies Reviewed in *Update 1998*			
Gambini et al., 1997	Italian rice growers	27	1.1 (0.7–1.6)
Kogevinas et al., 1997	IARC cohort		
	Workers exposed to TCDD (or higher-chlorinated dioxins)	52	1.0 (0.8–1.3)

TABLE 7-2 Continued

Reference	Study Population	Exposed Cases[a]	Estimated Risk (95% CI)[a]
	Workers not exposed to TCDD (or higher-chlorinated dioxins)	33	1.2 (0.8–1.6)
	Workers exposed to any phenoxy herbicide or chlorophenol	86	1.1 (0.8–1.3)
Becher et al., 1996	German chemical production workers		
	Plant I	2	0.4 (0.0–1.4)
	Plant II	0	
	Plant III	1	2.2 (0–12)
	Plant IV	0	
Ott and Zober, 1996	BASF cleanup workers	5	1.0 (0.3–2.3)[b]
	TCDD <0.1 µg/kg body wt	2	1.1 (0.1–3.9)[b]
	TCDD 0.1–0.99 µg/kg body wt	2	1.4 (0.2–5.1)[b]
	TCDD >1 µg/kg body wt	1	0.5 (0.0–3.0)[b]
Ramlow et al., 1996	Pentachlorophenol production workers		
	0-year latency	4	0.8 (0.2–2.1)
	15-year latency	4	1.0 (0.3–2.6)
Studies Reviewed in Update 1996			
Blair et al., 1993	U.S. farmers in 23 states		
	White males	2,291	1.0 (0.9–1.0)
Bueno de Mesquita et al., 1993	Phenoxy herbicide workers		NS
Collins et al., 1993	Monsanto 2,4-D production workers		NS
Studies Reviewed in VAO			
Ronco et al., 1992	Danish male self-employed farm workers	277	0.7 ($p < .05$)
Swaen et al., 1992	Dutch herbicide appliers	4	2.6 (0.7–6.5)
Fingerhut et al., 1991	NIOSH cohort	25	1.2 (0.8–1.8)
Manz et al., 1991	German production workers	8	0.9 (0.4–1.8)
Saracci et al., 1991	IARC cohort	41	1.1 (0.8–1.5)
Zober et al., 1990	BASF production workers—basic cohort	2	2.5 (0.4–14.1)[b]
Alavanja et al., 1989	USDA forest conservationists		1.4 (0.7–2.8)
	USDA soil conservationists		1.2 (0.7–2.0)
Henneberger et al., 1989	Paper and pulp workers	9	1.0 (0.5–2.0)
Solet et al., 1989	Paper and pulp workers	7	1.5 (0.6–3.0)
Alavanja et al., 1988	USDA agricultural extension agents		1.0 (0.7–1.5)
Bond et al., 1988	Dow 2,4-D production workers	4	2.1 (0.6–5.4)
Thomas, 1987	Flavor and fragrance chemical production workers		0.6
Coggon et al., 1986	British MCPA production workers	19	1.0 (0.6–1.6)
Hoar et al., 1986	Kansas residents		
	No herbicide use		1.6 (0.8–3.6)
	Herbicide use		1.5 (0.6–4.0)
Robinson et al., 1986	Paper and pulp workers	7	0.4 (0.2–0.9)
Lynge, 1985	Danish male production workers	10	1.0
Blair et al., 1983	Florida pesticide appliers	5	0.8
Wiklund, 1983	Swedish agricultural workers	1,332	0.8 (0.7–0.8)[c]
Thiess et al., 1982	BASF production workers		0.4

TABLE 7-2 Continued

Reference	Study Population	Exposed Cases[a]	Estimated Risk (95% CI)[a]
Burmeister, 1981	Farmers in Iowa	1,064	1.0 (NS)
Hardell, 1981	Residents of Sweden		
	Exposed to phenoxy acids	11	1.3 (0.6–2.8)
	Exposed to chlorophenols	6	1.8 (0.6–5.3)
ENVIRONMENTAL			
New Studies			
Bertazzi et al., 2001	Seveso residents—20-year follow-up		
	Zone A females	2	1.8 (0.4–7.0)
	Zone B males	10	1.2 (0.6–2.2)
	Zone B females	3	0.4 (0.1–1.3)
Bertazzi et al., 1998	Seveso residents—15-year follow-up		
	Zone A females	2	2.6 (0.6–10.5)
	Zone B males	5	0.8 (0.3–2.0)
	Zone B females	3	0.6 (0.2–1.9)
Studies Reviewed in *Update 1998*			
Bertazzi et al., 1997	Seveso residents—15-year follow-up		
	Zone A females	2	2.6 (0.3–9.4)
	Zone B males	5	0.8 (0.3–2.0)
	Zone B females	3	0.6 (0.1–1.8)
	Zone R males	34	0.8 (0.6–1.1)
	Zone R females	33	0.8 (0.6–1.1)
Svensson et al., 1995	Swedish fishermen, mortality		
	East coast	4	0.1 (0.0–0.7)
	West coast	58	1.0 (0.8–1.3)
	Swedish fishermen, incidence		
	East coast	5	0.4 (0.1–0.9)
	West coast	82	0.9 (0.8–1.2)
Studies Reviewed in *Update 1996*			
Bertazzi et al., 1993	Seveso residents—10-year follow-up, morbidity		
	Zone B males	2	0.5 (0.1–2.0)
	Zone B females	2	0.6 (0.1–2.3)
	Zone R males	32	1.1 (0.8–1.6)
	Zone R females	23	0.8 (0.5–1.3)
Studies Reviewed in *VAO*			
Lampi et al., 1992	Finnish community exposed to chlorophenol contamination	9	1.1 (0.7–1.8)
Pesatori et al., 1992	Seveso residents		
	Zones A, B males	3	0.6 (0.2–1.9)
	Zones A, B females	3	0.7 (0.2–2.2)
Bertazzi et al., 1989a	Seveso residents—10-year follow-up		
	Zones A, B, R males	20	1.0 (0.6–1.5)
	Zones A, B, R females	12	0.7 (0.4–2.2)

TABLE 7-2 Continued

Reference	Study Population	Exposed Cases[a]	Estimated Risk (95% CI)[a]
VIETNAM VETERANS			
New Studies			
AFHS, 2000	Air Force Ranch Hand veterans	7	1.5 (0.4–5.5)[b]
AIHW, 1999	Australian Vietnam veterans—male	188	221 expected (191–251)[b]
CDVA, 1998a	Australian Vietnam veterans—male	405[d]	117 expected (96–138)
CDVA, 1998b	Australian Vietnam veterans—female	1[d]	1 expected (0–5)
Studies Reviewed in *Update 1998*			
Crane et al., 1997a	Australian military Vietnam veterans	78	1.2 (1.0–1.5)
Crane et al., 1997b	Australian national service Vietnam veterans	6	0.6 (0.2–1.5)
Studies Reviewed in *Update 1996*			
Dalager et al., 1995	Women Vietnam veterans		2.8 (0.8–10.2)
	Nurses		5.7 (1.2–27.0)
Studies Reviewed in *VAO*			
Breslin et al., 1988	Army Vietnam veterans	209	1.0 (0.7–1.3)[e]
	Marine Vietnam veterans	33	1.3 (0.7–2.2)[e]
Anderson et al., 1986a	Wisconsin Vietnam veterans	4	—
Anderson et al., 1986b	Wisconsin Vietnam veterans	6	1.0 (0.4–2.2)

NOTE: MCPA = methyl-4-chlorophenoxyacetic acid; NS = not significant; USDA = United States Department of Agriculture.
[a] Given when available.
[b] Colon and rectal cancer results are combined in this study.
[c] 99% CI.
[d] Self-reported medical history. Answer to question: Since your first day of service in Vietnam, have you been told by a doctor that you have cancer of the colon?
[e] Intestinal and other GI cancer results are combined in this study.

TABLE 7-3 Selected Epidemiologic Studies—Rectal Cancer

Reference	Study Population	Exposed Cases[a]	Estimated Risk (95% CI)[a]
OCCUPATIONAL			
New Studies			
Steenland et al., 1999	U.S. chemical production workers	6	0.9 (0.3–1.9)
Hooiveld et al., 1998	Dutch chemical production workers	1	1.0 (0.0–5.6)
Rix et al., 1998	Danish paper mill workers	43	0.9 (0.6–1.2)
Studies Reviewed in *Update 1998*			
Kogevinas et al., 1997	IARC cohort		
	Workers exposed to TCDD (or higher-chlorinated dioxins)	29	1.3 (0.9–1.9)
	Workers not exposed to TCDD (or higher-chlorinated dioxins)	14	0.7 (0.4–1.2)

TABLE 7-3 *Continued*

Reference	Study Population	Exposed Cases[a]	Estimated Risk (95% CI)[a]
	Workers exposed to any phenoxy herbicide or chlorophenol	44	1.1 (0.8–1.4)
Becher et al., 1996	German chemical production workers		
	Plant I	6	1.8 (0.7–4.0)
	Plant II	0	
	Plant III	0	
	Plant IV	1	0.9 (0.0–4.9)
Ramlow et al., 1996	Pentachlorophenol production workers		
	0-year latency	0	
	15-year latency	0	
Studies Reviewed in *Update 1996*			
Blair et al., 1993	U.S. farmers in 23 states		
	White males	367	1.0 (0.9–1.1)
Bueno de Mesquita et al., 1993	Phenoxy herbicide workers		NS
Studies Reviewed in *VAO*			
Ronco et al., 1992	Danish male self-employed farmers	309	0.8 ($p < .05$)
Fingerhut et al., 1991	NIOSH cohort	5	0.9 (0.3–2.1)
Saracci et al., 1991	IARC cohort	24	1.1 (0.7–1.6)
Alavanja et al., 1989	USDA forest or soil conservationists	9	1.0 (0.5–1.9)
Henneberger et al., 1989	Paper and pulp workers	1	0.4 (0.0–2.1)
Alavanja et al., 1988	USDA agricultural extension agents	5	0.6 (0.2–1.3)
Bond et al., 1988	Dow 2,4-D production workers	1	1.7 (0.0–9.3)
Thomas, 1987	Flavor and fragrance chemical production workers		2.5
Coggon et al., 1986	British MCPA chemical workers	8	0.6 (0.3–1.2)
Lynge, 1985	Danish male production workers	14	1.5
Blair et al., 1983	Florida pesticide appliers	2	1.0
Wiklund, 1983	Swedish agricultural workers	1,083	0.9 (0.9–1.0)[b]
ENVIRONMENTAL			
New Studies			
Bertazzi et al., 2001	Seveso residents—20-year follow-up		
	Zone A males	1	2.2 (0.3–15.6)
	Zone B males	10	1.2 (0.6–2.2)
	Zone B females	3	1.3 (0.4–4.1)
Bertazzi et al., 1998	Seveso residents—15-year follow-up		
	Zone B males	7	2.9 (1.3–6.2)
	Zone B females	2	1.3 (0.3–5.1)
Studies Reviewed in *Update 1998*			
Bertazzi et al., 1997	Seveso residents—15-year follow-up		
	Zone B males	7	2.9 (1.2–5.9)
	Zone B females	2	1.3 (0.1–4.5)
	Zone R males	19	1.1 (0.7–1.8)
	Zone R females	12	0.9 (0.5–1.6)

TABLE 7-3 *Continued*

Reference	Study Population	Exposed Cases[a]	Estimated Risk (95% CI)[a]
Svensson et al., 1995	Swedish fishermen, mortality		
	East coast	4	0.7 (0.2–1.9)
	West coast	31	1.0 (0.7–1.5)
	Swedish fishermen, incidence		
	East coast	9	0.9 (0.4–1.6)
	West coast	59	1.1 (0.8–1.4)
Studies Reviewed in *Update 1996*			
Bertazzi et al., 1993	Seveso residents—10-year follow-up, morbidity		
	Zone B males	3	1.4 (0.4–4.4)
	Zone B females	2	1.3 (0.3–5.4)
	Zone R males	17	1.1 (0.7–1.9)
	Zone R females	7	0.6 (0.3–1.3)
Studies Reviewed in *VAO*			
Pesatori et al., 1992	Seveso residents		
	Zones A, B males	3	1.2 (0.4–3.8)
	Zones A, B females	2	1.2 (0.3–4.7)
Bertazzi et al., 1989a	Seveso residents—10-year follow-up		
	Zones A, B, R males	10	1.0 (0.5–2.0)
	Zones A, B, R females	7	1.2 (0.5–2.7)
Bertazzi et al., 1989b	Seveso residents—10-year follow-up		
	Zone B males	2	1.7 (0.4–7.0)
VIETNAM VETERANS			
New Studies			
AFHS, 2000	Air Force Ranch Hand veterans	7	1.5 (0.4–5.5)[c]
AIHW, 1999	Australian Vietnam veterans—male	188	221 expected (191–251)[c]
Studies Reviewed in *Update 1998*			
Crane et al., 1997a	Australian military Vietnam veterans	16	0.6 (0.4–1.0)
Crane et al., 1997b	Australian national service Vietnam veterans	3	0.7
Studies Reviewed in *VAO*			
Anderson et al., 1986a	Wisconsin Vietnam veterans	1	—
Anderson et al., 1986b	Wisconsin Vietnam veterans	1	—

NOTE: MCPA = methyl-4-chlorophenoxyacetic acid; NS = not significant; USDA = United States Department of Agriculture.

[a] Given when available.
[b] 99% CI.
[c] Colon and rectal cancer results are combined in this study.

TABLE 7-4 Selected Epidemiologic Studies—Pancreatic Cancer

Reference	Study Population	Exposed Cases[a]	Estimated Risk (95% CI)[a]
OCCUPATIONAL			
New Studies			
Ojajärvi et al., 2000	Meta-analysis of 161 populations		MRR = 1.0 (0.8–1.3)
Steenland et al., 1999	U.S. chemical production workers	16	1.0 (0.6–1.6)
Hooiveld et al., 1998	Dutch chemical production workers	4	2.5 (0.7–6.3)
Rix et al., 1998	Danish paper mill workers		
	Males	30	1.1 (0.8–1.7)
	Females	2	0.3 (0.0–1.1)
Studies Reviewed in *Update 1998*			
Gambini et al., 1997	Italian rice growers	7	0.9 (0.4–1.9)
Kogevinas et al., 1997	IARC cohort		
	Workers exposed to TCDD (or higher-chlorinated dioxins)	30	1.0 (0.7–1.4)
	Workers not exposed to TCDD (or higher-chlorinated dioxins)	16	0.9 (0.5–1.4)
	Workers exposed to any phenoxy herbicide or chlorophenol	47	0.9 (0.7–1.2)
Becher et al., 1996	German chemical production workers		
	Plant I	2	0.6 (0.1–2.3)
	Plant II	0	
	Plant III	0	
	Plant IV	2	1.7 (0.2–6.1)
Ramlow et al., 1996	Pentachlorophenol production workers		
	0-year latency	2	0.7 (0.1–2.7)
	15-year latency	2	0.9 (0.1–3.3)
Studies Reviewed in *Update 1996*			
Blair et al., 1993	U.S. farmers in 23 states		
	White males	1,133	1.1 (1.1–1.2)
Bueno de Mesquita et al., 1993	Phenoxy herbicide workers		NS
Studies Reviewed in *VAO*			
Ronco et al., 1992	Danish self-employed male farm workers	137	0.6 ($p < .05$)
Swaen et al., 1992	Dutch herbicide appliers	3	2.2 (0.4–6.4)
Fingerhut et al., 1991	NIOSH cohort	10	0.8 (0.4–1.6)
Saracci et al., 1991	NIOSH cohort	26	1.1 (0.7–1.6)
Alavanja et al., 1989	USDA forest conservationists		1.2 (0.4–3.4)
	USDA soil conservationists		1.1 (0.5–2.2)
Henneberger et al., 1989	Paper and pulp workers	9	1.9 (0.9–3.6)
Solet et al., 1989	Paper and pulp workers	1	0.4 (0.0–2.1)
Alavanja et al., 1988	USDA agricultural extension agents	21	1.3 (0.8–1.9)
Thomas, 1987	Flavor and fragrance chemical production workers		1.4
Coggon et al., 1986	British MCPA production workers	9	0.7 (0.3–1.4)
Robinson et al., 1986	Paper and pulp workers	4	0.3 (0.1–1.1)

TABLE 7-4 *Continued*

Reference	Study Population	Exposed Cases[a]	Estimated Risk (95% CI)[a]
Lynge, 1985	Danish male production workers	3	0.6
Blair et al., 1983	Florida pesticide appliers	4	1.0
Wiklund, 1983	Swedish agricultural workers	777	0.8 (0.8–0.9)[b]
Burmeister, 1981	Farmers in Iowa	416	1.1
ENVIRONMENTAL			
New Studies			
Bertazzi et al., 2001	Seveso residents—20-year follow-up		
	Zone A males	1	1.3 (0.2–9.5)
	Zone B males	3	0.6 (0.2–1.9)
	Zone B females	1	0.3 (0.0–2.4)
Bertazzi et al., 1998	Seveso residents—15-year follow-up		
	Zone A males	1	1.9 (0.3–13.5)
	Zone B males	2	0.6 (0.1–2.2)
	Zone B females	1	0.5 (0.1–3.9)
Studies Reviewed in *Update 1998*			
Bertazzi et al., 1997	Seveso residents—15-year follow-up		
	Zone A males	1	1.9 (0.0–10.5)
	Zone B males	2	0.6 (0.1–2.0)
	Zone B females	1	0.5 (0.0–3.1)
	Zone R males	20	0.8 (0.5–1.2)
	Zone R females	11	0.7 (0.4–1.3)
Svensson et al., 1995	Swedish fishermen mortality		
	East coast	5	0.7 (0.2–1.6)
	West coast	33	0.8 (0.6–1.2)
	Swedish fishermen incidence		
	East coast	4	0.6 (0.2–1.6)
	West coast	37	1.0 (0.7–1.4)
Studies Reviewed in *VAO*			
Pesatori et al., 1992	Seveso residents		
	Zones A, B males	2	1.0 (0.3–4.2)
	Zones A, B females	1	1.6 (0.2–12.0)
Bertazzi et al., 1989a	Seveso residents—10-year follow-up		
	Zones A, B, R males	9	0.6 (0.3–1.2)
	Zones A, B, R females	4	1.0 (0.3–2.7)
Bertazzi et al., 1989b	Seveso residents—10-year follow-up		
	Zone B males	2	1.1 (0.3–4.5)
VIETNAM VETERANS			
Studies Reviewed in *Update 1998*			
Crane et al., 1997a	Australian military Vietnam veterans	38	1.4 (1.0–1.9)
Crane et al., 1997b	Australian national service Vietnam veterans	6	1.5
Studies Reviewed in *Update 1996*			
Visintainer et al., 1995	Michigan Vietnam veterans		

TABLE 7-4 *Continued*

Reference	Study Population	Exposed Cases[a]	Estimated Risk (95% CI)[a]
Studies Reviewed in *VAO*			
Thomas et al., 1991	U.S. Vietnam veterans—women	5	2.7 (0.9–6.2)
Breslin et al., 1988	Army Vietnam veterans	82	0.9 (0.6–1.2)
	Marine Vietnam veterans	18	1.6 (0.5–5.8)
Anderson et al., 1986a	Wisconsin Vietnam veterans	6	5.5 (2.8–10.9)
Anderson et al., 1986b	Wisconsin Vietnam veterans	4	—

NOTE: MCPA = methyl-4-chlorophenoxyacetic acid; MRR = meta-risk ratio; NS = not significant; USDA = United States Department of Agriculture.

[a] Given when available.

[b] 99% CI.

HEPATOBILIARY CANCERS

Background

This category includes cancers of the liver (ICD·9 155.0, 155.2) and the hepatobiliary duct (ICD·9 155.1). According to American Cancer Society estimates, 10,000 men and 5,300 women will be diagnosed with liver cancer in the United States in 2000; 8,500 men and 5,300 women will die from the disease (ACS, 2000a).

In the United States, liver cancers account for about 1 percent of new cancer cases and 2.5 percent of cancer deaths. Misclassification of metastatic cancers as primary liver cancer can, however, lead to overreporting of deaths due to liver cancer (Percy et al., 1990). In developing countries, especially sub-Saharan Africa and Southeast Asia, liver cancers are common and are among the leading causes of death. The known risk factors for liver cancer include chronic infection with hepatitis B or C virus and exposure to the carcinogens aflatoxin and vinyl chloride. In the general population, the incidence of liver and intrahepatic bile duct cancer increases slightly with age, and remains greater for men than women and greater for African Americans than whites throughout ages 45–59 years.

Average Annual Cancer Incidence (per 100,000 individuals) in the United States[a]
Liver and Intrahepatic Bile Duct Cancers

	45–49 Years of Age			50–54 Years of Age			55–59 Years of Age		
	All Races	White	Black	All Races	White	Black	All Races	White	Black
Males	5.6	3.9	11.4	8.1	5.4	17.2	14.2	9.8	25.6
Females	1.5	1.0	2.0	2.6	1.8	4.5	4.1	3.5	4.0

[a] SEER nine standard registries, crude age-specific rate, 1993–1997.

Summary of *VAO*, *Update 1996*, and *Update 1998*

The committee responsible for *VAO* found there to be inadequate or insufficient information to determine whether an association existed between exposure to herbicides used in Vietnam or the contaminant dioxin and hepatobiliary cancers. Additional information available to the committees responsible for *Update 1996* and *Update 1998* did not change this finding. Table 7-5 provides summaries of the results of studies underlying these findings and a list of reports that contain details of the research.

Update of the Scientific Literature

Occupational Studies

The largest industrial cohort exposed to dioxins is the group of 5,132 U.S. workers known as the NIOSH cohort. This group was assembled from employees of 12 major chemical manufacturers that produced 2,4,5-trichlorophenol, 2,4,5-T, Silvex, Erbon, Ronnel, and hexachlorophene. Workers engaged in production and maintenance were exposed to TCDD as a contaminant in these chemicals. The first study of mortality through 1987 among these workers (Fingerhut, 1991) found excess cancer mortality for all cancers combined (SMR = 1.2, 1.0–1.3); however, no elevated risk was observed for cancers of the liver or hepatobiliary duct. This cohort has been updated through 1993, and an exposure–response analysis on a subcohort (approximately 69 percent of the population) has been conducted (Steenland et al., 1999). In that update, mortality from cancer of the liver and hepatobiliary duct (ICD·9 155–156) is not different from expected (0.9, 0.4–1.6). These cancers were not examined in the subcohort of 608 workers who had medical records reporting chloracne or in the more detailed exposure assessment conducted of workers employed in 8 (of a total of 12) plants that had sufficient information on the level of TCDD contamination in their products and detailed work histories.

In a study of a cohort of Danish paper mill workers, Rix et al. (1998) examined mortality from a wide range of causes. The likelihood of substantial dioxin exposure among these workers is unclear, since the three mills in the study never produced paper pulp themselves. Rather, they manufactured paper from imported bleached and unbleached pulp. There are no direct measures of exposure for these workers, and a qualitative assessment of chemicals used in paper manufacture by department does not include chlorinated organic compounds, although chlorine, chlorine dioxide, and hypochlorite were used. For two of the mills, the period of follow-up was January 1, 1943, to December 31, 1993, while for the third mill, follow-up started at January 1, 1965. Incident cancer cases were identified from the Danish Cancer Register, and the expected numbers of cases was calculated using the rates for the total Danish population by gender, 5-year age group, and calendar time. For cancer sites of specific interest, Poisson regression models were used to analyze by duration and years since first employment and by department of employment. For liver cancer, an SIR of 1.1 (0.5–2.0, 10 cases) was found for men. For women, the SIR was 0.6 (0.0–3.2, 1 case). No excess was seen when male workers were stratified by department of work.

Environmental Studies

In a review of early, mid-term, and long-term health effects, Bertazzi et al. (1998) continued the follow-up of people environmentally exposed to TCDD in the Seveso accident. The events that led to the exposure and the methods used to study this population have been fully described in Chapter 6. Their 1998 report reviews the full range of indicators of exposure and effects on animal and human health. In the case of hepatobiliary cancer mortality (ICD·9 155–156), the report does not appear to add any new information to Bertazzi et al. (1997), which was reviewed in *Update 1998*. After 15 years' follow-up (1976–1991), death from hepatobiliary cancer was not reported for zone A. Zones A and B showed lower than expected mortality, except in zone B where women had a nonsignificant elevation (RR = 1.1, 0.4–3.1, 4 cases).

In another report, Bertazzi et al. (2001) extended the mortality analysis through the end of 1996. They examined mortality from hepatobiliary cancer (ICD·9 155–156) and generally found no evidence of excess risk, similar to that seen in their earlier studies of the Seveso population. In this study, there were no cases of hepatobiliary cancer mortality in zone A, and no excess was observed in zone B. No important pattern emerged when the study population was stratified by gender, latency, and zone of residence. An RR of 2.1 (0.7–6.7, 3 cases) was observed for hepatobiliary cancer for zone B women in the 10–14-year latency group.

Vietnam Veteran Studies

In the Air Force Health Study final report (AFHS, 2000), the small number of subjects with a malignant neoplasm of the liver (2 cases among 861 Ranch Hand veterans) resulted in a very limited analysis for this outcome. The percentage of Ranch Hands in the high-dioxin category with a malignant neoplasm of the liver was greater than the percentage of comparisons, resulting in a nonsignificant adjusted RR of 7.1 (0.7–71.3).

Model 4 analysis (Ranch Hand 1987 dioxin category) found a positive association between 1987 dioxin levels and a malignant neoplasm of the liver; after adjustment for covariates, the risk was 2.5-fold higher for each doubling of the 1987 measured blood dioxin level (1.0–6.2).

Synthesis

VAO and subsequent reports found that there were relatively few occupational, environmental, or veteran studies of hepatobiliary cancer (Table 7-5). The updated analysis of mortality among U.S. chemical workers did not find any elevation in liver cancer mortality, nor did a study of Danish paper mill workers. Updates of the Seveso cohort mortality studies did not add any new information on hepatobiliary cancer. Among the studies of Vietnam veterans, the recent study of Air Force personnel (AFHS, 2000) provides a suggestion of an association between herbicide exposure and liver cancer; however, when considered with the overall body of evidence, this finding is not sufficient to change the conclusion that there is inadequate or insufficient evidence of an association.

Conclusions

Strength of Evidence in Epidemiologic Studies

The result of this update is no change in the conclusion of inadequate or insufficient evidence to determine whether an association exists between exposure to herbicides (2,4-D, 2,4,5-T and its contaminant TCDD, cacodylic acid, and picloram) and hepatobiliary cancer. The evidence regarding association is drawn from occupational and other studies in which subjects were exposed to a variety of herbicides and herbicide components. Though several of these studies involve sizable cohorts, hepatobiliary cancers are rare, and as a result, the number of expected cases is fairly small. Additionally, the NIOSH cohort study and Seveso investigations have not adjusted for life-style factors.

Biologic Plausibility

Rats and mice orally administered TCDD for 2 years were evaluated for development of cancer (NTP, 1982). Neoplastic nodules in the liver of female rats were significantly increased in the high-TCDD-dose group, while a significant increase of hepatocellular carcinomas was noted in high-dose-treated male and female mice. It is interesting to note that the high dose of TCDD that increased the incidence of neoplasia in these studies also increased the incidence of toxic hepatitis in both sexes of rats and mice. A summary of the biologic plausibility for the carcinogenicity of TCDD and the herbicides in general is presented in the conclusion to this chapter. A discussion of toxicological studies that concern biologic plausibility is contained in Chapter 3.

Increased Risk of Disease Among Vietnam Veterans

There are insufficient data to determine whether Vietnam veterans are at an elevated risk for liver cancer.

TABLE 7-5 Selected Epidemiologic Studies—Hepatobiliary Cancer

Reference	Study Population	Exposed Cases[a]	Estimated Risk (95% CI)[a]
OCCUPATIONAL			
New Studies			
Steenland et al., 1999	U.S. chemical production workers	7	0.9 (0.4–1.6)
Rix et al., 1998	Danish paper mill workers		
	Males	10	1.1 (0.5–2.0)
	Females	1	0.6 (0.0–3.2)
Studies Reviewed in *Update 1998*			
Gambini et al., 1997	Italian rice growers	7	1.3 (0.5–2.6)
Kogevinas et al., 1997	IARC cohort		
	Workers exposed to TCDD (or higher-chlorinated dioxins)	12	0.9 (0.4–1.5)
	Workers not exposed to TCDD (or higher-chlorinated dioxins)	3	0.4 (0.1–1.2)
	Workers exposed to any phenoxy herbicide or chlorophenol	15	0.7 (0.4–1.2)
Becher et al., 1996	German chemical production workers	1	1.2 (0.0–6.9)
Ott and Zober, 1996	BASF cleanup workers	2	2.1 (0.3–8.0)
	TCDD <0.1 µg/kg body wt	1	2.8 (0.1–15.5)
	TCDD 0.1–0.99 µg/kg body wt	0	
	TCDD >1 µg/kg body wt	1	2.8 (0.1–15.5)
Ramlow et al., 1996	Pentachlorophenol production workers		
	0-year latency	0	
	15-year latency	0	
Studies Reviewed in *Update 1996*			
Asp et al., 1994	Finnish herbicide appliers	2	0.6 (0.1–2.2)
Blair et al., 1993	U.S. farmers in 23 states	326	1.0 (0.9–1.1)
Collins et al., 1993	Monsanto 2,4-D production workers	2	1.4 (0.2–5.2)
Studies Reviewed in *VAO*			
Ronco et al., 1992	Danish and Italian farm workers		
	Danish male self-employed farmers	23	0.4
	Employees of Danish farmers	9	0.8
	Female family workers	5	0.5
Fingerhut et al., 1991	NIOSH cohort	6	1.2 (0.4–2.5)
	20-year latency	1	0.6 (0.0–3.3)
Saracci et al., 1991	IARC cohort	4	0.4 (0.1–1.1)
Solet et al., 1989	Paper and pulp workers	2	2.0 (0.2–7.3)
Bond et al., 1988	Dow 2,4-D production workers		1.2
Lynge, 1985	Danish production workers	3	1.0
Hardell et al., 1984	Male residents of northern Sweden	102	1.8 (0.9–4.0)
Wiklund, 1983	Swedish agricultural workers	103	0.3 (0.3–0.4)[b]
Zack and Suskind, 1980	Monsanto production workers	0	—
ENVIRONMENTAL			
New Studies			
Bertazzi et al., 2001	Seveso residents—20-year follow-up		
	Zone B males	6	0.5 (0.2–1.2)
	Zone B females	7	1.2 (0.6–2.6)

TABLE 7-5 *Continued*

Reference	Study Population	Exposed Cases[a]	Estimated Risk (95% CI)[a]
Bertazzi et al., 1998	Seveso residents—15-year follow-up		
	Zone B males	4	0.6 (0.2–1.5)
	Zone B females	4	1.1 (0.4–3.1)
	Zone R males	35	0.7 (0.5–1.0)
	Zone R females	25	0.8 (0.6–1.3)
Studies Reviewed in *Update 1998*			
Bertazzi et al., 1997	Seveso residents—15-year follow-up		
	Zone B males	4	0.6 (0.2–1.4)
	Zone B females	4	1.1 (0.3–2.9)
	Zone R males	35	0.7 (0.5–1.0)
	Zone R females	25	0.8 (0.5–1.3)
Svensson et al., 1995	Swedish fishermen, mortality		
	East coast	1	0.5 (0.0–2.6)
	West coast	9	0.9 (0.4–1.7)
	Swedish fishermen, incidence		
	East coast	6	1.3 (0.5–2.8)
	West coast	24	1.0 (0.6–1.5)
Studies Reviewed in *Update 1996*			
Bertazzi et al., 1993	Seveso residents—10-year follow-up, morbidity		
	Zone B males	5	1.8 (0.7–4.4)
	Zone B females	5	3.3 (1.3–8.1)
	Zone R males	11	0.5 (0.3–1.0)
	Zone R females	12	0.9 (0.5–1.7)
Cordier et al., 1993	Military service in South Vietnam for ≥10 years after 1960	11	8.8 (1.9–41.0)
Studies Reviewed in *VAO*			
Pesatori et al., 1992	Seveso residents		
	Zones A, B males	4	1.5 (0.5–4.0)
	Zones A, B females	1	1.2 (0.2–9.1)
Bertazzi et al., 1989b	Seveso residents—10-year follow-up		
	Zone B males	3	1.2 (0.4–3.8)
	Zone R males	7	0.4 (0.2–0.8)
Hoffman et al., 1986	Residents of Quail Run Mobile Home Park	0	—
Stehr et al., 1986	Missouri residents	0	—
VIETNAM VETERANS			
New Studies			
AFHS, 2000	Air Force Ranch Hand veterans	2	1.6 (0.2–11.4)
Studies Reviewed in *Update 1998*			
Crane et al., 1997a	Australian military Vietnam veterans	8	0.6 (0.3–1.2)
Crane et al., 1997b	Australian national service Vietnam veterans	1	—
Studies Reviewed in *VAO*			
CDC, 1990	U.S. men born between 1921 and 1953	8	1.2 (0.5–2.7)
Breslin et al., 1988	Army Vietnam veterans	34	1.0 (0.8–1.4)
	Marine Vietnam veterans	6	1.2 (0.5–2.8)
Anderson et al., 1986a,b	Wisconsin Vietnam veterans	0	—

[a] Given when available.
[b] 99% CI.

NASAL AND NASOPHARYNGEAL CANCER

Background

There are many types of nasal (ICD·9 160.0–160.9) and nasopharyngeal (ICD·9 147.0–147.9) cancers, although undifferentiated carcinoma, squamous cell carcinoma, and lymphomas account for the vast majority of malignancies. The epithelium of the nasal and nasopharyngeal cavities is partly squamous, partly columnar, and partly ciliated pseudostratified columnar. There are also serous and mucous glands and lymphoid aggregates in close association with the epithelium.

The American Cancer Society (ACS) estimates that approximately 3,900 men and 1,300 women will be diagnosed with nasal, pleural, tracheal, and other respiratory system cancers in the United States in 2000 and that some 700 men and 400 women will die from the diseases (ACS, 2000a). Roughly speaking, nasal and nasopharyngeal cancers account for between one-third and one-half of these totals. ACS (2000a) estimates suggest that approximately 6,500 men and 2,100 women will be diagnosed with cancers of the pharynx (including nasopharynx, tonsil, oropharynx, hypopharynx, and buccal cavity) and that 1,500 men and 600 women will die from them. Nasopharyngeal cancers make up approximately one in five of these cancers. The incidence rates reported below show that men are at a greater risk than women for these diseases and that incidence increases with age, although the very small number of cases indicates that care should be exercised in interpreting the numbers.

Nasopharyngeal cancer is relatively common in China and Southeast Asia. It is also more common in Chinese and Vietnamese Americans than in whites, African Americans, or other groups, suggesting that genetic factors may play a role in this disease (Miller et al., 1996). There is no similar association for nasal cancer. Reported risk factors for nasal cancer include occupational exposure to nickel and chromium compounds (Hayes, 1997), wood dust (Demers et al., 1995), and formaldehyde (Blair and Kazerouni, 1997). Studies of nasopharyngeal cancer have reported associations with the consumption of salt-preserved foods (Miller et al., 1996), cigarette smoking (Zhu et al., 1995), and Epstein-Barr virus (Mueller, 1995).

Average Annual Cancer Incidence (per 100,000 individuals) in the United States[a]
Nasal and Nasopharyngeal Cancers

	45–49 Years of Age			50–54 Years of Age			55–59 Years of Age		
	All Races	White	Black	All Races	White	Black	All Races	White	Black
Nose, Nasal Cavity, and Mid-ear									
Males	0.9	0.7	1.6	1.2	1.2	1.1	1.7	1.6	2.5
Females	0.4	0.4	0.7	0.7	0.7	0.6	0.8	0.8	1.2
Nasopharynx									
Males	1.5	0.4	2.3	2.1	1.0	1.9	3.5	2.2	3.5
Females	0.8	0.3	0.7	0.6	0.4	0.3	0.6	0.4	1.6

[a] SEER nine standard registries, crude age-specific rate, 1993–1997.

Summary of *VAO*, *Update 1996*, and *Update 1998*

The committee responsible for *VAO* found there to be inadequate or insufficient information to determine whether an association existed between exposure to herbicides used in Vietnam or the contaminant dioxin and nasal or nasopharyngeal cancer. Additional information available to the committees responsible for *Update 1996* and *Update 1998* did not change this finding. Table 7-6 provides summaries of the results of the studies underlying these findings and a list of reports that contain details of the research.

Update of the Scientific Literature

Occupational Studies

Caplan et al. (2000) evaluated exposures among cases with nasal cancer identified in population-based cancer registries in five metropolitan areas and three states, ensuring diversity of risk factors. The cancers were a mixed group that included mostly nasopharyngeal carcinomas (more squamous than adenocarcinomas), some sarcomas, and lymphomas. This heterogeneity makes attribution of nasopharyngeal carcinoma to particular risk factors difficult. Compared to controls, cases overall showed increased odds of 2.5 (1.1–5.3) of having smoked cigarettes and having worked in jobs that involved herbicide exposure (odds ratio [OR] = 2.2, 1.2–3.7) such as lawn care, highway right-of-way maintenance, and forestry. However, subjects with nasal cancer were not more likely to have reported known exposure to herbicides or pesticides or to have worked on a farm. In this community-derived sample, cases also did not show increased odds of exposure to certain known risk factors such as wood dust. However, population-based case-control studies have low power to detect occupational risks when the exposure prevalence is low (Hu et al., 1999); therefore the lack of association with a known risk factor (wood dust) does not constitute evidence of an invalid study, relative to that study's herbicide findings. The implication of these findings for the risk of Vietnam era veterans is unclear.

Environmental Studies

Chapter 3 of *Update 1998* addressed the possibility that TCDD-induced metabolism of procarcinogens may alter cancer risk at various tissues, but there was no empirical evidence to confirm or refute this assertion. Hildesheim et al. (1997) have identified an allele of the gene expressing one form of cytochrome P450 (*CYP2E1*) among Chinese subjects that may be associated with a risk of nasopharyngeal cancer. This allelic form, called *c2c2*, was strongly associated with risk for nasopharyngeal carcinoma among nonsmoking Chinese but not Chinese who smoke. Among Chinese who smoke, the risk for nasopharyngeal

CANCER   275

carcinoma was associated with the allelic form *c1c1*. This raises the possibility that selective induction of cytochromes by TCDD in epithelial cells of the nasal and sinus mucosa may play a role in increasing susceptibility to the effects of cancer initiators in complex ways. Studies are under way by this author and by Aparaso (2000) to resolve these and related issues.

Bertazzi et al. (2001) did not identify any nasopharyngeal carcinomas in their population of TCDD-exposed residents of Seveso.

Vietnam Veteran Studies

Ranch Hand participants do not show an excess risk of nasopharyngeal cancer or other cancers of the head and neck, nor was there an exposure–response relationship among those cancers that did occur (AFHS, 2000).

Synthesis

Nasal and nasopharyngeal cancers are relatively rare in the United States and thus difficult to study epidemiologically. Newly available studies do not change the committee's belief that scientific evidence on the association between herbicide exposure and nasopharyngeal cancer is too sparse to draw conclusions. Information on other cancers of the respiratory tract does not affect the evaluation of nasal and nasopharyngeal cancers because they have different etiologies.

Conclusions

Strength of Evidence in Epidemiologic Studies

There is no information contained in the research reviewed for this report to change the conclusion that there is inadequate or insufficient evidence to determine whether an association exists between exposure to herbicides (2,4-D, 2,4,5-T and its contaminant TCDD, cacodylic acid, and picloram) and nasopharyngeal cancer.

Biologic Plausibility

No animal studies have found an increased incidence of nasal or nasopharyngeal cancer. A summary of the biologic plausibility for the carcinogenicity of TCDD and the herbicides used in Vietnam is presented in the conclusion to this chapter. A discussion of toxicological studies that concern biologic plausibility is contained in Chapter 3.

Increased Risk of Disease Among Vietnam Veterans

The available data on Vietnam veterans do not suggest there is an association between TCDD or herbicide exposure and nasal or nasopharyngeal cancer.

TABLE 7-6 Selected Epidemiologic Studies—Nasal and Nasopharyngeal Cancer

Reference	Study Population	Exposed Cases[a]	Estimated Risk (95% CI)[a]
OCCUPATIONAL			
New Studies			
Caplan et al., 2000	Men selected from population-based cancer registries who have nasal cancer	70	2.2 (1.2–3.7)
Studies Reviewed in *Update 1998*			
Kogevinas et al., 1997	IARC cohort		
	Oral cavity and pharynx cancer (ICD-9 140–149)	26	1.1 (0.7–1.6)
	Nose and nasal sinuses cancer (ICD-9 160)	3	1.6 (0.3–4.7)
Studies Reviewed in *Update 1996*			
Asp et al., 1994	Finnish herbicide applicators	1	0.5 (0.0–2.9)
Studies Reviewed in *VAO*			
Ronco et al., 1992	Danish and Italian farm workers		0.6 (NS)
Saracci et al., 1991	IARC cohort	3	2.9 (0.6–8.5)
Coggon et al., 1986	British MCPA production workers	3	4.9 (1.0–14.4)
Robinson et al., 1986	Paper and pulp workers	0	—
Wiklund, 1983	Swedish agricultural workers	64	0.8 (0.6–1.2)
Hardell et al., 1982	Residents of northern Sweden		
	Phenoxy acid exposure	8	2.1 (0.9–4.7)
	Chlorophenol exposure	9	6.7 (2.8–16.2)
ENVIRONMENTAL			
Studies Reviewed in *VAO*			
Bertazzi et al., 1993	Seveso residents—10-year follow-up, morbidity		
	Zone R females	2	2.6 (0.5–13.3)
VIETNAM VETERANS			
New Studies			
AFHS, 2000	Air Force Ranch Hand veterans	9	1.0 (0.4–2.8)
Studies Reviewed in *Update 1998*			
Crane et al., 1997a	Australian military Vietnam veterans		
	Nasal cancer	2	1.2 (0.2–4.4)
	Nasopharyngeal cancer	2	0.5 (0.1–1.9)
Crane et al., 1997b	Australian national service Vietnam veterans		
	Nasal cancer	0	0 (0.0–>10)
	Nasopharyngeal cancer	1	1.3 (0.0–>10)
Studies Reviewed in *VAO*			
CDC, 1990	U.S. men born between 1921 and 1953		
	Vietnam veterans	2	0.7 (0.1–3.0)

NOTE: MCPA = methyl-4-chlorophenoxyacetic acid; NS = not significant.

[a] Given when available.

LARYNGEAL CANCER

Background

According to American Cancer Society estimates, 8,100 men and 2,000 women will be diagnosed with cancer of the larynx (ICD·9 161.0–161.9) in the United States in 2000, and 3,100 men and 800 women will die from the disease (ACS, 2000a). These numbers represent approximately 1 percent of new cancer diagnoses and deaths. Cancer of the larynx is more common in men than women, with an overall ratio in the United States of about 5:1. Incidence also increases with age in the 45–59 age group.

Risk factors include tobacco and alcohol, which act individually and synergistically. Research suggests that gastroesophageal reflux, human papillomavirus, a weakened immune system, and occupational exposure to asbestos and certain chemicals and dusts may also increase incidence (ACS, 1998).

Average Annual Cancer Incidence (per 100,000 individuals) in the United States[a]
Laryngeal Cancer

	45–49 Years of Age			50–54 Years of Age			55–59 Years of Age		
	All Races	White	Black	All Races	White	Black	All Races	White	Black
Males	5.0	4.5	11.6	11.3	10.5	23.2	19.7	18.7	42.2
Females	1.3	1.2	3.3	2.6	2.7	3.5	4.6	4.3	9.7

[a] SEER nine standard registries, crude age-specific rate, 1993–1997.

Summary of *VAO*, *Update 1996*, and *Update 1998*

The committee responsible for *VAO* found there to be limited or suggestive evidence of an association between exposure to herbicides used in Vietnam or the contaminant dioxin and laryngeal cancers. Additional information available to the committees responsible for *Update 1996* and *Update 1998* did not change this finding. Table 7-7 provides summaries of the results of the studies underlying these findings and a list of reports that contain details of the research.

Update of the Scientific Literature

Occupational Studies

The NIOSH cohort mortality study of 5,132 TCDD-exposed U.S. chemical workers at 12 plants demonstrated a relative risk of 2.2 (1.1–4.1, based on 10 deaths), confirming earlier reports from this cohort (Steenland et al., 1999) and consistent with the conclusion that a general pattern of elevated risk was observed in the studies available to previous committees. Further evidence of an association arises from the demonstration of an exposure–response relationship, with a higher relative risk of 2.5 (0.3–9.1, based on 2 cases) observed in the subgroup of workers with chloracne.

Environmental Studies

Laryngeal cancer was not elevated in the one study population for which exposure to TCDD was not occupational. Bertazzi and colleagues (Bertazzi et al., 1998; Pesatori et al., 1998) reported on 15 years of follow-up of residents of Seveso, Italy, who were exposed to relatively pure TCDD in the industrial incident of 1976. They did not separate laryngeal cancer from all respiratory cancers because of the small number and found only lung cancer cases in zone A, the high-exposure area, where the population was much smaller. However, in zone B—the area of medium exposure—the number of observations allowed a more detailed examination by site. In this zone, the relative risk of 1.2 for all respiratory cancers among males (0.9–1.7, 40 deaths) was exactly the same as for lung cancer alone ($N = 34$). This suggests a proportionate increase in risk at sites in the respiratory tract other than lung, even though statistical significance was not achieved. The relative risk for females was not elevated (RR = 0.5, 0.1–2.0, 2 cases observed). The relative risk for males in zone R, the uncontaminated area, was 0.9 (0.8–1.1, 208 cases observed), and the relative risk for females was 1.1 (0.8–1.5, 35 cases observed). These relative risks and even confidence intervals are exactly the same as those for lung cancer for males in zone R and differ by one-tenth from those for females, although lung cancer cases represented about 81 percent of all respiratory cancers. Thus, it can be concluded that the increase in risk for laryngeal cancers, which would constitute all or the great majority of the rest of the respiratory cancers, was about the same. This is weak but suggestive evidence that the findings in the Seveso study do not contradict the several positive occupational studies. Incidence rates at 20 years were essentially unchanged and showed no pattern in the incidence rate over time (Bertazzi et al., 2001).

Vietnam Veteran Studies

Ranch Hand participants have not shown an excess risk of laryngeal carcinoma or an exposure–response relationship among those cases that have occurred (AFHS, 2000).

Synthesis

Studies published since *Update 1998* in general continue to support the conclusion that there is limited/suggestive evidence of an association between laryngeal cancer and exposure to the herbicides of concern in this report. A conclusion that there is sufficient evidence cannot be reached at this time because the most important risk factors for cancer of the larynx are not controlled in any of these studies and may confound the relationship to the extent that they could produce the slight elevation observed in most positive studies. There are also well-designed studies of considerable statistical power that do not show such an association, although weak internal evidence suggests that there may be some effect even in the negative study from Seveso. The evidence for an association continues to rest exclusively on occupational studies.

Conclusions

Strength of Evidence in Epidemiologic Studies

There is no information contained in the research reviewed for this report to change the conclusion that there is limited or suggestive evidence of an association between exposure to herbicides (2,4-D, 2,4,5-T and its contaminant TCDD, cacodylic acid, and picloram) and laryngeal cancer.

Biologic Plausibility

No animal studies have found an increased incidence of laryngeal cancer. A summary of the biologic plausibility for the carcinogenicity of TCDD and the herbicides in general is presented in the conclusion to this chapter. A discussion of toxicological studies that concern biologic plausibility is contained in Chapter 3.

Increased Risk of Disease Among Vietnam Veterans

The AFHS did not find an excess risk of laryngeal cancer among the veterans it studied. The committee's conclusion of limited/suggestive evidence is based on data from other groups of individuals exposed to herbicides or TCDD.

TABLE 7-7 Selected Epidemiologic Studies—Laryngeal Cancer

Reference	Study Population	Exposed Cases[a]	Estimated Risk (95% CI)[a]
OCCUPATIONAL			
Studies Reviewed in *Update 1998*			
Gambini et al., 1997	Italian rice growers	7	0.9 (0.4–1.9)
Kogevinas et al., 1997	IARC cohort	21	1.6 (1.0–2.5)
	Workers exposed to TCDD (or higher-chlorinated dioxins)	12	1.7 (1.0–2.8)
Ramlow et al., 1996	Pentachlorophenol production workers	2	2.9 (0.3–10.3)
Studies Reviewed in *Update 1996*			
Blair et al., 1993	U.S. farmer in 23 states		
	White males	162	0.7 (0.6–0.8)
	Nonwhite males	32	1.1 (0.8–1.5)
Studies Reviewed in *VAO*			
Fingerhut et al., 1991	NIOSH cohort		
	1-year exposure, 20-year latency	3	2.7 (0.6–7.8)
Manz et al., 1991	German production workers	2	2.0 (0.2–7.1)
Saracci et al., 1991	IARC cohort—exposed subcohort	8	1.5 (0.6–2.9)
Bond et al., 1988	Dow 2,4-D production workers	1	3.0 (0.4–16.8)
Coggon et al., 1986	British MCPA production workers	4	2.3 (0.5–4.5)
ENVIRONMENTAL			
New Studies			
Bertazzi et al., 2001	Seveso residents—20-year follow-up		
	Zone B males	55	1.3 (1.0–1.6)[b]
	Zone B females	5	0.8 (0.3–1.9)[b]
Bertazzi et al., 1998	Seveso residents—15-year follow-up		
	Zone B males	40	1.2 (0.9–1.7)[b]
	Zone B females	2	0.5 (0.1–2.0)[b]
	Zone R males	208	0.9 (0.8–1.1)[b]
	Zone R females	35	1.1 (0.8–1.5)[b]
Pesatori et al., 1998	Seveso residents—15-year follow-up		
	Zone A males	5	2.4 (1.0–5.7)[b]
	Zone A females	2	1.3 (0.3–5.3)[b]
	Zone B males	13	0.7 (0.4–1.3)[b]
	Zone B females	8	0.9 (0.4–1.7)[b]
	Zone R males	122	1.0 (0.9–1.3)[b]
	Zone R females	71	0.8 (0.7–1.1)[b]
VIETNAM VETERANS			
New Studies			
AFHS, 2000	Air Force Ranch Hand veterans	4	0.6 (0.2–2.4)
Studies Reviewed in *Update 1998*			
Crane et al., 1997a	Australian military Vietnam veterans	12	1.3 (0.7–2.3)
Crane et al., 1997b	Australian national service Vietnam veterans	0	0 (0 to >10)
Watanabe and Kang, 1996	Army Vietnam veterans	50	1.3
	Marine Vietnam veterans	4	0.7

NOTE: MCPA = methyl-4-chlorophenoxyacetic acid.

[a] Given when available.

[b] This report did not separate laryngeal from lung and other respiratory cancers.

LUNG CANCER

Background

Lung cancer (carcinomas of the lung and bronchus, ICD·9 162.2–162.9) is the leading cause of cancer death in the United States. According to American Cancer Society estimates, 89,500 men and 74,600 women will be diagnosed with this cancer in the United States in 2000, and approximately 89,300 men and 67,600 women will die from the disease (ACS, 2000a). These numbers represent roughly 13 percent of new cancer diagnoses and 28 percent of cancer deaths in 2000. The principal types of lung neoplasms are identified collectively as bronchogenic carcinoma ("bronchus" is the term used to describe either of the two main branches of the trachea) or carcinoma of the lung. The lung is also a common site for the development of metastatic cancer.

Lung cancer incidence can vary greatly in the age groups that describe most Vietnam veterans. For men and women, the incidence of lung cancer increases rapidly beginning about age 40. The incidence in 50–54-year-olds is double that of 45–49-year-olds, and it doubles again for 55–59-year-olds. The rate for African-American males is consistently higher than for females or white males.

The American Cancer Society estimates that more than 90 percent of lung cancers in males are the result of tobacco smoking (ACS, 1998). Tobacco smoke may include both tumor initiators and promoters. Among the other risk factors are occupational exposure to asbestos, chromium, nickel, aromatic hydrocarbons, and radioactive ores.

Average Annual Cancer Incidence (per 100,000 individuals) in the United States[a]
Lung and Bronchus Cancer

	45–49 Years of Age			50–54 Years of Age			55–59 Years of Age		
	All Races	White	Black	All Races	White	Black	All Races	White	Black
Males	33.0	30.0	66.8	79.1	72.7	163.7	154.2	145.9	298.4
Females	27.3	27.1	41.0	58.6	58.6	83.3	104.1	108.8	115.8

[a] SEER nine standard registries, crude age-specific rate, 1993–1997.

Summary of *VAO*, *Update 1996*, and *Update 1998*

The committee responsible for *VAO* found there to be limited or suggestive evidence of an association between exposure to herbicides used in Vietnam or the contaminant dioxin and lung or bronchus cancer. Additional information available to the committees responsible for *Update 1996* and *Update 1998* did not change this finding. Table 7-8 provides summaries of the results of the studies underlying these findings and a list of reports that contain details of the research.

Update of the Scientific Literature

Occupational Studies

The largest U.S. study of workers exposed to TCDD has provided evidence of an elevated risk among those most exposed and of an exposure–response relationship. This study has been conducted by NIOSH on U.S. chemical plant workers exposed to TCDD. Steenland et al. (1999) evaluated mortality following an interval of, or lagged by, 15 years among 5,132 chemical workers in 12 U.S. plants where TCDD exposure had been documented. The relative risk for lung cancer, alone, was 1.1 (0.9–1.3, 125 deaths observed). However, the subgroup of workers that developed chloracne, who were suspected to have high exposure, showed a relative risk of 1.5 (1.0–2.1, 30 observed). The subgroup scoring in the highest two exposure septiles (the highest two-sevenths) showed a relative risk for respiratory cancers of 1.7 (1.2–2.3, 19 observed). An exposure–response relationship was demonstrable for most of the exposure range. Higher septiles showed a higher risk compared to lower septiles of exposure, but the highest septile showed less risk than the second highest. This may be a statistical anomaly, or it could be an indication that persons who were most heavily exposed and who therefore were at the highest risk died of other TCDD-related causes before getting lung cancer. The phenomenon is known as competing mortality. Whether competing mortality is acting in the exposed population remains speculation. These findings do clearly indicate a statistically significant risk for those in the highest-exposure group, suggest a general exposure–response relationship, and also suggest that other confounders, such as cigarette smoking, do not fully account for the effect.

Environmental Studies

Bertazzi and colleagues (Bertazzi et al., 1998; Pesatori et al., 1998) reported on mortality patterns among residents of Seveso, Italy, 15 years following the 1976 industrial incident that contaminated the area with relatively pure TCDD. Lung cancer rates were not conspicuously or significantly elevated, nor were all respiratory cancers, which followed the same pattern as lung cancer. Lung cancer rates at 15 years, which follow, showed no suggestion of an exposure–response relationship or predisposition by sex. Residents in zone A, the area most heavily contaminated, showed a relative risk for males of 1.0 (0.4–2.6, 4 cases observed), but no cases were observed in females. Residents of zone B, the middle-level contaminated area, showed a relative risk for males of 1.2 (0.9–1.7, 34 cases observed) and for females of 0.6 (0.1–2.3, 2 cases observed). Residents of zone R, an area of low contamination, showed a relative risk for males of 0.9 (0.8–1.1, 176 cases observed). Incidence rates at 20 years were essentially unchanged and showed no pattern in the incidence rate over time (Bertazzi et al., 2001).

These findings are in contrast to the observation that nonmalignant respiratory disorders, which are also associated with cigarette smoking, did show a statistically significant elevation in this population for some subgroups. At present, only 20 years of follow-up are available for the Seveso population. This may not be enough time to evaluate the effect on an outcome whose latency is usually measured in decades. Subsequent studies of lung cancer incidence in this cohort should provide a more complete picture.

Smoking undoubtedly plays a critical role as a risk factor for these cancers as with most lung cancers, and it is likely that almost all of the lung cancers are found in smokers in these exposed populations. The incidence of lung cancers among smokers in the exposed populations, however, may be elevated compared to other populations that include a high percentage of smokers. Comparisons of smoking prevalence among these exposed populations may reveal other explanations for the excess risk.

Vietnam Veteran Studies

In the Air Force Health Study final report (AFHS, 2000), researchers reported 10 cases of lung cancer among Ranch Hands and 3 cases among comparisons (RR = 3.7, 0.8–17.1; Model 1, adjusted). Ranch Hand subjects do not show an exposure–response relationship with indicators of dioxin, exposure, or history of job assignment having an opportunity for herbicide exposure, however. Some or all of the cases may be attributable to cigarette consumption patterns in this population. The unique Ranch Hand population shows a lifetime prevalence of cigarette smoking of 72 percent, with a mean consumption among smokers of 17.3 pack-years; 46 percent of smokers have a history exceeding 10 pack-years. Confounding any association with herbicide exposure, cigarette smoking covaries with 1987 dioxin levels, as do insecticide exposure and exposure to ionizing radiation.

The government of Australia's mail surveys of approximately 50,000 male and female nationals who served in Vietnam (CDVA, 1998a,b) reported that 120 male veterans and no female veterans indicated a doctor had told them they had lung cancer since their first day of service in Vietnam. This was in excess of the number expected for males, which was 65 (49–89). However, further analysis during the validation study (AIHW, 1999) estimated that there were 46 validated cases of lung cancer, indicating a significantly lower prevalence of lung cancer in veterans than in an Australian community standard.

Synthesis

Recent studies, extending previous observations on the NIOSH cohort, do not support a change in the conclusion that there is limited/suggestive evidence for an association between herbicides of concern in this report and risk of lung cancer. Evidence for an exposure–response relationship has been slightly strengthened since *Update 1998* but still does not support a conclusion of sufficient evidence.

Although the Seveso study does not show an excess, it remains early in the follow-up of this cohort for the characterization of cancers with latencies of decades.

Conclusions

Strength of Evidence in Epidemiologic Studies

A growing body of research supports the conclusion that there is limited/suggestive evidence of an association between exposure to herbicides (2,4-D, 2,4,5-T and its contaminant TCDD, cacodylic acid, and picloram) and cancer of the lung, bronchus, and trachea. Although the absence of data on smoking limits the usefulness of available studies, evidence from studies of individuals occupationally exposed to TCDD and phenoxy herbicides increasingly suggests that smoking alone is not the only factor and that these workplace chemicals are associated with an increased risk of neoplasms at these sites.

In response to a request from the Department of Veterans Affairs, the committee responsible for *Update 1998* addressed cancer latency issues related to Agent Orange. A review of the literature provided some information on how long the effects of herbicide or TCDD exposures might last. The evidence reviewed by that committee suggested that if respiratory cancer does result from exposures to the herbicides used in Vietnam, the greatest relative risk might be in the first decade after exposure, but until further follow-up had been carried out for some of the cohorts it was not possible to put an upper limit on the length of time these herbicides could exert their effect. There is nothing in the most recent literature that changes this conclusion.

Biologic Plausibility

In a two-year study, an increased incidence of squamous cell carcinomas occurred in the lung of rats administered 0.1 µg of TCDD/kg/day (Kociba et al., 1978). That increase, however, has not been seen in other studies, including studies by the National Toxicology Program. The finding by Kociba et al. (1978), nevertheless, does suggest an association between exposure to TCDD and cancer of the lung in Sprague Dawley rats. A summary of the biologic plausibility for the carcinogenicity of TCDD and the herbicides in general is presented in the conclusion to this chapter. A discussion of toxicological studies that concern biologic plausibility is contained in Chapter 3.

Increased Risk of Disease Among Vietnam Veterans

Although Ranch Hand participants show a markedly elevated risk of lung cancer, the extent to which this excess risk may be attributable to herbicide or TCDD exposure is not clear.

TABLE 7-8 Selected Epidemiologic Studies—Lung/Bronchus Cancer

Reference	Study Population	Exposed Cases[a]	Estimated Risk (95% CI)[a]
OCCUPATIONAL			
New Studies			
Steenland et al., 1999	U.S. chemical workers who developed chloracne	30	1.5 (1.0–2.1)
	Two highest cumulative exposure septiles	19	1.7 (1.2–2.3)
Studies Reviewed in *Update 1998*			
Gambini et al., 1997	Italian rice growers	45	0.8 (0.6–1.1)
Kogevinas et al., 1997	Phenoxy herbicides: 36 cohorts		
	Exposed to TCDD or higher PCDD	225	1.1 (1.0–1.3)
	Exposed to no or lower PCDD	148	1.0 (0.9–1.2)
Becher et al., 1996	German chemical production workers	47	1.4 (1.1–1.9)
Ott and Zober, 1996	BASF cleanup workers	6	3.1 (1.1–6.7)
Ramlow et al., 1996	Pentachlorophenol production workers	18	1.0 (0.6–1.5)
Studies Reviewed in *Update 1996*			
Asp et al., 1994	Finnish herbicide appliers	37	1.0 (0.7–1.4)
Blair et al., 1993	U.S. farmers from 23 states		
	White males	6,473	0.9 (0.9–0.9)
	Nonwhite males	664	1.0 (0.9–1.1)
Bloemen et al., 1993	Dow 2,4-D production workers	9	0.8 (0.4–1.5)
Kogevinas et al., 1993	Female herbicide spraying and production workers	2	1.4 (0.2–4.9)
Lynge, 1993	Danish male production workers	13	1.6 (0.9–2.8)
Studies Reviewed in *VAO*			
Bueno de Mesquita et al., 1993	Phenoxy herbicide workers	9	1.7 (0.5–6.3)
Swaen et al., 1992	Herbicide appliers	12	1.1 (0.6–1.9)
Coggon et al., 1991	Phenoxy herbicide production workers	19	1.3 (0.8–2.1)
		14	1.2 (0.7–2.1)
Fingerhut et al., 1991	TCDD-exposed workers	89	1.1 (0.9–1.4)
	≥1-year exposure; ≥20 years' latency	40	1.4 (1.0–1.9)
Green, 1991	Herbicide sprayers in Ontario	5	1.1 (0.4–2.5)
Manz et al., 1991	Phenoxy herbicide production workers	26	1.7 (1.1–2.4)
Saracci et al., 1991	Herbicide spraying and production workers	173	1.0 (0.9–1.2)
	Probably exposed subgroup	11	2.2 (1.1–4.0)
McDuffie et al., 1990	Saskatchewan farmers applying herbicides	103	0.6
Zober et al., 1990	BASF production workers	6	1.6
	High exposure	4	2.0 (0.6–5.2)
	Chloracne	6	1.8 (0.7–4.0)
Wiklund et al., 1989a	Pesticide appliers in Sweden	38	0.5 (0.4–0.7)
Bond et al., 1988	Dow 2,4-D production workers		
	(15-year latency)	9	1.2 (0.6–2.3)
	Low cumulative exposure	1	0.7
	Medium cumulative exposure	2	1.0
	High cumulative exposure	5	1.7

TABLE 7-8 Continued

Reference	Study Population	Exposed Cases[a]	Estimated Risk (95% CI)[a]
Coggon et al., 1986	MCPA production workers	101	1.2 (1.0–1.4)
	Background exposure	39	1.0 (0.7–1.4)
	Low-grade exposure	35	1.1 (0.8–1.6)
	High-grade exposure	43	1.3 (1.0–1.8)
Lynge, 1985	Danish production workers		
	Males	38	1.2
	Females	6	2.2
	Manufacture and packing only—males	11	2.1 (1.0–3.7)
Blair et al., 1983	Licensed pesticide appliers in Florida, lawn and ornamental herbicides only	7	0.9 (0.4–1.9)
Axelson et al., 1980	Herbicide sprayers in Sweden	3	1.4 (0.3–4.0)
Bender et al., 1989	Herbicide sprayers in Minnesota	54	0.7 (0.5–0.9)
ENVIRONMENTAL			
New Studies			
Bertazzi et al., 2001	Seveso residents—20-year follow-up		
	Zone A males	9	1.5 (0.8–3.0)
	Zone B males	48	1.3 (0.9–1.7)
	Zone B females	4	0.7 (0.3–2.0)
Bertazzi et al., 1998	Seveso residents—15-year follow-up		
	Zone A males	4	1.0 (0.4–2.6)
	Zone B males	34	1.2 (0.9–1.7)
	Zone B females	2	0.6 (0.1–2.3)
	Zone R males	176	0.9 (0.8–1.1)
	Zone R females	29	1.0 (0.7–1.6)
Pesatori et al., 1998	Seveso (respiratory)—15-year follow-up		
	Zone A males	5	2.4 (1.0–5.7)
	Zone A females	2	1.3 (0.3–5.3)
	Zone B males	13	0.7 (0.4–1.3)
	Zone B females	8	0.9 (0.4–1.7)
	Zone R males	122	2.0 (0.9–1.3)
	Zone R females	71	0.8 (0.7–1.1)
Studies Reviewed in *Update 1998*			
Bertazzi et al., 1997	Seveso residents—15-year follow-up		
	Zone A males	4	1.0 (0.3–2.5)
	Zone B males	34	1.2 (0.9–1.7)
	Zone B females	2	0.6 (0.1–2.1)
	Zone R males	176	0.9 (0.8–1.0)
	Zone R females	29	1.0 (0.7–1.5)
Svensson et al., 1995	Swedish fishermen, mortality		
	East coast	16	0.8 (0.5–1.3)
	West coast	77	0.9 (0.7–1.1)
Studies Reviewed in *VAO*			
Bertazzi et al., 1993	Seveso residents—10-year follow-up, morbidity		
	Zone A males	2	0.8 (0.2–3.4)

TABLE 7-8 Continued

Reference	Study Population	Exposed Cases[a]	Estimated Risk (95% CI)[a]
	Zone B males	18	1.1 (0.7–1.8)
	Zone R males	96	0.8 (0.7–1.0)
	Zone R females	16	1.5 (0.8–2.5)
VIETNAM VETERANS			
New Studies			
AFHS, 2000	Air Force Ranch Hand veterans	10	3.7 (0.8–17.1)
AIHW, 1999	Australian Vietnam veterans—male	46	65 expected (49–81)
CDVA, 1998a	Australian Vietnam veterans—male	120[b]	65 expected (49–81)
CDVA, 1998b	Australian Vietnam veterans—female	0[b]	—
Studies Reviewed in *Update 1998*			
Crane et al., 1997a	Australian military Vietnam veterans	212	1.3 (1.1–1.5)
Crane et al., 1997b	Australian national service Vietnam veterans	27	2.2 (1.1–4.3)
Dalager and Kang, 1997	Army Chemical Corps veterans	11	1.4 (0.4–5.4)
Mahan et al., 1997	Case-control	111	1.4 (1.0–1.9)
Watanabe and Kang, 1996	Vietnam service Army	1,139	1.1
	Non-Vietnam	1,141	1.1
	Vietnam service Marines	215	1.2
	Non-Vietnam	77	0.9
Watanabe and Kang, 1995	Vietnam service Marines vs. non-Vietnam	42	1.3 (0.8–2.1)

NOTE: MCPA = methyl-4-chlorophenoxyacetic acid; PCDD = polychlorinated dioxins.

[a] Given when available.

[b] Self-reported medical history. Answer to question: Since your first day of service in Vietnam, have you been told by a doctor that you have lung cancer?

BONE CANCER

Background

According to the American Cancer Society, approximately 1,500 men and 1,000 women will be diagnosed with bone or joint cancer (ICD·9 170.0–170.9) in the United States in 2000, and 800 men and 600 women will die as a result of this cancer (ACS, 2000a). Primary bone cancers are among the least common malignancies. The bones are, however, frequent sites for secondary tumors of other cancers that have metastasized (i.e., have spread from another site). Only the primary cancers are considered here.

Bone cancer is more common in teenagers than adults. The incidence among individuals in the age groups that characterize most Vietnam veterans is quite low, and care should be exercised when interpreting the numbers presented below.

Among the risk factors for adults contracting bone and joint cancer are exposure to ionizing radiation from treatment for other cancers and a history of certain noncancerous bone diseases.

Average Annual Cancer Incidence (per 100,000 individuals) in the United States[a]
Bone and Joint Cancer

	45–49 Years of Age			50–54 Years of Age			55–59 Years of Age		
	All Races	White	Black	All Races	White	Black	All Races	White	Black
Males	0.7	0.7	0.5	0.7	0.8	0.8	1.3	1.4	1.5
Females	0.8	0.9	0.5	0.8	0.7	1.0	0.7	0.8	[b]

[a] SEER nine standard registries, crude age-specific rate, 1993–1997.
[b] Insufficient data to provide meaningful incidence rate.

Summary of *VAO*, *Update 1996*, and *Update 1998*

The committee responsible for *VAO* found there to be inadequate or insufficient information to determine whether an association existed between exposure to herbicides used in Vietnam or the contaminant dioxin and bone cancer. Additional information available to the committees responsible for *Update 1996* and *Update 1998* did not change this finding. Table 7-9 provides summaries of the results of the studies underlying these findings and a list of reports that contain details of the research.

Update of the Scientific Literature

Occupational Studies

The update of the industrial cohort exposed to dioxins known as the NIOSH cohort (Steenland, 1999) did not report results for bone cancer.

In a study of a cohort of Danish paper mill workers, Rix et al. (1998) examined mortality from a wide range of causes. The likelihood of substantial dioxin exposure among these workers is unclear, since the three mills in the study never produced paper pulp themselves. Rather, they manufactured paper from imported bleached and unbleached pulp. There are no direct measures of exposure for these workers, and a qualitative assessment of chemicals used in paper manufacture by department does not include chlorinated organic compounds, although chlorine, chlorine dioxide, and hypochlorite were used. For two of the mills, the period of follow-up was January 1, 1943, to December 31, 1993, while for the third mill, follow-up started at January 1, 1965. Incident cancer cases were identified from the Danish Cancer Register, and expected numbers of cases were calculated using the rates for the total Danish population by gender, 5-year age group, and calendar time. For cancer sites of specific interest, Poisson regression models were used to analyze by duration and years since first employment and by department of employment. For bone cancer, only one case was found, yielding an SIR of 0.5 (0.0–2.7) for men, and no cases were seen among women in the cohort.

Environmental Studies

In a review of early, mid-term, and long-term health effects, Bertazzi et al. (1998) continued the follow-up of people environmentally exposed to TCDD in the Seveso accident. The events that led to the exposure and the methods used to study this population have been fully described previously. In the case of bone cancer mortality, the report does not appear to add any new information to Bertazzi et al. (1997), which was reviewed in *Update 1998*. After 15 years' follow-up (1976–1991), there were no deaths from bone cancer among residents of zone A and only one case in zone B, which occurred in a woman (RR = 2.6, 0.3–19.4). Men in zone R (considered to be the low-exposure region) had an RR of 0.5 (0.1–2.0, 2 cases), while women in zone R had a significant elevation (RR = 2.4, 1.0–5.7, 7 cases).

In another report, Bertazzi et al. (2001) extended the mortality analysis through the end of 1996; however mortality from bone cancer is not mentioned.

Vietnam Veteran Studies

In the Air Force Health Study final report (AFHS, 2000), bone cancer was not reported as one of the health outcomes of interest.

Synthesis

The committee found little new information to add to the sparse existing data set. There is no evidence to indicate a change from the conclusion that there is inadequate or insufficient evidence to determine whether an association exists between exposure to the herbicides 2,4-D, 2,4,5-T and its contaminant TCDD, cacodylic acid, and picloram and bone cancer.

Conclusions

Strength of Evidence in Epidemiologic Studies

There is no information contained in the research reviewed for this report to change the conclusion that there is inadequate or insufficient evidence to determine whether an association exists between exposure to herbicides (2,4-D, 2,4,5-T and its contaminant TCDD, cacodylic acid, and picloram) and bone cancer. The evidence regarding an association is drawn from occupational and environmental studies in which the subjects were exposed to a variety of herbicides and herbicide compounds.

Biologic Plausibility

No animal studies have found an increased incidence of bone cancer. A summary of the biologic plausibility for the carcinogenicity of TCDD and the herbicides in general is presented in the conclusion to this chapter. A discussion of toxicological studies that concern biologic plausibility is contained in Chapter 3.

Increased Risk of Disease Among Vietnam Veterans

There are no data on which to base a conclusion concerning whether Vietnam veterans may or may not be at increased risk for bone cancer due to exposure to herbicides or TCDD.

TABLE 7-9 Selected Epidemiologic Studies—Bone Cancer

Reference	Study Population	Exposed Cases[a]	Estimated Risk (95% CI)[a]
OCCUPATIONAL			
New Studies			
Rix et al., 1998	Danish paper mill workers		
	Males	1	0.5 (0.0–2.7)
	Females	0	
Studies Reviewed in *Update 1998*			
Gambini et al., 1997	Italian rice growers	1	46 (0.6–255.2)
Hertzman et al., 1997	British Columbia sawmill workers		
	Mortality	5	1.3 (0.5–2.7)
	Incidence	4	1.1 (0.4–2.4)
Kogevinas et al., 1997	IARC cohort	5	1.2 (0.4–2.8)
	Workers exposed to TCDD		
	(or higher-chlorinated dioxins)		1.1
	Workers not exposed to TCDD		
	(or higher-chlorinated dioxins)		1.4
Ramlow et al., 1996	Pentachlorophenol production workers	0	
Studies Reviewed in *Update 1996*			
Blair et al., 1993	U.S. farmers in 23 states	49	1.3 (1.0–1.8)
Collins et al., 1993	Monsanto 2,4-D production workers	2	5.0 (0.6–18.1)
Studies Reviewed in *VAO*			
Ronco et al., 1992	Danish male self-employed farm workers	9	0.9
Fingerhut et al., 1991	NIOSH cohort	2	2.3 (0.3–8.2)
Zober et al., 1990	BASF production workers	0	— (0.0–70.0)
Bond et al., 1988	Dow 2,4-D production workers	0	— (0.0–31.1)
Coggon et al., 1986	British MCPA production workers	1	0.9 (0.0–5.0)
Wiklund, 1983	Swedish agricultural workers	44	1.0 (0.6–1.4)[b]
Burmeister, 1981	Farmers in Iowa	56	1.1 (NS)

TABLE 7-9 *Continued*

Reference	Study Population	Exposed Cases[a]	Estimated Risk (95% CI)[a]
ENVIRONMENTAL			
New Studies			
Bertazzi et al., 1998	Seveso residents—15-year follow-up		
	Zone B females	1	2.6 (0.3–19.4)
	Zone R males	2	0.5 (0.1–2.0)
	Zone R females	7	2.4 (1.0–5.7)
Studies Reviewed in *Update 1998*			
Bertazzi et al., 1997	Seveso residents—15-year follow-up		
	Zone B females	1	2.6 (0.0–14.4)
	Zone R males	2	0.5 (0.1–1.7)
	Zone R females	7	2.4 (1.0–4.9)
VIETNAM VETERANS			
Studies Reviewed in *Update 1998*			
Clapp, 1997	Massachusetts Vietnam veterans	4	0.9 (0.1–11.3)
AFHS, 1996	Air Force Ranch Hand veterans	0	
Studies Reviewed in *VAO*			
Breslin et al., 1988	Army Vietnam veterans	27	0.8 (0.4–1.7)
	Marine Vietnam veterans	11	1.4 (0.1–21.5)
Anderson et al., 1986a	Wisconsin Vietnam veterans	1	—
Anderson et al., 1986b	Wisconsin Vietnam veterans	1	—
Lawrence et al., 1985	New York Vietnam veterans	8	1.0 (0.3–3.0)

NOTE: MCPA = methyl-4-chlorophenoxyacetic acid; NS = not significant.
[a] Given when available.
[b] 99% CI.

SOFT-TISSUE SARCOMAS

Background

Soft-tissue sarcoma (STS) (ICD·9 171.0–171.9, 164.1) arises in the soft somatic tissues that occur within and between organs. Three of the most common types of STS—liposarcoma, fibrosarcoma, and rhabdomyosarcoma—occur in similar numbers in men and women. Because of the diverse characteristics of STS, accurate diagnosis and classification can be difficult. The American Cancer Society estimates that 4,300 men and 3,800 women will be diagnosed with STS, and 2,200 men and 2,400 women will die from these cancers in the United States in 2000 (ACS, 2000a).

There is no consistent pattern to the incidence of STS over the age groups that describe most Vietnam veterans.

Among the risk factors for these cancers are exposure to ionizing radiation from treatment for other cancers and certain inherited conditions including Gardner's syndrome, Li-Fraumeni syndrome, and neurofibromatosis. Several chemical exposures have also been identified as possible risk factors (Zahm and Fraumeni, 1997).

Average Annual Cancer Incidence (per 100,000 individuals) in the United States[a]
Soft-Tissue Sarcomas (including malignant neoplasms of the heart)

	45–49 Years of Age			50–54 Years of Age			55–59 Years of Age		
	All Races	White	Black	All Races	White	Black	All Races	White	Black
Males	3.2	3.0	4.1	4.1	4.1	5.2	4.4	4.3	5.5
Females	2.2	2.2	3.1	3.3	3.0	5.7	3.4	3.3	3.6

[a] SEER nine standard registries, crude age-specific rate, 1993–1997.

Summary of *VAO*, *Update 1996*, and *Update 1998*

The committee responsible for *VAO* found there to be sufficient information to determine that an association existed between exposure to herbicides used in Vietnam or the contaminant dioxin and soft-tissue sarcoma. Additional information available to the committees responsible for *Update 1996* and *Update 1998* did not change this finding. Table 7-10 provides summaries of the results of the studies underlying these findings and a list of reports that contain details of the research.

Update of the Scientific Literature

Occupational Studies

The largest industrial cohort exposed to dioxins is the group of 5,132 U.S. workers known as the NIOSH cohort. This group was assembled from employees of 12 major chemical manufacturers that produced 2,4,5–trichlorophenol, 2,4,5–T, Silvex, Erbon, Ronnel, and hexachlorophene. Workers engaged in production and maintenance were exposed to TCDD as a contaminant of these chemicals. The first study of mortality through 1987 among these workers (Fingerhut, 1991) found excess cancer mortality for all cancers combined (SMR = 1.2, 1.0–1.3), and elevated risk was observed for STS (SMR = 9.2, 1.9–27.0). This cohort has been updated through 1993, and an exposure–response analysis on a subcohort (approximately 69 percent of the population) has been conducted (Steenland et al., 1999). In that report, results for STS are not presented, and the only mention is a note in the discussion that no new soft-tissue sarcomas were observed.

In a study of a cohort of Danish paper mill workers, Rix et al. (1998) examined mortality from a wide range of causes. The likelihood of substantial dioxin exposure among these workers is unclear, since the three mills in the study never produced paper pulp themselves. Rather, they manufactured paper from imported bleached and unbleached pulp. There are no direct measures of exposure for these workers, and a qualitative assessment of chemicals used in paper manufacture by department does not include chlorinated organic compounds, although chlorine, chlorine dioxide, and hypochlorite were used. For two of the mills, the period of follow-up was January 1, 1943, to December 31, 1993, while for the third mill, follow-up started at January 1, 1965. Incident cancer cases were identified from the Danish Cancer Register, and expected numbers of cases were calculated using the rates for the total Danish population by gender, 5-year age group, and calendar time. For cancer sites of specific interest, Poisson regression models were used to analyze by duration and years since first employment and by department of employment. For STS, a significant excess was observed in women in plants 1 and 2 (the two older plants) with an SIR of 2.3 (1.1–4.4, 9 cases). When the third mill (which started in 1965) was included, the SIR for women was 2.6 (1.3–4.7, 11 cases). For women employed in sorting and packing, the SIR was 4.0 (1.7–7.8, 8 cases), with no trend reported by length of employment or latency. For men, the SIR was 1.2 (0.6–2.0, 12 cases). The authors speculated that the only chemical noted to be present in the sorting and packing jobs the women held was organic glue and that exposure to chlorinated organic compounds was expected to be low among this group.

Hooiveld et al. (1998) reported on an update of a mortality study of workers at two chemical factories in the Netherlands. This group is included in the multinational IARC study of cancer and exposure to organochlorine compounds. This update of the Dutch cohort added 6.5 years of follow-up to a previous study of these workers (Bueno de Mesquita et al., 1993) and included analysis by estimated maximum TCDD serum level. This value was estimated for each member of the cohort by measuring serum TCDD levels for 144 subjects, including production workers known to be exposed to dioxins, workers in herbicide production, nonexposed production workers, and workers known to be exposed as a result of an accident that occurred in 1963. By assuming first-order TCDD elimination with an estimated half-life of 7.1 years, $TCDD_{max}$ was extrapolated for a group of 47 workers, and a regression model was constructed to estimate the effect of exposure as a result of the accident, duration of employment in the main production department, and time of first exposure before (or after) 1970 on the estimated $TCDD_{max}$ for each cohort member. No STS deaths were observed among the workers exposed to phenoxy herbicides or chlorophenols in this study population.

Environmental Studies

In a review of early, mid-term, and long-term health effects, Bertazzi et al. (1998) continued the follow-up of people environmentally exposed to TCDD in the Seveso accident. The events that led to the exposure and the methods used to study this population have been fully described previously. Their 1998 report reviews the full range of indicators of exposure and effects on animal and human health. For STS, the report does not appear to add any new information to Bertazzi et al. (1997), which was reviewed in *Update 1998*. After 15 years' follow-up (1976–1991), death from STS was not reported for residents of zone A, and there were no cases among residents of zone B. In zone R, there were no cases among women (1.5 expected), and the RR for men was 2.1 (0.6–5.4, 4 cases).

In another report, Bertazzi et al. (2001) extended the mortality analysis through the end of 1996; however no cases of STS were observed.

Viel et al. (2000) reported on an investigation of apparent clusters of STS and non-Hodgkin's lymphoma (NHL) cases in the vicinity of a municipal solid waste incinerator in Doubs, France. Series of incident NHL and STS cases from 1980 to 1995 were obtained from a cancer registry that included Doubs. Incident cases of Hodgkin's disease (HD) were also obtained for the same period. The reason for including Hodgkin's disease was to provide a check on possible selection bias by including a disease that the investigators considered to not be consistently associated with dioxin exposure. (In *VAO* and its updates, the committees have concluded that there is evidence of a positive association between dioxin exposure and HD.) The presumptive source of dioxin in this region is a municipal solid waste incinerator in the Besançon electoral ward in the west of Doubs. A measurement of dioxin emissions from the incinerator showed a level of 16.3 ng international toxic equivalency factor (I-TEQ)/m^3, far in excess of the European Union (EU) standard of 0.1 ng I-TEQ/m^3. In addition, measurements of dioxin in cow's milk from three farms near the incinerators suggested that the dioxin content of the milk was highest at the farm closest to the incinerator. These measurements were all well below the guideline of 6 ng I-TEQ/kg of fat, however. The authors do not provide any direct evidence of human exposure.

Analysis was conducted by looking for spatial clusters around the incinerator and a focused space–time scan test. Expected numbers of cases were calculated for each canton using the incidence rates for the entire department, stratified by gender and 5-year age interval. For STS, a statistically significant spatial cluster (SIR = 1.4, p = .004, 45 cases observed) was found in Besançon (where the incinerator is located) and Audeux (which borders it to the west). A similar result was obtained when the only spatial criterion was the canton, not proximity to the incinerator. In the focused space–time test, a significant excess was found for 1994–1995 in Besançon and Audeux (SIR = 3.4, p = .008, 12 cases). Excess cases of NHL were also observed in these same two cantons; however, there were no spatial or space–time clusters observed for HD. Despite the strengths of the study, limitations include an unclear route of dioxin exposure and the fact that coexposures to chemicals other than dioxin from the incinerator could be responsible for the observed clusters.

Vietnam Veteran Studies

In the Air Force Health Study (AFHS, 2000), the small number of cases of malignant neoplasm of the connective or other soft tissues limited the analysis. One case was identified among the 861 Ranch Hand veterans, and two cases among the comparison population of 1,249. All results from the analyses performed were nonsignificant.

The government of Australia's mail surveys of approximately 50,000 male nationals who served in Vietnam (CDVA, 1998a) reported that 398 male veterans indicated a doctor had told them they had soft-tissue sarcoma since their first day of service in Vietnam. This was much higher than the number expected for this population, 27 (17–37). The authors report that it is likely that errors occurred in reporting this condition because STS is a rare condition that may be confused with similar sounding conditions such as Ewing's sarcoma, lymphosarcoma, myoma, and lipoma. A follow-up to this study, conducted to medically confirm selected conditions reported in the survey (AIHW, 1999), determined there were 14 cases that could be validated, suggesting a significantly lower prevalence of soft-tissue sarcoma in veterans than in the Australian community. For female veterans, 3 cases were reported, which was within the range of 0–4 expected (CDVA, 1998b).

Synthesis

As noted in previous updates, the evidence of an association between STS and dioxin exposure is found in a small number of studies. The studies reviewed for this report continue a pattern of mixed findings. The update of the NIOSH cohort did not provide any new information on STS, since no new cases were observed. A study of Danish paper mill workers found some excess of STS among three different plants. Although the finding was quite stable among women, the link with dioxin exposure was not well established. An update of a cohort of Dutch chemical workers found no STS deaths among workers exposed to phenoxy herbicides or chlorophenols. Updates of the Seveso population did not add any new information on STS. In another study, apparent clusters of STS and NHL cases in the vicinity of a municipal solid waste incinerator found a statistically significant spatial cluster; however, concerns over poor exposure characterization lessen confidence in these findings. The study of Vietnam veterans provided no new information on STS.

Conclusions

Strength of Evidence in Epidemiologic Studies

There is no information contained in the research reviewed for this report to change the conclusion that there is sufficient evidence to conclude that an association exists between exposure to herbicides (2,4-D, 2,4,5-T and its contaminant TCDD, cacodylic acid, and picloram) and soft-tissue sarcoma.

Biologic Plausibility

No animal studies have found an increased incidence of soft-tissue sarcoma. A summary of the biologic plausibility for the carcinogenicity of TCDD and the herbicides in general is presented in the conclusion to this chapter. A discussion of toxicological studies that concern biologic plausibility is contained in Chapter 3.

Increased Risk of Disease Among Vietnam Veterans

The available data on Vietnam veterans do not permit a conclusion on whether they are at an elevated risk for soft-tissue sarcomas.

TABLE 7-10 Selected Epidemiologic Studies—Soft-Tissue Sarcoma

Reference	Study Population	Exposed Cases[a]	Estimated Risk (95% CI)[a]
OCCUPATIONAL			
New Studies			
Steenland et al., 1999	U.S. chemical production workers	0	—
Hooiveld et al., 1998	Dutch chemical production workers	0	—
Rix et al., 1998	Danish paper mill workers		
	Women in plants 1 and 2	9	2.3 (1.1–4.4)
	Women in plants 1, 2, and 3	11	2.6 (1.3–4.7)
	Women employed in sorting and packing	8	4.0 (1.7–7.8)
	Men employed in sorting and packing	12	1.2 (0.6–2.0)
Studies Reviewed in *Update 1998*			
Hertzman et al., 1997	Canadian sawmill workers	11	1.0 (0.6–1.7)
Kogevinas et al., 1997	IARC cohort		
	Workers exposed to TCDD (or higher-chlorinated dioxins)	6	2.0 (0.8–4.4)
	Workers not exposed to TCDD (or higher-chlorinated dioxins)	2	1.4
	Workers exposed to any phenoxy herbicide or chlorophenol	9	2.0 (0.9–3.8)
Ott and Zober, 1996	Workers exposed in 1953 accident	0	0.2 expected
Ramlow et al., 1996	Pentachlorophenol production workers	0	0.2 expected
Studies Reviewed in *Update 1996*			
Kogevinas et al., 1995	IARC cohort	11	—
Mack, 1995	U.S. cancer registry data (SEER program) review		
	Male	3,526	—
	Female	2,886	—
Blair et al., 1993	U.S. farmers from 23 states (white males)	98	0.9 (0.8–1.1)
Lynge, 1993	Danish male production workers	5	2.0 (0.7–4.8)
Kogevinas et al., 1992	IARC cohort (10–19 years after first exposure)	4	6.1 (1.7–15.5)

TABLE 7-10 Continued

Reference	Study Population	Exposed Cases[a]	Estimated Risk (95% CI)[a]
Studies Reviewed in *VAO*			
Bueno de Mesquita et al., 1993	Phenoxy herbicide workers	0	—
Hansen et al., 1992	Danish gardeners	3	5.3 (1.1–15.4)
Smith and Christophers, 1992	Male residents of Australia	30	1.0 (0.3–3.1)
Fingerhut et al., 1991	NIOSH cohort	4	3.4 (0.9–8.7)
	Those with 20 years' latency and 1 year of exposure	3	9.2 (1.9–27.0)
Manz et al., 1991	German production workers	0	—
Saracci et al., 1991	IARC cohort	4	2.0 (0.6–5.2)
Zober et al., 1990	German production workers	0	—
Alavanja et al., 1989	Forest or soil conservationists	2	1.0 (0.1–3.6)
Bond et al., 1988	Dow 2,4-D production workers	0	—
Wiklund et al., 1988, 1989b	Swedish agricultural workers	7	0.9 (0.4–1.9)
Woods et al., 1987	Male residents of Washington State		
	High phenoxy exposure		0.9 (0.4–1.9)
	Those with self-reported chloracne		3.3 (0.8–14.0)
Coggon et al., 1986	British MCPA chemical workers	1	—
Hoar et al., 1986	Kansas residents		0.9 (0.5–1.6)
Vineis et al., 1986	Italian rice growers	66	
	Among all living women	5	2.4 (0.4–16.1)
Smith et al., 1983, 1984; Smith and Pearce, 1986	New Zealand workers exposed to herbicides		1.6 (0.7–3.8)
Lynge, 1985	Danish male production workers	5	2.7 (0.9–6.3)
Balarajan and Acheson, 1984	Agricultural workers in England	42	
	Overall		1.7 (1.0–2.9)
	Those under age 75		1.4 (0.8–2.6)
Blair et al., 1983	Florida pesticide appliers	0	—
Hardell, 1981	Swedish workers	52	
	Phenoxy herbicide exposure		5.5 (2.2–13.8)
Eriksson et al., 1979, 1981	Swedish workers		5.1 matched (2.2–10.2)
ENVIRONMENTAL			
New Studies			
Bertazzi et al., 2001	Seveso—20-year follow-up	0	—
Viel et al., 2000	Residents located near a French solid waste incinerator		
	Spatial cluster	45	1.4 ($p = .004$)
	1994–1995	12	3.4 ($p = .008$)
Bertazzi et al., 1998	Seveso—15-year follow-up	0	—

TABLE 7-10 *Continued*

Reference	Study Population	Exposed Cases[a]	Estimated Risk (95% CI)[a]
Studies Reviewed in *Update 1998*			
Bertazzi et al., 1997	Seveso residents—15-year follow-up		
	Zone R males	4	2.1 (0.6–5.4)
Gambini et al., 1997	Rice-growing farmers	1	0.3 expected
Svensson et al., 1995	Swedish fishermen, incidence		
	West coast	3	0.5 (0.1–1.4)
Studies Reviewed in *Update 1996*			
Bertazzi et al., 1993	Seveso residents—10-year follow-up, morbidity		
	Zone R males	6	2.8 (1.0–7.3)
	Zone R females	2	1.6 (0.3–7.4)
Studies Reviewed in *VAO*			
Lampi et al., 1992	Finnish town	6	1.6 (0.7–3.5)
Bertazzi et al., 1989a	Seveso residents—10-year follow-up		
	Zone A, B, R males	2	5.4 (0.8–38.6)
	Zone A, B, R females	1	2.0 (0.2–1.9)
Bertazzi et al., 1989b	Seveso residents—10-year follow-up		
	Zone R males	2	6.3 (0.9–45.0)
	Zone B females	1	17.0 (1.8–163.6)
VIETNAM VETERANS			
New Studies			
AFHS, 2000	Air Force Ranch Hand veterans	1	0.8 (0.1–12.8)
AIHW, 1999	Australian Vietnam veterans—male	14	27 expected (17–37)
CDVA, 1998a	Australian Vietnam veterans—male	398[b]	27 expected (17–37)
CDVA, 1998b	Australian Vietnam veterans—female	2[b]	0 expected (0–4)
Studies Reviewed in *Update 1998*			
Clapp, 1997	Massachusetts Vietnam Veterans	18	1.6 (0.5–5.4)
Crane et al., 1997a	Australian military Vietnam veterans	0–9	<1
Crane et al., 1997b	Australian national service Vietnam veterans	4	0.7
	Comparison group	2	—
AFHS, 1996	Ranch Hand veterans	1	—
	Comparisons	1	—
Visintainer et al., 1995	Vietnam veterans	8	1.1 (0.5–2.2)
Watanabe and Kang, 1995	U.S. Marines in Vietnam	0	—
Studies Reviewed in *Update 1996*			
Kogan and Clapp, 1988	Vietnam veterans in Massachusetts	9	5.2 (2.4–11.1)
Kang et al., 1986	Vietnam veterans		
	Comparing those who served with those who did not		0.8 (0.6–1.1)
Lawrence et al., 1985	Vietnam veterans in New York	2	1.1 (0.2–6.7)
Greenwald et al., 1984	New York State Vietnam veterans		0.5 (0.2–1.3)

TABLE 7-10 *Continued*

Reference	Study Population	Exposed Cases[a]	Estimated Risk (95% CI)[a]
Studies Reviewed in *VAO*			
Watanabe et al., 1991	Marine Vietnam veterans	8	1.1
Bullman et al., 1990	Army veterans serving in I Corps	10	0.9 (0.4–1.6)
Michalek et al., 1990	Ranch Hand veterans	1	—
	Comparisons	1	—
Breslin et al., 1988	Army Vietnam veterans	30	1.0
Fett et al., 1987	Australian Vietnam veterans	1	1.3 mortality rate, age-adjusted (0.1–20.0)
Anderson et al., 1986a,b	Wisconsin Vietnam veterans	5	1.5 (0.6–3.5)
Breslin et al., 1986	Vietnam veterans in Massachusetts	2	3.8 (0.5–13.8)

NOTE: MCPA = methyl-4-chlorophenoxyacetic acid.

[a] Given when available.

[b] Self-reported medical history. Answer to question: Since your first day of service in Vietnam, have you been told by a doctor that you have soft-tissue sarcoma?

SKIN CANCERS—ALL TYPES

Background

Skin cancers are generally divided into two broad categories: neoplasms that develop from melanocytes (malignant melanoma) and those that do not. The common nonmelanocytic skin cancers, which include basal and squamous cell carcinomas, have a far higher incidence than malignant melanoma but are considered less aggressive and therefore more treatable. In *VAO* and *Update 1996*, all skin cancers were assessed together. However, beginning with *Update 1998*, the committee chose to address studies assessing malignant melanoma separately from those assessing nonmelanocytic cancers (basal and squamous cell carcinoma). Because nonmelanocytic cancers are highly treatable, studies of these cancers have been divided further into those that discuss mortality and those that discuss incidence. Many studies report results by combining all types of skin cancers or do not specify the type of skin cancers assessed. These are also listed in Tables 7-11 and 7-12 in the interest of completeness.

According to American Cancer Society estimates, 27,300 men and 20,400 women will be diagnosed with cutaneous melanoma (ICD·9 172.0–172.9) in the United States in 2000, and 4,800 men and 2,900 women will die of this cancer (ACS, 2000a). Approximately 1,300,000 cases of nonmelanocytic skin cancers (ICD·9 173.0–173.9), primarily basal cell and squamous cell carcinomas, are diagnosed in the United States each year (ACS, 2000a). Since it is not required to report these cancers to registries, the data regarding the numbers of cases are not as precise as for other cancers. The American Cancer Society estimates that approximately 1,900 individuals will die from these diseases in 2000.

Skin cancers are far more likely to occur in fair-skinned individuals; the risk for whites is roughly 20 times that for dark-skinned African Americans. Incidence also increases with age, although more strikingly for males than females. Other risk factors for melanoma include the presence of certain moles on the skin, a suppressed immune system, and excessive exposure to ultraviolet (UV) radiation, typically from the sun. A family history of the disease has been identified as a risk factor, but it is unclear whether this is due to genetic factors or to similarities in skin type and sun exposure patterns.

Excessive exposure to UV radiation is the single most important risk factor for nonmelanocytic skin cancers. Certain skin diseases and chemical exposures have also been identified as potential risk factors. SEER incidence data are not available for nonmelanocytic skin cancers.

Average Annual Cancer Incidence (per 100,000 individuals) in the United States[a]
Melanomas of the Skin

	45–49 Years of Age			50–54 Years of Age			55–59 Years of Age		
	All Races	White	Black	All Races	White	Black	All Races	White	Black
Males	24.6	28.0	0.8	32.8	37.0	2.2	38.6	43.4	3.0
Females	20.1	23.2	1.6	20.3	23.3	0.6	23.5	27.0	2.0

[a] SEER nine standard registries, crude age-specific rate, 1993–1997.

Many studies report results by combining all types of cancers or do not specify the type of skin cancer assessed. Studies such as these are listed in Tables 7-11 and 7-12 according to the *VAO* report in which they appeared.

TABLE 7-11 Selected Epidemiologic Studies—All (or unspecified) Skin Cancer Mortality

Reference	Study Population	Exposed Cases[a]	Estimated Risk (95% CI)[a]
OCCUPATIONAL			
Studies Reviewed in *VAO*			
Fingerhut et al., 1991	NIOSH cohort	4	0.8 (0.2–2.1)
Saracci et al., 1991	IARC cohort	3	0.3 (0.1–0.9)
Alavanja et al., 1988	USDA agricultural extension agents	5	1.1 (0.5–2.6)
Burmeister, 1981	Farmers in Iowa	105	1.1 (NS)

TABLE 7-11 *Continued*

Reference	Study Population	Exposed Cases[a]	Estimated Risk (95% CI)[a]
VIETNAM VETERANS			
Studies Reviewed in *Update 1998*			
Dalager and Kang, 1997	Army Chemical Corps veterans	4	1.5 (0.3–8.6)
Watanabe and Kang, 1996	Army Vietnam veterans	234	1.0
	Marine Vietnam veterans	73	1.3 (1.0–1.6)
Studies Reviewed in *VAO*			
Anderson et al., 1986a	Wisconsin Vietnam veterans	6	0.9 (0.4–2.0)
Anderson et al., 1986b	Wisconsin Vietnam veterans	5	1.3 (0.4–3.1)

NOTE: NS = not significant; USDA = United States Department of Agriculture.
[a] Given when available.

TABLE 7-12 Selected Epidemiologic Studies—All (or unspecified) Skin Cancer Morbidity

Reference	Study Population	Exposed Cases[a]	Estimated Risk (95% CI)[a]
OCCUPATIONAL			
Studies Reviewed in *Update 1998*			
Ott and Zober, 1996	German BASF trichlorophenol production workers	5	1.2 (0.4–2.8)
Studies Reviewed in *VAO*			
Hansen et al., 1992	Danish gardeners	32	1.1 (0.8–1.6)
Lynge, 1985	Danish male production workers	14	0.7
Suskind and Hertzberg, 1984	Monsanto production workers	8	1.6
VIETNAM VETERANS			
New Studies			
AFHS, 2000	Air Force Ranch Hand veterans	325	1.3 (1.1–1.6)
Ketchum et al., 1999	Ranch Hand (RH) veterans and comparisons through June 1997		
	Comparisons	158	(control group)
	Background-exposure RH veterans	57	1.0 (0.7–1.5)
	Low-exposure RH veterans	44	1.3 (0.8–2.0)
	High-exposure RH veterans	22	0.8 (0.5–1.4)
Studies Reviewed in *VAO*			
Wolfe et al., 1990	Air Force Ranch Hand veterans	88	1.5 (1.1–2.0)
CDC, 1988	Army enlisted Vietnam veterans	15	0.8 (0.4–1.7)

[a] Given when available.

SKIN CANCER—MELANOMA

Summary of *VAO*, *Update 1996*, and *Update 1998*

The committee responsible for *VAO* found that there was inadequate or insufficient information to determine whether an association existed between exposure to herbicides used in Vietnam or the contaminant dioxin and skin cancer. Additional information available to the committee responsible for *Update 1996* did not change this finding. The *Update 1998* committee considered separately the literatures regarding malignant melanoma and nonmelanocytic skin cancers. It found that there was inadequate or insufficient information to determine whether an association existed between exposure to herbicides used in Vietnam or the contaminant dioxin and melanoma. Tables 7-13 and 7-14 provide summaries of the results of the studies underlying these findings and a list of reports that contain details of the research.

Update of the Scientific Literature

Occupational Studies

Hooiveld et al. (1998) conducted a retrospective cohort study of Dutch production and contract workers exposed to phenoxy herbicides, chlorophenols, and contaminants between 1950 and 1976. Of the 1,129 workers identified in the original cohort, 549 exposed and 482 unexposed male workers were included in this study. One death was attributed to malignant melanoma, leading to an SMR of 2.9 (0.1–15.9).

Environmental Studies

Bertazzi et al. (1998) conducted a review of the effects of dioxin exposure following a 1976 industrial accident in Seveso, examining mortality in the population 15 years after the incident. Extensive monitoring of soil levels and measurements of a limited number of human blood samples allowed for classification of the exposed population into three categories: zone A—high exposure, zone B—medium exposure, and zone R—lowest level of exposure. Few deaths were attributed to melanoma. In the high-exposure (A) zone, there were no melanoma deaths observed in males; for females, 1 death was reported when 0.1 was expected (RR = 9.4, 1.3–68.8). There were no deaths attributed to melanoma in zone B. Among males in zone R, 3 deaths were reported when 2.8 were expected (RR = 1.1, 0.3–3.7); among females, there were 3 deaths when 5.0 were expected (RR = 0.6, 0.2–2.0).

A later study (Bertazzi et al., 2001) extends the mortality analysis to 20 years following the event for zones A and B only. For zone A, there was no change in melanoma mortality. The 1 reported death (0.2 expected) for females resulted in a relative risk of 6.6 (0.9–47.7). In zone B, there was 1 death among males where 0.6 was expected (RR = 1.7, 0.2–12.5) and 1 death among females where 1.0 was expected (RR = 1.0, 0.1–7.4).

Schreinemachers' (2000) examination of cancer mortality over the years 1980–1989 in four northern wheat-producing states used wheat acreage per county as a surrogate for exposure to chlorophenoxy herbicides (including 2,4-D). There was an inconsistent pattern of age-standardized mortality rate ratios for malignant melanoma for white males and females. None of the values were statistically significant.

Vietnam Veteran Studies

The Air Force Health Study (AFHS) is a long-term longitudinal study of the health of veterans who participated in Operation Ranch Hand and were thus responsible for the majority of aerial spraying of herbicides in Vietnam. A matched cohort consisting of Air Force veterans who served in Southeast Asia but were not occupationally exposed to herbicides is used as the comparison group in these studies. More details on this study are contained in Chapter 6.

The latest in the series of AFHS reports describes the results of the 1997 physical examination of Ranch Hand veterans and their comparison cohort (AFHS, 2000). The authors evaluated the incidence of basal cell carcinomas (overall and at four specific sites), squamous cell carcinomas, nonmelanoma (basal cell carcinomas, squamous cell carcinomas, and malignant epithelial neoplasms not otherwise specified), and melanoma. Skin cancer analyses, except for the analyses of benign neoplasms, were limited to nonblacks because blacks have been observed to exhibit only benign skin neoplasms in all phases of the study to date. Participants with skin neoplasms that predated their service in Southeast Asia were also excluded. Factors that might influence or be correlated with the incidence of skin cancers—age, military occupation, skin color, hair color, eye color, skin reaction to sun after the first exposure, skin reaction to sun after repeated exposure, lifetime exposure to ionizing radiation and industrial chemicals (yes or no), average lifetime residential history, and measures of serum dioxin level—were statistically controlled for in some analyses.

Significantly more Ranch Hands (325 of 805) than comparisons (402 of 1,168) experienced some form of skin cancer since their service in Southeast Asia (RR = 1.3, 1.1–1.6; Model 1, adjusted). However, analyses that examined dioxin concentrations in blood and/or that controlled for confounding variables yielded inconsistent results. Ranch Hand veterans in the "low"-dioxin category showed higher incidence levels than those in the "high" or "background" categories or the comparisons, and one model showed a statistically significant inverse relationship between dioxin category and skin cancer.

There was a higher incidence of melanoma in Ranch Hands (16 of 805) than in comparisons (13 of 1,168), but the difference was not statistically significant (RR = 1.8, 0.8–3.8; Model 1, adjusted) and the highest incidence of melanoma was observed in low-dioxin-category Ranch Hands. None of the models that used categories of dioxin concentration or that adjusted for confounding variables produced statistically significant results.

A 1999 paper by Ketchum and colleagues reports the results of an earlier analysis of data available through July 1997 (not including the 1997 physical examination) on the Ranch Hand and comparison cohorts. Analyses were limited to nonblack veterans and were controlled for the factors listed above. This analysis found no association between a categorical measure of serum dioxin levels and the incidence of melanoma or skin cancers in general. Ranch Hand veterans in the low-exposure category had a higher incidence of skin cancers and melanoma than those in the background- or high-exposure categories, but the difference was not statistically significant. There was also no association between dioxin category and time to onset.

The Air Force Health Studies are notable for their attempts to control for confounding factors, something absent from many studies of this health outcome. The small number of melanoma cases, however, limits the informativeness of the results.

Results from the government of Australia's mail surveys of approximately 50,000 male and female nationals who served in Vietnam (CDVA, 1998a,b) found an excess of melanoma among both male and female veterans when comparing the number of Vietnam veterans responding yes to the question, *Since your first day of service in Vietnam, have you been told by a doctor that you have melanoma?* to expected national rates. Seven percent (2,689 of 40,030) of the male veterans responded yes compared to the expected 1 percent (380; 95% CI 342–418) (CDVA, 1998a). This translates to an observed–expected ratio of ~7.1. The report suggested that the indicated prevalence might be overstated because prudent physicians often remove possible melanomas and this may leave the impression that such lesions are malignant. A separate study of female veterans reported that 7 (3 percent) responded yes, while 3 (expected range 1–8) were expected, for an observed–expected ratio of 2.3 (CDVA, 1998b). One strength of these surveys is their relatively high response rates. Weaknesses include the use of self-reported cases with no validation through medical record reviews or other means, the inability to control for important confounders, and the use of a nonmilitary control group. Results for females were based on a very small number of subjects.

The follow-up validation study (AIHW, 1999) estimated that there were 483 validated cases of melanoma among respondents. This was much smaller than the reported number of cases but still in excess of the expected number, 380 (342–418).

CANCER   305

Synthesis

Studies reviewed for the first time in *Update 2000* add to the body of knowledge by providing additional morbidity data and mortality analyses to account for factors that confound the evaluation of melanoma incidence in groups with exposure to chemical agents. The occupational and Seveso studies have too few cases to be informative. The studies of veterans in Australia and of the Ranch Hand cohort provide some important new data; however, the information is not strong enough to lead the committee to change its prior finding. The committee continues to encourage researchers to make an effort to control confounding from UV (sunlight) exposures and acknowledges the efforts of AFHS researchers in this area.

Conclusions

Strength of Evidence in Epidemiologic Studies

There is no information contained in the research reviewed for this report to change the conclusion that there is inadequate or insufficient evidence to determine whether an association exists between exposure to herbicides (2,4-D, 2,4,5-T and its contaminant TCDD, cacodylic acid, and picloram) and melanoma. The evidence regarding association is drawn from occupational, environmental, and veteran studies in which subjects were exposed to herbicides and herbicide components.

Biologic Plausibility

Mice were treated topically (applied to skin surface) for 2 years with TCDD. Under the conditions of the bioassay, fibrosarcomas occurred in the integumentary system of female mice (Huff et al., 1991). Therefore, continuous dermal exposure to TCDD can induce skin tumors (fibrosarcomas, not squamous cell carcinomas) in laboratory mice. Mechanistic data from in vitro and animal studies also support a role for TCDD as a promoter in the carcinogenic process. A summary of the biologic plausibility for the carcinogenicity of TCDD and the herbicides in general is presented in the conclusion to this chapter. A discussion of toxicological studies that concern biologic plausibility is contained in Chapter 3.

Increased Risk of Disease Among Vietnam Veterans

Studies of U.S. and Australian veterans have reported a higher incidence of melanoma among male, nonblack veterans than comparison groups. However, analyses controlling for factors that might influence or be correlated with the incidence of skin cancers do not show a relationship between measures of exposure to the herbicides used in Vietnam and this health outcome. The highest melanoma incidence in the AFHS reports was observed in veterans in the low-dioxin category, which would not be expected if there was an association between exposure and the outcome. The strongest evidence to date comes from the medical validation study of Australian Vietnam veterans. The estimated expected number of cases is considerably lower than the number of reported cases that were validated. However, adjustments for potentially important confounders were not carried out. Overall, data from those who served in Vietnam are not adequate to infer an association between malignant melanoma and exposure to herbicides used in Vietnam.

TABLE 7-13 Selected Epidemiologic Studies—Melanoma Mortality

Reference	Study Population	Exposed Cases[a]	Estimated Risk (95% CI)[a]
OCCUPATIONAL			
New Studies			
Hooiveld et al., 1998	Dutch production workers	1	2.9 (0.1–15.9)
Studies Reviewed in Update 1998			
Hertzman et al., 1997	Sawmill workers	17	1.4 (0.9–2.0)
Kogevinas et al., 1997	IARC cohort		
	Workers exposed to TCDD		
	(or higher-chlorinated dioxins)	5	0.5 (0.2–3.2)
	Workers not exposed to TCDD		
	(or higher-chlorinated dioxins)	4	1.0 (0.3–2.4)
Svensson et al., 1995	Swedish fishermen		
	East coast	0	0.0 (0.0–1.7)
	West coast	6	0.7 (0.2–1.5)
Studies Reviewed in Update 1996			
Blair et al., 1993	U.S. farmers in 23 states (white male)	244	1.0 (0.8–1.1)
Studies Reviewed in VAO			
Wigle et al., 1990	Saskatchewan farmers	24	1.1 (0.7–1.6)
Wiklund, 1983	Swedish agricultural workers	268	0.8 (0.7–1.0)[b]
ENVIRONMENTAL			
New Studies			
Bertazzi et al., 2001	Seveso residents—20-year follow-up		
	Zone A females	1	6.6 (0.9–47.7)
	Zone B males	1	1.7 (0.2–12.5)
	Zone B females	1	1.0 (0.1–7.4)
Schreinemachers, 2000	Rural or farm residents of Minnesota, Montana, and North and South Dakota		
	Males—counties with wheat acreage 23,000–110,999	50	0.8 (0.6–1.1)
	Males—counties with wheat acreage >111,000	41	0.8 (0.6–1.1)

TABLE 7-13 Continued

Reference	Study Population	Exposed Cases[a]	Estimated Risk (95% CI)[a]
	Females—counties with wheat acreage 23,000–110,999	59	1.2 (0.9–1.8)
	Females—counties with wheat acreage >111,000	29	0.7 (0.5–1.2)
Bertazzi et al., 1998	Seveso residents—15-year follow-up		
	Zone A females	1	9.4 (1.3–68.8)
	Zone R males	3	1.1 (0.3–3.7)
	Zone R females	3	0.6 (0.2–2.0)
Studies Reviewed in *Update 1998*			
Bertazzi et al., 1997	Seveso residents—15-year follow-up		
	Zone R males	3	1.1 (0.2–3.2)
	Zone R females	3	0.6 (0.1–1.8)
Studies Reviewed in *VAO*			
Bertazzi et al., 1989a	Seveso residents—10-year follow-up		
	Zones A, B, R males	3	3.3 (0.8–13.9)
VIETNAM VETERANS			
Studies Reviewed in *Update 1998*			
Crane et al., 1997a	Australian military Vietnam veterans	51	1.3 (1.0–1.8)
Crane et al., 1997b	Australian national service Vietnam veterans	16	0.5 (0.2–1.3)
Studies Reviewed in *VAO*			
Breslin et al., 1988	Army Vietnam veterans	145	1.0 (0.9–1.1)
	Marine Vietnam veterans	36	0.9 (0.6–1.5)

NOTE: NS = not significant.
[a] Given when available.
[b] 99% CI.

TABLE 7-14 Selected Epidemiologic Studies—Melanoma Morbidity

Reference	Study Population	Exposed Cases[a]	Estimated Risk (95% CI)[a]
OCCUPATIONAL			
Studies Reviewed in *Update 1998*			
Hertzman et al., 1997	Sawmill workers	38	1.0 (0.7–1.2)
Svensson et al., 1995	Swedish fishermen		
	East coast	0	0 (0.0–0.7)
	West coast	20	0.8 (0.5–1.2)
Studies Reviewed in *Update 1996*			
Lynge, 1993	Danish male production workers	4	4.3 (1.2–10.9)
Studies Reviewed in *VAO*			
Ronco et al., 1992	Danish self-employed farmers	72	0.7 ($p < .05$)

TABLE 7-14 Continued

Reference	Study Population	Exposed Cases[a]	Estimated Risk (95% CI)[a]
VIETNAM VETERANS			
New Studies			
AFHS, 2000	Air Force Ranch Hand veterans	16	1.8 (0.8–3.8)
AIHW, 1999	Australian Vietnam veterans—male	483	380 expected (342–418)
Ketchum et al., 1999	Ranch Hand (RH) veterans and comparisons through June 1997		
	Comparisons	9	(control group)
	Background-exposure RH veterans	4	1.1 (0.3–4.5)
	Low-exposure RH veterans	6	2.6 (0.7–9.1)
	High-exposure RH veterans	2	0.9 (0.2–5.6)
CDVA, 1998a	Australian Vietnam veterans—male	2,689[b]	380 expected (342–418)
CDVA, 1998b	Australian Vietnam veterans—female	7[b]	3 expected (1–8)
Studies Reviewed in *Update 1998*			
Clapp, 1997	Massachusetts Vietnam veterans	21	1.4 (0.7–2.9)
Studies Reviewed in *VAO*			
Wolfe et al., 1990	Air Force Ranch Hand veterans	4	1.3 (0.3–5.2)

NOTE: NS = not significant.
[a] Given when available.
[b] Self-reported medical history. Answer to question: Since your first day of service in Vietnam, have you been told by a doctor that you have melanoma?

SKIN CANCER—BASAL AND SQUAMOUS CELL (NONMELANOMA)

Summary of *VAO*, *Update 1996*, and *Update 1998*

The committee responsible for *VAO* found that there was inadequate or insufficient information to determine whether an association existed between exposure to herbicides used in Vietnam or the contaminant dioxin and skin cancer. Additional information available to the committee responsible for *Update 1996* did not change this finding. The *Update 1998* committee considered separately the literatures regarding malignant melanoma and nonmelanocytic skin cancers. It found that there was inadequate or insufficient information to determine whether an association existed between exposure to the herbicides used in Vietnam or the contaminant dioxin and basal or squamous cell cancers. Tables 7-15 and 7-16 provide summaries of the results of the studies underlying these findings and a list of reports that contain details of the research.

Update of the Scientific Literature

Occupational Studies

A thorough review of the new published material did not reveal any relevant occupational studies.

Environmental Studies

A thorough review of the new published material did not reveal any relevant environmental studies.

Vietnam Veteran Studies

The AFHS is a long-term longitudinal study of the health of the group of veterans who participated in Operation Ranch Hand herbicide spray missions and a matched cohort consisting of Air Force veterans who served in Southeast Asia but were not occupationally exposed to herbicides. More details on this study series are contained in Chapter 3. The discussion of melanoma above contains more information on the methodology used in the AFHS to evaluate skin cancers.

Several analyses of nonmelanoma skin cancers were conducted: basal cell carcinomas of the ear, face, head, and neck; basal cell carcinomas of the trunk; basal cell carcinomas of the upper extremities; basal cell carcinomas of the lower extremities; all basal cell carcinoma sites combined; squamous cell carcinomas; and an all-nonmelanoma category consisting of all basal cell carcinomas, squamous cell carcinomas, and malignant epithelial neoplasms not otherwise specified.

A slightly greater proportion of Ranch Hands (15 percent; 121 of 805) than comparisons (13.3 percent; 155 of 1,168) experienced a basal cell carcinoma (BCC) after their service in Southeast Asia (RR = 1.2, 0.9–1.6; Model 1, adjusted) (AFHS, 2000). An analysis that controlled for confounding variables found a statistically significant excess of BCC in Ranch Hands in the low-dioxin category (RR = 1.6, 1.1–2.4), but the same analysis found no excess for Ranch Hands in the high-dioxin category (RR = 1.0, 0.6–1.6). As the estimated initial serum dioxin levels in Ranch Hands increased, the percentage of participants with BCC decreased—there was a statistically significant inverse association found between initial dioxin and any basal cell carcinoma in an analysis that controlled for confounders (RR = 0.7, p = .014; Model 2, adjusted). Other models yielded nonsignificant results. Analyses that separated BCC by location generated inconsistent but generally nonsignificant results, as might be expected from the small number of cases examined.

There were relatively few squamous cell carcinomas among Ranch Hands (20 of 805) and comparisons (22 of 1,168) (RR = 1.5, 0.8–2.8; Model 1, adjusted). None of the analyses of this outcome yielded statistically significant results. The analysis of all nonmelanomas identified 134 (out of 805) in Ranch Hands and 176 (out of 1,168) in comparisons, for a relative risk of 1.2 (0.9–1.5; Model 1, adjusted). Basal cell carcinomas make up approximately 90 percent of these, and results are similar to those reported for that outcome.

A paper by Ketchum and colleagues (1999) reports the results of an earlier analysis of data available through July 1997 (not including the 1997 physical examination) on the Ranch Hand and comparison cohorts. Analyses were limited to nonblack veterans and were controlled for the same confounding variables outlined in the melanoma section. This analysis found no association between a categorical measure of serum dioxin levels and the incidence of basal or squamous cell carcinomas. Ranch Hand veterans in the low-exposure category had a higher incidence of skin cancers and melanoma than those in the background- or high-exposure categories or the comparison group, but the differences were not statistically significant. There was also no association between dioxin category and time to onset for either cancer.

As stated in the discussion of melanoma, the Air Force Health Studies are notable for their attempts to control for confounding factors, something absent from many studies of this health outcome. The small number of cases, however, limits the informativeness of the results.

The government of Australia conducted mail surveys of all individuals with Vietnam service, which included those involved in combat, medical teams, war correspondents, entertainers, and philanthropy workers (CDVA, 1998a,b). Questionnaires were mailed to 49,944 male veterans (80 percent response rate) and 278 female veterans (81 percent response rate).

Seventeen percent of both male (6,936) and female (37) respondents reported having been told by a doctor that they had a basal cell or squamous cell carcinoma since their first day of service in Vietnam (CDVA, 1998a,b). There was no estimate made of the expected number of cases or the range of expected numbers. The authors state that such skin lesions are often removed without pathological confirmation and their prevalence is not monitored by cancer registries, so proper comparisons are not calculable. The strengths of these surveys include their relatively high response rates. Weaknesses include the use of self-reported cases and the inability to control for important confounders. Results for females were based on a very small number of subjects.

Synthesis

There are relatively few studies that examine nonmelanomas and fewer that separate basal and squamous cell carcinomas, even though there are differences in the etiologies of these outcomes. Studies of U.S. and Australian Vietnam veterans reviewed for the first time in this report provide new morbidity data for these outcomes, with AFHS studies accounting for factors that confound the

CANCER   *311*

evaluation of nonmelanoma incidence in groups with exposure to chemical agents. As was true for the evaluation of melanomas, these studies do not provide information that would lead the committee to change its prior findings. The committee continues to encourage researchers to make an effort to control confounding from UV (sunlight) exposures and acknowledges the efforts of AFHS researchers in this area.

Conclusions

Strength of Evidence in Epidemiologic Studies

There is no information contained in the research reviewed for this report to change the conclusion that there is inadequate or insufficient evidence to determine whether an association exists between exposure to herbicides (2,4-D, 2,4,5-T and its contaminant TCDD, cacodylic acid, and picloram) and basal or squamous cell cancers.

Biologic Plausibility

Mice were treated topically (applied to skin surface) for 2 years with TCDD (Huff et al., 1991). Under the conditions of the bioassay, fibrosarcomas occurred in the integumentary system of female mice. Therefore, continuous, dermal exposure to TCDD can induce skin tumors (fibrosarcomas, not squamous cell carcinomas) in laboratory mice. Mechanistic data from in vitro and animal studies also support a role for TCDD as a promoter in the carcinogenic process. A summary of the biologic plausibility for the carcinogenicity of TCDD and the herbicides in general is presented in the conclusion to this chapter. A discussion of toxicological studies that concern biologic plausibility is contained in Chapter 3.

Increased Risk of Disease Among Vietnam Veterans

The AFHS report a higher incidence of nonmelanomas among male, nonblack veterans than in the comparison group. However, analyses controlling for factors that might influence or be correlated with the incidence of skin cancers do not show a relationship between measures of exposure to the herbicides used in Vietnam and these health outcomes.

TABLE 7-15 Selected Epidemiologic Studies—Other Nonmelanoma (basal and squamous cell) Skin Cancer Mortality

Reference	Study Population	Exposed Cases[a]	Estimated Risk (95% CI)[a]
OCCUPATIONAL			
Studies Reviewed in *Update 1998*			
Hertzman et al., 1997	Sawmill workers	38	1.0 (0.7–1.2)
Kogevinas et al., 1997	IARC cohort		
	Workers exposed to TCDD		
	(or higher-chlorinated dioxins)	4	1.2 (0.3–3.2)
	Workers not exposed to TCDD		
	(or higher-chlorinated dioxins)	0	—
Svensson et al., 1995	Swedish fishermen		
	East coast	0	0.0 (0.0–15.4)
	West coast	5	3.0 (1.0–7.1)
Studies Reviewed in *Update 1996*			
Blair et al., 1993	U.S. farmers in 23 states (white male)	425	1.1 (1.0–1.2)
Studies Reviewed in *VAO*			
Coggon et al., 1986	British MCPA chemical workers	3	3.1 (0.6–9.0)
Wiklund, 1983	Swedish agricultural workers	708	1.1 (1.0–1.2)[b]

NOTE: MCPA = methyl-4-chlorophenoxyacetic acid.
[a] Given when available.
[b] 99% CI.

TABLE 7-16 Selected Epidemiologic Studies—Other Nonmelanoma (basal and squamous cell) Skin Cancer Morbidity

Reference	Study Population	Exposed Cases[a]	Estimated Risk (95% CI)[a]
OCCUPATIONAL			
Studies Reviewed in *Update 1998*			
Zhong and Rafnsson, 1996	Icelandic pesticide users	5	2.8 (0.9–6.6)
Svensson et al., 1995	Swedish fishermen		
	East coast	22	2.3 (1.4–3.5)
	West coast	69	1.1 (0.9–1.4)
Studies Reviewed in *VAO*			
Ronco et al., 1992	Danish self-employed farmers	493	0.7 ($p < .05$)
ENVIRONMENTAL			
Studies Reviewed in *Update 1998*			
Gallagher et al., 1996	Alberta, Canada, residents—squamous cell carcinoma		
	All herbicide exposure	79	1.5 (1.0–2.3)
	Low herbicide exposure	33	1.9 (1.0–3.6)

TABLE 7-16 Continued

Reference	Study Population	Exposed Cases[a]	Estimated Risk (95% CI)[a]
	High herbicide exposure	46	3.9 (2.2–6.9)
	All fungicide exposure	96	1.4 (0.9–2.1)
	Low fungicide exposure	40	0.8 (0.4–1.4)
	High fungicide exposure	56	2.4 (1.4–4.0)
	Alberta, Canada, residents—basal cell carcinoma		
	All herbicide exposure	70	1.1 (0.8–1.7)
	All fungicide exposure	76	0.9 (0.6–1.3)
Studies Reviewed in *Update 1996*			
Bertazzi et al., 1993	Seveso residents—10-year follow-up, morbidity		
	Zone A males	1	2.4 (0.3–17.2)
	Zone B males	2	0.7 (0.2–2.9)
	Zone R males	20	1.0 (0.6–1.6)
Studies Reviewed in *VAO*			
Pesatori et al., 1992	Seveso residents		
	Zones A, B males	3	1.0 (0.3–3.0)
	Zones A, B females	3	1.5 (0.5–4.9)
VIETNAM VETERANS			
New Studies			
AFHS, 2000	Air Force Ranch Hand veterans		
	Basal cell carcinoma (BCC)	121	1.2 (0.9–1.6)
	Squamous cell carcinoma (SCC)	20	1.5 (0.8–2.8)
CDVA, 1998a	Australian Vietnam veterans—male	6,936[b]	—
CDVA, 1998b	Australian Vietnam veterans—female	37[b]	—
Studies Reviewed in *VAO*			
Wolfe et al., 1990	Air Force Ranch Hand veterans		
	Basal cell carcinoma	78	1.5 (1.0–2.1)
	Squamous cell carcinoma	6	1.6 (0.5–5.1)

[a] Given when available.

[b] Self-reported medical history. Answer to question: Since your first day of service in Vietnam, have you been told by a doctor that you have other skin cancers (BCC and SCC)?

BREAST CANCER

Background

Breast cancer (ICD·9 174.0–174.9 for females) is the single most common cancer among women in the United States, excluding nonmelanocytic skin cancers. The American Cancer Society estimates that 182,800 women will be diagnosed with breast cancer in the United States in 2000 and that 40,800 will die from the disease (ACS, 2000a). Overall, these numbers represent approximately 30 percent of the incidence of new cancers and 15 percent of cancer deaths among women. Among women aged 40–55, breast cancer is the leading cause of cancer death.

Breast cancer incidence generally increases with age. In the age groups that characterize most Vietnam veterans, the incidence for whites is slightly higher than that for African Americans. Risk factors other than aging include a personal or family history of breast cancer and certain characteristics of one's reproductive history (specifically, early onset of menarche, late onset of menopause, and either no pregnancies or first full-term pregnancy after 30 years of age). A pooled analysis of six large-scale prospective studies of invasive breast cancer found that alcohol consumption was associated with a linear increase in incidence in women over the range of consumption reported by most women (Smith-Warner et al., 1998). The potential role of other personal behavioral and environmental factors in breast cancer incidence is being studied extensively.

The majority of women Vietnam veterans who were exposed to Agent Orange are now approaching or have reached menopause and will experience an increasing risk of breast cancer. It is therefore predictable on the basis of demographics alone that breast cancer will be a conspicuous and significant cause of death.

Average Annual Cancer Incidence (per 100,000 individuals) in the United States[a]
Breast Cancer in Females

45–49 Years of Age			50–54 Years of Age			55–59 Years of Age		
All Races	White	Black	All Races	White	Black	All Races	White	Black
198.5	201.0	199.3	263.7	272.4	243.5	305.0	312.9	290.2

[a] SEER nine standard registries, crude age-specific rate, 1993–1997.

Summary of *VAO*, *Update 1996*, and *Update 1998*

The committee responsible for *VAO* found there to be inadequate or insufficient information to determine whether an association existed between exposure to herbicides used in Vietnam or the contaminant dioxin and breast cancer. Additional information available to the committees responsible for *Update 1996* and *Update 1998* did not change this finding. Table 7-17 provides summaries of the results of the studies underlying these findings and a list of reports that contain details of the research.

Update of the Scientific Literature

Occupational Studies

A thorough review of the new published material did not reveal any relevant occupational studies.

Environmental Studies

Since *Update 1998*, there has been elaboration on the experience of a non-occupationally exposed population that, unlike most extant occupational studies, has included sufficient numbers of women to report statistically stable risk estimates.

Since *Update 1998*, Bertazzi and colleagues have reported on 15 years (Bertazzi et al., 1998) and 20 years (Bertazzi et al., 2001) of observation of residents of Seveso, Italy, who experienced relatively pure TCDD exposure in the 1976 industrial incident. No elevations in mortality from breast cancer were found. Among residents of zone A, the area of highest contamination, the relative risk for females was 0.6 (0.1–3.9, 1 death observed), and there were no deaths from this cause among males. Among residents of zone B, the medium-exposure area, the relative risk for females was 0.8 (0.4–1.5, 9 deaths observed), and there were no deaths from this cause among males. As reported in Bertazzi et al. (1998), among residents of zone R, the area of low contamination, the relative risk for females was 0.8 (0.6–1.0, 67 deaths observed), and there were no deaths from this cause among males.

Several studies conducted in the late 1990s examined exposure to organochlorine compounds. The largest and most complete of these was conducted by Bagga et al. (2000), who examined cumulative exposure to organochlorines as reflected by levels of DDT and its metabolites in breast adipose tissue and found no difference in levels of women with breast cancer compared to women undergoing reduction mammoplasty. Age, body mass index, menopausal status at the time of diagnosis, and family history of breast cancer were taken into account in this study.

Similarly, Demers et al. (2000) reported on a large study from hospitals in Quebec in which total and 25 specific organochlorine levels did not differ between women with and without breast cancer. This study did report that among women with breast cancer, those with lymph node involvement, indicating spread of the tumor, and those with larger tumors had higher tissue organochlorine levels than those with more limited disease, after adjusting for age and other factors.

Høyer et al. (2000) studied 195 women in Copenhagen in a community survey who had provided blood samples in 1976–1978, and again in 1981–1983, and who subsequently developed breast cancer. The blood was analyzed for organochlorine compounds. Higher dieldrin levels, but not levels of other organochlorines tested such as total polychlorinated biphenyls (PCBs), were associated with markedly reduced survival times after diagnosis, demonstrating a dose–response relationship. The increased risk of dying from breast cancer in women with higher dieldrin levels was associated with more aggressive tumor behavior, such as high-grade malignancies, earlier metastases, and advanced disease at the time of diagnosis. Among the organochlorines, dieldrin is strongly estrogenic, meaning that it binds to estrogen receptors and duplicates the effects of hormones. This hormonal mimicry may have an effect on tumor promotion and cancer cell growth, or even on the aggressiveness of the cancer, which is suggested by the evidence. The phenoxyacetic herbicides, dioxins, furans, and PCBs may act differently.

Organochlorine herbicides were not specifically and separately examined in these studies, however. Duell et al. (2000) studied women who were exposed to organochlorine pesticides, including but not limited to herbicides, while living and working on farms in North Carolina. Consistent with earlier, similar studies, no excess risk of breast cancer was found overall, and the results were compatible with a reduced risk in proportion to duration of farming. However, investigators could not rule out an increased risk in a subgroup of farming women who directly handled pesticides on farms.

Vietnam Veteran Studies

The government of Australia's mail survey of approximately 278 female veterans yielded 223 responses. When asked if a doctor had told them they had breast cancer since their first day of service in Vietnam, 17 females responded in the affirmative. This is in excess of the 5 cases that were expected and beyond the expected range of 2-11 cases. Although there is a statistically significant excess of breast cancer in this study population, there are non-war-related risk factors that may be confounding the findings. Such factors include low number of pregnancies, childlessness, or mothers giving birth to their first children at an older age. Based on these data, it is difficult to interpret whether environmental exposures in Vietnam contributed to the excess of breast cancer reported.

Synthesis

Much available evidence suggests that exposure to TCDD, and probably the herbicides of concern in this report, exerts a protective effect for women against the risk of developing breast cancer. This finding is supported by the known antiestrogenic activity of TCDD, which may be expected to antagonize endogenous estrogen effects and does reduce the incidence of mammary tumors in treated animals. Animal studies also suggest a reduction in the frequency of breast cancer following exposure to TCDD. It is thus biologically plausible that exposure to TCDD, whatever its other effects, may reduce the risk of breast cancer experienced by women with comparable reproductive history.

Contradicting this interpretation of the literature are earlier studies of Australian Vietnam veterans (Crane et al., 1997a) and one very large occupational cohort (Kogevinas et al., 1997) that do show an excess risk among males; the occupational cohort also demonstrated a significant elevation among women. Overall, the data are not conclusive in supporting a protective effect or an association between exposure to the herbicides of concern in this report and the risk of breast cancer. The significance of these findings for Vietnam era veterans who may have experienced different patterns of organochlorine exposure, reflecting the herbicides of concern, is not known.

Although there appears to be limited evidence to suggest that there is an epidemiologically defined protective effect of exposure to TCDD in reducing the overall incidence of breast cancer, this should be understood as limited to the narrow context of frequency of new disease. The term "protective" is used here in a narrow technical sense of exposure being associated with a reduction in risk. The effect is not necessarily a benefit, because it remains possible that exposure to TCDD and Agent Orange may affect lethality, distribution of tissue type, rate of progression, and invasiveness. There is limited evidence that this may be the case for organochlorine exposure in general (Demers et al., 2000), but the data of Høyer et al. (2000) suggest that the effect is very specific in terms of compound. It is not known whether compounds relevant to Agent Orange exposure have this effect.

The possibility that TCDD may exert a significant biological effect means that there is a possibility that exposure could adversely affect the natural history of tumors that do arise. Limited evidence, as yet unconfirmed, suggests that there may be adverse effects from organochlorine exposure on the natural history of the cancers that occur. Of concern is the finding from Quebec (Demers et al., 2000) that markers for higher organochlorine exposure are associated with more invasive and progressive disease at the time of diagnosis, once a cancer does develop. In Danish women studied by Høyer et al. (2000), higher levels of one organochlorine were associated with poorer prognosis of breast cancer, but the relevance to women exposed to Agent Orange is uncertain.

Importantly, there is no evidence from which to evaluate the possibility that exposure to organochlorines may modify the natural history if exposure takes place at certain sensitive periods during the development of breast tissue, such as puberty and pregnancy.

Conclusions

Strength of Evidence in Epidemiologic Studies

There is no information contained in the research reviewed for this report to change the conclusion that there is inadequate or insufficient evidence to determine whether an association exists between exposure to herbicides (2,4-D, 2,4,5-T and its contaminant TCDD, cacodylic acid, and picloram) and risk of breast cancer. Some current evidence suggests that there may be an inverse correlation with incidence of tumors, but the evidence is limited and unconfirmed.

Biologic Plausibility

No animal studies have found an increased incidence of breast cancer. A summary of the biologic plausibility for the carcinogenicity of TCDD and the herbicides in general is presented in the conclusion to this chapter. A discussion of toxicological studies that concern biologic plausibility is contained in Chapter 3.

Increased Risk of Disease Among Vietnam Veterans

There are no data on which to base a conclusion concerning whether Vietnam veterans may or may not be at increased risk for breast cancer due to exposure to herbicides or TCDD.

TABLE 7-17 Selected Epidemiologic Studies—Breast Cancer

Reference	Study Population	Exposed Cases[a]	Estimated Risk (95% CI)[a]
OCCUPATIONAL			
New Studies			
Duell et al., 2000	Used pesticides in the garden	228	2.3 (1.7–3.1)
	Laundry for pesticide user	119	4.1 (2.8–5.9)
Studies Reviewed in *Update 1998*			
Kogevinas et al., 1997	IARC cohort, female; identical to Manz et al. (1991)	9	2.2 (1.0–4.1)
	IARC cohort, male	2	2.6 (0.3–9.3)
Studies Reviewed in *Update 1996*			
Blair et al., 1993	Female U.S. farmers from 23 states		
	White	71	1.0 (0.8–1.3)
	Nonwhite	30	0.7 (0.5–1.0)
Kogevinas et al., 1993	Female herbicide spraying and production workers	7	0.9 (0.4–1.9)
	Probably exposed to TCDD	1	0.9 (0.0–4.8)

TABLE 7-17 Continued

Reference	Study Population	Exposed Cases[a]	Estimated Risk (95% CI)[a]
Studies Reviewed in *VAO*			
Ronco et al., 1992	Danish family farm workers	429	0.8 ($p < .05$)
Manz et al., 1991	German production workers	9	2.2 (1.0–4.1)
Saracci et al., 1991	IARC cohort	1	0.3 (0.0–1.7)
Lynge, 1985	Danish production workers	13	0.9
Wiklund, 1983	Swedish agricultural workers	444	0.8 (0.7–0.9)[b]
ENVIRONMENTAL			
New Studies			
Bertazzi et al., 2001	Seveso residents—20-year follow-up		
	Zone A females	2	0.8 (0.2–3.1)
	Zone B females	12	0.7 (0.4–1.3)
Bagga et al., 2000	Women receiving medical care in Woodland Hills, California	73	NS
Demers et al., 2000	Women in Quebec City newly diagnosed	315	NS
Høyer et al., 2000	Female participants of Copenhagen City Heart Study	195	Overall survival RR 2.8 (1.4–5.6)
Bertazzi et al., 1998	Seveso residents—15-year follow-up		
	Zone A females	1	0.6 (0.1–3.9)
	Zone B females	9	0.8 (0.4–1.5)
	Zone R females	67	0.8 (0.6–1.0)
Studies Reviewed in *Update 1998*			
Bertazzi et al., 1997	Seveso residents—15-year follow-up		
	Zone A females	1	0.6 (0.0–3.1)
	Zone B females	9	0.8 (0.4–1.5)
	Zone R females	67	0.8 (0.6–1.0)
Studies Reviewed in *Update 1996*			
Bertazzi et al., 1993	Seveso residents—10-year follow-up, morbidity		
	Zone A females	1	0.5 (0.1–3.3)
	Zone B females	10	0.7 (0.4–1.4)
	Zone R females	106	1.1 (0.9–1.3)
Studies Reviewed in *VAO*			
Bertazzi et al., 1989b	Seveso residents—10-year follow-up		
	Zone B females	5	0.9 (0.4–2.1)
	Zone R females	28	0.6 (0.4–0.9)
VIETNAM VETERANS			
New Studies			
CDVA, 1998b	Australian Vietnam veterans—female	17[c]	5 expected (2–11)
Studies Reviewed in *Update 1998*			
Crane et al., 1997a	Australian military Vietnam veterans	3	5.5 (1.1–16.1)
Studies Reviewed in *Update 1996*			
Dalager et al., 1995	Women Vietnam veterans	26	1.0 (0.6–1.8)

TABLE 7-17 *Continued*

Reference	Study Population	Exposed Cases[a]	Estimated Risk (95% CI)[a]
Studies Reviewed in *VAO*			
Thomas et al., 1991	Women Vietnam veterans	17	1.2 (0.6–2.5)

NOTE: NS = not significant.
[a] Given when available.
[b] 99% CI.
[c] Self-reported medical history. Answer to question: Since your first day of service in Vietnam, have you been told by a doctor that you have breast cancer?

CANCERS OF THE FEMALE REPRODUCTIVE SYSTEM

Background

This section addresses cancers of the cervix (ICD·9 180.0–180.9), endometrium (also referred to as the corpus uteri, ICD·9 182.0–182.1, 182.8), and ovaries (ICD·9 183.0). Statistics for other cancers of the female reproductive system are presented as well. The American Cancer Society estimated the following numbers of new female reproductive system cancers in the United States for 2000 (ACS, 2000a):

Site	New Cases	Deaths
Cervix	12,800	4,600
Endometrium	36,100	6,500
Ovary	23,100	14,000
Other female genital	5,500	1,400

Taken together, these numbers represent roughly 6 percent of new cancer diagnoses and 5 percent of cancer deaths in women.

Incidence patterns and risk factors vary for these diseases. Cervical cancers occur more often in African-American women than in whites, whereas whites are more likely to develop endometrial and ovarian cancers. The incidence of endometrial and ovarian cancer also depends on age, with older women at greater risk. Other risk factors for these cancers vary. Human papillomavirus infection is the most important risk factor for cervical cancer. Diet, a family history of the disease, and breast cancer are among the risk factors for endometrial and ovarian cancers.

Average Annual Cancer Incidence (per 100,000 individuals) in the United States[a]
Female Genital System Cancers

	45–49 Years of Age			50–54 Years of Age			55–59 Years of Age		
	All Races	White	Black	All Races	White	Black	All Races	White	Black
Cervix	16.7	15.1	21.9	15.8	13.9	22.9	15.6	12.7	28.3
Endometrium	24.7	24.9	12.0	45.8	47.4	27.0	66.0	69.6	39.6
Ovary	22.8	24.2	12.9	29.8	30.9	20.7	35.6	38.4	21.4
Other genital	3.1	3.1	3.8	4.9	5.0	3.8	5.4	5.4	6.0
Overall	67.3	67.3	50.6	96.3	97.2	74.4	122.6	126.1	95.3

[a] SEER nine standard registries, crude age-specific rate, 1993–1997.

Summary of *VAO*, *Update 1996*, and *Update 1998*

The committee responsible for *VAO* found there to be inadequate or insufficient information to determine whether an association existed between exposure to herbicides used in Vietnam or the contaminant dioxin and female reproductive cancers. Additional information available to the committees responsible for *Update 1996* and *Update 1998* did not change this finding. Tables 7-18, 7-19, and 7-20 provide summaries of the results of the studies underlying these findings and a list of reports that contain details of the research.

Update of the Scientific Literature

Occupational Studies

Very few new data have appeared in the literature that relate exposures to 2,3,7,8-TCDD to uterine, ovarian, or cervical cancers. In a study of herbicides and adjuvants (i.e., additives to herbicides), levels of FSH (follicle-stimulating hormone) and free testosterone were elevated postapplication compared to pre-application in male appliers (Sweeney et al., 1997/98). Whether these findings (e.g., the associations with FSH) generalize to females is unknown.

Environmental Studies

A publication by Bertazzi et al. (1998) on the Seveso population indicates no increases in female reproductive cancers among those exposed in any of the three zones. In zone A, which had the highest exposures, no uterine cancer deaths are reported; 1 ovarian cancer death occurred where 0.4 was expected (RR = 2.3, 0.3–16.5). In zone B, with the second-highest exposures, the numbers of deaths from uterine and ovarian cancers were both less than expected. In zone R, where exposures were lower, but still above those not exposed to the accident, there were 27 uterine cancer deaths, with 23.7 expected, for a relative risk of 1.1 (0.8–1.7) and 21 ovarian cancer deaths, with 20.7 expected (RR = 1.0, 0.6–1.6).

The latest follow-up on cancer incidence in Seveso, which includes diagnoses made between 1976 and 1996 (20-year follow-up), shows 1 case of ovarian cancer in zone A and 2 in zone B (Bertazzi et al., 2001). When combined, these three represent a relative risk of 0.7 (0.2–2.0). An earlier paper (Pesatori et al., 1993) had shown 2 cases among young women (<19 years of age) during the period 1977–1986, where 0.0 were expected, both from zone R. The latest update also indicates 2 cases of uterine cancer in zone B, where 3.8 were expected, for a relative risk of 0.5 (0.1–2.1).

A case-control study of endometrial cancer was conducted in Sweden (Weiderpass et al., 2000). There were 154 cases and 205 eligible controls frequency-matched on age; women who had had a hysterectomy or had ever taken hormone replacement therapy were excluded. The authors measured 10 organochlorine pesticides and 10 PCB congeners. TCDD was not measured, although it can be assumed to have been present as a contaminant. Statistical analyses were conducted for individual compounds and for groups based on estrogenic or anti-androgenic activity. Cases had higher mean concentrations of p,p'-DDT, p,p'-DDE (dichlorodiphenyldichloroethylene), hexachlorobenzene, and β-HCH (hexachlorocyclohexane). However, after adjustment for age and body mass index, no pesticides were associated with endometrial cancer case status.

The biologic plausibility that TCDD may interact with endometrial tissue was investigated by Kuchenhoff et al. (1999). Endometrial tissue was collected from 86 premenopausal women, and expression of the aryl hydrocarbon receptor (AhR) mRNA and protein were measured. In 43 percent of the women, the endometria showed AhR expression; receptor protein was exclusively in the apical part of the cytoplasm of epithelial cells in the endometrial glands. AhR mRNA was expressed in the cytoplasm of endometrial epithelial cells. AhR expression was maximal at the time of ovulation.

Vietnam Veterans Studies

A study of female Vietnam veterans from Australia used a mail survey to obtain information on health conditions, reproductive histories, and conditions of their children (CDVA, 1998b). Out of 484 veterans, only 278 were successfully traced, and 223 responded. Tracing is more difficult for women who marry and change their name. As a result, the respondents were far less likely to be married, and they reported only half as many children as a comparable community group. There appeared to be an excess of all cancers combined. There were 4 cases of uterine cancer (1 expected) and 8 cases of cervical cancer (1 expected). One case of ovarian cancer (zero expected) and no cases of vaginal cancer (zero expected) were observed. The numbers are small, and since the authors did not stratify or adjust for marital status, these comparisons may be confounded. Because the health status of unmarried adults is generally worse than that of married adults of the same age, results may be biased toward

CANCER   323

greater differences between the veterans and the comparison group. Stratification or adjustment in multivariate models for marital status could be used to eliminate this confounding bias. Nevertheless, the findings can be viewed as indicating a possibility that service in Vietnam may have an association with some reproductive cancers in females.

Synthesis

The epidemiologic studies regarding female reproductive tract cancers are summarized in Tables 7-18, 7-19, and 7-20. The evidence from these studies remains inconclusive, in spite of some strong associations with ovarian and uterine cancers, largely because most of the published studies include a small number of cases and/or have poor exposure characterization or too short a follow-up period. The committee concludes that more research is needed on populations of women with documented exposure to herbicides and TCDD.

Conclusions

Strength of Evidence in Epidemiologic Studies

There is no information contained in the research reviewed for this report to change the conclusion that there is inadequate or insufficient evidence to determine whether an association exists between exposure to herbicides (2,4-D, 2,4,5-T and its contaminant TCDD, cacodylic acid, and picloram) and uterine, ovarian, or cervical cancers. The evidence regarding association is drawn from occupational and environmental studies in which subjects were exposed to a variety of herbicides and herbicide components and from a study of Australian female Vietnam veterans.

Biologic Plausibility

No animal studies have found an increased incidence of female reproductive cancer; however, recent work has demonstrated that TCDD interacts with the AhR in endometrial tissue. A summary of the biologic plausibility for the carcinogenicity of TCDD and the herbicides in general is presented in the conclusion to this chapter. A discussion of toxicological studies that concern biologic plausibility is contained in Chapter 3.

Increased Risk of Disease Among Vietnam Veterans

The limited data on increased risk for female reproductive cancers in Vietnam veterans come from an Australian study. Although the proportion of women with uterine and cervical cancers was higher than expected, the small number of cases and the possibility of confounding from marital status preclude drawing definitive conclusions. An ongoing study in female U.S. veterans of the Vietnam era may shed further light on this issue.

TABLE 7-18 Selected Epidemiologic Studies—Cancers of the Cervix

Reference	Study Population	Exposed Cases[a]	Estimated Risk (95% CI)[a]
OCCUPATIONAL			
Studies Reviewed in *Update 1998*			
Kogevinas et al., 1997	IARC cohort	0	—
Studies Reviewed in *Update 1996*			
Blair et al., 1993	U.S. farmers in 23 states		
	Whites	6	0.9 (0.3–2.0)
	Nonwhites	21	2.0 (0.3–3.1)
Studies Reviewed in *VAO*			
Ronco et al., 1992	Danish farmers		
	Self-employed farmers	7	0.5
	Family workers	100	0.5
	Employees	12	0.8
Wiklund, 1983	Swedish agricultural workers	82	0.6
VIETNAM VETERANS			
New Studies			
CDVA, 1998b	Australian Vietnam veterans—female	8[b]	1 expected (0–5)

[a] Given when available.
[b] Self-reported medical history. Answer to question: Since your first day of service in Vietnam, have you been told by a doctor that you have cancer of the cervix?

TABLE 7-19 Selected Epidemiologic Studies—Cancers of the Uterus

Reference	Study Population	Exposed Cases[a]	Estimated Risk (95% CI)[a]
OCCUPATIONAL			
Studies Reviewed in *Update 1998*			
Kogevinas et al., 1997	IARC cohort (includes cancers of the endometrium)	3	3.4 (0.7–10.0)
Studies Reviewed in *VAO*			
Blair et al., 1993	U.S. farmers in 23 states		
	Whites	15	1.2

TABLE 7-19 *Continued*

Reference	Study Population	Exposed Cases[a]	Estimated Risk (95% CI)[a]
	Nonwhites	17	1.4
Ronco et al., 1992	Danish farmers		
	Self-employed farmers	8	0.6
	Family workers	103	0.8
	Employees	9	0.9
Wiklund, 1983	Swedish agricultural workers	135	0.9
ENVIRONMENTAL			
New Studies			
Bertazzi et al., 2001	Seveso residents—20-year follow-up		
	Zone B females	2	0.5 (0.1–2.1)
Weiderpass et al., 2000	Swedish females	154	1.0 (0.6–2.0)
Bertazzi et al., 1998	Seveso residents—15-year follow-up		
	Zone B females	1	0.3 (0.0–2.4)
Studies Reviewed in *Update 1998*			
Bertazzi et al., 1997	Seveso residents—15-year follow-up		
	Zone B females	1	0.3 (0.0–1.9)
	Zone R females	27	1.1 (0.8–1.7)
VIETNAM VETERANS			
New Studies			
CDVA, 1998b	Australian Vietnam veterans—female	4[b]	1 expected (0–5)
Studies Reviewed in *Update 1996*			
Dalager et al., 1995	Women Vietnam veterans	4	2.1 (0.6–5.4)

[a] Given when available.
[b] Self-reported medical history. Answer to question: Since your first day of service in Vietnam, have you been told by a doctor that you have uterine cancer?

TABLE 7-20 Selected Epidemiologic Studies—Ovarian Cancer

Reference	Study Population	Exposed Cases[a]	Estimated Risk (95% CI)[a]
OCCUPATIONAL			
Studies Reviewed in *Update 1998*			
Kogevinas et al., 1997	IARC cohort	0	—
Studies Reviewed in *Update 1996*			
Kogevinas et al., 1993	IARC cohort	1	0.7
Lynge, 1993	Danish female production workers	7	3.2
Studies Reviewed in *VAO*			
Ronco et al., 1992	Danish farmers		
	Self-employed farmers	12	0.9
	Family workers	104	0.8
	Employees	5	0.5
Donna et al., 1984	Female residents near Alessandria, Italy	18	4.4 (1.9–16.1)

TABLE 7-20 *Continued*

Reference	Study Population	Exposed Cases[a]	Estimated Risk (95% CI)[a]
ENVIRONMENTAL			
New Studies			
Bertazzi et al., 2001	Seveso residents—20-year follow-up		
	Zone A females	1	1.6 (0.2–11.2)
	Zone B females	2	0.5 (0.1–2.0)
Bertazzi et al., 1998	Seveso residents—15-year follow-up		
	Zone A females	1	2.3 (0.3–16.5)
Studies Reviewed in *Update 1998*			
Bertazzi et al., 1997	Seveso residents—15-year follow-up		
	Zone A females	1	2.3 (0.0–12.8)
	Zone R females	21	1.0 (0.6–1.6)
VIETNAM VETERANS			
New Studies			
CDVA, 1998b	Australian Vietnam veterans—female	1[b]	0 expected (0–4)

[a] Given when available.
[b] Self-reported medical history. Answer to question: Since your first day of service in Vietnam, have you been told by a doctor that you have ovarian cancer?

PROSTATE CANCER

Background

According to American Cancer Society estimates, 180,400 new cases of prostate cancer (ICD·9 185) will be diagnosed in the United States in 2000, and 31,900 men will die from the disease (ACS, 2000a). This makes prostate cancer the most common cancer among men, excluding nonmelanocytic skin cancers. Among men it is expected to account for approximately 29 percent of new diagnoses and 11 percent of cancer deaths in 2000.

Prostate cancer incidence varies dramatically as a function of age and race. The risk increases fivefold between 45–49 and 50–54 years of age, and nearly triples between 50–54 and 55–59 years of age. As a group, African-American men have the highest recorded incidence of prostate cancer in the world (Miller et al., 1996). Their risk is roughly twice that of whites in the United States, 4 times higher than Alaskan natives, and nearly 7.5 times higher than Korean Americans.

Little is known about the causes of prostate cancer. Other than race and age, risk factors include a family history of the disease and a diet high in fats.

Average Annual Cancer Incidence (per 100,000 individuals) in the United States[a]
Prostate Cancer

45–49 Years of Age			50–54 Years of Age			55–59 Years of Age		
All Races	White	Black	All Races	White	Black	All Races	White	Black
26.6	23.8	61.2	111.4	104.4	224.6	284.4	273.0	522.0

[a] SEER nine standard registries, crude age-specific rate, 1993–1997.

Summary of *VAO, Update 1996,* and *Update 1998*

The committee responsible for *VAO* found there to be limited or suggestive evidence to determine whether an association existed between exposure to herbicides used in Vietnam or the contaminant dioxin and prostate cancer. Additional information available to the committees responsible for *Update 1996* and *Update 1998* did not change this finding. Table 7-21 provides summaries of the results of the studies underlying these findings and a list of reports that contain details of the research.

Update of the Scientific Literature

Since *Update 1998*, a few new published papers have reported data on prostate cancer mortality or incidence in populations with possible or documented exposures to TCDD. Several of these involved occupational exposures (Dich and Wiklund, 1998; Fleming et al., 1999a,b; Steenland et al., 1999; Sharma-Wagner et al., 2000), two reports concern the Seveso cohort (Bertazzi et al., 1998, 2001), and data are reported from the Ranch Hand study (AFHS, 2000) and the Australian Vietnam veterans Validation Study (AIHW, 1999).

Occupational Studies

Three occupational studies provide data on mortality from prostate cancer. In the NIOSH study of 5,132 production workers with known exposure to 2,3,7,8-TCDD, Steenland et al. (1999) examined mortality from prostate cancer. A total of 28 such deaths were observed, yielding an SMR of 1.2 (0.8–1.7). No further analyses by dose or using internal comparisons were reported for this outcome.

A study of cancer mortality in pesticide appliers was conducted in Florida. Fleming et al. (1999a) followed 33,658 appliers age 20 or more, licensed by the Florida Department of Agriculture and Consumer Services between January 1, 1975, and December 31, 1993. Ninety percent were male ($N = 30,155$), and the total number of person-years of follow-up was 290,791 (an average of just less than 10 years per person). The mean age at first license, among men, was 39.5 (standard deviation [SD] = 13.3), and the mean years licensed was 7.1 (SD = 4.4). There were 64 deaths from prostate cancer, for an SMR of 2.4 (1.8–3.0). The authors state that there was a decreasing trend with later years of license (data not shown). There is reference to, but no documentation of, similar findings for incidence. The authors also note a current theory that postulates vitamin D exposure to be protective for prostate cancer; if true, those working outdoors might be at lower risk than the general population, which spends a considerable portion of time indoors, even in Florida.

A second study focused on pesticide appliers, but examined prostate cancer incidence. Dich and Wiklund (1998) carried out a cohort study for incident cases of prostate cancer among 20,025 pesticide appliers in agriculture, licensed between 1965 (when licensing was begun) and 1976 in Sweden. The most commonly used pesticides were phenoxyacetic acid herbicides, organochlorine compounds, mercury, and organophosphorous compounds. Cases were identified through the Swedish Cancer Registry. The follow-up period was through December 31, 1991, and the mean follow-up for this cohort was 21.3 years. In this cohort, there were 401 cases compared with 355 expected, for a standardized incidence ratio of 1.1 (1.0–1.2). Among those born later than 1935, the SIR was 2.0 (0.8–4.2), while for those born earlier, it was 1.1 (1.0–1.2). The authors noted that besides pesticides, the environment of farmers and pesticide appliers includes other potential carcinogens, such as exhaust fumes, solvents, fuel oils, and exposure to animals and consequently zoonotic viruses. The authors speculate about cadmium and cadmium compounds, which are present in pesticides and also occur as impurities in fertilizers; however, it should be noted that an early finding of an excess of prostate cancer among workers exposed to cadmium (Lemen et al., 1976) was not confirmed in the numerous later studies conducted with improved exposure assessment (e.g., Armstrong and Kazantzis, 1983; Sorahan and Waterhouse, 1983). The small excess incidence of prostate cancer in pesticide appliers found by Dich and Wiklund is particularly interesting given an earlier follow-up of this same cohort to 1982 (Wiklund et al., 1989a), which found no increased risk: the SIR was 1.0 (0.8–1.2). In other words, all of the excess occurred in the last 9 or 10 years of follow-up.

In an exploratory study, Sharma-Wagner et al. (2000) linked the National Swedish Cancer Registry to the 1960 National Census using the 10-digit personal ID codes assigned to every Swedish citizen to examine prostate cancer incidence rates by industry and occupation. The authors included cases diagnosed from 1961 through 1979 and derived the expected numbers of cases from national rates for 5-year birth cohorts. Slightly elevated SIRs were found for farmers, fishermen, and hunters, who had an SIR of 1.0 (1.0–1.1), while employment in agriculture had an SIR of 1.1 (1.0–1.1). Slight excesses were again seen when these broad groups were divided into specific categories: the SIR for actual agriculture and stock raising was 1.1; similarly, farmers, foresters, and gardeners showed a 10 percent excess. This study lacked data on smoking or duration of employment and had no exposure information for the specific industries or occupations examined. Also, prostate cancer incidence was reduced among paper mill workers (SIR = 0.9, 0.8–1.0), but elevated for pulp grinding (SIR = 1.4, 1.0–1.9). The magnitude of dioxin exposures in these occupations or industries is unknown.

Environmental Studies

The Seveso cohort had been followed through 1991, and its mortality compared with people living in the surrounding areas of Lombardy (Bertazzi et al., 1998). In this 15-year period, among males, there were no cases in 5,541 person-years for the small group having the highest exposure (i.e., those in zone A), with 0.7 expected; 6 observed in 42,219 person-years for those in the medium-exposure zone B, with 4.8 expected for a relative risk of 1.2 (0.6–2.8); and 39 observed during 265,408 person-years for those in the low-exposure zone R, with 33 expected for an RR of 1.2 (0.8–1.7).

A further follow-up of the Seveso cohort evaluated the latency between the chemical accident that led to widespread TCDD exposure and the occurrence of various cancers from 1976 to 1996. In these 20 years of follow-up, 8 cases of prostate cancer occurred in zone B, with 3 of these in the first 4 years after exposure. Although the RR in the first 4 years is 2.2, the 95% CI is quite wide (0.7–7.1) (Bertazzi et al., 2001).

Vietnam Veterans Studies

Two studies of men who served in Vietnam examined prostate cancer incidence. The Air Force Health Study 1997 follow-up of Ranch Hand personnel did not reveal any excess of prostate cancer cases (AFHS, 2000). Ranch Hand personnel did not have higher risks than the comparison cohort, nor was the risk of prostate cancer seen to rise with increasing blood dioxin levels. Analyses of PSA (prostate-specific antigen), a biological marker of increased risk for prostate cancer, were also reported for this cohort. Most of the analyses showed no significant differences. The only analysis that showed a significant finding was one in which higher initial dioxin levels were associated with a lower prevalence of abnormally high PSA levels (AFHS, 2000).

In contrast, Australia's Vietnam veterans did show an excess risk of prostate cancer compared to the number expected based on an Australian community standard: 212 observed versus 147 expected cases (AIHW, 1999).

Synthesis

As with previous updates, the new data are not entirely consistent, and studies focusing on mortality may have insufficient power or suffer from biases related to health care access and utilization. Among the three mortality studies, the two cohorts showing nonsignificant excesses of prostate cancer of about 20 percent (Bertazzi et al., 1998; Steenland et al., 1999) had the highest-quality exposure information; however, when observed associations are this weak, biases could have induced artifactually elevated risks. It is unclear what these biases may be in such varied populations involving quite different types of exposure scenarios. Generally, in studies using mortality as an outcome, detection bias is unlikely to explain any elevated risks.

On the other hand, factors that increase incidence might not be the same as those related to subsequent mortality among those with the disease. The recent introduction and widespread adoption of PSA for screening purposes has led to increased incidence rates in the United States; the long-term impact of screening on incidence or mortality rates is difficult to predict for any country or population and will depend on the rapidity with which the screening tool is adopted, its differential use across various ages of men, and the aggressiveness of tumors detected early by this test (Gann, 1997). Differences among countries in the rate of use of PSA could produce more variable, less consistent results in studies of exogenous exposures and prostate cancer.

Since prostate cancer tends not to be fatal in the overwhelming majority of cases, studies of mortality may be unable to detect an increased incidence of this disease. For this reason, a positive finding in a mortality study should be examined closely to determine whether the exposed group might have had poorer access to treatments that would decrease the likelihood of death. For example, is it possible that pesticide appliers in Florida would have had less access to medical care than their counterparts of the same ages in the general population? The finding of an excess of prostate cancer incidence would tend to weigh against this explanation, but further details on the incidence data are not available.

Similarly, weak findings in mortality studies should be viewed skeptically since these studies provide little information about the incidence of the disease. One might consider whether the exposed population had better access to care, hence reducing its risk of mortality. Is it possible that in Seveso, for example, those in the exposed zones receive more close surveillance or more aggressive medical care than those in the unexposed region? Similarly, although we do not have information on TCDD production workers, those with employment in manufacturing are more likely to have health insurance than the general U.S. population, potentially reducing the likelihood of death from an incident case of prostate cancer. The true association would then be stronger than that observed.

The excess prostate cancer incidence in the study from Sweden, the strong association in the study of Florida's pesticide appliers, and the reference of Fleming et al. (1999b) to positive findings for incidence in the Florida cohort are all suggestive of a positive association, but unfortunately, the exposure in these cohorts is not well defined. Therefore, these studies provide some evidence that pesticide application is a risk factor for prostate cancer; they do not provide direct evidence that 2,3,7,8-TCDD or the herbicides used in Vietnam are carcinogenic to the prostate. The clear excess observed in Australia's Vietnam veterans supports an association between prostate cancer and exposures incurred in Vietnam, under the assumption that the veterans are not receiving better health surveillance than the general population of the same age in that country. In contrast, the null findings among Ranch Hand personnel run counter to this conclusion. Since the Ranch Hand and comparison cohorts receive similar surveillance within the AFHS, diagnostic issues would not be expected to bias the results.

The plausibility of a causal relationship could be argued on the basis that this organ is hormonally responsive, and TCDD has been shown to be an endocrine disrupter (i.e., a chemical that alters the production or metabolism of hormones). Data concerning the effect of TCDD on hormone levels in occupationally exposed men are therefore relevant. Sweeney et al. (1997/98) examined 281 workers at two production facilities from the NIOSH study and found a trend toward elevated serum levels of follicle-stimulating hormone and luteinizing hormone (LH), and a trend for lower testosterone levels, according to the serum concentration of lipid-adjusted TCDD. These findings were from models adjusted for age, alcohol, smoking, and diabetes mellitus, and the models for LH and testosterone were also adjusted for body mass index. They suggest that exposures of workers, particularly to greater than 20 pg/g, are associated with alterations in male reproductive hormone concentrations. The prostate may be a target organ for hormonally active xenobiotics, lending biologic plausibility to an association with TCDD exposure.

Prostate cancer is a very common condition in older men. For this reason, it is likely that there are multiple factors responsible for its development. Still, even a small relative risk can mean a large number of cases. Thus, if the observed 13 percent increased incidence among Swedish pesticide appliers was due solely to exposure to dioxin, it could translate into a large number of cases. Generally speaking, for common conditions such as prostate cancer and cardiovascular disease, relative risks are not expected to be high for any particular causative factor since the background rates are already high. This situation is in contrast to that for rare diseases, where one tends to observe higher RRs.

Although the data are generally mixed, it should also be kept in mind that most Vietnam veterans have not yet reached the age at which this cancer tends to appear and that morbidity is likely to represent a more sensitive outcome than mortality for this site of cancer. Further follow-up of the Ranch Hand cohort will be particularly valuable for the assessment of this outcome.

Conclusions

Strength of Evidence in Epidemiologic Studies

There is limited/suggestive evidence of an association between exposure to herbicides (2,4-D, 2,4,5-T and its contaminant TCDD, cacodylic acid, and picloram) and prostate cancer. Although the associations are not large, there are a number of studies providing evidence suggestive of a small increase in either morbidity or mortality from prostate cancer. The evidence regarding association is drawn from occupational studies in which subjects were exposed to a variety of pesticides, herbicides, and herbicide components and is also based on data from studies of Vietnam veterans. A major consideration is the fact that prostate cancer tends not to be fatal; thus, mortality studies have lower statistical power to detect a comparable effect than a similar-sized morbidity (incidence) study would have. In incidence and mortality studies, comparisons of exposed and unexposed populations may be biased by differences in health care seeking behavior, access to care, and quality of care received. The high incidence of this disease in older men suggests that multiple factors are responsible for its occurrence and therefore that relative risks will not be expected to be high, even if the absolute numbers of cases are substantial.

Biologic Plausibility

No animal studies have found an increased incidence of prostate cancer. A summary of the biologic plausibility for the carcinogenicity of TCDD and the herbicides in general is presented in the conclusion to this chapter. A discussion of toxicological studies that concern biologic plausibility is contained in Chapter 3.

Increased Risk of Disease Among Vietnam Veterans

Studies that have been conducted in Vietnam veterans have had a low likelihood of detecting an increased risk of prostate cancer, if service in Vietnam is actually associated with this cancer, because of weak study design and the relatively young age of Vietnam veterans. Continued follow-up of the Ranch Hand cohort for both biologic monitoring of PSA levels and verification of prostate cancer incidence will be important for determining prostate cancer risk. The statistically significant elevated prostate cancer SMRs for Australian male Vietnam veterans is suggestive that U.S. Vietnam veterans may be at increased risk. Further follow-up that includes, in particular, studies of morbidity among living veterans would help to define the risk.

TABLE 7-21 Selected Epidemiologic Studies—Prostate Cancer

Reference	Study Population	Exposed Cases[a]	Estimated Risk (95% CI)[a]
OCCUPATIONAL			
New Studies			
Sharma-Wagner et al., 2000	Swedish citizens		
	Agriculture and stock raising	6,080	1.1
	Farmers, foresters, and gardeners	5,219	1.1
	Paper mill workers	304	0.9 (0.8–1.0)
	Pulp grinding	39	1.4 (1.0–1.9)
Fleming et al., 1999a	Florida pesticide appliers	353	1.9 (1.7–2.1)
Fleming et al., 1999b	Florida pesticide appliers	64	2.4 (1.8–3.0)
Steenland et al., 1999	NIOSH cohort	28	1.2 (0.8–1.7)
Dich and Wiklund, 1998	Swedish pesticide appliers	401	1.1 (1.0–1.2)
	Born 1935 or later	7	2.0 (0.8–4.2)
	Born before 1935	394	1.1 (1.0–1.2)
Studies Reviewed in *Update 1998*			
Gambini et al., 1997	Italian rice growers	19	1.0 (0.6–1.5)
Hertzman et al., 1997	Canadian sawmill workers		
	Mortality	282	1.0 (0.9–1.1)
	Morbidity for male genital tract cancers	116	1.2 (1.0–1.4)
Kogevinas et al., 1997	IARC cohort	43	1.1 (0.8–1.5)
Becher et al., 1996	German chemical production workers	9	1.3
Ott and Zober, 1996	BASF cleanup workers	4	1.1 (0.3–2.8)
Zhong and Rafnsson, 1996	Icelandic pesticide users	10	0.7 (0.3–1.2)
Studies Reviewed in *Update 1996*			
Asp et al., 1994	Finnish herbicide appliers	5	0.8 (0.3–1.8)
Blair et al., 1993	U.S. farmers in 23 states		
	Whites	3,765	1.2 (1.1–1.2)
	Nonwhites	564	1.1 (1.1–1.2)
Bueno de Mesquita et al., 1993	Dutch production workers	3	2.6 (0.5–7.7)
Collins et al., 1993	Monsanto 2,4-D production workers	9	1.6 (0.7–3.0)
Studies Reviewed in *VAO*			
Morrison et al., 1993	Canadian farmers, age 45–69 years, no employees, or custom workers, sprayed ≥250 acres	20	2.2 (1.3–3.8)
Ronco et al., 1992	Danish self-employed farm workers	399	0.9 ($p < .05$)
Swaen et al., 1992	Dutch herbicide appliers	1	1.3 (0.0–7.3)
Fingerhut et al., 1991	NIOSH cohort	17	1.2 (0.7–2.0)
	20-year latency, 1-year exposure	9	1.5 (0.7–2.9)
Manz et al., 1991	German production workers	7	1.4 (0.6–2.9)
Saracci et al., 1991	IARC cohort	30	1.1 (0.8–1.6)
Zober et al., 1990	BASF production workers	0	— (0.0–7.5)
Alavanja et al., 1989	USDA forest conservationists		1.6 (0.9–3.0)
	Soil conservationists		1.0 (0.6–1.8)
Henneberger et al., 1989	Paper and pulp workers	9	1.0 (0.7–2.0)
Solet et al., 1989	Paper and pulp workers	4	1.1 (0.3–2.9)

TABLE 7-21 *Continued*

Reference	Study Population	Exposed Cases[a]	Estimated Risk (95% CI)[a]
Alavanja et al., 1988	USDA agricultural extension agents		1.0 (0.7–1.5)
Bond et al., 1988	Dow 2,4-D production workers	1	1.0 (0.0–5.8)
Coggon et al., 1986	British MCPA production workers	18	1.3 (0.8–2.1)
Robinson et al., 1986	Paper and pulp workers	17	1.2 (0.7–2.0)
Lynge, 1985	Danish production workers	9	0.8
Blair et al., 1983	Florida pesticide appliers	2	0.5
Burmeister et al., 1983	Iowa residents		1.2 ($p < .05$)
Wiklund, 1983	Swedish agricultural workers	3,890	1.0 (0.9–1.0)[b]
Burmeister, 1981	Iowa farmers	1,138	1.1 ($p < .01$)
ENVIRONMENTAL			
New Studies			
Bertazzi et al., 2001	Seveso residents—20-year follow-up		
	Zone B males	8	1.2 (0.6–2.4)
Bertazzi et al., 1998	Seveso residents—15-year follow-up		
	Zone B males	6	1.2 (0.6–2.8)
Studies Reviewed in *Update 1998*			
Bertazzi et al., 1997	Seveso residents—15-year follow-up		
	Zone B males	6	1.2 (0.5–2.7)
	Zone R males	39	1.2 (0.8–1.6)
Svensson et al., 1995	Swedish fishermen, mortality	12	1.0 (0.5–1.8)
	Swedish fishermen, incidence	38	1.1 (0.8–1.5)
Studies Reviewed in *Update 1996*			
Bertazzi et al., 1993	Seveso residents—10-year follow-up, morbidity		
	Zone R males	16	0.9 (0.5–1.5)
Studies Reviewed in *VAO*			
Pesatori et al., 1992	Seveso residents		
	Zones A, B males	4	1.4 (0.5–3.9)
Bertazzi et al., 1989a	Seveso residents—10-year follow-up		
	Zones A, B, R males	19	1.6 (1.0–2.7)
Bertazzi et al., 1989b	Seveso residents—10-year follow-up		
	Zone B males	3	2.2 (0.7–6.9)
VIETNAM VETERANS			
New Studies			
AFHS, 2000	Air Force Ranch Hand veterans	26	0.7 (0.4–1.3)
AIHW, 1999	Australian Vietnam veterans—male	212	147 expected (123–171)
CDVA, 1998a	Australian Vietnam veterans—male	428[c]	147 expected (123–171)
Studies Reviewed in *Update 1998*			
Clapp, 1997	Massachusetts Vietnam veterans		
	Exposed cancers	15	0.8 (0.4–1.6)

TABLE 7-21 *Continued*

Reference	Study Population	Exposed Cases[a]	Estimated Risk (95% CI)[a]
Crane et al., 1997a	Australian military Vietnam veterans	36	1.5 (1.1–2.1)
	Army	26	1.6 (1.1–2.4)
	Navy	8	2.2 (0.9–4.3)
	Air Force	2	0.5 (0.1–1.9)
AFHS, 1996	Air Force Ranch Hand veterans	2	4.0
Watanabe and Kang, 1996	Army Vietnam veterans	58	0.9
	16+ years after discharge		1.1
Studies Reviewed in *Update 1996*			
Visintainer et al., 1995	Michigan Vietnam veterans	19	1.1 (0.6–1.7)
Studies Reviewed in *VAO*			
Breslin et al., 1988	Army Vietnam veterans	30	0.9 (0.6–1.2)
	Marine Vietnam veterans	5	1.3 (0.2–10.3)
Anderson et al., 1986b	Wisconsin Vietnam veterans	2	—

NOTE: MCPA = methyl-4-chlorophenoxyacetic acid; USDA = United States Department of Agriculture.

[a] Given when available.
[b] 99% CI.
[c] Self-reported medical history. Answer to question: Since your first day of service in Vietnam, have you been told by a doctor that you have prostate cancer?

TESTICULAR CANCER

Background

The American Cancer Society estimates that 6,900 men will be diagnosed with testicular cancer (ICD·9 186.0–186.9) in the United States in 2000 and that 300 will die from the disease (ACS, 2000a).

Testicular cancer is far more likely in men younger than 40 than in those who are older. On a lifetime basis, the risk for white men is about four times greater than for African Americans. Cryptorchidism, or undescended testicles, is a major risk factor for testicular cancer. Family history of the disease also appears to play a role. Several other hereditary and environmental factors have been suggested, but research regarding them is inconsistent (Bosl and Motzer, 1997).

Average Annual Cancer Incidence (per 100,000 individuals) in the United States[a]
Testicular Cancer

45–49 Years of Age			50–54 Years of Age			55–59 Years of Age		
All Races	White	Black	All Races	White	Black	All Races	White	Black
5.6	6.3	1.3	3.6	4.1	0.4	2.1	2.3	1.0

[a] SEER nine standard registries, crude age-specific rate, 1993–1997.

Summary of *VAO, Update 1996,* and *Update 1998*

The committee responsible for *VAO* found that there was inadequate or insufficient information to determine whether an association existed between exposure to herbicides used in Vietnam or the contaminant dioxin and testicular cancer. Additional information available to the committees responsible for *Update 1996* and *Update 1998* did not change this finding. Table 7-22 provides summaries of the results of the studies underlying these findings and a list of reports that contain details of the research.

Update of the Scientific Literature

Occupational Studies

A case-control study of occupational risk factors for testicular cancer was conducted by Hardell et al. (1998). The researchers identified cases between 30 and 75 years of age from the Swedish Cancer Registry over the period 1989–1992. Controls were age matched, with two identified for each case. There were 4 cases of testicular cancer among cases with self-reported occupational exposure to herbicides and 24 cases among controls, leading to an OR of 0.3 (0.1–1.0).

Fleming et al. (1999b) examined cancer incidence over the years 1975–1993 in a cohort of licensed pesticide appliers in Florida. Phenoxy herbicides were among the exposures for this cohort. Age-matched incidence data for the Florida general population were used for comparison. The researchers found a statistically significant elevation in testicular cancer (SIR = 2.5, 1.6–3.7; based on 23 cases) in the pesticide appliers.

Environmental Studies

The 15-year follow-up of people environmentally exposed to TCDD in a 1976 industrial accident in Seveso, Italy (Bertazzi et al., 1998), did not report testicular cancer separately, but instead subsumed it into a category called "genitourinary cancers" (ICD·9 179–189). No deaths among males were recorded in this category in zone A, the high-exposure area. In zone B, the medium-exposure area, 10 deaths were observed where 10.5 were expected (RR = 1.0, 0.5–1.8); in the low-exposure zone, R, 73 deaths were observed where 72.3 were expected (1.0, 0.8–1.3). A later study (Bertazzi et al., 2001) extending the mortality analysis to 20 years following the event reported 1 genitourinary cancer death in zone A (0.5, 0.1–3.7) and 16 in zone B (1.1, 0.7–1.8).

Vietnam Veteran Studies

The 15-year update of the Ranch Hand study (AFHS, 2000) reported 3 cases of testicular neoplasms: 1 in the low initial dioxin category and 2 in the medium.

No cases were found among the comparison population. The small number of cases did not permit meaningful statistical analysis of this outcome.

The government of Australia conducted mail surveys of 49,944 male veterans (80 percent response rate) who served in Vietnam, including those involved in combat, medical teams, war correspondents, entertainers, and philanthropy workers (CDVA, 1998a). The self-report data that were gathered were compared with age-matched Australian national data. Of the veterans, 151 indicated that they been told by a doctor that they had cancer of the testis since their first day of service in Vietnam. This was significantly in excess of the expected number of cases, 110 (expected range = 89–131). However, it was noted that there was a potential for benign tumors of the testis, scrotum, and epididymis to have been misreported as testicular cancer. A follow-up to this study was conducted to medically confirm selected conditions reported in the survey (AIHW, 1999). Sources used to validate reported conditions included clinicians, several Australian morbidity and mortality data bases, DVA data, and documentation provided by the veterans. Based on these data, the authors estimated that there were 59 validated cases of cancer of the testis among respondents, fewer than the expected number.

Synthesis

The relatively low incidence of testicular cancer reported in the studies reviewed by the committee complicates their evaluation. Among the studies reviewed in this report, only Fleming et al. (1999b) reported a statistically significant difference between the observed and expected number of cases. However, the pesticide appliers studied by these researchers were likely exposed to a wide variety of chemicals, making it difficult to ascribe any effect to a particular compound. Studies with either large numbers of cases or known TCDD exposures do not show an increased risk among males exposed to the herbicides used in Vietnam or dioxin.

Conclusions

Strength of Evidence in Epidemiologic Studies

There is no information contained in the research reviewed for this report to change the conclusion that there is inadequate or insufficient evidence to determine whether an association exists between exposure to herbicides (2,4-D, 2,4,5-T and its contaminant TCDD, cacodylic acid, and picloram) and testicular cancer.

Biologic Plausibility

No animal studies have found an increased incidence of testicular cancer. A summary of the biologic plausibility for the carcinogenicity of TCDD and the herbicides in general is presented in the conclusion to this chapter. A discussion of toxicological studies that concern biologic plausibility is contained in Chapter 3.

Increased Risk of Disease Among Vietnam Veterans

There are insufficient data on testicular cancer in Vietnam veterans to draw a specific conclusion as to whether or not they are at increased risk.

TABLE 7-22 Selected Epidemiologic Studies—Testicular Cancer

Reference	Study Population	Exposed Cases[a]	Estimated Risk (95% CI)[a]
OCCUPATIONAL			
New Studies			
Fleming et al., 1999	Florida pesticide appliers	23	2.5 (1.6–3.7)
Hardell et al., 1998	Workers exposed to herbicides	4	0.3 (0.1–1.0)
Studies Reviewed in *Update 1998*			
Hertzman et al., 1997	British Columbia sawmill workers		
	Mortality	116[b]	1.0 (0.8–1.1)
	Incidence	18	1.0 (0.6–1.4)
Kogevinas et al., 1997	IARC cohort	7	1.3 (0.5–2.7)
Ramlow et al., 1996	Pentachlorophenol production workers	0	—
Studies Reviewed in *Update 1996*			
Blair et al., 1993	U.S. farmers in 23 states		
	White males	32	0.8 (0.6–1.2)
	Nonwhite males	6	1.3 (0.5–2.9)
Studies Reviewed in *VAO*			
Ronco et al., 1992	Danish self-employed farm workers	74	0.9
Saracci et al., 1991	IARC cohort	7	2.3 (0.9–4.6)
Bond et al., 1988	Dow 2,4-D production workers	1	4.6 (0.0–25.7)
Coggon et al., 1986	British MCPA production workers	4	2.2 (0.6–5.7)
Wiklund, 1983	Swedish agricultural workers	101	1.0 (0.7–1.2)[c]
ENVIRONMENTAL			
New Studies			
Bertazzi et al., 2001	Seveso residents—20-year follow-up		
	Zone A males	1	0.5 (0.1–3.7)
	Zone B males	16	1.1 (0.7–1.8)
Bertazzi et al., 1998	Seveso residents—15-year follow-up		
	Zone B males	10	1.0 (0.5–1.8)
	Zone R males	73	1.0 (0.8–1.3)
Studies Reviewed in *Update 1998*			
Zhong and Rafnsson, 1996			
	Icelandic pesticide users	2	1.2 (0.1–4.3)
Studies Reviewed in *Update 1996*			
Bertazzi et al., 1993	Seveso residents—10-year follow-up, morbidity		
	Zone B males	1	1.0 (0.1–7.5)
	Zone R males	9	1.4 (0.7–3.0)
Studies Reviewed in *VAO*			
Pesatori et al., 1992	Seveso residents		
	Zones A, B males	1	0.9 (0.1–6.7)
	Zone R males	9	1.5 (0.7–3.0)

TABLE 7-22 Continued

Reference	Study Population	Exposed Cases[a]	Estimated Risk (95% CI)[a]
VIETNAM VETERANS			
New Studies			
AFHS, 2000	Air Force Ranch Hand veterans	3	—
AIHW, 1999	Australian Vietnam veterans—male	59	110 expected (89–131)
CDVA, 1998a	Australian Vietnam veterans—male	151[d]	110 expected (89–131)
Studies Reviewed in *Update 1998*			
Clapp, 1997	Massachusetts Vietnam veterans—incidence	30	1.2 (0.4–3.3)
Crane et al., 1997a	Australian military Vietnam veterans	4	NS
Crane et al., 1997b	Australian national service Vietnam veterans	4	1.3
Dalager and Kang, 1997	Army Chemical Corps veterans	2	4.0 (0.5–14.5)
Watanabe and Kang, 1996	Vietnam service, Army		1.1
	Vietnam service, Marines		1.0
Studies Reviewed in *Update 1996*			
Bullman et al., 1994	Navy veterans	12	2.6 (1.1–6.2)
Studies Reviewed in *VAO*			
Tarone et al., 1991	Patients at three Washington, D.C., area hospitals		2.3 (1.0–5.5)
Watanabe et al., 1991	Army Vietnam veterans	109	1.2
	Marine Vietnam veterans	28	0.8
Breslin et al., 1988	Army Vietnam veterans	90	1.1 (0.8–1.5)
	Marine Vietnam veterans	26	1.3 (0.5–3.6)
Anderson et al., 1986a	Wisconsin Vietnam veterans	11	1.0 (0.5–1.7)
Anderson et al., 1986b	Wisconsin Vietnam veterans	9	1.0 (0.5–1.9)

NOTE: MCPA = methyl-4-chlorophenoxyacetic acid; NS = not significant.

[a] Given when available.

[b] "Male genital cancers."

[c] 99% CI.

[d] Self-reported medical history. Answer to question: Since your first day of service in Vietnam, have you been told by a doctor that you have cancer of the testis?

URINARY BLADDER CANCER

Background

Urinary bladder cancer (ICD·9 188.0–188.9) is the most common of the genitourinary tract cancers. According to American Cancer Society estimates, 38,300 men and 14,900 women will be diagnosed with this cancer in the United States in 2000, and 8,100 men and 4,100 women will die from the disease (ACS, 2000a). In males, where this cancer is about three times more likely to occur than in females, these numbers represent approximately 6 percent of new cancer diagnoses and 3 percent of deaths. Overall, bladder cancer is the fifth most common cancer and the fifth leading cause of cancer death in the United States.

Among males in the age groups that characterize most Vietnam veterans, bladder cancer incidence is about twice as high in whites as in African Americans. Rates are slightly higher in white women than in African-American women. Bladder cancer incidence increases greatly with age for individuals older than 40. For the age groups shown below, the incidence rate in each 5-year grouping is roughly double that of the age group before it.

The most important known risk factor for bladder cancer is smoking. About half of bladder cancers in men and one-third in women are thought to be due to smoking (Miller et al., 1996). Occupational exposures to aromatic amines (also called arylamines), polycyclic aromatic hydrocarbons (PAHs), and certain other organic chemicals used in the rubber, leather, textile, paint products, and printing industries are also associated with higher incidence. High-fat diets have been implicated as risk factors, along with exposure to the parasite *Schistosoma haematobium*.

Average Annual Cancer Incidence (per 100,000 individuals) in the United States[a]
Urinary Bladder Cancer

	45–49 Years of Age			50–54 Years of Age			55–59 Years of Age		
	All Races	White	Black	All Races	White	Black	All Races	White	Black
Males	13.8	15.1	8.3	27.1	29.1	16.5	49.9	53.7	30.1
Females	4.1	4.7	2.9	9.1	10.2	5.1	14.7	16.3	8.5

[a] SEER nine standard registries, crude age-specific rate, 1993–1997.

Summary of *VAO*, *Update 1996*, and *Update 1998*

The committees responsible for *VAO* and *Update 1996* found that there was limited or suggestive evidence of *no* association between exposure to herbicides used in Vietnam or the contaminant dioxin and urinary bladder cancer. Additional information available to the committee responsible for *Update 1998* led it to change this conclusion to that of inadequate or insufficient information regarding an association. Table 7-23 provides summaries of the results of the studies underlying these findings and a list of reports that contain details of the research.

Update of Scientific Literature

Occupational Studies

Hooiveld et al. (1998) conducted a retrospective cohort study of 549 exposed and 482 unexposed male Dutch production and contract workers exposed to phenoxy herbicides, chlorophenols, and contaminants between 1950 and 1976. Four deaths attributed to bladder cancer were identified, leading to a marginally significant standardized mortality ratio of 3.7 (1.0–9.5). A separate analysis of 140 male workers exposed to TCDD as a result of an accident recorded one death due to bladder cancer (SMR = 2.8, 0.1–15.5).

In an updated analysis of cohorts involved in the NIOSH study, Steenland et al. (1999) performed mortality analyses involving 5,132 chemical workers at 12 U.S. plants by use of life table techniques (U.S. population referent) and Cox regression (internal referent). The SMR for bladder cancer was based on 16 deaths (6 in the high-exposure group) and was 2.0 (1.1–3.2) for the total cohort and 3.0 (1.4–8.5) for the chloracne cohort. Although the case numbers among the high-exposure cohort were relatively few and the authors did not comment specifically on this organ site, the SMR associated with bladder cancer in individuals with high exposure was the second highest among all diagnostic categories. However, the authors point out that this association is complicated by the fact that the observed elevation in bladder cancer cases was largely due to an excess at only a single plant (which accounted for 10 of the 16 deaths) where there was also exposure to 4-aminobiphenyl, an arylamine that is a well-established human bladder carcinogen (IARC, 1987).

Environmental Studies

The follow-up of people environmentally exposed to TCDD in a 1976 industrial accident in Seveso, Italy, continues. The events that led to the exposure and the methods used to study this population are described in earlier reports and in Chapter 6. Bertazzi et al. (1998) updated the analysis after 15 years' follow-up. There were no deaths from bladder cancers among females in zones A (high-exposure area) or B (medium-exposure area). The numbers of deaths observed among females in zone R (low-exposure area) and among males in all three zones were not statistically different from the numbers expected. A later study (Bertazzi et al., 2001) extends the mortality analysis to 20 years following the event for zones A and B. Two additional deaths were observed in zone B, but the overall results were again statistically indistinguishable from expected numbers.

Schreinemachers' (2000) examination of cancer mortality over the years 1980–1989 in four northern wheat-producing states combined the analysis of bladder cancer with other cancers of the urinary organs (ICD·9 189.3). This analysis, which used wheat acreage per county as a surrogate for exposure to chlorophenoxy herbicides (including 2,4-D), found slightly lower than expected age-standardized mortality rate ratios (SRRs) for these cancers for white males and slightly higher than expected SRRs for white females. None of the values were statistically significant.

Vietnam Veteran Studies

In their 15-year update of the Ranch Hand study, AFHS (2000) researchers reported a relatively sparse number of malignant neoplasms of the kidney or bladder combined among Ranch Hands (11 of 861) and comparisons (6 of 1,249) (RR = 3.1, 0.9–11.0; Model 1, adjusted). After adjustment for covariates, the incidence in Ranch Hands in the low-dioxin category (5 cases) was higher than in comparisons, but the confidence interval is quite wide (RR = 4.4, 1.0–19.0; Model 3, adjusted). All other comparisons based on occupation, rank, and dioxin category did not show significant elevated risk for Ranch Hands.

Synthesis

Various factors complicate the interpretation of the newest studies of urinary bladder cancer. Coexposure to TCDD and the known bladder carcinogen 4-aminobiphenyl in one plant examined in the Steenland et al. (1999) study makes it very difficult to discern whether dioxin exposure affected the observed incidence. Bladder and kidney cancers—data which were combined for analysis in AFHS (2000)—have a common association with smoking but are otherwise etiologically distinct diseases, weakening the informativeness of the AFHS results. Other studies are hampered by the small number of bladder cancer cases identified.

Nonetheless, the recent research on urinary bladder and kidney cancer raises questions about the possibility of an association with herbicide or dioxin exposure. The committee encourages further follow-up on the AFHS and occupational cohorts and urges researchers to separate kidney and bladder cancers in their analyses and to fully control for exposure to other potential or known bladder carcinogens in the occupational setting.

Conclusions

Strength of Evidence in Epidemiologic Studies

There is no information contained in the research reviewed for this report to change the conclusion that there is inadequate or insufficient evidence to determine whether an association exists between exposure to herbicides (2,4-D, 2,4,5-T and its contaminant TCDD, cacodylic acid, and picloram) and urinary bladder cancer.

Biologic Plausibility

No animal studies have found an increased incidence of urinary bladder cancer. A summary of the biologic plausibility for the carcinogenicity of TCDD and the herbicides in general is presented in the conclusion to this chapter. A discussion of toxicological studies that concern biologic plausibility is contained in Chapter 3.

Increased Risk of Disease Among Vietnam Veterans

Although limited data available on Vietnam veterans do suggest they may be at an elevated risk for urinary bladder cancer, the estimated risk ratios are very unstable. Further studies of Ranch Hand Air Force veterans may clarify whether exposures incurred in Vietnam, or dioxin in particular, are associated with altered risks for bladder cancer.

TABLE 7-23 Selected Epidemiologic Studies—Urinary Bladder Cancer

Reference	Study Population	Exposed Cases[a]	Estimated Risk (95% CI)[a]
OCCUPATIONAL			
New Studies			
Steenland et al., 1999	U.S. chemical production workers		
	Total cohort	16	2.0 (1.1–3.2)
	High-exposure cohort	6	3.0 (1.4–8.5)
Hooiveld et al., 1998	Male Dutch production and contract workers		
	Total cohort	4	3.7 (1.0–9.5)
	Accidentally exposed subcohort	1	2.8 (0.1–15.5)
Studies Reviewed in *Update 1998*			
Hertzman et al., 1997	British Columbia sawmill workers		
	Mortality	33	0.9 (0.7–1.2)
	Incidence	94	1.0 (0.8–1.2)
Kogevinas et al., 1997	IARC cohort		
	Workers exposed to TCDD		
	(or higher-chlorinated dioxins)	24	1.4 (0.9–2.1)
	Workers exposed to any phenoxy		
	herbicide or chlorophenol	34	1.0 (0.7–1.5)
Studies Reviewed in *Update 1996*			
Asp et al., 1994	Finnish herbicide appliers—incidence	12	1.6 (0.8–2.8)
Bueno de Mesquita et al., 1993	Dutch production workers	1	1.2 (0.0–6.7)
Collins et al., 1993	Monsanto 2,4-D production workers	16[b]	6.8 (3.9–11.1)
Studies Reviewed in *VAO*			
Ronco et al., 1992	Danish male self-employed farmers	300	0.6 ($p < .05$)
Fingerhut et al., 1991	NIOSH cohort	9	1.6 (0.7–3.0)
	20-year latency	4	1.9 (0.5–4.8)
Green, 1991	Herbicide sprayers in Ontario	1	1.0 (0.0–5.6)
Saracci et al., 1991	IARC cohort	13	0.8 (0.2–1.4)
Zober et al., 1990	BASF production workers	0	— (0.0–15.0)
Alavanja et al., 1989	USDA forest or soil conservationists	8	0.8 (0.3–1.6)

TABLE 7-23 *Continued*

Reference	Study Population	Exposed Cases[a]	Estimated Risk (95% CI)[a]
Henneberger et al., 1989	Mortality among paper and pulp workers	4	1.2 (0.3–3.2)
Alavanja et al., 1988	USDA agricultural extension agents	8	0.7 (0.4–1.4)
Bond et al., 1988	Dow 2,4-D production workers	0	— (0.0–7.2)
Coggon et al., 1986	British MCPA production workers	8	0.9 (0.4–1.7)
Robinson et al., 1986	Paper and pulp workers	8	1.2 (0.6–2.6)
Lynge, 1985	Danish male production workers	11	0.8
Blair et al., 1983	Florida pesticide appliers	3	1.6
Burmeister, 1981	Farmers in Iowa	274	0.9 (NS)
ENVIRONMENTAL			
New Studies			
Bertazzi et al., 2001	Seveso residents—20-year follow-up		
	Zone A males	1	1.7 (0.2–12.0)
	Zone B males	5	1.1 (0.5–2.8)
Schreinemachers, 2000	Rural or farm residents of Minnesota, Montana, North Dakota, and South Dakota		
	Males—counties with wheat acreage 23,000–110,999	147	0.8 (0.7–1.0)
	Males—counties with wheat acreage >111,000	129	0.9 (0.7–1.1)
	Females—counties with wheat acreage 23,000–110,999	67	1.1 (0.8–1.5)
	Females—counties with wheat acreage >111,000	59	1.1 (0.8–1.6)
Bertazzi et al., 1998	Seveso residents—15-year follow-up		
	Zone A males	1	2.4 (0.3–16.8)
	Zone B males	3	0.9 (0.3–3.0)
	Zone R males	21	0.9 (0.6–1.5)
	Zone R females	4	0.6 (0.2–1.8)
Studies Reviewed in *Update 1998*			
Gambini et al., 1997	Italian rice growers	12	1.0 (0.5–1.8)
Ott and Zober, 1996	BASF cleanup workers	2	1.4 (0.4–3.2)
Svensson et al., 1995	Swedish fishermen, mortality		
	East coast		1.3 (0.4–3.1)
	West coast		1.0 (0.6–1.6)
	Swedish fishermen, incidence		
	East coast		0.7 (0.4–1.3)
	West coast		0.9 (0.7–1.1)
Studies Reviewed in *VAO*			
Pesatori et al., 1992	Seveso residents		
	Zones A, B males	10	1.6 (0.9–3.1)
	Zones A, B females	1	0.9 (0.1–6.8)
Lampi et al., 1992	Finnish community exposed to chlorophenols		1.0 (0.6–1.9)

TABLE 7-23 Continued

Reference	Study Population	Exposed Cases[a]	Estimated Risk (95% CI)[a]
VIETNAM VETERANS			
New Studies			
AFHS, 2000	Air Force Ranch Hand veterans	11	3.1 (0.9–11.0)
Studies Reviewed in *Update 1998*			
Clapp, 1997	Massachusetts Vietnam veterans	80	0.6 (0.2–1.3)
Crane et al., 1997a	Australian military Vietnam veterans	11	1.1 (0.6–2.0)
Crane et al., 1997b	Australian national service Vietnam veterans	1	0.6
Studies Reviewed in *VAO*			
Breslin et al., 1988	Army Vietnam veterans	9	0.6 (0.3–1.2)
	Marine Vietnam veterans	4	2.4 (0.1–66.4)
Anderson et al., 1986a	Wisconsin Vietnam veterans	0	—
Anderson et al., 1986b	Wisconsin Vietnam veterans	1	—

NOTE: MCPA = methyl-4-chlorophenoxyacetic acid; NS = not significant; USDA = United States Department of Agriculture.

[a] Given when available.
[b] Many of the employees studied were also exposed to 4-aminobiphenyl, a known bladder carcinogen.

RENAL CANCER

Background

Cancers of the kidney (ICD·9 189.0) and renal pelvis (ICD·9 189.1) are often grouped together in epidemiologic studies; cancer of the ureter (ICD·9 189.2) may also be aggregated with these. Although the diseases of these organs have different characteristics and may have different risk factors, there is logic to this aggregation because these structures are all exposed to filterable compounds, such as polycyclic aromatic hydrocarbons, that appear in urine. The American Cancer Society estimates that 18,800 men and 12,400 women will be diagnosed with renal cancers (ICD·9 189.0, 189.1) in the United States in 2000 and that 7,300 men and 4,600 women will die from the disease (ACS, 2000a). These figures represent between 2 and 3 percent of all new cancer diagnoses and deaths.

Renal cancer is twice as common in men as in women. In the age groups that represent most Vietnam veterans, African-American men have a slightly higher incidence than white men; African-American and white women have roughly the same rate of the disease. With the exception of Wilm's tumor (which is more likely to occur in children), renal cancer is more common in individuals older than 50 years of age.

Smoking is a well-established risk factor for renal cancer. Phenacetin-containing analgesic abuse has also been implicated. Individuals with certain rare syndromes—notably, von Hippel-Lindau syndrome and tuberous sclerosis—are at higher risk. Other potential factors include diet, weight, and occupational exposure to asbestos and cadmium. Firefighters, who are routinely exposed to numerous pyrolysis products, are a known higher-risk group.

Average Annual Cancer Incidence (per 100,000 individuals) in the United States[a]
Kidney and Renal Pelvis Cancer

	45–49 Years of Age			50–54 Years of Age			55–59 Years of Age		
	All Races	White	Black	All Races	White	Black	All Races	White	Black
Males	12.9	12.2	21.2	23.0	22.5	37.4	32.8	32.7	41.7
Females	5.7	5.6	8.0	10.6	10.5	13.7	15.6	16.0	19.4

[a] SEER nine standard registries, crude age-specific rate, 1993–1997.

Summary of *VAO, Update 1996,* and *Update 1998*

The committee responsible for *VAO* found that there was inadequate or insufficient information to determine whether an association existed between exposure to herbicides used in Vietnam or the contaminant dioxin and renal cancer. Additional information available to the committees responsible for *Update 1996* and *Update 1998* did not change this finding. Table 7-24 provides summaries of the results of the studies underlying these findings and a list of reports that contain details of the research.

Update of the Scientific Literature

Occupational Studies

Hooiveld et al. (1998) conducted a retrospective cohort study of 549 exposed and 482 unexposed male Dutch production and contract workers exposed to phenoxy herbicides, chlorophenols, and contaminants between 1950 and 1976. Four deaths attributed to kidney cancer were identified, leading to a statistically significant standardized mortality ratio of 4.1 (1.1–10.4). A "urinary organs" category combining bladder and kidney cancer produced an SMR of 3.9 (1.7–7.6), based on 8 deaths. No kidney cancer deaths were recorded in a separate analysis of 140 male workers exposed to TCDD as a result of an accident.

In the update of the industrial cohort exposed to dioxins known as the NIOSH cohort, Steenland et al. (1999) performed mortality analyses involving 5,132 chemical workers at 12 U.S. plants by use of life table techniques (U.S. population referent) and Cox regression (internal referent). The SMR for kidney cancer

CANCER   347

was 1.6 (0.8–2.7), based on 13 deaths. No Cox regression analysis was conducted for renal cancer.

Environmental Studies

Bertazzi and colleagues' (2001) most recent follow-up of people environmentally exposed to TCDD in a 1976 industrial accident in Seveso, Italy, extends the mortality analysis to 20 years following the event. Details of this ongoing study are given in Chapter 6. There were no deaths from kidney cancers among individuals in zone A, the high-exposure area. Three deaths each were reported for males (RR = 0.9, 0.3–3.0) and females (RR = 2.1, 0.7–6.7) in zone B, the medium-exposure area. These figures were not distinguishable from the expected numbers of deaths.

Schreinemachers' (2000) examination of cancer mortality over the years 1980–1989 in four northern wheat-producing states combined kidney and ureter cancer for analysis (ICD·9 189 excluding 189.3). This analysis, which used wheat acreage per county as a surrogate for exposure to chlorophenoxy herbicides (including 2,4-D), reported age-standardized mortality rate ratios near unity for white males and females. A trend of increasing SMR as a function of acreage per county was noted for males.

Vietnam Veteran Studies

In their 15-year update of the Ranch Hand study, AFHS (2000) researchers reported a relatively sparse number of malignant neoplasms of the kidney or bladder combined among Ranch Hands (11 of 861) and comparisons (6 of 1,249) (RR = 3.1, 0.9–11.0; Model 1, adjusted). After adjustment for covariates, there was a marginally significant difference in incidence between Ranch Hands in the low-dioxin category (5 cases) and comparisons (RR = 4.4, 1.0–19.0; Model 3, adjusted). All other comparisons based on occupation, rank, and dioxin category did not achieve statistical significance.

Synthesis

Studies of renal cancer published since *Update 1998* continue the pattern of equivocal results seen previously. The informativeness of the Hooiveld et al. (1998) results is limited by the lack of control for smoking—a known confounder. Cigarette smoking also covaried with the indicators of herbicide exposure used by AFHS researchers, confounding their analyses. The elevated incidence observed in the AFHS cohort was seen in Ranch Hands in the low-dioxin category but not the high-dioxin category, which would not be expected if an association existed between exposure and the outcome.

Conclusions

Strength of Evidence in Epidemiologic Studies

There is no information contained in the research reviewed for this report to change the conclusion that there is inadequate or insufficient evidence to determine whether an association exists between exposure to herbicides (2,4-D, 2,4,5-T and its contaminant TCDD, cacodylic acid, and picloram) and renal cancer.

Biologic Plausibility

No animal studies have found an increased incidence of renal cancer. A summary of the biologic plausibility for the carcinogenicity of TCDD and the herbicides in general is presented in the conclusion to this chapter. A discussion of toxicological studies that concern biologic plausibility is contained in Chapter 3.

Increased Risk of Disease Among Vietnam Veterans

The limited data available on Vietnam veterans do not suggest they are at an elevated risk for renal cancer.

TABLE 7-24 Selected Epidemiologic Studies—Renal Cancer

Reference	Study Population	Exposed Cases[a]	Estimated Risk (95% CI)[a]
OCCUPATIONAL			
New Studies			
Steenland et al., 1999	U.S. chemical production workers	13	1.6 (0.8–2.7)
Hooiveld et al., 1998	Male Dutch production and contract workers		
	Total cohort—kidney cancer	4	4.1 (1.1–10.4)
	Total cohort—"urinary organs"	8	3.9 (1.7–7.6)
	Accidentally exposed subcohort	0	—
Studies Reviewed in *Update 1998*			
Kogevinas et al., 1997	IARC cohort		
	Workers exposed to TCDD (or higher-chlorinated dioxins)	26	1.6 (1.1–2.4)
	Workers exposed to any phenoxy herbicide or chlorophenol		1.1 (0.7–1.6)
Studies Reviewed in *Update 1996*			
Mellemgaard et al., 1994	Danish Cancer Registry patients		
	Occupational herbicide exposure among males	13	1.7 (0.7–4.3)
	Occupational herbicide exposure among females	3	5.7 (0.6–5.8)

TABLE 7-24 *Continued*

Reference	Study Population	Exposed Cases[a]	Estimated Risk (95% CI)[a]
Blair et al., 1993	U.S. farmers in 23 states		
	White males	522	1.1 (1.0–1.2)
	Nonwhite males	30	—
	White females	6	—
	Nonwhite females	6	—
Studies Reviewed in *VAO*			
Ronco et al., 1992	Danish male self-employed farm workers	141	0.6 ($p < .05$)
Fingerhut et al., 1991	NIOSH cohort	8	1.4 (0.6–2.8)
Manz et al., 1991	German production workers	3	1.6 (0.3–4.6)
Saracci et al., 1991	IARC cohort	11	1.0 (0.5–1.7)
Alavanja et al., 1989	USDA forest conservationists		1.7 (0.5–5.5)
	Soil conservationists		2.4 (1.0–5.9)
Henneberger et al., 1989	Paper and pulp workers	3	1.5 (0.3–4.4)
Alavanja et al., 1988	USDA agricultural extension agents		1.7 (0.9–3.3)
Bond et al., 1988	Dow 2,4-D production workers	0	— (0.0–6.2)
Robinson et al., 1986	Paper and pulp workers	6	1.2 (0.5–3.0)
Coggon et al., 1986	British MCPA production workers	5	1.0 (0.3–2.3)
Lynge, 1985	Danish male production workers	3	0.6
Wiklund, 1983	Swedish agricultural workers	775	0.8 (0.7–0.9)[b]
Blair et al., 1983	Florida pesticide appliers	1	0.5
Burmeister, 1981	Farmers in Iowa	178	1.1 (NS)
ENVIRONMENTAL			
New Studies			
Bertazzi et al., 2001	Seveso residents—20-year follow-up		
	Zone B males	3	0.9 (0.3–3.0)
	Zone B females	3	2.1 (0.7–6.7)
Schreinemachers, 2000	Rural or farm residents of Minnesota, Montana, North Dakota, and South Dakota		
	Males—counties with wheat acreage 23,000–110,999	147	1.0 (0.8–1.2)
	Males—counties with wheat acreage >111,000	129	1.0 (0.8–1.3)
	Females—counties with wheat acreage 23,000–110,999	85	0.9 (0.7–1.2)
	Females—counties with wheat acreage >111,000	90	1.1 (0.8–1.4)
Studies Reviewed in *Update 1996*			
Bertazzi et al., 1993	Seveso residents—10-year follow-up, morbidity		
	Zone R males	10	0.9 (0.4–1.7)
	Zone R females	7	1.2 (0.5–2.7)
Studies Reviewed in *VAO*			
Pesatori et al., 1992	Seveso residents		
	Zones A, B males	0	—
	Zones A, B females	1	1.1 (0.2–8.1)

TABLE 7-24 Continued

Reference	Study Population	Exposed Cases[a]	Estimated Risk (95% CI)[a]
VIETNAM VETERANS			
New Studies			
AFHS, 2000	Air Force Ranch Hand veterans	11	3.1 (0.9–11.0)
Studies Reviewed in *Update 1998*			
Crane et al., 1997a	Australian military Vietnam veterans	22	1.2 (0.8–1.9)
Crane et al., 1997b	Australian national service Vietnam veterans	3	3.9
Studies Reviewed in *Update 1996*			
Visintainer et al., 1995	Michigan Vietnam veterans	21	1.4 (0.9–2.2)
Studies Reviewed in *VAO*			
Breslin et al., 1988	Army Vietnam veterans	55	0.9 (0.5–1.5)
	Marine Vietnam veterans	13	0.9 (0.5–1.5)
Kogan and Clapp, 1988	Massachusetts Vietnam veterans	9	1.8 (1.0–3.5)
Anderson et al., 1986a	Wisconsin Vietnam veterans	1	—
Anderson et al., 1986b	Wisconsin Vietnam veterans	2	—

NOTE: MCPA = methyl-4-chlorophenoxyacetic acid; NS = not significant; USDA = United States Department of Agriculture.
[a] Given when available.
[b] 99% CI.

BRAIN TUMORS

Background

According to the American Cancer Society, approximately 9,500 men and 7,000 women will be diagnosed with new cases of brain and other nervous system cancers (ICD·9 191.0–191.9, 192.0–192.3, 192.8–192.9) in the United States in 2000, and 7,100 men and 5,900 women will die from these cancers (ACS, 2000a). These numbers represent approximately 1.4 percent of new cancer diagnoses and 2.4 percent of all cancer deaths.

For individuals in the United States age 45–59, brain cancer is slightly more common in males than females and slightly more common in whites than African Americans.

Exposure to ionizing radiation is an established risk factor for brain cancer. Several other potential factors have been examined, but the American Cancer Society notes that the majority of brain cancers are not associated with any known risk factors.

Average Annual Cancer Incidence (per 100,000 individuals) in the United States[a]
Brain and Other Nervous System Cancers

	45–49 Years of Age			50–54 Years of Age			55–59 Years of Age		
	All Races	White	Black	All Races	White	Black	All Races	White	Black
Males	6.6	6.9	4.1	10.4	11.7	4.1	14.1	15.1	10.1
Females	4.6	5.0	2.7	6.8	7.6	3.2	9.5	10.3	8.5

[a] SEER nine standard registries, crude age-specific rate, 1993–1997.

Summary of *VAO*, *Update 1996*, and *Update 1998*

The committee responsible for *VAO* found that there was limited or suggestive evidence of *no* association between exposure to herbicides used in Vietnam or the contaminant dioxin and brain cancer. Additional information available to the committees responsible for *Update 1996* and *Update 1998* did not change this finding. Table 7-25 provides summaries of the results of the studies underlying these findings and a list of reports that contain details of the research.

Update of Scientific Literature

Occupational Studies

Hooiveld and colleagues' (1998) retrospective cohort study of Dutch production and contract workers exposed to phenoxy herbicides, chlorophenols, and contaminants found no deaths due to brain cancer between 1950 and 1976 in the cohort of 1,031 males.

In the update of the industrial cohort exposed to dioxins known as the NIOSH cohort, Steenland et al. (1999) performed mortality analyses involving 5,132 chemical workers at 12 U.S. plants by use of life table techniques (U.S. population referent) and Cox regression (internal referent). The SMR for brain and nervous system cancers was 0.8 (0.4–1.6), based on 8 deaths.

Environmental Studies

The follow-up of people environmentally exposed to TCDD in a 1976 industrial accident in Seveso, Italy, continues. The events that led to the exposure and the methods used to study this population are described in earlier reports and in Chapter 6. Bertazzi et al. (1998) update the population after 15 years' follow-up. There were no deaths from brain cancers among males or females in zone A, the high-exposure area. In zone B, the medium-exposure area, 1 death was observed among males where 1.3 were expected (0.8, 0.1–5.5). For females, 3 deaths were observed where 0.9 was expected, leading to a marginally significant SMR of 3.2 (1.0–10.3). For zone R, the low-exposure area, 12 deaths were attributed to brain cancer in males where 8 were expected (1.3, 0.7–2.5); for females, 8 deaths were reported where 7.2 were expected (1.1, 0.5–2.4).

A later study (Bertazzi et al., 2001) extends the mortality analysis to 20 years following the event for zones A and B. No new deaths occurred in either zone, leading to lower SMRs than those reported above because of the additional years included.

Schreinemachers' (2000) examination of cancer mortality over the years 1980–1989 in four northern wheat-producing states used wheat acreage per county as a surrogate for exposure to chlorophenoxy herbicides, including 2,4-D. The analysis found slightly lower than expected age-standardized mortality rate ratios for these cancers among white males and females in counties with between 23,000 and 110,999 acres of wheat and slightly higher than expected SRRs for individuals in counties with 111,000 or more acres of wheat. None of the values were statistically significant.

Vietnam Veteran Studies

In their 15-year update of the Ranch Hand study, AFHS (2000) researchers reported the presence of only one malignant brain neoplasm and thus performed no statistical analysis.

Synthesis

The studies reviewed for the first time in this report, like those reviewed in earlier *Veterans and Agent Orange* reports, found small numbers of cases of brain tumors and risk estimates fairly evenly distributed around 1.0.

Conclusions

Strength of Evidence in Epidemiologic Studies

Based on its evaluation of the epidemiologic evidence reviewed in this and previous *Veterans and Agent Orange* reports, the committee finds there is limited/suggestive evidence of *no* association between exposure to herbicides (2,4-D, 2,4,5-T and its contaminant TCDD, cacodylic acid, and picloram) and brain tumors.

Biologic Plausibility

No animal studies have found an increased incidence of brain tumors. A summary of the biologic plausibility for the carcinogenicity of TCDD and the herbicides in general is presented in the conclusion to this chapter. A discussion of toxicological studies that concern biologic plausibility is contained in Chapter 3.

Increased Risk of Disease Among Vietnam Veterans

The limited data available on Vietnam veterans do not suggest they are at an elevated risk for brain tumors.

TABLE 7-25 Selected Epidemiologic Studies—Brain Tumors

Reference	Study Population	Exposed Cases[a]	Estimated Risk (95% CI)[a]
OCCUPATIONAL			
New Studies			
Steenland et al., 1999	U.S. chemical production workers	8	0.8 (0.4–1.6)
Studies Reviewed in *Update 1998*			
Gambini et al., 1997	Italian rice growers	4	0.9 (0.2–2.3)
Kogevinas et al., 1997	IARC cohort		
	Workers exposed to TCDD (or higher-chlorinated dioxins)	12	0.6 (0.3–1.1)
	Workers not exposed to TCDD (or higher-chlorinated dioxins)	10	0.8 (0.4–1.5)
	Workers exposed to any phenoxy herbicide or chlorophenol	22	0.7 (0.4–1.0)
Becher et al., 1996	German chemical production workers		
	Subcohort I	3	2.3 (0.5–6.8)
Ramlow et al., 1996	Pentachlorophenol production workers		
	0-year latency	1	—
	15-year latency	1	—
Studies Reviewed in *Update 1996*			
Asp et al., 1994	Finnish herbicide appliers	3	1.2 (0.3–3.6)
Dean, 1994	Irish farmers and farm workers		
	Males	195	—
	Females	72	—
Blair et al., 1993	U.S. farmers in 23 states		
	White males	447	1.2 (1.1–1.3)
	Nonwhite males	16	1.0 (0.6–1.6)
	White females	9	1.1 (0.5–2.1)
	Nonwhite females	1	0.4 (0.0–2.1)
Studies Reviewed in *VAO*			
Morrison et al., 1992	Farmers in Canadian prairie province		
	250+ acres sprayed with herbicides	24	0.8 (0.5–1.2)
Ronco et al., 1992	Danish male self-employed farm workers	194	1.1
Swaen et al., 1992	Dutch herbicide appliers	3	3.2 (0.6–9.3)
Fingerhut et al., 1991	NIOSH cohort	5	0.7 (0.2–1.6)
Saracci et al., 1991	IARC cohort	6	0.4 (0.1–0.8)
Wigle et al., 1990	Saskatchewan farmers	96	1.0 (0.8–1.3)
Alavanja et al., 1989	USDA forest or soil conservationists	6	1.7 (0.6–3.7)
Henneberger et al., 1989	Paper and pulp workers	2	1.2 (0.1–4.2)
Alavanja et al., 1988	USDA agricultural extension agents		1.0 (0.4–2.4)
Bond et al., 1988	Dow 2,4-D production workers	0	— (0.0–4.1)

TABLE 7-25 Continued

Reference	Study Population	Exposed Cases[a]	Estimated Risk (95% CI)[a]
Musicco et al., 1988	Men and women in the Milan, Italy, area	61	1.6 (1.1–2.4)
Coggon et al., 1986	British MCPA production workers	11	1.2 (0.6–2.2)
Robinson et al., 1986	Paper and pulp workers	4	0.6 (0.2–2.1)
Lynge, 1985	Danish male production workers	4	0.7
Blair et al., 1983	Florida pesticide appliers	5	2.0
Burmeister, 1981	Farmers in Iowa	111	1.1 (NS)
ENVIRONMENTAL			
New Studies			
Bertazzi et al., 2001	Seveso residents—20-year follow-up		
	Zone B males	1	0.5 (0.1–3.5)
	Zone B females	3	2.2 (0.7–7.0)
Schreinemachers, 2000	Rural or farm residents of Minnesota, Montana, North Dakota, and South Dakota		
	Males—counties with wheat acreage 23,000–110,999	131	0.9 (0.8–1.2)
	Males—counties with wheat acreage >111,000	130	1.1 (0.9–1.4)
	Females—counties with wheat acreage 23,000–110,999	94	1.0 (0.7–1.2)
	Females—counties with wheat acreage >111,000	95	1.2 (0.9–1.5)
Bertazzi et al., 1998	Seveso residents—15-year follow-up		
	Zone B males	1	0.8 (0.1–5.5)
	Zone B females	3	3.2 (1.0–10.3)
	Zone R males	12	1.3 (0.7–2.5)
	Zone R females	8	1.1 (0.5–2.4)
Studies Reviewed in *Update 1998*			
Bertazzi et al., 1997	Seveso residents—15-year follow-up		
	Zone B males	1	0.8 (0.0–4.2)
	Zone B females	3	3.2 (0.6–9.4)
	Zone R males	12	1.3 (0.7–2.3)
	Zone R females	8	1.1 (0.5–2.2)
Svensson et al., 1995	Swedish fishermen, mortality		
	East coast	2	0.6 (0.1–2.1)
	West coast	15	1.0 (0.6–1.7)
	Swedish fishermen, incidence		
	East coast	3	0.5 (0.1–1.4)
	West coast	24	0.9 (0.6–1.4)
Studies Reviewed in *Update 1996*			
Bertazzi et al., 1993	Seveso residents—10-year follow-up, morbidity		
	Zone R males	6	0.6 (0.3–1.4)
	Zone R females	6	1.4 (0.6–3.4)
Studies Reviewed in *VAO*			
Pesatori et al., 1992	Seveso residents		
	Zones A, B females	1	1.5 (0.2–11.3)

TABLE 7-25 *Continued*

Reference	Study Population	Exposed Cases[a]	Estimated Risk (95% CI)[a]
Bertazzi et al., 1989a	Seveso residents—10-year follow-up		
	Zones A, B, R males	5	1.2 (0.4–3.1)
	Zones A, B, R females	5	2.1 (0.8–5.9)
VIETNAM VETERANS			
New Studies			
AFHS, 2000	Air Force Ranch Hand veterans	1	—
Studies Reviewed in *Update 1998*			
Crane et al., 1997a	Australian military Vietnam veterans	39	1.1 (0.8–1.5)
Crane et al., 1997b	Australian national service Vietnam veterans	13	1.4
Dalager and Kang, 1997	Army Chemical Corps veterans	2	1.9[b]
Studies Reviewed in *Update 1996*			
Dalager et al., 1995	Women Vietnam veterans	4	1.4 (0.4–3.7)
Visintainer et al., 1995	Michigan Vietnam veterans	36	1.1 (0.8–1.5)
Boyle et al., 1987	Vietnam Experience Study	3	—
Studies Reviewed in *VAO*			
Thomas and Kang, 1990	Army Chemical Corps Vietnam veterans	2	5.0
Breslin et al., 1988	Army Vietnam veterans	116	1.0 (0.3–3.2)
	Marine Vietnam veterans	25	1.1 (0.2–7.1)
Anderson et al., 1986a	Wisconsin Vietnam veterans	13	1.6 (0.9–2.7)
Anderson et al., 1986b	Wisconsin Vietnam veterans	8	0.8 (0.3–1.5)
Lawrence et al., 1985	New York Vietnam veterans	4	0.5 (0.2–1.5)

NOTE: MCPA = methyl-4-chlorophenoxyacetic acid; NS = not significant; USDA = United States Department of Agriculture.

[a] Given when available.

[b] Crude rate ratio of Vietnam to non-Vietnam veterans.

NON-HODGKIN'S LYMPHOMA

Background

Non-Hodgkin's lymphoma (ICD·9 200.0–200.8, 202.0–202.2, 202.8–202.9) is the more common of the two primary types of cancer of the lymphatic system. The American Cancer Society estimates that 31,700 men and 23,200 women will be diagnosed with this disease in the United States in 2000 and that 13,700 men and 12,400 women will die from it (ACS, 2000a). Collectively, lymphomas (which also include Hodgkin's disease) are the fifth most common form of cancer in the United States and the sixth leading cause of cancer death.

NHL incidence is uniformly higher in males than females and, in most age groups, higher in whites than African Americans. In the cohorts that characterize most Vietnam veterans, rates increase with age for whites and vary inconsistently for African Americans.

The causes of NHL are poorly understood. Individuals with suppressed or compromised immune systems are known to be at higher risk, and some studies show increased incidence in individuals with HIV, human T-cell lymphotropic virus (HTLV), Epstein-Barr virus, and gastric *Helicobacter pylori* infections. A number of behavioral, occupational, and environmental risk factors have also been proposed (Blair et al., 1997).

Average Annual Cancer Incidence (per 100,000 individuals) in the United States[a]
Non-Hodgkin's Lymphoma

	45–49 Years of Age			50–54 Years of Age			55–59 Years of Age		
	All Races	White	Black	All Races	White	Black	All Races	White	Black
Males	23.1	22.9	32.0	29.6	29.3	36.6	37.2	38.8	33.2
Females	12.3	12.8	11.2	18.6	18.7	18.4	27.8	28.9	15.3

[a] SEER nine standard registries, crude age-specific rate, 1993–1997.

Summary of *VAO*, *Update 1996*, and *Update 1998*

The committee responsible for *VAO* found that there was sufficient information to determine that an association existed between exposure to herbicides used in Vietnam or the contaminant dioxin and non-Hodgkin's lymphoma. Additional information available to the committees responsible for *Update 1996* and *Update 1998* did not change this finding. Table 7-26 provides summaries of the results of the studies underlying these findings and a list of reports that contain details of the research.

Update of the Scientific Literature

Occupational Studies

Hooiveld et al. (1998) conducted a retrospective cohort study of 549 exposed and 482 unexposed male Dutch production and contract workers exposed to phenoxy herbicides, chlorophenols, and contaminants between 1950 and 1976. Three deaths were attributed to NHL, leading to a standardized mortality ratio of 3.8 (0.8–11.0).

In an update and expansion of cohorts involved in the NIOSH study, Steenland et al. (1999) performed mortality analyses involving 5,132 chemical workers at 12 U.S. plants by use of life table techniques (U.S. population referent) and Cox regression (internal referent). The standardized mortality ratio for NHL was 1.1, based on 12 deaths since 1960 (0.6–1.9).

Environmental Studies

An ongoing study of people environmentally exposed to TCDD in Seveso, Italy, as the result of a 1976 industrial accident is detailed in Chapter 6. The 15-year follow-up reported by Bertazzi et al. (1998) found no deaths due to NHL in the high-exposure area, zone A. The observed numbers of deaths in the medium-exposure area—zone B—and the low-exposure area—zone R—were in line with the expected numbers. An extension of the mortality analysis to 20 years following the event for zones A and B (Bertazzi et al., 2001) found that 1 NHL death each had occurred among the male (RR = 3.2, 0.4–23.0) and female (RR = 3.3, 0.5–23.7) residents of zone A. No additional NHL deaths were reported for males in zone B (0.9, 0.2–3.8; based on 2 deaths); 3 deaths were recorded for females (RR = 1.6, 0.5–4.9).

Viel et al. (2000) examined whether there were cancer clusters in an area surrounding a municipal solid waste incinerator located near Doubs, France. High-dioxin emissions (16.3 ng I-TEQ/m^3, far in excess of the EU standard of 0.1 ng I-TEQ/m^3) had been measured from the incinerator, and elevated levels were detected in the milk from cows that grazed near the facility. Data from a general population cancer registry over the years 1980–1995 were combined with demographic information for the analysis. A statistically significant excess of NHL was observed in residents in an area near the incinerator (SIR = 1.3, $p = .00003$; based on 286 cases). When the analysis was confined to 1991–1994, the SIR increased to 1.8 ($p = .00003$; based on 109 cases). However, the authors do not provide any direct evidence of human exposure.

Schreinemachers (2000) examined cancer mortality in white males and females over the years 1980–1989 in four northern wheat-producing states, using wheat acreage per county as a surrogate for exposure to chlorophenoxy herbicides (including 2,4-D). NHL mortality was not analyzed separately but was instead subsumed into a category labeled "lymphosarcoma, reticulum cell sarcoma including other lymphoma." Age-standardized mortality rate ratios for this category were slightly below unity for males and females. None of the values were statistically significant.

Vietnam Veteran Studies

Air Force Health Study researchers (AFHS, 2000), in their 15-year update of the Ranch Hand study, reported 1 case among Ranch Hand veterans and 3 cases among comparisons (RR = 0.2, 0.0–2.6; Model 1, adjusted). None of the limited analyses of these data yielded statistically significant results.

The government of Australia's mail surveys of approximately 50,000 male and female nationals who served in Vietnam (CDVA, 1998a,b) reported that 137 male veterans indicated a doctor had told them they had NHL since their first day of service in Vietnam. This was significantly in excess of the 48 cases expected (range 34–62) given age-standardized rates (CDVA, 1998a). The authors observed that although it was possible there was some error in the responses, such errors were unlikely to explain the excess number of cases reported. However, a follow-up conducted to medically confirm selected conditions reported by males in the survey study (AIHW, 1999) estimated that there were 62 validated cases of NHL among respondents, at the limit of the expected number. For female veterans, 2 cases were reported, which was within the range of 0–4 expected (CDVA, 1998b).

Synthesis

Some but not all of the studies of NHL published since the release of *Update 1998* show elevated incidence or mortality in populations exposed to dioxin or phenoxy herbicides. Studies of a population living near a solid waste incinerator shown to have high dioxin emissions (Viel et al., 2000) and of male Vietnam veterans from Australia (CDVA, 1998a) reported elevated incidence rates. The latest Seveso cohort study showed a threefold increased risk of NHL for the group most heavily exposed, although this was based on very small numbers. A mortality study in areas where chlorophenoxy herbicides may have been used (Schreinemachers, 2000) observed rates similar to those expected in the general population. The NIOSH occupational study surprisingly showed no excess in NHL mortality, while the exposed Dutch workers showed a nonsignificant but nearly fourfold increased risk. The committee considered these results in light of the body of the literature reviewed in earlier reports, which includes several well-conducted studies showing increased incidence.

Conclusions

Strength of Evidence in Epidemiologic Studies

There is sufficient evidence to conclude that an association exists between exposure to herbicides (2,4-D, 2,4,5-T and its contaminant TCDD, cacodylic acid, and picloram) and non-Hodgkin's lymphoma. The evidence regarding association is drawn from occupational and other studies in which subjects were exposed to a variety of herbicides and herbicide components.

Biologic Plausibility

No animal studies have found an increased incidence of non-Hodgkin's lymphoma. A summary of the biologic plausibility for the carcinogenicity of TCDD and the herbicides in general is presented in the conclusion to this chapter. A

Increased Risk of Disease Among Vietnam Veterans

Because of the few numbers of veterans with non-Hodgkin's lymphoma in the Ranch Hand study, analysis was limited and no conclusions could be drawn. However, data from a survey study of male Vietnam veterans from Australia indicated a possibly elevated risk of non-Hodgkin's lymphoma.

TABLE 7-26 Selected Epidemiologic Studies—Non-Hodgkin's Lymphoma

Reference	Study Population	Exposed Cases[a]	Estimated Risk (95% CI)[a]
OCCUPATIONAL			
New Studies			
Steenland et al., 1999	U.S. chemical production workers	12	1.1 (0.6–1.9)
Hooiveld et al., 1998	Male Dutch production and contract workers	3	3.8 (0.8–11.0)
Studies Reviewed in *Update 1998*			
Gambini et al., 1997	Italian rice growers		1.3 (0.3–3.3)
Keller-Byrne et al., 1997	Farmers in the central United States		1.3 (1.2–1.6)
Kogevinas et al., 1997	IARC cohort		
	Workers exposed to TCDD (or higher-chlorinated dioxins)	24	1.4 (0.9–2.1)
	Workers exposed to any phenoxy herbicide or chlorophenol	9	1.0
Becher et al., 1996	German chemical production workers	6	3.3 (1.2–7.1)
Nanni et al., 1996	Italian farming and animal-breeding workers	23[b]	1.8 (1.2–2.6)
Ramlow et al., 1996	Pentachlorophenol production workers	[c]	1.3 (0.4–3.1)
Amadori et al., 1995	Italian farming and animal-breeding workers	164	1.8 (1.2–2.6)
Studies Reviewed in *Update 1996*			
Kogevinas et al., 1995	IARC cohort diagnosed with NHL		
	Exposed to 2,4,5-T		1.9 (0.7–4.8)
	Exposed to TCDD		1.9 (0.7–5.1)
Asp et al., 1994	Finnish herbicide appliers	1	0.4 (0.0–2.0)
Dean, 1994	Irish farmers and farm workers		
	Males	244[b]	—
	Females	84[b]	—
Hardell et al., 1994	Male residents of northern Sweden		
	Exposure to phenoxy herbicides	25	5.5 (2.7–11.0)
	Exposure to chlorophenols	35	4.8 (2.7–8.8)

TABLE 7-26 *Continued*

Reference	Study Population	Exposed Cases[a]	Estimated Risk (95% CI)[a]
Morrison et al., 1994	Farm operators in three Canadian provinces		
	All farm operators		0.8 (0.7–0.9)
	Highest quartile of herbicides sprayed	19	2.1 (1.1–3.9)
	Highest quartile of herbicides sprayed relative to no spraying	6	3.0 (1.1–8.1)
Blair et al., 1993	U.S. farmers from 23 states (white males)	843	1.2 (1.1–1.3)
Bloemen et al., 1993	Dow 2,4-D production workers	2	2.0 (0.2–7.1)
Bueno de Mesquita et al., 1993	Dutch production workers		
	Workers exposed to phenoxy herbicides	2	3.0 (0.4–10.8)
Lynge, 1993	Danish male production workers	10	1.7 (0.5–4.5)
Persson et al., 1993	Swedish NHL patients		
	Exposure to phenoxy herbicides		2.3 (0.7–7.2)
	Occupation as a lumberjack		6.0 (1.1–31.0)
Zahm et al., 1993	Females in eastern Nebraska farms		1.0 (0.7–1.4)
Kogevinas et al., 1992	IARC cohort		
	Workers exposed to any phenoxy herbicide or chlorophenol	11	1.0 (0.5–1.7)
Studies Reviewed in *VAO*			
Hansen et al., 1992	Danish gardeners—men and women	8	2.0 (0.9–3.9)
Ronco et al., 1992	Danish farm workers—self-employed and employees	147	1.0
	Italian farm workers—self-employed and employees	14	1.3
Smith and Christophers, 1992	Male residents of Australia		
	Exposure >1 day	15	1.5 (0.6–3.7)
	Exposure >30 days	7	2.7 (0.7–9.6)
Swaen et al., 1992	Dutch herbicide appliers	0	—
Vineis et al., 1991	Residents of selected Italian provinces		
	Male residents of contaminated areas		2.2 (1.4–3.5)
Wigle et al., 1990	Canadian farmers		
	All farmers	103	0.9 (0.8–1.1)
	Farmers spraying herbicides on 250+ acres	10	2.2 (1.0–4.6)
Zahm et al., 1990	White male residents of Nebraska		
	Ever done farm work	147	0.9 (0.6–1.4)
	Ever mixed or applied 2,4-D	43	1.5 (0.9–2.5)
Alavanja et al., 1989	USDA soil conservationists		1.8 (0.7–4.1)
	USDA forest conservationists		2.5 (1.0–6.3)
Corrao et al., 1989	Italian farmers licensed to apply pesticides		
	Licensed pesticide users and nonusers	45[d]	1.4 (1.0–1.9)
	Farmers in arable land areas	31	1.8 (1.2–2.5)
LaVecchia et al., 1989	Residents of the Milan, Italy, area		
	Agricultural occupations		2.1 (1.3–3.4)
Persson et al., 1989	Orebro Hospital		
	Exposed to phenoxy acids	6	4.9 (1.0–27.0)

TABLE 7-26 *Continued*

Reference	Study Population	Exposed Cases[a]	Estimated Risk (95% CI)[a]
Wiklund et al., 1989b	Swedish pesticide appliers	27	1.1 (0.7–1.6)
Alavanja et al., 1988	USDA extension agents		1.2 (0.7–2.3)
Dubrow et al., 1988	Ohio residents	15	1.6 (0.8–3.4)
Olsson and Brandt, 1988	Lund Hospital patients		
	Exposed to herbicides		1.3 (0.8–2.1)
	Exposed to chlorophenols		1.2 (0.7–2.0)
Wiklund et al., 1988	Swedish agricultural and forestry workers		
	Workers in land or animal husbandry		1.0 (0.9–1.1)
	Timber cutters		0.9 (0.7–1.1)
Pearce et al., 1987	Male residents of New Zealand		
	Farming occupations		1.0 (0.7–1.5)
	Fencing work		1.4 (0.9–2.2)
Woods et al., 1987	Male residents of Washington State		
	Phenoxy herbicide use		1.1 (0.8–1.4)
	Chlorophenol use		1.0 (0.8–1.2)
	Farming occupations		1.3 (1.0–1.7)
	Forestry herbicide appliers		4.8 (1.2–19.4)
Hoar et al., 1986	Kansas residents		
	Farmers compared to nonfarmers	133	1.4 (0.9–2.1)
	Farmers using herbicides >20 days/year	7	6.0 (1.9–19.5)
Pearce et al., 1986	Male residents of New Zealand		
	Agricultural sprayers	19[e]	1.5 (0.7–3.3)
Pearce et al., 1985	Male residents of New Zealand		
	Agricultural occupations, ages 20–64		1.4 (0.9–2.0)
Burmeister et al., 1983	Iowa residents		
	Farmers		1.3
	Farmers in 33 counties with highest herbicide use		
	Born before 1890		3.4
	Born 1890–1900		2.2
	Born after 1900		1.3
Riihimiki et al., 1982	Finnish herbicide appliers	0	—
Wiklund, 1983	Swedish agricultural workers		1.1 (0.9–1.2)
Cantor, 1982	Wisconsin residents	175	1.2 (1.0–1.5)
Hardell et al., 1980	Umea Hospital patients		
	Exposed to phenoxy acids	41	4.8 (2.9–8.1)[d]
	Exposed to chlorophenols	50	4.3 (2.7–6.9)[d]
ENVIRONMENTAL			
New Studies			
Bertazzi et al., 2001	Seveso residents—20-year follow-up		
	Zone A males	1	3.2 (0.4–23.0)
	Zone A females	1	3.3 (0.5–23.7)
	Zone B males	2	0.9 (0.2–3.8)
	Zone B females	3	1.6 (0.5–4.9)

TABLE 7-26 *Continued*

Reference	Study Population	Exposed Cases[a]	Estimated Risk (95% CI)[a]
Schreinemachers, 2000	Rural or farm residents of Minnesota, Montana, North Dakota, and South Dakota		
	Males—counties with wheat acreage 23,000–110,999	186	0.8 (0.7–1.0)
	Males—counties with wheat acreage >111,000	176	0.9 (0.8–1.1)
	Females—counties with wheat acreage 23,000–110,999	202	1.0 (0.8–1.2)
	Females—counties with wheat acreage >111,000	162	1.0 (0.8–1.2)
Viel et al., 2000	Residents near a French municipal solid waste incinerator	286	1.3 ($p = .00003$)
Bertazzi et al., 1998	Seveso residents—15-year follow-up		
	Zone B males	2	1.5 (0.4–6.0)
	Zone R males	10	1.1 (0.5–2.1)
	Zone R females	8	0.9 (0.4–1.8)
Studies Reviewed in *Update 1998*			
Bertazzi et al., 1997	Seveso residents—15-year follow-up		
	Zone B males	2	1.5 (0.2–5.3)
Studies Reviewed in *Update 1996*			
Bertazzi et al., 1993	Seveso residents—10-year follow-up, morbidity		
	Zone B males	3	2.3 (0.7–7.4)
	Zone B females	1	0.9 (0.1–6.4)
	Zone R males	12	1.3 (0.7–2.5)
	Zone R females	10	1.2 (0.6–2.3)
Studies Reviewed in *VAO*			
Lampi et al., 1992	Finnish community exposed to chlorophenols		
	Compared to two uncontaminated municipalities		2.8 (1.4–5.6)
	Compared to cancer control region		2.1 (1.3–3.4)
Pesatori et al., 1992	Seveso residents		
	Zones A, B males	3	
	Zones A, B females	1	
	Zone R males	13	
	Zone R females	10	
Bertazzi et al., 1989b	Seveso residents—10-year follow-up		
	Zone B females	2	1.0 (0.3–4.2)
	Zone R males	3	1.0 (0.3–3.4)
	Zone R females	4	1.6 (0.5–4.7)
VIETNAM VETERANS			
New Studies			
AFHS, 2000	Air Force Ranch Hand veterans	1	0.2 (0.0–2.6)
AIHW, 1999	Australian Vietnam veterans	62	48 expected (34–62)

TABLE 7-26 Continued

Reference	Study Population	Exposed Cases[a]	Estimated Risk (95% CI)[a]
CDVA, 1998a	Australian Vietnam veterans—male	137[f]	48 expected (34–62)
CDVA, 1998b	Australian Vietnam veterans—female	2[f]	0 expected (0–4)
Studies Reviewed in *Update 1998*			
Crane et al., 1997a	Australian military Vietnam veterans		1.3 (0.5–3.5)
Watanabe and Kang, 1996	Marine Vietnam veterans		1.7 (1.2–2.2)
Studies Reviewed in *Update 1996*			
Visintainer et al., 1995	Michigan Vietnam veterans	32	1.5 (1.0–2.1)
Studies Reviewed in *VAO*			
Clapp et al., 1991	Massachusetts Vietnam veterans		1.2 (0.6–2.4)
Dalager et al., 1991	Vietnam veterans diagnosed with NHL	100	1.0 (0.7–1.8)
O'Brien et al., 1991	Army enlisted Vietnam veterans	7[g]	1.8
Thomas et al., 1991	Women Vietnam veterans	3	1.3 (0.3–1.8)
Watanabe et al., 1991	Army Vietnam veterans compared to Vietnam era Army veterans	140	0.8
	Army Vietnam veterans compared to combined Army and Marine Vietnam era veterans	140	0.9
	Marine Vietnam veterans compared to Vietnam era veterans	42	1.8
	Marine Vietnam veterans compared to combined Army and Marine Vietnam era veterans	42	1.2
CDC, 1990	U.S. men born between 1921 and 1953		
	Vietnam veterans	99	1.5 (1.1–2.0)
	Army Vietnam veterans	45	1.2 (0.8–1.8)
	Marine Vietnam veterans	10	1.8 (0.8–4.3)
	Air Force Vietnam veterans	12	1.0 (0.5–2.2)
	Navy Vietnam veterans	32	1.9 (1.1–3.2)
	Blue-water Navy Vietnam veterans	28	2.2 (1.2–3.9)
Michalek et al., 1990	Air Force Ranch Hand veteran mortality	0	
Wolfe et al., 1990	Air Force Ranch Hand veteran morbidity	1	
Breslin et al., 1988	Army Vietnam veterans	108	0.8 (0.6–1.0)
	Marine Vietnam veterans	35	2.1 (1.2–3.8)
Garland et al., 1988	Navy enlisted personnel 1974–1983		0.7
Burt et al., 1987	Army combat Vietnam veterans	39	1.1 (0.7–1.5)
	Marine combat Vietnam veterans	17	3.2 (1.4–7.4)
	Army Vietnam veterans (service 1967–1969)	64	0.9 (0.7–1.3)
	Marine Vietnam veterans (service 1967–1969)	17	2.5 (1.1–5.8)
Fett et al., 1987	Australian Vietnam veterans	4	1.8 (0.4–8.0)
Anderson et al., 1986a	Wisconsin Vietnam veterans		
	Wisconsin Vietnam veterans compared to Wisconsin nonveterans	13	0.7
	Wisconsin Vietnam veterans compared to non-Vietnam era veterans	13	0.6

TABLE 7-26 *Continued*

Reference	Study Population	Exposed Cases[a]	Estimated Risk (95% CI)[a]
	Wisconsin Vietnam veterans compared to Vietnam era veterans	13	1.0
Anderson et al., 1986b	Wisconsin Vietnam veterans compared to general population	24	0.7
	Wisconsin Vietnam veterans compared to Wisconsin veterans	24	1.1
Holmes et al., 1986	West Virginia Vietnam veterans compared to West Virginia Vietnam era veterans	2	1.1
Lawrence et al., 1985	New York Vietnam veterans	10[d]	1.0 (0.4–2.2)

NOTE: USDA = United States Department of Agriculture.

[a] Given when available.
[b] Includes NHL and chronic lymphocytic leukemia combined.
[c] Includes all lymphomas combined.
[d] Includes both NHL and Hodgkin's disease.
[e] Only NHL other than lymphosarcoma and reticulosarcoma (ICD·9 202).
[f] Self-reported medical history. Answer to question: Since your first day of service in Vietnam, have you been told by a doctor that you have NHL?
[g] NHL, 4 living cases and 3 deaths listed by Boyle et al. (1987).

HODGKIN'S DISEASE

Background

Hodgkin's disease (ICD·9 201.0–201.9) is distinct from NHL in its cell of origin, demographics, and genetics. According to American Cancer Society estimates, 4,200 men and 3,200 women will be diagnosed with the disease in the United States in 2000, and 700 men and an equal number of women will die from it (ACS, 2000a).

HD is less common in individuals in the age groups that characterize most Vietnam veterans than in individuals both younger and older. For individuals older than 40, the incidence rate for males generally exceeds that for females and the rate for whites exceeds that for African Americans. However, the very small numbers of cases indicates that care should be exercised when interpreting the figures.

The potential infectious nature of HD has been a topic of discussion since its earliest description. Increased incidence in individuals with a history of infectious mononucleosis has been observed in some studies, and a link with Epstein-Barr virus has been proposed. In addition to the occupational associations discussed below, higher rates of the disease have been observed in individuals with suppressed or compromised immune systems.

Average Annual Cancer Incidence (per 100,000 individuals) in the United States[a]
Hodgkin's Disease

	45–49 Years of Age			50–54 Years of Age			55–59 Years of Age		
	All Races	White	Black	All Races	White	Black	All Races	White	Black
Males	3.5	3.6	3.6	3.3	3.6	2.2	3.7	3.8	5.5
Females	1.7	1.8	1.6	1.9	2.1	1.9	2.0	2.2	1.2

[a] SEER nine standard registries, crude age-specific rate, 1993–1997.

Summary of *VAO*, *Update 1996*, and *Update 1998*

The committee responsible for *VAO* found there was sufficient information to determine that an association existed between exposure to herbicides used in Vietnam or the contaminant dioxin and Hodgkin's disease. Additional information available to the committees responsible for *Update 1996* and *Update 1998* did not change this finding. Table 7-27 provides summaries of the results of the studies underlying these findings and a list of reports that contain details of the research.

Update of the Scientific Literature

Occupational Studies

Hooiveld and colleagues' (1998) retrospective cohort study of 549 exposed and 482 unexposed male Dutch production and contract workers exposed to phenoxy herbicides, chlorophenols, and contaminants between 1950 and 1976 reported 1 death from HD in the cohorts under examination (SMR = 3.2, 0.1–17.6).

Rix et al. (1998) examined mortality in a cohort of 14,362 male and female Danish paper mill workers, an occupation with presumed exposure to chlorinated organic compounds including dioxins. Incident cancer cases were identified from the Danish Cancer Register, and expected numbers of cases were calculated using the rates for the total Danish population by gender, 5-year age group, and calendar time. Poisson regression models were used to analyze by duration and years since first employment and by department of employment. The authors report a statistically significant elevation in HD incidence in males (SIR = 2.0, 1.2–3.2; based on 18 cases) but not females (SIR = 1.0, 0.1–3.8; based on 2 cases). Most of the males diagnosed with HD were involved in storage and transport (SIR = 4.1).

Steenland et al. (1999), in an update and expansion of cohorts involved in the

NIOSH study, performed mortality analyses involving 5,132 chemical workers at 12 U.S. plants. The 3 deaths attributed to HD were consistent with the number anticipated (SMR = 1.1, 0.2–3.2).

Environmental Studies

The highest documented environmental exposure to TCDD continues to be the Seveso cohort. Details of this ongoing study are given in Chapter 6. The 15-year update (Bertazzi et al., 1998, 1999) did not report any HD deaths in the high-exposure area, zone A. There was elevated HD mortality for both men (RR = 3.3, 0.8–14.0; based on 2 deaths) and women (RR = 6.5, 1.5–29.0; based on 2 deaths) in zone B, the medium-exposure area. The low-exposure area, zone R, reported no deaths from this cancer for males and 4 for females (RR = 1.9, 0.6–5.8). A later study (Bertazzi et al., 2001) extended the mortality analysis to 20 years following the event for zones A and B. No additional HD deaths were reported in either zone, leading to lowered calculated relative risks for males (3.0, 0.7–12.4) and females (4.3, 1.0–18.3) in zone B in this latest follow-up.

Viel et al. (2000) examined whether there were cancer clusters in an area surrounding a municipal solid waste incinerator located near Doubs, France. High-dioxin emissions (16.3 ng I-TEQ/m^3, far in excess of the EU standard of 0.1 ng I-TEQ/m^3), had been measured from the incinerator, and elevated levels were detected in the milk from cows that grazed near the facility. Data from a general population cancer registry over the years 1980–1995 were combined with demographic information for the analysis. Hodgkin's disease incidence exhibited no specific spatial distribution. When the analysis time frame was limited to 1992–1993, an elevated SIR of 1.5 was observed in the area around the incinerator, but this was based on 9 cases and did not reach statistical significance (p = .9). However, the authors do not provide any direct evidence of human exposure.

Schreinemachers (2000) examined cancer mortality in white males and females over the years 1980–1989 in four northern wheat-producing states, using wheat acreage per county as a surrogate for exposure to chlorophenoxy herbicides (including 2,4-D). There was a statistically significant elevation in the age-standardized mortality rate ratio for males in counties with 23,000–110,999 acres under wheat cultivation (SRR = 1.8, 1.1–2.9; based on 32 deaths). HD mortality for females in these counties and for both males and females in counties with greater than 111,000 acres under wheat cultivation was the expected numbers of cases.

Vietnam Veteran Studies

In the most recently published 15-year update of the Ranch Hand study, AFHS (2000) researchers report that the incidence of Hodgkin's disease among the Ranch Hand (1 case among 861 subjects) and comparison (3 cases among

1,249 subjects) populations was limited (RR = 0.3, 0.0–3.2; Model 1, adjusted). Given the small numbers of cases, all analyses were nonsignificant.

Synthesis

The relatively low incidence of HD complicates the evaluation of epidemiologic studies addressing this lymphoreticular tumor. Newly published studies report small numbers of cases and are imprecise, although the pattern is one of excess risk in nearly all exposed study populations. However, earlier studies carried out in Sweden (for example, the work of Hardell and colleagues) were well conducted, based on good exposure characterization, and have not been contradicted by later work. The committee believes that data available for review in this report, when combined with information available to previous *Veterans and Agent Orange* committees, demonstrate a pattern of elevated mortality and morbidity risk. Although not as clearly demonstrated as for NHL, biologic plausibility also exists for a positive association between TCDD and the development of HD due to their common lymphoreticular origin and association with common risk factors.

Conclusions

Strength of Evidence in Epidemiologic Studies

Based on its evaluation of the epidemiologic evidence reviewed in this and previous *Veterans and Agent Orange* reports, the committee finds there is sufficient evidence to conclude that an association exists between exposure to herbicides (2,4-D, 2,4,5-T and its contaminant TCDD, cacodylic acid, and picloram) and Hodgkin's disease.

Biologic Plausibility

No animal studies have found an increased incidence of Hodgkin's disease. A summary of the biologic plausibility for the carcinogenicity of TCDD and the herbicides in general is presented in the conclusion to this chapter. A discussion of toxicological studies that concern biologic plausibility is contained in Chapter 3.

Increased Risk of Disease Among Vietnam Veterans

The available data on Hodgkin's disease in Vietnam veterans are too limited to form the basis of a conclusion regarding increased risk.

TABLE 7-27 Selected Epidemiologic Studies—Hodgkin's Disease

Reference	Study Population	Exposed Cases[a]	Estimated Risk (95% CI)[a]
OCCUPATIONAL			
New Studies			
Steenland et al., 1999	U.S. chemical production workers	3	1.1 (0.2–3.2)
Hooiveld et al., 1998	Dutch chemical production workers	1	3.2 (0.1–17.6)
Rix et al., 1998	Danish paper mill workers		
	Men	18	2.0 (1.2–3.2)
	Women	2	1.1 (0.1–3.8)
Studies Reviewed in *Update 1998*			
Gambini et al., 1997	Italian rice growers	1	0.7 (0.1–3.6)
Kogevinas et al., 1997	IARC cohort		1.0 (0.5–1.8)
Becher et al., 1996	German chemical production workers		NS
Ramlow et al., 1996	Pentachlorophenol production workers		NS
Waterhouse et al., 1996	Residents of Tecumseh, Michigan		2.9 (1.1–3.4)
Studies Reviewed in *Update 1996*			
Asp et al., 1994	Finnish herbicide appliers	2	1.7 (0.2–6.0)
Blair et al., 1993	U.S. farmers from 23 states—white males	56	1.0 (0.8–1.3)
Kogevinas et al., 1993	IARC cohort—females	1	
Persson et al., 1993	Swedish NHL patients		
	Exposure to phenoxy herbicides	5	7.4 (1.4–40.0)[b]
Kogevinas et al., 1992	IARC cohort	3	0.6 (0.1–1.7)
Studies Reviewed in *VAO*			
Eriksson et al., 1992	Swedish Cancer Registry patients		
	Male sawmill workers	10	2.2
	Male farmers	97	1.2
	Male forestry workers	35	1.2
	Male horticulture workers	11	1.2
Ronco et al., 1992	Danish and Italian farm workers		
	Male Danish farmers—self-employed	27	0.6
	Male Italian farmers—self-employed	10	2.9
	Male Italian farmers—employees	1	0.4
	Male Italian farmers—self-employed and employees	11	1.9
	Female Italian farmers—self-employed	1	1.9
Swaen et al., 1992	Dutch herbicide appliers	1	3.3
Fingerhut et al., 1991	NIOSH cohort	3	1.2 (0.3–3.5)
	20-year latency, 1+ years of exposure	1	—
Green, 1991	Ontario herbicide sprayers	0	—
Saracci et al., 1991	IARC cohort	2	0.4 (0.1–1.4)
Zober et al., 1990	BASF production workers	0	—
Alavanja et al., 1989	USDA forest or soil conservationists	4	2.2 (0.6–5.6)
LaVecchia et al., 1989	Residents of the Milan, Italy, area		
	Agricultural occupations		2.1 (1.0–3.8)
	Chemical industry occupations		4.3 (1.4–10.2)
Persson et al., 1989	Orebro Hospital patients		
	Farming	6	1.2 (0.4–3.5)
	Exposed to phenoxy acids	4	3.8 (0.5–35.2)
Wiklund et al., 1989b	Swedish pesticide appliers	15	1.5 (0.8–2.4)

TABLE 7-27 *Continued*

Reference	Study Population	Exposed Cases[a]	Estimated Risk (95% CI)[a]
Alavanja et al., 1988	USDA agricultural extension agents		
	PMR analysis	6	2.7 (1.2–6.3)
	Case-control analysis	6	1.1 (0.3–3.5)
Bond et al., 1988	Dow workers with chloracne	1	
Dubrow et al., 1988	Ohio residents	3	2.7
Wiklund et al., 1988	Swedish agricultural and forestry workers		
	Workers in land or animal husbandry	242	1.0 (0.9–1.2)
	Workers in silviculture	15	2.3 (1.3–3.7)
Hoar et al., 1986	Kansas residents		
	All farmers	71	0.8 (0.5–1.2)
	Farm use of herbicides (phenoxy acids and others)		0.9 (0.5–1.5)
	Farmers using herbicides >20 days/year	3	1.0 (0.2–4.1)
	Farmers using herbicides >15 years	10	1.2 (0.5–2.6)
Pearce et al., 1985	Male residents of New Zealand		
	Agricultural occupations, ages 20–64		1.0 (0.6–2.0)
Burmeister et al., 1983	Iowa residents		1.4
Hardell and Bengtsson, 1983	Umea Hospital patients		
	Exposed to phenoxy acids	6	5.0 (2.4–10.2)
	Exposed to high-grade chlorophenols	9	6.5 (2.7–19.0)
	Exposed to low-grade chlorophenols	5	2.4 (0.9–6.5)
Riihimaki et al., 1982	Finnish herbicide appliers	0	—
Wiklund, 1983	Swedish agricultural workers	226	1.0 (0.9–1.2)[c]
Burmeister, 1981	Farmers in Iowa		1.2
Hardell et al., 1980	Umea Hospital patients		
	Exposed to phenoxy acids	41	4.8 (2.9–8.1)[d]
	Exposed to chlorophenols	50	4.3 (2.7–6.9)[d]
ENVIRONMENTAL			
New Studies			
Bertazzi et al., 2001	Seveso residents—20-year follow-up		
	Zone B males	2	3.0 (0.7–12.4)
	Zone B females	2	4.3 (1.0–18.3)
Schreinemachers, 2000	Rural or farm residents of Minnesota, Montana, North Dakota, and South Dakota		
	Males—counties with wheat acreage 23,000–110,999	32	1.8 (1.1–2.9)
	Males—counties with wheat acreage >111,000	14	0.8 (0.4–1.5)
	Females—counties with wheat acreage 23,000–110,999	19	1.0 (0.6–1.9)
	Females—counties with wheat acreage >111,000	14	0.9 (0.4–1.7)

TABLE 7-27 Continued

Reference	Study Population	Exposed Cases[a]	Estimated Risk (95% CI)[a]
Viel et al., 2000	Residents around a French municipal solid waste incinerator	9	1.5
Bertazzi et al., 1998	Seveso residents—15-year follow-up		
	Zone B males	2	3.3 (0.8–14.0)
	Zone B females	2	6.5 (1.5–29.0)
	Zone R females	4	1.9 (0.6–5.8)
Studies Reviewed in *Update 1998*			
Bertazzi et al., 1997	Seveso residents—15-year follow-up		
	Zone B males	2	3.3 (0.4–11.9)
	Zone B females	2	6.5 (0.7–23.5)
	Zone R females	4	1.9 (0.5–4.9)
Studies Reviewed in *Update 1996*			
Bertazzi et al., 1993	Seveso residents—10-year follow-up, morbidity		
	Zone B males	1	1.7 (0.2–12.8)
	Zone B females	1	2.1 (0.3–15.7)
	Zone R males	4	1.1 (0.4–3.1)
	Zone R females	3	1.0 (0.3–3.2)
VIETNAM VETERANS			
New Studies			
AFHS, 2000	Air Force Ranch Hand veterans	1	0.3 (0.0–3.2)
Studies Reviewed in *Update 1998*			
Watanabe and Kang, 1996	Marine and Army Vietnam veterans		1.9 (1.2–2.7)
Studies Reviewed in *Update 1996*			
Visintainer et al., 1995	Michigan Vietnam veterans	20	1.1 (0.7–1.8)
Studies Reviewed in *VAO*			
Watanabe et al., 1991	Army Vietnam veterans compared to Vietnam era Army veterans	116	1.0
	Marine Vietnam veterans compared to Vietnam era veterans	25	1.9
	Army Vietnam veterans compared to Vietnam era veterans	116	1.1
	Marine Vietnam veterans compared to Vietnam era veterans	25	1.0
CDC, 1990	U.S. men born between 1921 and 1953		
	Vietnam veterans	28	1.2 (0.7–2.4)
	Army Vietnam veterans	12	1.0 (0.5–2.0)
	Marine Vietnam veterans	4	1.7 (0.5–5.9)
	Air Force Vietnam veterans	5	1.7 (0.6–4.9)
	Navy Vietnam veterans	7	1.1 (0.4–2.6)
Michalek et al., 1990; Wolfe et al., 1990	Air Force Ranch Hand veteran mortality	0	—
Breslin et al., 1988	Army Vietnam veterans compared to Vietnam era Army veterans	92	1.2 (0.7–1.9)
	Marine Vietnam veterans compared to Marine Vietnam era veterans	22	1.3 (0.7–2.6)

TABLE 7-27 *Continued*

Reference	Study Population	Exposed Cases[a]	Estimated Risk (95% CI)[a]
Boyle et al., 1987	Vietnam Experience Study	0	—
Fett et al., 1987	Australian Vietnam veterans	0	—
Anderson et al., 1986a	Wisconsin Vietnam veterans compared to Wisconsin nonveterans	6	0.5 (0.2–1.2)
	Wisconsin Vietnam veterans compared to non-Vietnam era veterans	6	1.0 (0.4–2.2)
	Wisconsin Vietnam veterans compared to Vietnam era veterans	6	1.0 (0.4–2.1)
Anderson et al., 1986b	Wisconsin Vietnam veterans	4	—
Holmes et al., 1986	West Virginia Vietnam veterans compared to West Virginia Vietnam era veterans	5	8.3 (2.7–19.5)
Lawrence et al., 1985	New York Vietnam veterans compared to New York Vietnam era veterans	10[c]	1.0 (0.4–2.2)

NOTE: USDA = United States Department of Agriculture.
[a] Given when available.
[b] 90% CI.
[c] 99% CI.
[d] Includes both NHL and HD.

MULTIPLE MYELOMA

Background

Multiple myeloma (MM) (ICD·9 203.0, 203.2–203.8) is characterized by the proliferation of bone marrow stem cells that results in an excess of neoplastic plasma cells and the production of excess abnormal proteins, usually immunoglobulins. The American Cancer Society estimates that 7,300 men and 6,300 women in the U.S. will be diagnosed with this disease in 2000 and that 5,800 men and 5,400 women will die from it (ACS, 2000a).

MM incidence is highly age dependent, with a relatively low rate in individuals under 40 and most cases occurring between 55 and 70 years of age. Rates for African Americans are about twice those for whites. Incidence in males is slightly higher than in females, with the difference becoming more pronounced with age.

Increased incidence of MM has been observed in several occupational groups, including farmers and agricultural workers and those with workplace exposure to rubber, leather, paint, and petroleum (Riedel et al., 1991). Individuals with high exposure to ionizing radiation are also at greater risk. Evidence regarding other risk factors is mixed.

Average Annual Cancer Incidence (per 100,000 Individuals) in the United States[a]
Multiple Myeloma

	45–49 Years of Age			50–54 Years of Age			55–59 Years of Age		
	All Races	White	Black	All Races	White	Black	All Races	White	Black
Males	3.3	2.8	6.7	7.3	6.4	15.7	12.1	10.5	28.1
Females	2.6	2.1	7.1	5.0	4.0	15.9	6.9	5.9	17.0

[a] SEER nine standard registries, crude age-specific rate, 1993–1997.

Summary of *VAO*, *Update 1996*, and *Update 1998*

The committee responsible for *VAO* found that there was limited or suggestive evidence to determine whether an association existed between exposure to herbicides used in Vietnam or the contaminant dioxin and multiple myeloma. Additional information available to the committees responsible for *Update 1996* and *Update 1998* did not change this finding. Table 7-28 provides summaries of the results of the studies underlying these findings and a list of reports that contain details of the research.

Update of the Scientific Literature

Occupational Studies

Hooiveld and colleagues' (1998) retrospective cohort study of 549 exposed and 482 unexposed male Dutch production and contract workers exposed to phenoxy herbicides, chlorophenols, and contaminants between 1950 and 1976 did not identify any deaths from MM in the cohorts under examination.

In an update and expansion of cohorts involved in the NIOSH study, Steenland et al. (1999) performed mortality analyses involving 5,132 chemical workers at 12 U.S. plants by use of life table techniques (U.S. population referent) and Cox regression (internal referent). The SMR for MM, based on 10 deaths since 1960, was 2.1 (1.0–3.8). Although the case numbers for multiple myeloma were relatively low and the authors did not comment specifically on this diagnosis, this SMR was the fourth highest among the total study cohort.

Environmental Studies

Bertazzi et al. (1998) continue the follow-up of people environmentally exposed to TCDD in Seveso, Italy. Details of this ongoing study are given in Chapter 6. Their 1998 paper updates the population after 15 years' follow-up. There were no deaths due to MM in zone A, the high-exposure area. The number of deaths for males in the medium-exposure area—zone B—was equal to that expected (RR = 1.1, 0.2–8.2; based on 1 death). However, the 4 deaths observed in zone B females were significantly in excess of the 0.6 expected (RR = 6.6, 2.3–18.5). In zone R, where residents had much lower potential exposure to TCDD than in zones A and B, the observed number of deaths was close to the expected number for both males (0.8, 0.3–2.0; based on 5 deaths) and females (1.0, 0.4–2.5; based on 5 deaths).

A later study (Bertazzi et al., 2001) extended the mortality analysis to 20 years following the event for zones A and B. No additional MM deaths were reported in either zone, leading to lowered calculated relative risks for males (RR = 0.7, 0.1–5.0) and females (3.7, 1.3–10.2).

Schreinemachers (2000) examined cancer mortality over the years 1980–1989 in four northern wheat-producing states, using wheat acreage per county as a surrogate for exposure to chlorophenoxy herbicides (including 2,4-D). The analysis of MM yielded age-standardized mortality rate ratios near unity for white males and females. None of the values were statistically significant.

Vietnam Veteran Studies

In their 15-year update of the Ranch Hand study, AFHS (2000) researchers reported a relatively sparse number of "other malignant neoplasms of lymphoid and histiocytic tissue"—a diagnostic category that includes the leukemias and multiple myeloma—among Ranch Hands (2 of 861) and comparisons (4 of 1,249) (RR = 0.7, 0.1–5.0; Model 1, adjusted). These numbers were too limited to permit meaningful analyses.

Synthesis

As previous reports have stated, the low incidence of MM among the various cohorts that have been studied makes it difficult to draw firm conclusions from every study. Of the studies reviewed for the first time in this report, only Steenland et al. (1999) has both a sufficient number of cases and data that clearly point to exposure to the herbicides and contaminants most relevant to Vietnam veterans. A twofold increased risk was observed, based on 10 cases (1.0–3.8).

Conclusions

Strength of Evidence in Epidemiologic Studies

There is limited/suggestive evidence of an association between exposure to herbicides (2,4-D, 2,4,5-T and its contaminant TCDD, cacodylic acid, and picloram) and multiple myeloma. The evidence regarding association is drawn from earlier occupational and other studies in which subjects were exposed to a variety of herbicides and herbicide components.

Biologic Plausibility

No animal studies have found an increased incidence of multiple myeloma. A summary of the biologic plausibility for the carcinogenicity of TCDD and the herbicides in general is presented in the conclusion to this chapter. A discussion of toxicological studies that concern biologic plausibility is contained in Chapter 3.

Increased Risk of Disease among Vietnam Veterans

There are insufficient data on multiple myeloma in Vietnam veterans to draw a specific conclusion as to whether or not they are at increased risk.

TABLE 7-28 Selected Epidemiologic Studies—Multiple Myeloma

Reference	Study Population	Exposed Cases[a]	Estimated Risk (95% CI)[a]
OCCUPATIONAL			
New Studies			
Steenland et al., 1999	U.S. chemical production workers	10	2.1 (1.0–3.8)
Hooiveld et al., 1998	Dutch chemical production workers	0	—
Studies Reviewed in *Update 1998*			
Gambini et al., 1997	Italian rice growers	0	—
Kogevinas et al., 1997	IARC cohort		
	Workers exposed to TCDD		
	(or higher-chlorinated dioxins)		1.2 (0.6–2.3)
	Workers not exposed to TCDD		
	(or higher-chlorinated dioxins)		1.6 (0.7–3.1)
	Workers exposed to any phenoxy		
	herbicide or chlorophenol	17	1.3 (0.8–2.1)
Becher et al., 1996	German chemical production workers—Plant I	3	5.4 (1.1–15.9)
Studies Reviewed in *Update 1996*			
Asp et al., 1994	Finnish herbicide appliers	3	2.6 (0.5–7.7)
Dean, 1994	Irish farmers and farm workers	170	1.0
Semenciw et al., 1994	Farmers in Canadian prairie provinces	160	0.8 (0.7–1.0)
Blair et al., 1993	U.S. farmers from 23 states		
	White males	413	1.2 (1.0–1.3)
	White females	14	1.8 (1.0–3.0)
	Nonwhite males	51	0.9 (0.7–1.2)
	Nonwhite females	11	1.1 (0.6–2.0)
	Farmers in central U.S. states		
	White males	233	1.2
	White females	12	2.6

TABLE 7-28 Continued

Reference	Study Population	Exposed Cases[a]	Estimated Risk (95% CI)[a]
Brown et al., 1993	Iowa male users of pesticides or herbicides	111	1.2 (0.8–1.7)
Lynge, 1993	Danish production workers		
	Male	0	—
	Female	2	12.5 (1.5–45.1)
Zahm et al., 1992	Eastern Nebraska users of herbicides		
	Male	8	0.6 (0.2–1.7)
	Female	10	2.3 (0.8–7.0)
	Eastern Nebraska users of insecticides		
	Male	11	0.6 (0.2–1.4)
	Female	21	2.8 (1.1–7.3)
Studies Reviewed in *VAO*			
Eriksson and Karlsson, 1992	Residents of northern Sweden	20	2.2 (1.0–5.7)
Swaen et al., 1992	Dutch herbicide appliers	3	8.2 (1.6–23.8)
Fingerhut et al., 1991	NIOSH cohort	5	1.6 (0.5–3.9)
	20-year latency, 1+ years of exposure	3	2.6 (0.5–7.7)
Saracci et al., 1991	IARC cohort	4	0.7 (0.2–1.8)
Alavanja et al., 1989	USDA forest or soil conservationists		1.3 (0.5–2.8)
Boffetta et al., 1989	ACS Prevention Study II subjects	12	2.1 (1.0–4.2)
	Farmers using herbicides or pesticides	8	4.3 (1.7–10.9)
LaVecchia et al., 1989	Residents of the Milan, Italy, area		
	Agricultural employment		2.0 (1.1–3.5)
Morris et al., 1986	Residents of four SEER areas		2.9 (1.5–5.5)
Pearce et al., 1986	Male residents of New Zealand		
	Use of agricultural spray	16	1.3 (0.7–2.5)
	Likely sprayed 2,4,5-T	14	1.6 (0.8–3.1)
Cantor and Blair, 1984	Wisconsin residents		
	Farmers in counties with highest herbicide usage		1.4 (0.8–2.3)
Burmeister et al., 1983	Iowa residents (farmers in counties with highest herbicide usage)		
	Born 1890–1900		2.7 ($p < .05$)
	Born after 1900		2.4 ($p < .05$)
Riihimaki et al., 1982	Finnish herbicide appliers	1	2.5 (0.3–14.0)
ENVIRONMENTAL			
New Studies			
Bertazzi et al., 2001	Seveso residents—20-year follow-up		
	Zone B males	1	0.7 (0.1–5.0)
	Zone B females	4	3.7 (1.3–10.2)
Schreinemachers, 2000	Rural or farm residents of Minnesota, Montana, North Dakota, and South Dakota		
	Males—counties with wheat acreage 23,000–110,999	108	1.0 (0.8–1.3)
	Males—counties with wheat acreage >111,000	75	0.8 (0.6–1.0)

TABLE 7-28 Continued

Reference	Study Population	Exposed Cases[a]	Estimated Risk (95% CI)[a]
	Females—counties with wheat acreage 23,000–110,999	91	1.0 (0.8–1.3)
	Females—counties with wheat acreage >111,000	77	1.0 (0.7–1.3)
Bertazzi et al., 1998	Seveso residents—15-year follow-up		
	Zone B males	1	1.1 (0.2–8.2)
	Zone B females	4	6.6 (2.3–18.5)
	Zone R males	5	0.8 (0.3–2.0)
	Zone R females	5	1.0 (0.4–2.5)
Studies Reviewed in *Update 1998*			
Bertazzi et al., 1997	Seveso residents—15-year follow-up		
	Zone B females	4	6.6 (1.8–16.8)
Studies Reviewed in *Update 1996*			
Bertazzi et al., 1993	Seveso residents—10-year follow-up, morbidity		
	Zone B males	2	3.2 (0.8–13.3)
	Zone B females	2	5.3 (1.2–22.6)
	Zone R males	1	0.2 (0.0–1.6)
	Zone R females	2	0.6 (0.2–2.8)
Studies Reviewed in *VAO*			
Pesatori et al., 1992	Seveso residents		
	Zones A, B males	2	2.7 (0.6–11.3)
	Zones A, B females	2	4.4 (1.0–18.7)
	Zone R males	1	0.2 (0.0–1.5)
	Zone R females	3	0.9 (0.3–3.1)
VIETNAM VETERANS			
New Studies			
AFHS, 2000	Air Force Ranch Hand veterans	2	0.7 (0.1–5.0)
Studies Reviewed in *Update 1998*			
Crane et al., 1997a	Australian military Vietnam veterans	6	0.6 (0.2–1.4)
Crane et al., 1997b	Australian military Vietnam veterans	0	
Watanabe and Kang, 1996	Army Vietnam veterans		0.9
	Marine Vietnam veterans		0.6
Studies Reviewed in *VAO*			
Breslin et al., 1988	Army Vietnam veterans		0.8 (0.2–2.5)
	Marine Vietnam veterans	2	0.5 (0.0–17.1)

NOTE: USDA = United States Department of Agriculture.
[a] Given when available.

LEUKEMIA

Background

There are four primary types of leukemia (ICD·9 202.4, 203.1, 204.0–204.9, 205.0–205.9, 206.0–206.9, 207.0–207.2, 207.8, 208.0–208.9): the acute and chronic forms of lymphocytic leukemia and the acute and chronic forms of myeloid (or granulocytic) leukemia. According to American Cancer Society estimates, 16,900 men and 13,900 women will be diagnosed with some form of the disease in the United States in 2000, and 12,100 men and 9,600 women will die from it (ACS, 2000a). Collectively, leukemias were expected to account for 2.5 percent of all new cancer diagnoses and nearly 4 percent of cancer deaths in 2000.

The different forms of leukemia have different patterns of incidence and, in some cases, different risk factors.

Acute lymphocytic leukemia (ALL) is a disease of the young and of individuals older than 70, and plays a rather small role in the age groups that characterize most Vietnam veterans. The lifetime incidence of ALL is slightly higher in whites than African Americans and in males than females. Exposure to high doses of ionizing radiation is a known risk factor for this form of leukemia; evidence for other factors is inconsistent.

Acute myeloid leukemia (AML) is the most common leukemia among adults—the incidence increasing steadily with age for individuals older than 40. In the Vietnam veteran age groups, AML accounts for roughly one out of every four leukemias in men and one out of three in women. Overall, this leukemia is slightly more common in males than females. White males have a higher incidence than white females; the lifetime incidence in African-American males and females is roughly equal. Risk factors associated with an increased risk of AML include high doses of ionizing radiation, occupational exposure to benzene, and some medications used in cancer chemotherapy (melphalan, for example). Genetic disorders including Fanconi's anemia and Down's syndrome are associated with an increased risk of AML, and tobacco smoking has been suggested as a risk factor.

Chronic lymphocytic leukemia (CLL) is the most common of the four primary types of leukemia in men. It is largely a disease of individuals older than 40, and incidence doubles every 5 years for individuals in the three age groups that characterize most Vietnam veterans. Over a lifetime, CLL is nearly twice as common in whites than African Americans and more common in men than women. Some occupational groups, notably farmers, appear to have a higher incidence of CLL than would otherwise be expected. A family history of the disease and a compromised immune system are among additional suspected risk factors. Unlike the other primary forms of leukemia, exposure to ionizing radiation does not appear to be associated with increased incidence of CLL.

The incidence of chronic myeloid leukemia (CML) increases steadily with age for individuals over 30. Lifetime incidence is roughly equal in whites and African Americans and is slightly higher in males than females. For individuals in the age groups that characterize most Vietnam veterans, CML accounts for approximately one in five leukemias. CML is associated with an acquired chromosomal abnormality known as the "Philadelphia chromosome." Exposure to high doses of ionizing radiation is a known risk factor for this abnormality; other factors are under study.

Little is known about the risk factors associated with other forms of leukemia. However, two human retroviruses have been linked to human leukemias: HTLV-1 appears to cause adult T-cell leukemia or lymphoma, whereas the data linking HTLV-2 to hairy cell leukemia are less definitive.

Average Annual Cancer Incidence (per 100,000 individuals) in the United States[a]
Leukemias

	45–49 Years of Age			50–54 Years of Age			55–59 Years of Age		
	All Races	White	Black	All Races	White	Black	All Races	White	Black
All Leukemias									
Males	8.2	8.3	7.7	14.5	14.9	13.1	18.8	19.4	15.6
Females	5.7	5.3	7.4	9.4	10.0	5.1	11.8	12.1	8.5
Acute Lymphocytic Leukemia									
Males	0.7	0.6	1.0	0.9	0.9	[b]	0.8	0.8	1.0
Females	0.2	0.3	0.2	0.5	0.4	[b]	0.5	0.5	0.8
Chronic Lymphocytic Leukemia									
Males	2.4	2.5	2.6	5.2	5.1	6.0	7.6	7.9	7.5
Females	1.1	1.1	1.1	2.3	2.6	1.3	3.8	4.1	0.4
Acute Myeloid Leukemia									
Males	2.0	2.0	2.1	3.1	3.3	3.0	4.2	4.7	2.0
Females	2.3	2.1	3.6	3.5	3.7	2.5	3.7	3.8	3.2
Chronic Myeloid Leukemia									
Males	1.5	1.4	1.3	2.2	2.3	3.4	2.9	2.8	4.0
Females	1.1	1.0	1.1	1.7	1.8	1.0	1.8	1.7	2.4
All Other Leukemias[c]									
Males	1.1	1.2	0.5	2.3	2.5	0.8	2.5	2.6	1.0
Females	0.7	0.7	0.5	0.7	0.8	0.3	1.5	1.5	0.8

[a] SEER nine standard registries, crude age-specific rate, 1993–1997.
[b] Insufficient data to provide a meaningful incidence rate.
[c] Includes leukemic reticuloendotheliosis (hairy cell), plasma cell, monocytic, and acute and chronic erythremia and erythroleukemia.

Summary of *VAO*, *Update 1996*, and *Update 1998*

The committee responsible for *VAO* found there to be inadequate or insufficient information to determine whether an association existed between exposure to herbicides used in Vietnam or the contaminant dioxin and leukemia. Additional information available to the committees responsible for *Update 1996* and *Update 1998* did not change this finding. Table 7-29 provides summaries of the

Update of the Scientific Literature

Occupational Studies

Hooiveld and colleagues' (1998) retrospective cohort study of 549 exposed and 482 unexposed male Dutch production and contract workers exposed to phenoxy herbicides, chlorophenols, and contaminants between 1950 and 1976 reported 1 death attributed to leukemia (SMR = 1.0, 0.0–5.7).

A study of cancer incidence among workers in three paper production plants in Denmark by Rix et al. (1998) reviewed cancer registry data over the years 1943–1990. Among men, 20 cases were observed while 25.4 were expected, leading to an SIR of 0.8 (0.5–1.2). For women, 7 cases were observed for women while 5.4 were expected (SIR = 1.3, 0.5–2.7).

In the update of the industrial cohort exposed to dioxins known as the NIOSH cohort, Steenland et al. (1999) performed mortality analyses involving 5,132 chemical workers at 12 U.S. plants by use of life table techniques (U.S. population referent) and Cox regression (internal referent). The SMR for leukemia was 0.8 (0.4–1.5), based on 10 deaths.

Environmental Studies

Bertazzi et al. (1998, 1999) continue the follow-up of people environmentally exposed to TCDD in Seveso, Italy. Details of this ongoing study are given in Chapter 6. These papers update the population after 15 years' follow-up. There were no deaths due to leukemia in zone A, the high-exposure area. Among men in the medium-exposure area—zone B—there were 7 deaths (RR = 3.1, 1.4–6.7); among women, 1 death (RR = 0.6, 0.1–4.0). In zone R, where residents had much lower potential exposure to TCDD than in zones A and B, there were 12 deaths from leukemia each in men (0.8, 0.4–1.5) and women (0.9, 0.5–1.6).

A later study (Bertazzi et al., 2001) extends the mortality analysis to 20 years following the event for zones A and B only. There was no change in leukemia mortality in zone A. In zone B, 9 deaths were reported for males where 3.8 were expected, for a statistically significant relative risk of 2.4 (1.2–4.7). Of these deaths, 5 were attributed to myeloid leukemias (RR = 3.8, 1.5–9.6). The 3 observed deaths among females were comparable to the 2.7 expected (RR = 1.1, 0.4–3.5).

Schreinemachers (2000) examined cancer mortality over the years 1980–1989 in four northern wheat-producing states, using wheat acreage per county as a surrogate for exposure to chlorophenoxy herbicides (including 2,4-D). The leukemia analysis yielded age-standardized mortality rate ratios near unity for white males and females. None of the values were statistically significant.

Vietnam Veteran Studies

In their 15-year update of the Ranch Hand study, AFHS (2000) researchers reported a relatively sparse number of "other malignant neoplasms of lymphoid and histiocytic tissue"—a diagnostic category that includes the leukemias and multiple myeloma—among Ranch Hands (2 of 861) and comparisons (4 of 1,249) (RR = 0.7, 0.1–5.0; Model 1, adjusted). Given the small number of cases, all analyses led to nonsignificant results.

The government of Australia conducted mail surveys of approximately 50,000 male and female nationals who served in Vietnam, including those involved in combat, medical teams, war correspondents, entertainers, and philanthropy workers (CDVA, 1998a,b). The self-report data gathered were compared with age-matched Australian national data. The authors found an excess of male veterans reporting that a doctor had told them they had leukemia since their first day of service in Vietnam, compared to age-standardized expected rates; 64 cases were report where 26 were expected (range 16–36) (CDVA, 1998a). One case was reported by a female veteran, within the range of 0–4 expected (CDVA, 1998b). A follow-up was conducted to medically confirm selected conditions reported by males in the survey study (AIHW, 1999). Sources used to validate reported conditions included clinicians, several Australian morbidity and mortality data bases, CDVA data, and documentation provided by veterans. Based on these data, the authors estimated that there were 27 validated cases of leukemia among respondents, approximately equal to the expected number.

Synthesis

Studies of leukemia reviewed for the first time in this report continue the pattern of those examined in previous *Veterans and Agent Orange* reports, with risks fairly evenly distributed around the null.

Conclusions

Strength of Evidence in Epidemiologic Studies

There is no information contained in the research reviewed for this report to change the conclusion that there is inadequate or insufficient evidence to determine whether an association exists between exposure to herbicides (2,4-D, 2,4,5-T and its contaminant TCDD, cacodylic acid, and picloram) and leukemia.

Biologic Plausibility

No animal studies have found an increased incidence of leukemia. A summary of the biologic plausibility for the carcinogenicity of TCDD and the herbi-

CANCER

cides in general is presented in the conclusion to this chapter. A discussion of toxicological studies that concern biologic plausibility is contained in Chapter 3.

Increased Risk of Disease Among Vietnam Veterans

The limited data available on Vietnam veterans do not suggest they are at an elevated risk for leukemia.

TABLE 7-29 Selected Epidemiologic Studies—Leukemia

Reference	Study Population	Exposed Cases[a]	Estimated Risk (95% CI)[a]
OCCUPATIONAL			
New Studies			
Steenland et al., 1999	U.S. chemical production workers	10	0.8 (0.4–1.5)
Hooiveld et al., 1998	Dutch chemical production workers	1	1.0 (0.0–5.7)
Rix et al., 1998	Danish paper mill workers		
	Males	20	0.8 (0.5–1.2)
	Females	7	1.3 (0.5–2.7)
Studies Reviewed in *Update 1998*			
Gambini et al., 1997	Italian rice growers		0.6 (0.2–1.7)
Kogevinas et al., 1997	IARC cohort	34	1.0 (0.7–1.4)
Becher et al., 1996	German chemical production workers		1.8 (0.5–4.1)
Ramlow et al., 1996	Pentachlorophenol production workers		1.0 (0.1–3.6)
Waterhouse et al., 1996	Residents of Tecumseh, Michigan		1.4 (1.0–1.9)
Amadori et al., 1995	Italian farming and animal-breeding workers		1.8 (1.2–2.6)
Studies Reviewed in *Update 1996*			
Asp et al., 1994	Finnish herbicide appliers	2	—
Semenciw et al., 1994	Farmers in Canadian prairie provinces	357	0.9 (0.8–1.0)
Blair et al., 1993	U.S. farmers in 23 states	1,072	1.3 (1.2–1.4)
Kogevinas et al., 1993	Female herbicide-spraying and production workers	1	—
Studies Reviewed in *VAO*			
Bueno de Mesquita et al., 1993	Dutch production workers Workers exposed to phenoxy herbicides	2	2.2 (0.3–7.9)
Hansen et al., 1992	Danish gardeners		
	All gardeners—CLL	6	2.5 (0.9–5.5)
	All gardeners—all other types of leukemia	3	1.2 (0.3–3.6)
	Male gardeners—CLL	6	2.8 (1.0–6.0)
	Male gardeners—all other types of leukemia	3	1.4 (0.3–4.2)
Ronco et al., 1992	Danish and Italian farm workers		
	Danish self-employed farmers		0.9
	Danish male farmers		1.0
	Italian self-employed farmers		0.7
	Italian male farmers		0.9

TABLE 7-29 *Continued*

Reference	Study Population	Exposed Cases[a]	Estimated Risk (95% CI)[a]
Fingerhut et al., 1991	U.S. chemical workers	6	0.7 (0.2–1.5)
Saracci et al., 1991	Chemical workers		
	Exposed	18	
	Probably exposed	0	—
	Nonexposed	3	0.9 (0.2–2.6)
	Unknown exposure	0	—
Brown et al., 1990	Residents of Iowa and Minnesota		
	All types of leukemia, ever farmed		1.2 (1.0–1.5)
	CLL, ever farmed		1.4 (1.1–1.9)
	All types of leukemia, any herbicide use		1.2 (0.9–1.6)
	CLL, any herbicide use		1.4 (1.0–2.0)
	Herbicide users, phenoxy acid use		1.2 (0.9–1.6)
	All types of leukemia, 2,4-D use		1.2 (0.9–1.6)
	All types of leukemia, 2,4,5-T use		1.3 (0.7–2.2)
Wigle et al., 1990	Saskatchewan farmers	138	0.9 (0.7–1.0)
Zober et al., 1990	BASF production workers		
	Second additional cohort	1	5.2 (0.4–63.1)
Alavanja et al., 1988	USDA agricultural extension agents		1.9 (1.0–3.5)
Bond et al., 1988	Dow workers with chloracne	2	3.6 (0.4–13.0)
Blair and White, 1985	Residents of Nebraska		
	All cases, all leukemia—farming		1.3
Burmeister et al., 1982	Residents of Iowa		
	CLL in white, male farmers		1.9 (1.2–3.1)
ENVIRONMENTAL			
New Studies			
Bertazzi et al., 2001	Seveso residents—20-year follow-up		
	Zone B males	9	2.4 (1.2–4.7)
	Zone B females	3	1.1 (0.4–3.5)
Schreinemachers, 2000	Rural or farm residents of Minnesota, Montana, North Dakota, and South Dakota		
	Males—counties with wheat acreage 23,000–110,999	246	1.0 (0.8–1.1)
	Males—counties with wheat acreage >111,000	248	1.1 (1.0–1.3)
	Females—counties with wheat acreage 23,000–110,999	183	1.0 (0.8–1.2)
	Females—counties with wheat acreage >111,000	146	0.9 (0.8–1.2)
Bertazzi et al., 1998	Seveso residents—15-year follow-up		
	Zone B males	7	3.1 (1.4–6.7)
	Zone B females	1	0.6 (0.1–4.0)
	Zone R males	12	0.8 (0.4–1.5)
	Zone R females	12	0.9 (0.5–1.6)

TABLE 7-29 Continued

Reference	Study Population	Exposed Cases[a]	Estimated Risk (95% CI)[a]
Studies Reviewed in *Update 1998*			
Bertazzi et al., 1997	Seveso residents—15-year follow-up		
	Zone B males	7	3.1 (1.3–6.4)
	Zone B females	1	0.6 (0.0–3.1)
Studies Reviewed in *Update 1996*			
Bertazzi et al., 1993	Seveso residents—10-year follow-up, morbidity		
	Zone B males	2	1.6 (0.4–6.5)
	Zone B females	2	1.8 (0.4–7.3)
Studies Reviewed in *VAO*			
Bertazzi et al., 1992	Seveso residents—10-year follow-up		
	Zones A, B, R males	4	2.1 (0.7–6.9)
	Zones A, B, R females	1	2.5 (0.2–27.0)
VIETNAM VETERANS			
New Studies			
AFHS, 2000	Air Force Ranch Hand veterans	2	0.7 (0.1–5.0)
AIHW, 1999	Australian Vietnam veterans	27	26 expected (16–36)
CDVA, 1998a	Australian Vietnam veterans—male	64[b]	26 expected (16–36)
CDVA, 1998b	Australian Vietnam veterans—female	1[b]	0 expected (0–4)
Studies Reviewed in *Update 1998*			
Dalager and Kang, 1997	Army Chemical Corps veterans		1.0 (0.1–3.8)
Crane et al., 1997b	Australian military Vietnam veterans		0.5 (0.1–3.0)
Studies Reviewed in *Update 1996*			
Visintainer et al., 1995	Michigan Vietnam veterans	30	1.0 (0.7–1.5)

NOTE: USDA = United States Department of Agriculture.

[a] Given when available.

[b] Self-reported medical history. Answer to question: Since your first day of service in Vietnam, have you been told by a doctor that you have leukemia?

SUMMARY

Based on the occupational, environmental, and veteran studies reviewed, the committee has reached one of four standard conclusions about the strength of the evidence regarding association between an exposure to herbicides and/or TCDD and each of the cancers studied. As explained in Chapter 4, these distinctions reflect the committee's judgment that if an association between exposure and an outcome were "real," it would be found in a large, well-designed epidemiologic study in which exposure to herbicides or dioxin was sufficiently high, well characterized, and appropriately measured on an individual basis. Consistent with the charge to the committee by the Secretary of Veterans Affairs in Public Law 102-

4 and with accepted standards for scientific reviews, the distinctions between these standard conclusions are based on statistical association, not on causality. The committee used the same criteria to categorize diseases by the strength of the evidence as were used in *VAO*, *Update 1996*, and *Update 1998*.

Health Outcomes with Sufficient Evidence of an Association

In *VAO, Update 1996*, and *Update 1998*, the committees found sufficient evidence of an association between exposure to herbicides and/or TCDD and three cancers: soft-tissue sarcoma, non-Hodgkin's lymphoma, and Hodgkin's disease. The scientific literature continues to support the classification of these three cancers in the category of sufficient evidence. Based on the literature, there are no additional cancers that satisfy the criteria necessary for this category.

For diseases in this category, a positive association between herbicides and the outcome must be observed in studies in which chance, bias, and confounding can be ruled out with reasonable confidence. The committee also regarded evidence from several small studies that are free from bias and confounding, and show an association that is consistent in magnitude and direction, as sufficient evidence for an association.

Health Outcomes with Limited/Suggestive Evidence of Association

In *VAO, Update 1996*, and *Update 1998*, the committees found limited/suggestive evidence of an association between herbicide or dioxin exposure and the following cancers: larynx, lung, bronchus (trachea), prostate, and multiple myeloma. The scientific literature continues to support the classification of these diseases in the category of limited/suggestive evidence. Based on the literature, there are no additional cancers that satisfy the criteria necessary for this category.

For outcomes in this category, the evidence must be suggestive of an association between herbicides and the outcome, but may be limited because chance, bias, or confounding could not be ruled out with confidence. Typically, at least one high-quality study indicates a positive association, though most frequently several studies provide positive results, but the results of other studies may be inconsistent.

Health Outcomes with Inadequate/Insufficient Evidence to Determine Whether an Association Exists

The scientific data for many of the cancers reviewed by the committee were inadequate or insufficient to determine whether an association exists. For these cancers, the available studies are of insufficient quality, consistency, or statistical power to permit a conclusion regarding the presence or absence of an association. For example, studies fail to control for confounding or have inadequate exposure assessment. This category includes hepatobiliary cancers (cancers of the liver and intrahepatic bile duct), nasal and nasopharyngeal cancer, bone cancer, skin cancers (including basal cell carcinoma, squamous cell carcinoma, and nonmelanocytic skin cancers), breast cancer, cancers of the female reproductive system (including cervix, endometrium, and ovaries), testicular cancer, urinary bladder cancer, renal cancer (cancers of the kidney and renal pelvis), and leukemias.

Health Outcomes with Limited/Suggestive Evidence of *No* Association

In *VAO, Update 1996,* and *Update 1998,* the committees found a sufficient number and variety of well-designed studies to conclude that there is limited/suggestive evidence of *no* association between a small group of cancers and exposure to TCDD or herbicides. This group includes gastrointestinal tumors (colon, rectal, stomach, and pancreatic) and brain tumors. The most recent scientific evidence continues to support the classification of such cancers in this category. Based on an evaluation of the whole of the scientific literature, there are no additional cancers that satisfy the criteria necessary for this category.

For outcomes in this category, several adequate studies covering the full range of levels of exposure that human beings are known to encounter are mutually consistent in not showing a positive association between exposure to herbicides and the outcome at any level of exposure. These studies have relatively narrow confidence intervals. A conclusion of "no association" is inevitably limited to the conditions, level of exposure, and length of observation covered by the available studies. In addition, the possibility of a very small elevation in risk at the levels of exposure studied can never be excluded.

Biologic Plausibility

This section summarizes the biologic plausibility, on the basis of data from animal and cellular studies, of a connection between exposure to dioxin or herbicides and various forms of cancer. Details of the committee's evaluation of data from these studies are presented in Chapter 3. Some of the preceding discussions of cancer outcomes include references to papers relevant to specific types of cancer.

Although evidence suggests that TCDD is not genotoxic, data in animals indicate that TCDD has carcinogenic activity. A number of animal species, including strains of rats, mice, and hamsters, have been exposed to TCDD and examined for increases in tumor incidence and cancer. These have included studies in which TCDD was fed to animals, applied to their skin, injected under their skin, or injected into the abdominal cavity. This research indicates that TCDD can both cause cancers or tumors and act as a promoter (i.e., enhancing the incidence of certain cancers or tumors in the presence of known carcinogens). Increased cancer rates have been observed at several different sites in the body, notably the thyroid gland, skin, and lungs. Studies have demonstrated an increased incidence of liver cancer following TCDD exposure, but only after other adverse changes in the liver were observed. TCDD is also an extremely potent promoter of neoplasia in laboratory rats. Decreased rates of some cancers—including those of the uterus, pancreas, and pituitary and mammary glands—have also been reported. The sites at which effects were observed and the exposure levels needed to induce them varied considerably from species to species.

The mechanism by which TCDD exerts its carcinogenic effects is not established. TCDD has a wide range of effects on growth regulation, hormone systems, and other factors associated with the regulation of activities in normal cells; these effects could influence tumor formation. Data from female rats suggest that complex hormonal interactions are involved in TCDD-induced carcinogenesis.

Most studies are consistent with the hypothesis that the effects of TCDD are mediated by the AhR, a protein in animal and human cells to which TCDD can bind. Following the binding of TCDD, the TCDD–AhR complex has been shown to bind DNA, leading to changes in transcription (i.e., genes are differentially regulated). In many cases, this differential gene regulation leads to transformation of a normal cell into an abnormal cell. Furthermore, data from animals genetically modified not to express the AhR suggest that the AhR plays a role in normal growth, which supports the hypothesis that TCDD could affect cell growth.

The transcriptional alterations induced by TCDD result in alterations in some forms of cellular metabolism at a very basic level. For example, TCDD has been shown to significantly induce cytochrome P4501A1 (CYP1A1) mRNA levels and ethoxyresorufin O-deethylase (EROD) activity in several types of human cancer cells. These changes result in altered cell metabolism and could be involved in TCDD's carcinogenic activity. Experiments involving several strains of mice provide evidence that a functional AhR is required for TCDD induction of CYP1A1 and liver tumor promotion. CYP1A1 induction in various mice strains, however, was not directly related to the degree of tumor-promoting capability, suggesting that other undefined genetic factors also might play an important role. In addition, protective cellular mechanisms can affect the response to TCDD, further complicating the carcinogenic effects of TCDD.

There are differences among various experimental animals in susceptibility to TCDD-induced effects; the site at which tumors are induced also varies from species to species. Induction of P450s by TCDD is also highly specific for species and cell type. Differences in the induction of P450s could play a role in the different responses seen in different cell types and species.

Although structural differences in the AhR have been identified among different species, this receptor operates in a similar manner in animals and humans. Therefore, a common mechanism is likely to underlie the carcinogenic effects of TCDD in humans and animals, and data in animals support a biological basis for the carcinogenic effects of TCDD. Because of the many species and strain differences in TCDD responses, however, controversy remains regarding the TCDD exposure level that is carcinogenic.

Fewer studies have been conducted on the carcinogenicity of the other herbicides compared to TCDD. Several studies of the carcinogenicity of 2,4-D, 2,4,5-T, and picloram have been performed in laboratory animals. In general, negative results were seen. However, some studies do not meet present-day standards for cancer bioassays, and others produced equivocal results. Thus, it is not possible to have confidence in the conclusions regarding the carcinogenicity of these compounds at this time. With respect to genotoxicity, however, the majority of evidence indicates that 2,4-D is genotoxic only at very high concentrations. Although 2,4,5-T increased the formation of DNA adducts by cytochrome P450-derived metabolites of benzo[*a*]pyrene, most available evidence indicates that 2,4,5-T is genotoxic only at high levels.

There is some evidence that cacodylic acid (also known as dimethylarsinic acid, DMA) is carcinogenic. DMA may induce DNA modifications that sensitize it to free-radical injury. Other studies concluded that it is a promoter of urinary bladder, kidney, liver, and thyroid gland carcinogenesis in rats; causes pulmonary neoplasms in mice; and causes bladder hyperplasia and tumors in rats. Another exposure study in mice, however, produced negative results.

The foregoing evidence suggests that a connection between TCDD and cancer in humans is, in general, biologically plausible. However, differences in sensitivity and susceptibility across individual animals, strains, and species; the lack of strong evidence of organ-specific effects across species; and differences in route, dose, duration, and timing of exposure complicate any more definitive conclusions about the presence or absence of a mechanism for the induction of site-specific cancers by TCDD. Experiments on 2,4-D, 2,4,5-T, and picloram in animals and cells do not provide a biologic basis for any carcinogenic effects of these compounds. Information is emerging that there might be animal data supporting a carcinogenic effect of cacodylic acid, but these data alone are not sufficient to draw conclusions on the carcinogenicity of this compound in humans.

Considerable uncertainty remains about how to apply this information to the evaluation of potential health effects of herbicides or dioxin exposure in Vietnam veterans. Scientists disagree over the extent to which information derived from animals and cellular studies predicts human health outcomes and the extent to which the health effects resulting from high-dose exposure are comparable to those resulting from low-dose exposure. Investigating the biological mechanisms underlying TCDD's carcinogenic effects continues to be a very active area of research, and subsequent updates of this report might have more and better information on which to base conclusions, at least for that compound.

Increased Risk of Disease Among Vietnam Veterans

Under the Agent Orange Act of 1991, the committee is asked to determine (to the extent that available scientific data permit meaningful determinations) the increased risk of the diseases it studies among those exposed to herbicides during their service in Vietnam. Chapter 1 presents the committee's general findings regarding this charge. Where more specific information about particular health outcomes is available, this information can be found in the preceding discussions of those diseases.

REFERENCES

ACS (American Cancer Society). 1998. Cancer Facts and Figures. http://www.cancer.org/statistics/cff98/graphicaldata.html (accessed March 12).

ACS. 2000a. Cancer Facts and Figures. http://www3.cancer.org/cancerinfo/sitecenter.asp?ct=1&ctid=8&scp=8.3.10.40038&scs=4&scss=3&scdoc=41170&pnt=2&language=english.html (accessed October 20).

ACS. 2000b. Basic Facts. http://www3.cancer.org/cancerinfo/sitecenter.asp?ct=1&ctid=8&scp=8.3.1.40029&scs=4&scss=6&scdoc=40044&pnt=2&language=english.html (accessed December 21).

AFHS (Air Force Health Study). 1996. An Epidemiologic Investigation of Health Effects in Air Force Personnel Following Exposure to Herbicides. Mortality Update 1996. Brooks AFB, TX: Epidemiologic Research Division. Armstrong Laboratory. AL/AO-TR-1996-0068. 31 pp.

AFHS. 2000. An Epidemiologic Investigation of Health Effects in Air Force Personnel Following Exposure to Herbicides. 1997 Follow-up Examination and Results. Reston, VA: Science Application International Corporation. F41624–96–C1012.

AIHW (Australian Institute of Health and Welfare). 1999. Morbidity of Vietnam Veterans: A Study of the Health of Australia's Vietnam Veteran Community, Volume 3: Validation Study. Canberra.

Alavanja MC, Blair A, Merkle S, Teske J, Eaton B. 1988. Mortality among agricultural extension agents. American Journal of Industrial Medicine 14:167–176.

Alavanja MC, Merkle S, Teske J, Eaton B, Reed B. 1989. Mortality among forest and soil conservationists. Archives of Environmental Health 44:94–101.

Amadori D, Nanni O, Falcini F, Saragoni A, Tison V, Callea A, Scarpi E, Ricci M, Riva N, Buiatti E. 1995. Chronic lymphocytic leukaemias and non-Hodgkin's lymphomas by histological type in farming-animal breeding workers: a population case-control study based on job titles. Occupational and Environmental Medicine 52(6):374–379.

Anderson HA, Hanrahan LP, Jensen M, Laurin D, Yick W-Y, Wiegman P. 1986a. Wisconsin Vietnam Veteran Mortality Study: Proportionate Mortality Ratio Study Results. Madison: Wisconsin Division of Health.

Anderson HA, Hanrahan LP, Jensen M, Laurin D, Yick W-Y, Wiegman P. 1986b. Wisconsin Vietnam Veteran Mortality Study: Final Report. Madison: Wisconsin Division of Health.

Aparaso NE. 2000. Pharmacogenetic Studies. Bethesda, MD: Crisp Data Base, National Institutes of Health.

Armstrong BG, Kazantzis G. 1983. The mortality of cadmium workers. Lancet 1(8339):1425–1427.

Asp S, Riihimaki V, Hernberg S, Pukkala E. 1994. Mortality and cancer morbidity of Finnish chlorophenoxy herbicide applicators: an 18-year prospective follow-up. American Journal of Industrial Medicine 26:243–253.

Axelson O, Sundell L, Andersson K, Edling C, Hogstedt C, Kling H. 1980. Herbicide exposure and tumor mortality: an updated epidemiologic investigation on Swedish railroad workers. Scandinavian Journal of Work, Environment, and Health 6:73–79.

Bagga D, Anders KH, Wang HJ, Roberts E, Glaspy JA. 2000. Organochlorine pesticide content of breast adipose tissue from women with breast cancer and control subjects. Journal of the National Cancer Institute 92(9):750–753.

Balarajan R, Acheson ED. 1984. Soft tissue sarcomas in agriculture and forestry workers. Journal of Epidemiology and Community Health 38:113–116.

Becher H, Flesch-Janys D, Kauppinen T, et al. 1996. Cancer mortality in German male workers exposed to phenoxy herbicides and dioxins [see comments]. Cancer Causes and Control 7:312–321.

Bender AP, Parker DL, Johnson RA, Scharber WK, Williams AN, Marbury MC, Mandel JS. 1989. Minnesota highway maintenance worker study: cancer mortality. American Journal of Industrial Medicine 15:545–556.

Bertazzi PA, Zocchetti C, Pesatori AC, Guercilena S, Sanarico M, Radice L. 1989a. Mortality in an area contaminated by TCDD following an industrial incident. Medicina Del Lavoro 80:316–329.

Bertazzi PA, Zocchetti C, Pesatori AC, Guercilena S, Sanarico M, Radice L. 1989b. Ten-year mortality study of the population involved in the Seveso incident in 1976. American Journal of Epidemiology 129:1187–1200.

Bertazzi PA, Zocchetti C, Pesatori AC, Guercilena S, Consonni D, Tironi A, Landi MT. 1992. Mortality of a young population after accidental exposure to 2,3,7,8-tetrachlorodibenzodioxin. International Journal of Epidemiology 21:118–123.

Bertazzi A, Pesatori AC, Consonni D, Tironi A, Landi MT, Zocchetti C. 1993. Cancer incidence in a population accidentally exposed to 2,3,7,8-tetrachlorodibenzo-*para*-dioxin [see comments]. Epidemiology 4:398–406.

Bertazzi PA, Zochetti C, Guercilena S, Consonni D, Tironi A, Landi MT, Pesatori AC. 1997. Dioxin exposure and cancer risk: a 15-year mortality study after the "Seveso accident." Epidemiology 8(6):646–652.

Bertazzi PA, Bernucci I, Brambilla G, Consonni D, Pesatori AC. 1998. The Seveso studies on early and long-term effects of dioxin exposure: a review. Environmental Health Perspectives 106 (Suppl 2):625–633.

Bertazzi PA, Pesatori AC, Bernucci I, Landi MT, Consonni D. 1999. Dioxin exposure and human leukemias and lymphomas. Lessons from the Seveso accident and studies on industrial workers. Leukemia 13(Suppl 1):72–74.

Bertazzi PA, Consonni D, Bachetti S, Rubagotti M, Baccarelli A, Zocchetti C, Pesatori AC. 2001. Health effects of dioxin exposure: a 20-year mortality study. American Journal of Epidemiology 153(11):1031-1044.

Blair A, Kazerouni N. 1997. Reactive chemicals and cancer. Cancer Causes and Control 8(3):473–490.

Blair A, White DW. 1985. Leukemia cell types and agricultural practices in Nebraska. Archives of Environmental Health 40:211–214.

Blair A, Grauman DJ, Lubin JH, Fraumeni JF Jr. 1983. Lung cancer and other causes of death among licensed pesticide applicators. Journal of the National Cancer Institute 71:31–37.

Blair A, Mustafa D, Heineman EF. 1993. Cancer and other causes of death among male and female farmers from twenty-three states. American Journal of Industrial Medicine 23:729–742.

Blair A, Zahm SH, Cantor KP, Ward MH. 1997. Occupational and environmental risk factors for chronic lymphocytic leukemia and non-Hodgkin's lymphoma. In: Marti GE, Vogt RF, Zenger VE, eds. Proceedings of the USPHS Workshop on Laboratory and Epidemiologic Approaches to Determining the Role of Environmental Exposures as Risk Factors for B-Cell Chronic Lymphocytic and Other B-Cell Lymphoproliferative Disorders. U.S. Department of Health and Human Services, Public Health Service.

Bloemen LJ, Mandel JS, Bond GG, Pollock AF, Vitek RP, Cook RR. 1993. An update of mortality among chemical workers potentially exposed to the herbicide 2,4-dichlorophenoxyacetic acid and its derivatives. Journal of Occupational Medicine 35:1208–1212.

Boffetta P, Stellman SD, Garfinkel L. 1989. A case-control study of multiple myeloma nested in the American Cancer Society prospective study. International Journal of Cancer 43:554–559.

Bond GG, Wetterstroem NH, Roush GJ, McLaren EA, Lipps TE, Cook RR. 1988. Cause specific mortality among employees engaged in the manufacture, formulation, or packaging of 2,4-dichlorophenoxyacetic acid and related salts. British Journal of Industrial Medicine 45:98–105.

Bosl GJ, Motzer RJ. 1997. Testicular germ-cell cancer. New England Journal of Medicine 337(4): 242–253.

Boyle C, Decoufle P, Delaney RJ, DeStefano F, Flock ML, Hunter MI, Joesoef MR, Karon JM, Kirk ML, Layde PM, McGee DL, Moyer LA, Pollock DA, Rhodes P, Scally MJ, Worth RM. 1987. Postservice Mortality Among Vietnam Veterans. Atlanta: Centers for Disease Control. CEH 86-0076. 143 pp.

Breslin P, Kang H, Lee Y, Burt V, Shepard BM. 1988. Proportionate mortality study of U.S. Army and U.S. Marine Corps veterans of the Vietnam War. Journal of Occupational Medicine 30:412–419.

Brown LM, Blair A, Gibson R, Everett GD, Cantor KP, Schuman LM, Burmeister LF, Van Lier SF, Dick F. 1990. Pesticide exposures and other agricultural risk factors for leukemia among men in Iowa and Minnesota. Cancer Research 50:6585–6591.

Brown LM, Burmeister LF, Everett GD, Blair A. 1993. Pesticide exposures and multiple myeloma in Iowa men. Cancer Causes and Control 4:153–156.

Bueno de Mesquita HB, Doornbos G, van der Kuip DA, Kogevinas M, Winkelmann R. 1993. Occupational exposure to phenoxy herbicides and chlorophenols and cancer mortality in the Netherlands. American Journal of Industrial Medicine 23:289–300.

Bullman TA, Kang HK, Watanabe KK. 1990. Proportionate mortality among U.S. Army Vietnam veterans who served in Military Region I. American Journal of Epidemiology 132:670–674.

Bullman TA, Watanabe KK, Kang HK. 1994. Risk of testicular cancer associated with surrogate measures of Agent Orange exposure among Vietnam veterans on the Agent Orange Registry. Annals of Epidemiology 4:11–16.

Burmeister LF. 1981. Cancer mortality in Iowa farmers: 1971–1978. Journal of the National Cancer Institute 66:461–464.

Burmeister LF, Van Lier SF, Isacson P. 1982. Leukemia and farm practices in Iowa. American Journal of Epidemiology 115(5):720–728.

Burmeister LF, Everett GD, Van Lier SF, Isacson P. 1983. Selected cancer mortality and farm practices in Iowa. American Journal of Epidemiology 118:72–77.

Burt VL, Breslin PP, Kang HK, Lee Y. 1987. Non-Hodgkin's Lymphoma in Vietnam Veterans. Department of Medicine and Surgery, Veterans Administration, 33 pp.

Cantor KP. 1982. Farming and mortality from non-Hodgkin's lymphoma: a case-control study. International Journal of Cancer 29:239–247.

Cantor KP, Blair A. 1984. Farming and mortality from multiple myeloma: a case control study with the use of death certificates. Journal of the National Cancer Institute 72:251–255.

Caplan LS, Hall HI, Levine RS, Zhu K. 2000. Preventable risk factors for nasal cancer. Annals of Epidemiology 10:186–191.

CDC (Centers for Disease Control). 1988. Health status of Vietnam veterans. II. Physical health. Journal of the American Medical Association 259:2708–2714.

CDC. 1990. The association of selected cancers with service in the U.S. military in Vietnam. III. Hodgkin's disease, nasal cancer, nasopharyngeal cancer, and primary liver cancer. The Selected Cancers Cooperative Study Group [see comments]. Archives of Internal Medicine 150: 2495–2505.

CDVA (Commonwealth Department of Veterans' Affairs). 1998a. Morbidity of Vietnam Veterans: A Study of the Health of Australia's Vietnam Veteran Community. Volume 1: Male Vietnam Veterans Survey and Community Comparison Outcomes. Canberra: Department of Veterans' Affairs.

CDVA. 1998b. Morbidity of Vietnam Veterans: A Study of the Health of Australia's Vietnam Veteran Community. Volume 2: Female Vietnam Veterans Survey and Community Comparison Outcomes. Canberra: Department of Veterans' Affairs.

Clapp RW. 1997. Update of cancer surveillance of veterans in Massachusetts, USA. International Journal of Epidemiology 26(3):679–681.

Clapp RW, Cupples LA, Colton T, Ozonoff DM. 1991. Cancer surveillance of veterans in Massachusetts, 1982–1988. International Journal of Epidemiology 20:7–12.

Coggon D, Pannett B, Winter PD, Acheson ED, Bonsall J. 1986. Mortality of workers exposed to 2-methyl-4-chlorophenoxyacetic acid. Scandinavian Journal of Work, Environment, and Health 12:448–454.

Coggon D, Pannett B, Winter P. 1991. Mortality and incidence of cancer at four factories making phenoxy herbicides. British Journal of Industrial Medicine 48:173–178.

Collins JJ, Strauss ME, Levinskas GJ, Conner PR. 1993. The mortality experience of workers exposed to 2,3,7,8-tetrachlorodibenzo-p-dioxin in a trichlorophenol process accident. Epidemiology 4:7–13.

Corrao G, Caller M, Carle F, Russo R, Bosia S, Piccioni P. 1989. Cancer risk in a cohort of licensed pesticide users. Scandinavian Journal of Work, Environment, and Health 15:203–209.

Crane PJ, Barnard DL, Horsley KW, Adena MA. 1997a. Mortality of Vietnam Veterans: The Veteran Cohort Study. A Report of the 1996 Retrospective Cohort Study of Australian Vietnam Veterans. Canberra: Department of Veterans' Affairs.

Crane PJ, Barnard DL, Horsley KW, Adena MA. 1997b. Mortality of National Service Vietnam Veterans: A Report of the 1996 Retrospective Cohort Study of Australian Vietnam Veterans. Canberra: Department of Veterans' Affairs.

Dalager NA, Kang HK. 1997. Mortality among Army Chemical Corps Vietnam veterans. American Journal of Industrial Medicine 31:719–726.

Dalager NA, Kang HK, Burt VL, Weatherbee L. 1991. Non-Hodgkin's lymphoma among Vietnam veterans. Journal of Occupational Medicine 33:774–779.

Dalager NA, Kang HK, Thomas TL. 1995. Cancer mortality patterns among women who served in the military: the Vietnam experience. Journal of Occupational and Environmental Medicine 37:298–305.

Dean G. 1994. Deaths from primary brain cancers, lymphatic and haematopoietic cancers in agricultural workers in the Republic of Ireland. Journal of Epidemiology and Community Health 48:364–368.

Demers PA, Boffetta P, Kogevinas M, Blair A, Miller BA, Robinson CF, Roscoe RJ, Winter PD, Colin D, Matos E, et al. 1995. Pooled reanalysis of cancer mortality among five cohorts of workers in wood-related industries. Scandinavian Journal of Work, Environment and Health 21(3):179–190.

Demers A, Ayotte P, Brisson J, Dodin S, Robert J, Dewailly E. 2000. Risk and aggressiveness of breast cancer in relation to plasma organochlorine concentrations. Cancer Epidemiology, Biomarkers and Prevention 9:161–166.

Dich J, Wiklund K. 1998. Prostate cancer in pesticide applicators in Swedish agriculture. Prostate 34(2):100–112.

Donna A, Betta P-G, Robutti F, Crosignani P, Berrino F, Bellingeri D. 1984. Ovarian mesothelial tumors and herbicides: a case-control study. Carcinogenesis 5:941–942.

Dubrow R, Paulson JO, Indian RW. 1988. Farming and malignant lymphoma in Hancock County, Ohio. British Journal of Industrial Medicine 45:25–28.

Duell EJ, Millikan RC, Savitz DA, Newman B, Smith JC, Schell MJ, Sandler DP. 2000. A population-based case-control study of farming and breast cancer in North Carolina. Epidemiology 11(5):523–531.

Eriksson M, Karlsson M. 1992. Occupational and other environmental factors and multiple myeloma: a population based case-control study. British Journal of Industrial Medicine 49:95–103.

Eriksson M, Hardell L, Berg NO, Moller T, Axelson O. 1979. Case-control study on malignant mesenchymal tumor of the soft tissue and exposure to chemical substances. Lakartidningen 76:3872–3875.

Eriksson M, Hardell L, Berg NO, Moller T, Axelson O. 1981. Soft-tissue sarcomas and exposure to chemical substances: a case-referent study. British Journal of Industrial Medicine 38:27–33.

Fett MJ, Nairn JR, Cobbin DM, Adena MA. 1987. Mortality among Australian conscripts of the Vietnam conflict era. II. Causes of death. American Journal of Epidemiology 125:878–884.

Fingerhut MA, Halperin WE, Marlow DA, Piacitelli LA, Honchar PA, Sweeney MH, Greife AL, Dill PA, Steenland K, Suruda AJ. 1991. Cancer mortality in workers exposed to 2,3,7,8-tetrachlorodibenzo-p-dioxin. New England Journal of Medicine 324:212–218.

Fleming LE, Bean JA, Rudolph M, Hamilton K. 1999a. Mortality in a cohort of licensed pesticide applicators in Florida. Journal of Occupational and Environmental Medicine 56(1):14–21.

Fleming LE, Bean JA, Rudolph M, Hamilton K. 1999b. Cancer incidence in a cohort of licensed pesticide applicators in Florida. Journal of Occupational and Environmental Medicine 41(4):279–288.

Gallagher RP, Bajdik CD, Fincham S, Hill GB, Keefe AR, Coldman A, McLean DI. 1996. Chemical exposures, medical history, and risk of squamous and basal cell carcinoma of the skin. Cancer Epidemiology, Biomarkers and Prevention 5(6):419–424.

Gambini GF, Mantovani C, Pira E, Piolatto PG, Negri E. 1997. Cancer mortality among rice growers in Novara Province, northern Italy. American Journal of Industrial Medicine 31:435–441.

Gann PH. 1997. Interpreting recent trends in prostate cancer incidence and mortality. Epidemiology 8(2):117–120.

Garland FC, Gorham ED, Garland CF, Ferris JA. 1988. Non-Hodgkin's lymphoma in U.S. Navy personnel. Archives of Environmental Health 43:425–429.

Green LM. 1991. A cohort mortality study of forestry workers exposed to phenoxy acid herbicides. British Journal of Industrial Medicine 48:234–238.

Greenwald P, Kovasznay B, Collins DN, Therriault G. 1984. Sarcomas of soft tissues after Vietnam service. Journal of the National Cancer Institute 73:1107–1109.

Hansen ES, Hasle H, Lander F. 1992. A cohort study on cancer incidence among Danish gardeners. American Journal of Industrial Medicine 21:651–660.

Hardell L. 1981. Relation of soft-tissue sarcoma, malignant lymphoma and colon cancer to phenoxy acids, chlorophenols and other agents. Scandinavian Journal of Work, Environment, and Health 7:119–130.

Hardell L, Bengtsson NO. 1983. Epidemiological study of socioeconomic factors and clinical findings in Hodgkin's disease, and reanalysis of previous data regarding chemical exposure. British Journal of Cancer 48:217–225.

Hardell L, Eriksson M, Lenner P. 1980. Malignant lymphoma and exposure to chemical substances, especially organic solvents, chlorophenols, and phenoxy acids. Lakartidningen 77:208–210.

Hardell L, Johansson B, Axelson O. 1982. Epidemiological study of nasal and nasopharyngeal cancer and their relation to phenoxy acid or chlorophenol exposure. American Journal of Industrial Medicine 3:247–257.

Hardell L, Bengtsson NO, Jonsson U, Eriksson S, Larsson LG. 1984. Aetiological aspects on primary liver cancer with special regard to alcohol, organic solvents and acute intermittent porphyria: an epidemiological investigation. British Journal of Cancer 50:389–397.

Hardell L, Eriksson M, Degerman A. 1994. Exposure to phenoxyacetic acids, chlorophenols, or organic solvents in relation to histopathology, stage, and anatomical localization of non-Hodgkin's lymphoma. Cancer Research 54:2386–2389.

Hardell L, Nasman A, Ohlson CG, Fredrikson M. 1998. Case-control study on risk factors for testicular cancer. International Journal of Oncology 13(6):1299–1303.

Hayes RB. 1997. The carcinogenicity of metals in humans. Cancer Causes and Control 8(3):371–385.

Henneberger PK, Ferris BG Jr, Monson RR. 1989. Mortality among pulp and paper workers in Berlin, New Hampshire. British Journal of Industrial Medicine 46:658–664.

Hertzman C, Teschke K, Ostry A, Hershler R, Dimich-Ward H, Kelly S, Spinelli JJ, Gallagher RP, McBride M, Marion SA. 1997. Mortality and cancer incidence among sawmill workers exposed to chlorophenate wood preservatives. American Journal of Public Health 87(1):71–79.

Hildesheim A, Anderson LM, Chen CJ, Cheng YJ, Brinton LA, Daly AK, Reed CD, Chen IH, Caporaso NE, Hsu MM, Chen JY, Idle JR, Hoover RN, Yang CS, Chhabra SK. 1997. CYP2E1 genetic polymorphisms and risk of nasopharyngeal carcinoma in Taiwan. Journal of the National Cancer Institute 89(16):1207–1212.

Hoar SK, Blair A, Holmes FF, Boysen CD, Robel RJ, Hoover R, Fraumeni JF. 1986. Agricultural herbicide use and risk of lymphoma and soft-tissue sarcoma. Journal of the American Medical Association 256:1141–1147.

Hoffman RE, Stehr-Green PA, Webb KB, Evans RG, Knutsen AP, Schramm WF, Staake JL, Gibson BB, Steinberg KK. 1986. Health effects of long-term exposure to 2,3,7,8-tetrachlorodibenzo-p-dioxin. Journal of the American Medical Association 255:2031–2038.

Holmes AP, Bailey C, Baron RC, Bosanac E, Brough J, Conroy C, Haddy L. 1986. West Virginia Department of Health Vietnam-Era Veterans Mortality Study: Preliminary Report. Charlestown: West Virginia Health Department.

Hooiveld M, Heederik DJ, Kogevinas M, Boffetta P, Needham LL, Patterson DG Jr, Bueno de Mesquita HB. 1998. Second follow-up of a Dutch cohort occupationally exposed to phenoxy herbicides, chlorophenols, and contaminants. American Journal of Epidemiology 147(9):891–901.

Høyer AP, Jorgensen T, Brock JW, Grandjean P. 2000. Organochlorine exposure and breast cancer survival. Journal of Clinical Epidemiology 53(3):323–330.

Hu S-W, Hertz-Picciotto I, Siemiatycki J. 1999. When to be skeptical of negative studies: pitfalls in evaluating occupational risks in population-based case-control studies. Canadian Journal of Public Health 90(2):138–142.

Huff JE, Salmon AG, Hooper NK, Zeise L. 1991. Long-term carcinogenesis studies on 2,3,7,8-tetrachlorodibenzo-p-dioxin and hexachlorodibenzo-p-dioxins. Cell Biology and Toxicology 7(1): 67–94.

IARC (International Agency for Research on Cancer). 1987. 4-Aminobiphenyl. In Overall Evaluations of Carcinogenicity: An Updating of IARC Monographs Volumes 1 to 42. IARC Monographs on the Evaluation of the Carcinogenic Risk of Chemicals to Man, Supplement 7. Lyon, France: World Health Organization, IARC.

IOM (Institute of Medicine). 1994. Veterans and Agent Orange: Health Effects of Herbicides Used in Vietnam. Washington, DC: National Academy Press.

IOM. 1996. Veterans and Agent Orange: Update 1996. Washington, DC: National Academy Press.

IOM. 1999. Veterans and Agent Orange: Update 1998. Washington, DC: National Academy Press.

Kang HK, Weatherbee L, Breslin PP, Lee Y, Shepard BM. 1986. Soft tissue sarcomas and military service in Vietnam: a case comparison group analysis of hospital patients. Journal of Occupational Medicine 28:1215–1218.

Keller-Byrne JE, Khuder SA, Schaub EA, McAfee O. 1997. A meta-analysis of non-Hodgkin's lymphoma among farmers in the central United States. American Journal of Industrial Medicine 31(4):442–444.

Ketchum NS, Michalek JE, Burton JE. 1999. Serum dioxin and cancer in veterans of Operation Ranch Hand. American Journal of Epidemiology 149(7):630–639.

Kociba RJ, Keys DG, Beyer JE, Careon RM, Wade CE, Dittenber DA, Kalnins RP, Frauson LE, Park CN, Barnar SD, Hummel RA, Humiston CG. 1978. Results of a two-year chronic toxicity and oncogenicity study of 2,3,7,8-tetrachlorodibenzo-p-dioxin in rats. Toxicology and Applied Pharmacology 46:279–303.

Kogan MD, Clapp RW. 1988. Soft tissue sarcoma mortality among Vietnam veterans in Massachusetts, 1972 to 1983. International Journal of Epidemiology 17:39–43.

Kogevinas M, Saracci R, Bertazzi PA, Bueno De Mesquita BH, Coggon D, Green LM, Kauppinen T, Littorin M, Lynge E, Mathews JD, Neuberger M, Osman J, Pearce N, Winkelmann R. 1992. Cancer mortality from soft-tissue sarcoma and malignant lymphomas in an international cohort of workers exposed to chlorophenoxy herbicides and chlorophenols. Chemosphere 25:1071–1076.

Kogevinas M, Saracci R, Winkelmann R, Johnson ES, Bertazzi PA, Bueno de Mesquita HB, Kauppinen T, Littorin M, Lynge E, Neuberger M. 1993. Cancer incidence and mortality in women occupationally exposed to chlorophenoxy herbicides, chlorophenols, and dioxins. Cancer Causes and Control 4:547–553.

Kogevinas M, Kauppinen T, Winkelmann R, Becher H, Bertazzi PA, Bas B, Coggon D, Green L, Johnson E, Littorin M, Lynge E, Marlow DA, Mathews JD, Neuberger M, Benn T, Pannett B, Pearce N, Saracci R. 1995. Soft tissue sarcoma and non-Hodgkin's lymphoma in workers exposed to phenoxy herbicides, chlorophenols and dioxins: two nested case-control studies. Epidemiology 6:396–402.

Kogevinas M, Becher H, Benn T, Bertazzi PA, Boffetta P, Bueno de Mesquita HB, Coggon D, Colin D, Flesch-Janys D, Fingerhut M, Green L, Kauppinen T, Littorin M, Lynge E, Mathews JD, Neuberger M, Pearce N, Saracci R. 1997. Cancer mortality in workers exposed to phenoxy herbicides, chlorophenols, and dioxins. An expanded and updated international cohort study. American Journal of Epidemiology 145(12):1061–1075.

Kuchenhoff A, Seliger G, Klonisch T, Tscheudschilsuren G, Kaltwasser P, Seliger E, Buchmann J, Fischer B. 1999. Arylhydrocarbon receptor expression in the human endometrium. Fertility and Sterility 71(2):354–360.

Lampi P, Hakulinen T, Luostarinen T, Pukkala E, Teppo L. 1992. Cancer incidence following chlorophenol exposure in a community in southern Finland. Archives of Environmental Health 47:167–175.

LaVecchia C, Negri E, D'Avanzo B, Franceschi S. 1989. Occupation and lymphoid neoplasms. British Journal of Cancer 60:385–388.

Lawrence CE, Reilly AA, Quickenton P, Greenwald P, Page WF, Kuntz AJ. 1985. Mortality patterns of New York State Vietnam veterans. American Journal of Public Health 75:277–279.

Lemen RA, Lee JS, Wagoner JK, Blejer HP. 1976. Cancer mortality among cadmium production workers. Annals of the New York Academy of Sciences 271:273–279.

Lynge E. 1985. A follow-up study of cancer incidence among workers in manufacture of phenoxy herbicides in Denmark. British Journal of Cancer 52:259–270.

Lynge E. 1993. Cancer in phenoxy herbicide manufacturing workers in Denmark, 1947–87—an update. Cancer Causes and Control 4:261–272.

Mack TM. 1995. Sarcomas and other malignancies of soft tissue, retroperitoneum, peritoneum, pleura, heart, mediastinum, and spleen. Cancer 75:211–244.

Mahan CM, Bullman TA, Kang HK, Selvin S. 1997. A case-control study of lung cancer among Vietnam veterans. Journal of Occupational and Environmental Medicine 39(8):740–747.

Manz A, Berger J, Dwyer JH, Flesch-Janys D, Nagel S, Waltsgott H. 1991. Cancer mortality among workers in chemical plant contaminated with dioxin. Lancet 338:959–964.

McDuffie HH, Klaassen DJ, Dosman JA. 1990. Is pesticide use related to the risk of primary lung cancer in Saskatchewan? Journal of Occupational Medicine 32:996–1002.

Mellemgaard A, Engholm G, McLaughlin JK, Olsen JH. 1994. Occupational risk factors for renal-cell carcinoma in Denmark. Scandinavian Journal of Work, Environment, and Health 20:160–165.

Michalek JE, Wolfe WH, Miner JC. 1990. Health status of Air Force veterans occupationally exposed to herbicides in Vietnam. II. Mortality. Journal of the American Medical Association 264:1832–1836.

Miller BA, Kolonel LN, Bernstein L, Young JL Jr., Swanson GM, West D, Key CR, Liff JM, Glover CS, Alexander GA, et al. (eds). 1996. Racial/Ethnic Patterns of Cancer in the United States 1988–1992. Bethesda, MD: National Cancer Institute. NIH Pub. No. 96-4104.

Morris PD, Koepsell TD, Daling JR, Taylor JW, Lyon JL, Swanson GM, Child M, Weiss NS. 1986. Toxic substance exposure and multiple myeloma: a case-control study. Journal of the National Cancer Institute 76:987–994.

Morrison H, Semenciw RM, Morison D, Magwood S, Mao Y. 1992. Brain cancer and farming in western Canada. Neuroepidemiology 11:267–276.

Morrison H, Savitz D, Semenciw RM, Hulka B, Mao Y, Morison D, Wigle D. 1993. Farming and prostate cancer mortality. American Journal of Epidemiology 137:270–280.

Morrison HI, Semenciw RM, Wilkins K, Mao Y, Wigle DT. 1994. Non-Hodgkin's lymphoma and agricultural practices in the prairie provinces of Canada. Scandinavian Journal of Work, Environment, and Health 20:42–47.

Mueller N. 1995. Overview: viral agents and cancer. Environmental Health Perspectives 103(Suppl 8):259–261.

Musicco M, Sant M, Molinari S, Filippini G, Gatta G, Berrino F. 1988. A case-control study of brain gliomas and occupational exposure to chemical carcinogens: the risks to farmers. American Journal of Epidemiology 128:778–785.

Nanni O, Amadori D, Lugaresi C, Falcini F, Scarpi E, Saragoni A, Buiatti E. 1996. Chronic lymphocytic leukaemias and non-Hodgkin's lymphomas by histological type in farming-animal breeding workers: a population case-control study based on a priori exposure matrices. Occupational and Environmental Medicine 53(10):652–657.

NCI (National Cancer Institute). 2000. Surveillance, Epidemiology, and End Results (SEER) Program, Cancer Query System on the Web 1973–1997. http://www.seer.cancer.gov/Scientific Systems/Canques/spool/AAAfra434.html (accessed November 11).

NTP (National Toxicology Program). 1982. Technical Report Series No. 209. Carcinogenesis Bioassay of 2,3,7,8-Tetrachlorodibenzo-p-dioxin (CAS No. 1746-01-6) in Osborne-mendel Rats and B6c3F1 Mice (Gavage Study). NIH Publication No. 82-1765. 195 pp. National Toxicology Program, Research Triangle Park, NC, and Bethesda, MD.

O'Brien TR, Decoufle P, Boyle CA.1991. Non-Hodgkin's lymphoma in a cohort of Vietnam veterans. American Journal of Public Health 81:758–760.

Ojajärvi IA, Partanen TJ, Ahlbom A, Boffetta P, Hakulinen T, Jourenkova N, Kauppinen TP, Kogevinas M, Porta M, Vainio HU, Weiderpass E, Wesseling CH. 2000. Occupational exposures and pancreatic cancer: a meta-analysis. Occupational and Environmental Medicine 57:316–324.

Olsson H, Brandt L. 1988. Risk of non-Hodgkin's lymphoma among men occupationally exposed to organic solvents. Scandinavian Journal of Work, Environment, and Health 14:246–251.

Ott MG, Zober A. 1996. Cause specific mortality and cancer incidence among employees exposed to 2,3,7,8-TCDD after a 1953 reactor accident. Occupational and Environmental Medicine 53:606–612.

Pearce NE, Smith AH, Fisher DO. 1985. Malignant lymphoma and multiple myeloma linked with agricultural occupations in a New Zealand cancer registry-based sudy. American Journal of Epidemiology 121:225–237.

Pearce NE, Smith AH, Howard JK, Sheppard RA, Giles HJ, Teague CA. 1986. Non-Hodgkin's lymphoma and exposure to phenoxyherbicides, chlorophenols, fencing work, and meat works employment: a case control study. British Journal of Industrial Medicine 43:75–83.

Pearce NE, Sheppard RA, Smith AH, Teague CA. 1987. Non-Hodgkin's lymphoma and farming: an expanded case-control study. International Journal of Cancer 39:155–161.

Percy C, Ries GL, Van Holten VD. 1990. The accuracy of liver cancer as the underlying cause of death on death certificates. Public Health Reports 105:361–368.

Persson B, Dahlander AM, Fredriksson M, Brage HN, Ohlson CG, Axelson O. 1989. Malignant lymphomas and occupational exposures. British Journal of Industrial Medicine 46:516–520.

Persson B, Fredriksson M, Olsen K, Boeryd B, Axelson O. 1993. Some occupational exposures as risk factors for malignant lymphomas. Cancer 72:1773–1778.

Pesatori AC, Consonni D, Tironi A, Landi MT, Zocchetti C, Bertazzi PA. 1992. Cancer morbidity in the Seveso area, 1976–1986. Chemosphere 25:209–212.

Pesatori AC, Consonni D, Tironi A, Zocchetti C, Fini A, Bertazzi PA. 1993. Cancer in a young population in a dioxin-contaminated area. International Journal of Epidemiology 22(6):1010–1013.

Pesatori AC, Zocchetti C, Guercilena S, Consonni D, Turrini D, Bertazzi PA. 1998. Dioxin exposure and nonmalignant health effects: a mortality study. Occupational and Environmental Medicine 55(2):126–131.

Ramlow JM, Spadacene NW, Hoag SR, Stafford BA, Cartmill JB, Lerner PJ. 1996. Mortality in a cohort of pentachlorophenol manufacturing workers, 1940–1989. American Journal of Industrial Medicine 30:180–194.

Riedel D, Pottern LM, Blattner WA. 1991. Etiology and epidemiology of multiple myeloma. In: Wiernick PH, Camellos G, Kyle RA, Schiffer CA, eds. Neoplastic Disease of the Blood and Blood Forming Organs. New York: Churchill Livingstone.

Riihimaki V, Asp S, Hernberg S. 1982. Mortality of 2,4-dichlorophenoxyacetic acid and 2,4,5-trichlorophenoxyacetic acid herbicide applicators in Finland: first report of an ongoing prospective cohort study. Scandinavian Journal of Work, Environment, and Health 8:37–42.

Rix BA, Villadsen E, Engholm G, Lynge E. 1998. Hodgkin's disease, pharyngeal cancer, and soft tissue sarcomas in Danish paper mill workers. Journal of Occupational and Environmental Medicine 40(1):55–62.

Robinson CF, Waxweiler RJ, Fowler DP. 1986. Mortality among production workers in pulp and paper mills. Scandinavian Journal of Work, Environment, and Health 12:552–560.

Ronco G, Costa G, Lynge E. 1992. Cancer risk among Danish and Italian farmers. British Journal of Industrial Medicine 49:220–225.

Saracci R, Kogevinas M, Bertazzi PA, Bueno De Mesquita HB, Coggon D, Green LM, Kauppinen T, L'Abbe KA, Littorin M, Lynge E, Mathews JD, Neuberger M, Osman J, Pearce N, Winkelmann R. 1991. Cancer mortality in workers exposed to chlorophenoxy herbicides and chlorophenols. Lancet 338:1027–1032.

Schreinemachers DM. 2000. Cancer mortality in four northern wheat-producing states. Environmental Health Perspectives 108(9):873–881.

Semenciw RM, Morrison HI, Morison D, Mao Y. 1994. Leukemia mortality and farming in the prairie provinces of Canada. Canadian Journal of Public Health 85:208–211.

Sharma-Wagner S, Chokkalingam AP, Malker HS, Stone BJ, McLaughlin JK, Hsing AW. 2000. Occupation and prostate cancer risk in Sweden. Journal of Occupational and Environmental Medicine 42(5):517–525.

Smith AH, Pearce NE. 1986. Update on soft tissue sarcoma and phenoxyherbicides in New Zealand. Chemosphere 15:1795–1798.

Smith AH, Fisher DO, Giles HJ, Pearce NE. 1983. The New Zealand soft tissue sarcoma case-control study: interview findings concerning phenoxyacetic acid exposure. Chemosphere 12:565–571.

Smith AH, Pearce NE, Fisher DO, Giles HJ, Teague CA, Howard JK. 1984. Soft tissue sarcoma and exposure to phenoxyherbicides and chlorophenols in New Zealand. Journal of the National Cancer Institute 73:1111–1117.

Smith JG, Christophers AJ. 1992. Phenoxy herbicides and chlorophenols: a case control study on soft tissue sarcoma and malignant lymphoma. British Journal of Cancer 65:442–448.

Smith-Warner SA, Spiegelman D, Yaun SS, van den Brandt PA, Folsom AR, Goldbohm RA, Graham S, Holmberg L, Howe GR, Marshall JR, Miller AB, Potter JD, Speizer FE, Willett WC, Wolk A, Hunter DJ. 1998. Alcohol and breast cancer in women: a pooled analysis of cohort studies. Journal of the American Medical Association 279(7):535–540.

Solet D, Zoloth SR, Sullivan C, Jewett J, Michaels DM. 1989. Patterns of mortality in pulp and paper workers. Journal of Occupational Medicine 31:627–630.

Sorahan T, Waterhouse JA. 1983. Mortality study of nickel–cadmium battery workers by the method of regression models in life tables. British Journal of Industrial Medicine 40(3):293–300.

Steenland K, Piacitelli L, Deddens J, Fingerhut M, Chang LI. 1999. Cancer, heart disease, and diabetes in workers exposed to 2,3,7,8-tetrachlorodibenzo-p-dioxin. Journal of the National Cancer Institute 91(9):779–786.

Stehr PA, Stein G, Webb K, Schramm W, Gedney WB, Donnell HD, Ayres S, Falk H, Sampson E, Smith SJ. 1986. A pilot epidemiologic study of possible health effects associated with 2,3,7,8-tetrachlorodibenzo-p-dioxin contaminations in Missouri. Archives of Environmental Health 41:16–22.

Suskind RR, Hertzberg VS. 1984. Human health effects of 2,4,5-T and its toxic contaminants. Journal of the American Medical Association 251:2372–2380.

Svensson BG, Mikoczy Z, Stromberg U, Hagmar L. 1995. Mortality and cancer incidence among Swedish fishermen with a high dietary intake of persistent organochlorine compounds. Scandinavian Journal of Work, Environment and Health 21(2):106–115.

Swaen GMH, van Vliet C, Slangen JJM, Sturmans F. 1992. Cancer mortality among licensed herbicide applicators. Scandinavian Journal of Work, Environment, and Health 18:201–204.

Sweeney MH, Calvert GM, Egeland GA, Fingerhut MA, Halperin WE, Piacitelli LA. 1997/98. Review and update of the results of the NIOSH medical study of workers exposed to chemicals contaminated with 2,3,7,8-tetrachlorodibenzodioxin. Teratogenesis, Carcinogenesis, and Mutagenesis 17(4–5):241–247.

Tarone RE, Hayes HM, Hoover RN, Rosenthal JF, Brown LM, Pottern LM, Javadpour N, O'Connell KJ, Stutzman RE. 1991. Service in Vietnam and risk of testicular cancer. Journal of the National Cancer Institute 83:1497–1499.

Thiess AM, Frentzel-Beyme R, Link R. 1982. Mortality study of persons exposed to dioxin in a trichlorophenol-process accident that occurred in the BASF AG on November 17, 1953. American Journal of Industrial Medicine 3:179–189.

Thomas TL. 1987. Mortality among flavour and fragrance chemical plant workers in the United States. British Journal of Industrial Medicine 44:733–737.

Thomas TL, Kang HK. 1990. Mortality and morbidity among Army Chemical Corps Vietnam veterans: a preliminary report. American Journal of Industrial Medicine 18:665–673.

Thomas TL, Kang H, Dalager N. 1991. Mortality among women Vietnam veterans, 1973–1987. American Journal of Epidemiology 134:973–980.

U.S. Census. 1999. Statistical Abstract of the United States: 1999, 119th Edition. Washington, DC: U.S. Bureau of the Census.

Viel JF, Arveux P, Baverel J, Cahn JY. 2000. Soft-tissue sarcoma and non-Hodgkin's lymphoma clusters around a municipal solid waste incinerator with high dioxin emission levels. American Journal of Epidemiology 152(1):13–19.

Vineis P, Terracini B, Ciccone G, Cignetti A, Colombo E, Donna A, Maffi L, Pisa R, Ricci P, Zanini E, Comba P. 1986. Phenoxy herbicides and soft-tissue sarcomas in female rice weeders. A population-based case-referent study. Scandinavian Journal of Work, Environment, and Health 13:9–17.

Vineis P, Faggiano F, Tedeschi M, Ciccone G. 1991. Incidence rates of lymphomas and soft-tissue sarcomas and environmental measurements of phenoxy herbicides. Journal of the National Cancer Institute 83:362–363.

Visintainer PF, Barone M, McGee H, Peterson EL. 1995. Proportionate mortality study of Vietnam-era veterans of Michigan. Journal of Occupational and Environmental Medicine 37(4):423–428.

Watanabe KK, Kang HK. 1995. Military service in Vietnam and the risk of death from trauma and selected cancers. Annals of Epidemiology 5(5):407–412.

Watanabe KK, Kang HK. 1996. Mortality patterns among Vietnam veterans: a 24-year retrospective analysis. Journal of Occupational and Environmental Medicine 38(3):272–278.

Watanabe KK, Kang HK, Thomas TL. 1991. Mortality among Vietnam veterans: with methodological considerations. Journal of Occupational Medicine 33:780–785.

Waterhouse D, Carman WJ, Schottenfeld D, Gridley G, McLean S. 1996. Cancer incidence in the rural community of Tecumseh, Michigan: a pattern of increased lymphopoietic neoplasms. Cancer 77(4):763–770.

Weiderpass E, Adami HO, Baron JA, Wicklund-Glynn A, Aune M, Atuma S, Persson I. 2000. Organochlorines and endometrial cancer risk. Cancer Epidemiology, Biomarkers and Prevention 9:487–493.

Wigle DT, Semenciw RB, Wilkins K, Riedel D, Ritter L, Morrison HI, Mao Y. 1990. Mortality study of Canadian male farm operators: non-Hodgkin's lymphoma mortality and agricultural practices in Saskatchewan. Journal of the National Cancer Institute 82:575–582.

Wiklund K. 1983. Swedish agricultural workers: a group with a decreased risk of cancer. Cancer 51:566–568.

Wiklund K, Lindefors BM, Holm LE. 1988. Risk of malignant lymphoma in Swedish agricultural and forestry workers. British Journal of Industrial Medicine 45:19–24.

Wiklund K, Dich J, Holm LE, Eklund G. 1989a. Risk of cancer in pesticide applicators in Swedish agriculture. British Journal of Industrial Medicine 46:809–814.

Wiklund K, Dich J, Holm LE. 1989b. Risk of soft tissue sarcoma, Hodgkin's disease and non-Hodgkin's lymphoma among Swedish licensed pesticide applicators. Chemosphere 18:395–400.

Wolfe WH, Michalek JE, Miner JC, Rahe A, Silva J, Thomas WF, Grubbs WD, Lustik MB, Karrison TG, Roegner RH, Williams DE. 1990. Health status of Air Force veterans occupationally exposed to herbicides in Vietnam. I. Physical health. Journal of the American Medical Association 264:1824–1831.

Woods JS, Polissar L, Severson RK, Heuser LS, Kulander BG. 1987. Soft tissue sarcoma and non-Hodgkin's lymphoma in relation to phenoxy herbicide and chlorinated phenol exposure in western Washington. Journal of the National Cancer Institute 78:899–910.

Zack JA, Suskind RR. 1980. The mortality experience of workers exposed to tetrachlorodibenzodioxin in a trichlorophenol process accident. Journal of Occupational Medicine 22:11–14.

Zahm SH, Fraumeni JF Jr. 1997. The epidemiology of soft tissue sarcoma. Seminars in Oncology 24(5):504–514.

Zahm SH, Weisenburger DD, Babbitt PA, Saal RC, Vaught JB, Cantor KP, Blair A. 1990. A case-control study of non-Hodgkin's lymphoma and the herbicide 2,4-dichlorophenoxyacetic acid (2,4-D) in eastern Nebraska. Epidemiology 1:349–356.

Zahm SH, Blair A, Weisenburger DD. 1992. Sex differences in the risk of multiple myeloma associated with agriculture (2). British Journal of Industrial Medicine 49:815–816.

Zahm SH, Weisenburger DD, Saal RC, Vaught JB, Babbitt PA, Blair A. 1993. The role of agricultural pesticide use in the development of non-Hodgkin's lymphoma in women. Archives of Environmental Health 48:353–358.

Zhong Y, Rafnsson V. 1996. Cancer incidence among Icelandic pesticide users. International Journal of Epidemiology 25(6):1117–1124.

Zhu K, Levine RS, Brann EA, Gnepp DR, Baum MK. 1995. A population-based case-control study of the relationship between cigarette smoking and nasopharyngeal cancer (United States). Cancer Causes and Control 6(6):507–512.

Zober A, Messerer P, Huber P. 1990. Thirty-four-year mortality follow-up of BASF employees exposed to 2,3,7,8-TCDD after the 1953 accident. International Archives of Occupational and Environmental Health 62:139–157.

8

Reproductive Effects

INTRODUCTION

This chapter summarizes the scientific literature published since *Veterans and Agent Orange: Update 1998* (hereafter, *Update 1998*; IOM, 1999) on exposure to herbicides and adverse reproductive or developmental effects. The literature includes papers describing environmental, occupational, and Vietnam veteran studies that evaluated herbicide exposure and the risk of adverse outcomes, including spontaneous abortion, birth defects, stillbirths, neonatal and infant mortality, childhood cancer, low birthweight, and sperm quality and infertility. Besides studies of herbicides and 2,3,7,8-tetrachlorodibenzo-*p*-dioxin (TCDD), studies of populations exposed to polychlorinated biphenyls (PCBs) are also reviewed when relevant, since TCDD is a ubiquitous contaminant of PCBs.

The primary emphasis is on the potential adverse reproductive effects of herbicide exposure in males, because the vast majority of Vietnam veterans are men, but since approximately 8,000 women served in Vietnam (H. Kang, U.S. Department of Veterans Affairs, personal communication, December 14, 2000), findings relevant to female reproductive health are also included.

In addition to studies of specific health and developmental outcomes associated with reproduction, there have been several reports investigating reproductive hormones in relation to exposures to TCDD or related compounds such as PCBs, which are contaminated with TCDD when they occur in the human environment. Sweeney et al. (1998) measured several reproductive hormones, namely serum testosterone, luteinizing hormone (LH), and follicle-stimulating hormone (FSH) in workers exposed to TCDD through their involvement in chemical production. These authors found that among 479 male workers, as the serum concentration of 2,3,7,8-TCDD increased, so did the odds of having a high level of LH or FSH; the odds of having a low testosterone level also increased with the concentration of TCDD. A study of women from Seveso is in progress (Eskenazi et al., 2000). This investigation will examine serum TCDD concentration in relation to (1) endometriosis, (2) menstrual cycle characteristics, (3) age at menarche, (4) birth outcomes, (5) time to conception and infertility, and (6) age at menopause.

The following specific categories of reproductive effects have been reviewed in previous Veterans and Agent Orange (*VAO*) reports (IOM, 1994, 1996, 1999): fertility, sex ratio, spontaneous abortion, stillbirth and infant mortality, low birthweight and preterm delivery, and birth defects. New data since *Update 1998* are available for spontaneous abortion, sex ratio, birth defects, childhood cancer, low birthweight, and early postnatal growth.

BIRTH DEFECTS

Background

The March of Dimes defines a birth defect as "an abnormality of structure, function or metabolism, whether genetically determined or as the result of an environmental influence during embryonic or fetal life" (Bloom, 1981). Other terms often used interchangeably with birth defects are "congenital anomalies" and "congenital malformations." Major birth defects are usually defined as those abnormalities that are present at birth and severe enough to interfere with viability or physical well-being. Major birth defects are seen in approximately 2 to 3 percent of live births. An additional 5 percent of birth defects can be detected with follow-up through the first year of life. The cause of most birth defects is unknown. In addition to genetic factors, a number of other factors and exposures including medication, environmental, occupational, and life-style have long been implicated in the etiology of some birth defects (Kalter and Warkany, 1983). Historically, most etiologic research focused on the effect of maternal and fetal exposures, but work on paternal exposures is receiving increased attention. Paternal exposures could exert an effect through direct genetic damage to the male germ cell that is transmitted to the offspring and expressed as a birth defect; through transfer of chemicals via seminal fluid, with subsequent fetal exposure; or by indirect exposure from household contamination.

Summary of *VAO*, *Update 1996*, and *Update 1998*

The committee responsible for *VAO* found there to be inadequate or insufficient information to determine whether an association existed between exposure to herbicides used in Vietnam or the contaminant dioxin and birth defects among offspring. Additional information available to the committee responsible for *Update 1996* led it to conclude that there was limited or suggestive evidence of an association between the exposures and spina bifida in the children of veterans; there was no change in the conclusions regarding other birth defects. There was no change in these findings in *Update 1998*. Reviews of the studies underlying these findings may be found in the earlier reports.

Update of the Scientific Literature

Garcia et al. (1998) conducted a case-control study based on births in eight hospitals located in agricultural areas in Spain. Cases consisted of infants with any of the following malformations: nervous system defects, cardiovascular defects, epispadias or hypospadias, musculoskeletal defects, and unspecified defects. Some cases fell into more than one group. Controls were matched (1:1) with cases by hospital and date of birth. Interviews were conducted with parents of the cases and controls by telephone where possible and inperson otherwise. The questions covered potential confounders and activities that would involve potential exposure to pesticides. The critical exposure period for fathers was considered to be 3 months before conception through the first trimester of pregnancy, and for mothers, 1 month before conception through the first trimester. Interviewees who were involved in agricultural activities during this critical period were interviewed a second time to collect detailed information about their work and their potential exposures. Reliability and accuracy were assessed by gathering information from several sources, including employers and previously completed questionnaires. Several experts independently reviewed the interview information on exposures, and when discrepancies arose, a meeting was held to reach consensus. Overall, the adjusted odds ratio (OR) was 0.9 (95 percent confidence interval [95% CI] 0.3–2.7) for exposure to organochlorines. 2-Methyl-4-chlorophenoxyacetic acid (MCPA), a chlorophenoxy herbicide, showed an adjusted OR of 1.2 (0.4–3.8). When analyzed by a semiquantitative scale based on probability and intensity of exposure, the highest category of exposure to chlorophenoxy herbicides, compared to no exposure, showed an adjusted OR of 2.1 (0.5–9.8); the OR for MCPA was 2.6 (0.4–17.1). When analyzed according to an index based on months of work in agriculture and intensity of exposure, chlorophenoxy herbicides above the median had an OR of 3.1 (0.6–16.9), while for MCPA, the OR was 3.5 (0.6–21.8). When analyzed for involvement in pesticide treatments, those above the median level of exposure to chlorophenoxy herbicides had an OR of 0.6 (0.1–2.9), and a similar OR was seen for MCPA. Overall, this study provides little evidence for an association between herbicides chemically related to or potentially contaminated by TCDD and the risk of nervous system, cardiovascular, genital, musculoskeletal, or unspecified defects. However, because of the small number of exposed cases ($N = 21$), the statistical power and precision were poor.

In July 1998, the National Technical Information Service (NTIS) released a report that was apparently completed in 1984 regarding reproductive outcomes in Air Force personnel exposed to herbicides (Michalek et al., 1998a). The data concern the Ranch Hand cohort and a corresponding comparison group; comparisons are made for conceptions taking place in two time periods: pre- and post-Southeast Asia. The fathers were interviewed, and their reports of birth defects in their children were verified by reviewing birth and other medical records and birth and death certificates. The most common defects were of the musculoskeletal and the circulatory systems. About one-third of the reported defects had not been verified; this percentage was equal for Ranch Hands and comparisons. The analysis used only verified defects. No verification had been conducted for those responding that their children had no defects. In the pre-Southeast Asia period, those in the Ranch Hand group had a lower percentage of children with birth defects than the comparison group (OR = 0.7). In the post-Southeast Asia period, the percentage of children with birth defects was higher (OR = 1.5). These were significantly different; however, after adjustment for occupation; the test for homogeneity gave a p-value of 0.6. The differences between Ranch Hands and comparisons were found for the enlisted flying and enlisted ground crews but not for officers. When stratified by smoking, the strongest differences were found among children whose mothers smoked. Overall, this study suggests a possible association between service in Southeast Asia and birth defects but is limited because of the low verification of reported birth defects and the lack of verification of reports of no defects. The use of a heterogeneous group of defects could have reduced statistical power if exposure were associated with malformations in one system or of one type only.

The Australian Vietnam veterans Validation Study also examined spina bifida in the offspring of male Vietnam veterans (AIHW, 1999). In this study, an attempt was made to validate self-reported medical conditions. For each condition or disease, medical documents, physician certification, and records on disease or death registers were used. Three categories were created: (1) a condition was considered "validated" if sufficient information was found that confirmed the existence of the condition; (2) a condition was considered "not validated" if information from the validation source indicated that the condition did not or had not existed to the best of its knowledge; (3) a condition was considered "not able to be validated" when the source could not be contacted or accessed, or the source indicated was not able to confirm or deny the existence of the condition. The study made an adjustment to estimate the number that fell in the third category but would be expected to be validated based on information in reports in the first two categories. A total of 34 spina bifida cases were validated, and the adjustment brought this figure to an estimated 50. The expected number of cases, for comparison, was 33, for which a CI of 22–44 is given in the report. Thus, there appears to be a significant excess of spina bifida cases in children born to Australian Vietnam veterans. Cleft palate also showed an excess, with 94 estimated validated conditions, where 64 were expected.

Conclusions

Strength of Evidence in Epidemiologic Studies

The committee continues to believe that the available scientific literature provides limited/suggestive evidence of an association between exposure to herbicides (2,4-D, 2,4,5-T and its contaminant TCDD, cacodylic acid, and picloram) and spina bifida in offspring. The Australian veterans Validation Study lends further support to this conclusion. Given the limitations in this study, including the extrapolation of validation rates to cases with inadequate data, the information available is not strong enough to reclassify this outcome in the category of "sufficient evidence."

There is no information contained in the research reviewed for this report to change the conclusion that there is inadequate or insufficient evidence to determine whether an association exists between exposure to herbicides (2,4-D, 2,4,5-T and its contaminant TCDD, cacodylic acid, and picloram) and other birth defects.

Biologic Plausibility

Laboratory studies of potential male-mediated developmental toxicity of TCDD and herbicides, specifically with regard to birth defects, are too limited to permit conclusions. Research on chemical production workers with TCDD exposure suggests that some hormonal changes are associated with such exposure, but it is unclear whether these changes could be responsible for an increase in spina bifida or other birth defects.

A summary of the biologic plausibility for the reproductive effects of TCDD and the herbicides in general is presented in the conclusion to this chapter. A discussion of toxicological studies that concern biologic plausibility is contained in Chapter 3.

Increased Risk of Disease Among Vietnam Veterans

The new data from the Validation Study of Australian Vietnam veterans provides further evidence of an elevated risk for spina bifida among the offspring of men who served in Vietnam. Other data that have come to the attention of the committee are contained in a report from the Air Force Health Study, which indicates that among children conceived after service in Southeast Asia, birth defects may have been greater in the Ranch Hand group than in the comparison group. However, about one-third of reported birth defects were of unknown verification status, severely limiting the conclusions that can be drawn. Thus, the previous conclusion that there is limited/suggestive evidence for an increased risk of spina bifida among offspring of Vietnam veterans remains, but there are no changes with regard to other birth defects.

TABLE 8-1 Selected Epidemiologic Studies—Neural Tube Defects

Reference	Study Population	Exposed Cases[a]	Estimated Risk (95% CI)[a]
OCCUPATIONAL			
Studies reviewed in *Update 1998*			
Blatter et al., 1997	Offspring of Dutch farmers—spina bifida		
	Pesticide use		
	(moderate or heavy exposure)	9	1.7 (0.7–4.0)
	Herbicide use		
	(moderate or heavy exposure)	7	1.6 (0.6–4.0)
Kristensen et al., 1997	Offspring of Norwegian farmers—spina bifida		
	Tractor spraying equipment	28	1.6 (0.9–2.7)
	Tractor spraying equipment and orchards or greenhouses	5	2.8 (1.1–7.1)
Dimich-Ward et al., 1996	Sawmill workers		
	Spina bifida or anencephaly	22[b]	2.4 (1.1–5.3)
	Spina bifida	18[b]	1.8 (0.8–4.1)
Garry et al., 1996	Private pesticide appliers		
	Central nervous system defects	6	1.1 (0.5–2.4)
ENVIRONMENTAL[c]			
Studies Reviewed in *VAO*			
Stockbauer et al., 1988	TCDD soil contamination in Missouri		
	Central nervous system defects	3	3.0 (0.3–35.9)
Hanify et al., 1981	Spraying of 2,4,5-T in New Zealand		
	Anencephaly	10	1.4 (0.6–3.3)
	Spina bifida	13	1.1 (0.6–2.3)
VIETNAM VETERANS			
New Studies			
AIHW, 1999	Australian Vietnam veterans—Validation Study (spina bifida)	50	1.5 (NR)
Studies Reviewed in *Update 1996*			
Wolfe et al., 1995	Follow-up of Air Force Ranch Hands		
	Neural tube defects among Ranch Hands children[d]	4	
	Neural tube defects among comparison children	0	
Studies Reviewed in *VAO*			
CDC, 1989	Vietnam Experience Study		
	Spina bifida among Vietnam veterans' children	9	1.7 (0.6–5.0)
	Spina bifida among non-Vietnam veterans' children	5	
	Anencephaly among Vietnam veterans' children	3	
	Anencephaly among non-Vietnam veterans' children	0	

TABLE 8-1 *Continued*

Reference	Study Population	Exposed Cases[a]	Estimated Risk (95% CI)[a]
Erickson et al., 1984a,b	Birth Defects Study		
	Vietnam veterans: spina bifida	19	1.1 (0.6–1.7)
	Vietnam veterans: anencephaly	12	0.9 (0.5–1.7)
	EOI-5: spina bifida	19[c]	2.7 (1.2–6.2)
	EOI-5: anencephaly	7[c]	0.7 (0.2–2.8)
Australia Department of Veteran Affairs, 1983	Australian Vietnam veterans—Neural tube defects	16	0.9

NOTE: EOI = score based on interview; NR = not reported; 2,4,5-T = 2,4,5-trichlorophenoxyacetic acid.

[a] Given when available.

[b] Number of workers with maximal index of exposure (upper three quartiles) for any job held up to 3 months prior to conception.

[c] Either or both parents potentially exposed.

[d] Four neural tube defects among Ranch Hand offspring include two spina bifida (high dioxin level), one spina bifida (low dioxin), and one anencephaly (low dioxin). Denominator for Ranch Hand group is 792 and for comparison group 981.

[e] Number of Vietnam veterans fathering a child with a neural tube defect given any exposure opportunity index.

FERTILITY

Background

Male reproductive function is a complex system under the control of several components whose proper coordination is important for normal fertility. There are several components or end points related to male fertility, including reproductive hormones and sperm parameters. Only a brief description of male reproductive hormones is given here; more detailed reviews can be found elsewhere (Yen and Jaffe, 1991; Knobil et al., 1994). The reproductive neuroendocrine axis involves the central nervous system, the anterior pituitary gland, and the testis. The hypothalamus integrates neural inputs from the central and peripheral nervous systems and regulates gonadotropins (luteinizing hormone and follicle-stimulating hormone). Both of these hormones are necessary for normal spermatogenesis. Luteinizing hormone and follicle-stimulating hormone are secreted in episodic bursts by the anterior pituitary gland into the circulation. LH interacts with receptors on the Leydig cells, which leads to increased testosterone synthesis. FSH and testosterone from the Leydig cells interact with the Sertoli cells in the seminiferous tubule epithelium to regulate spermatogenesis. Several agents, such as lead and dibromochloropropane, have been shown to affect the neuroendocrine system and spermatogenesis (Bonde and Giwercman, 1995; Tas et al., 1996).

Summary of *VAO*, *Update 1996*, and *Update 1998*

The committee responsible for *VAO* found that there was inadequate or insufficient information to determine whether an association existed between exposure to the herbicides used in Vietnam or the contaminant dioxin and altered sperm parameters or infertility. Additional information available to the committees responsible for *Update 1996* and *Update 1998* did not change this finding. Reviews of the studies underlying these findings may be found in the earlier reports.

Update of the Scientific Literature

A few new studies have appeared in the literature in relation to fertility. A study of Danish farmers compared those who used pesticides with those who did not in relation to the "fecundability ratio (FR)" (Larsen et al., 1998). This ratio represents a means of assessing how long it takes a sexually active couple to achieve a pregnancy while not using any form of contraceptive. A low FR (i.e., an FR less than 1.0) suggests that it takes longer for the exposed group to achieve pregnancy. In this study, the farmers were questioned about their use of pesticides during the year before their youngest child was born. A specific list of pesticides with potential for spermatotoxicity was presented, which included 2,4-dichlorophenoxyacetic acid (2,4-D), benomyl, carbendazim, iprodione, isoproturon, atrazine, chlormequat chloride, glyphosate, deltamethrin, fenvalerate, dimethoate, mancozeb, manep, and dinoseb. Several variables were constructed that reflected farm practices known to be associated with exposure levels. Those exposed to pesticides at the start of unprotected coitus had similar fecundability to those who were not (i.e., pregnancies occurred at a similar rate for the two groups [FR = 1.0, 0.8–1.4]). A tendency toward reduced fecundability was observed for those who used three or more pesticides with spermatotoxic effects (FR = 0.9, 0.7–1.2), and similarly for those using a manually controlled sprayer (FR = 0.8, 0.6–1.1). The main weaknesses of the study were the relatively small number who were not using pesticides, the use of self-reported recall of pesticide use, and for the purposes of this report, the lack of information on TCDD level as a contaminant of the pesticides investigated. It should also be noted that studies limited to couples who achieve a pregnancy can be biased, because the most severe cases, those who are infertile, are excluded (Sallmén et al., 2000).

Abell et al. (2000) also report on fecundability, in an investigation of female greenhouse workers in Denmark. The study compared women members of the gardener's trade union who were employed in flower greenhouses with other members of the union and also evaluated different work activities or the use of protective gloves. Although it did not take longer for the flower greenhouse workers to become pregnant, those with higher exposures to pesticides did take longer. The FR was 0.7 (0.5–1.0) for those with more than 20 hours contact compared to those with less than 20 hours contact, 0.7 (0.5–1.0) for those who never used gloves versus those who used them always, and 0.6 (0.5–0.9) for those with high exposure based on several work practices versus those with low exposure. However, data on specific pesticide exposures or on TCDD contamination of such pesticides were not available.

Conclusions

Strength of Evidence in Epidemiologic Studies

There is no information contained in the research reviewed for this report to change the conclusion that there is inadequate or insufficient evidence to determine whether an association exists between exposure to herbicides (2,4-D, 2,4,5-T and its contaminant TCDD, cacodylic acid, and picloram) and altered hormone levels, decreased sperm count or quality, subfertility, or infertility.

Biologic Plausibility

Experimental animal evidence suggests that dioxin can alter testosterone synthesis, generally at relatively high doses, but does not provide direct clues as to the reproductive significance of alterations in hormone levels of the magnitude found in available studies.

A summary of the biologic plausibility for the reproductive effects of TCDD and the herbicides in general is presented in the conclusion to this chapter. A discussion of toxicological studies that concern biologic plausibility is contained in Chapter 3.

Increased Risk of Disease Among Vietnam Veterans

Given the large uncertainties that remain about the magnitude of exposures in Vietnam and about the potential risk, if any, for altered hormones, semen quality parameters, and subfertility or infertility, it is not possible for the committee to quantify the degree of risk for infertility likely to be experienced by Vietnam veterans because of their exposure to herbicides in Vietnam.

TABLE 8-2 Selected Epidemiologic Studies—Fertility

Reference	Study Population	Exposed Cases[a]	Estimated Relative Risk (95% CI)[a]
OCCUPATIONAL			
New Studies			
Abell et al., 2000[b]	Female greenhouse workers in Denmark		
	>20 hours manual contact per week	220	0.7 (0.5–1.0)
	Never used gloves	156	0.7 (0.5–1.0)
	High exposure	202	0.6 (0.5–0.9)
Larsen et al., 1998[b]	Danish farmers who used any potentially spermatotoxic pesticides, including		
	2,4-D	523	1.0 (0.8–1.4)
	Used three or more pesticides		0.9 (0.7–1.2)
	Used manual sprayer		0.8 (0.6–1.1)
Studies Reviewed in *Update 1998*			
Heacock et al., 1998	Workers at sawmills using chlorophenates	18,016 (births)	0.9 (0.8–0.9)
	Workers at sawmills using chlorophenates	18,016	0.7 (0.7–0.8)[c]
	Cumulative exposure (hours)		
	120–1,999	7,139	0.8 (0.8–0.9)
	2,000–3,999	4,582	0.9 (0.8–0.9)
	4,000–9,999	4,145	1.0 (0.9–1.1)
	≥10,000	1,300	1.1 (0.9–1.2)
Studies Reviewed in *Update 1996*			
Henriksen et al., 1996	Ranch Hands		
	Low testosterone		
	High dioxin (1992)	18	1.6 (0.9–2.7)
	High dioxin (1987)	3	0.7 (0.2–2.3)
	Low dioxin (1992)	10	0.9 (0.5–1.8)
	Low dioxin (1987)	10	2.3 (1.1–4.9)
	Background (1992)	9	0.5 (0.3–1.1)
	High FSH		
	High dioxin (1992)	8	1.0 (0.5–2.1)
	Low dioxin (1992)	12	1.6 (0.8–3.0)
	Background (1992)	16	1.3 (0.7–2.4)
	High LH		
	High dioxin (1992)	5	0.8 (0.3–1.9)
	Low dioxin (1992)	5	0.8 (0.5–3.3)
	Background (1992)	8	0.8 (0.4–1.8)
	Low sperm count		
	High dioxin	49	0.9 (0.7–1.2)
	Low dioxin	43	0.8 (0.6–1.0)
	Background	66	0.9 (0.7–1.2)

TABLE 8-2 *Continued*

Reference	Study Population	Exposed Cases[a]	Estimated Relative Risk (95% CI)[a]
VIETNAM VETERANS			
Studies Reviewed in *VAO*			
CDC, 1989	Vietnam Experience Study		
	Lower sperm concentration	42	2.3 (1.2–4.3)
	Proportion of abnormal sperm	51	1.6 (0.9–2.8)
	Reduced sperm motility	83	1.2 (0.8–1.8)
Stellman et al., 1988	American Legionnaires who served in Southeast Asia		
	Difficulty having children	349	1.3 ($p < .01$)

[a] Given when available.
[b] For this study, relative risk has been replaced with the fecundability ratio, for which a value less than 1.0 indicates an adverse effect.
[c] Standardized fertility ratio.

SPONTANEOUS ABORTION

Background

Spontaneous abortion refers to the expulsion of a nonviable fetus, generally before 20 weeks of gestation, not induced through physical or pharmacologic means. The background risk for recognized spontaneous abortion is generally around 7–15 percent (Hertz-Picciotto and Samuels, 1988), although it is established that many more pregnancies terminate before the woman is aware that she has become pregnant (Wilcox et al., 1988); the latter are known as subclinical pregnancy losses. Estimates of the risk of recognized spontaneous abortion will vary according to the design and method of analysis. Major types of study designs include cohorts of women asked retrospectively about their pregnancy history, cohorts of pregnant women, usually those receiving prenatal care, and cohorts of women who are monitored for future pregnancies. Retrospective reports may be limited by memory loss, particularly of spontaneous abortions that took place a long time before. Studies enrolling women who appear for prenatal care require the use of life tables and specialized statistical techniques to account for the varying times during pregnancy when women seek medical care. Enrollment of women before pregnancy provides the theoretically most valid estimate of risk, but because of very demanding protocols, this may attract nonrepresentative study groups.

Summary of *VAO*, *Update 1996*, and *Update 1998*

The committee responsible for *VAO* found that there was inadequate or insufficient information to determine whether an association existed between exposure to the herbicides used in Vietnam or the contaminant dioxin and spontaneous abortion. Additional information available to the committees responsible for *Update 1996* and *Update 1998* did not change this finding. Reviews of the studies underlying these findings may be found in the earlier reports.

Update of the Scientific Literature

A survey of women employed by the U.S. Forest Service assessed job exposures and reproductive outcomes (Driscoll, 1998). A mail questionnaire was sent to more than 10,000 women aged 18–52 who were full-time employees with at least a year of service. The questionnaire collected information on job duties and reproductive histories for a 10-year period. Questions inquired about use of herbicides, pesticides, and specific paints, as well as potential confounders including smoking, alcohol, hobbies, home pesticide applications, and so forth. A 59 percent response rate was achieved. The initial analysis showed foresters to have a greater proportion of pregnancies ending in miscarriage (18 percent) than non-foresters (14 percent), with an adjusted OR of 1.4 (1.1–1.9). When analyses were conducted for specific work exposures and adjusted for maternal age, self-reported strenuous work, smoking, and alcohol consumption, use of herbicides was associated with an increased risk of spontaneous abortion, OR = 2.0 (1.1–3.5). The primary weaknesses of this study were the low response rate with consequent possible selection bias and the lack of information regarding specific herbicides used.

Petrelli et al. (2000) conducted a small study of pregnancies among wives of pesticide appliers. Fifty-one workers were engaged in mixing pesticides manually, then applying them, with applications occurring for 6 hours daily. A comparison group consisted of food retailers, who had no direct exposure to pesticides through work or hobbies. Reproductive histories were collected by interviews. Pesticide appliers reported a greater proportion of spontaneous abortions among their wives' pregnancies, but the men were also less educated and more likely to smoke, although their wives were less likely to do so. Although multiple logistic regression analyses were conducted, education was not controlled and insufficient information was provided regarding models with interactions. Due to these weaknesses combined with the small sample size, the study provides little information relevant to this report. The list of pesticides applied during the period of employment of these workers included several that may have been contaminated by TCDD, but the published report did not address particular exposures.

A study of miscarriages among wives of Swedish fishermen, a group with a relatively high consumption of fish contaminated with PCBs, ascertained pregnancy outcomes by questionnaire (Axmon et al., 2000). After adjustment for numerous potential confounders, the women who consumed high quantities of fish had a lower risk of miscarriage than those with no fish consumption.

In a doctoral dissertation, Schwartz (1998) conducted an interview study with three groups of women: female veterans who served in Vietnam, female veterans of the Vietnam era who did not serve in Vietnam, and female civilians who were matched by age and occupation to the group who served in Vietnam. Ninety-five percent of the veterans were located, and a high response was achieved. The Vietnam era veterans differed markedly in age and occupation from the Vietnam veterans, who tended to be older and consisted mostly of nurses (84 percent versus 10 percent among Vietnam era veterans). Interviews were conducted, with questions taken from several sources, including the National Survey of the Vietnam Generation and the National Health Interview Survey. The former asked questions on demographics, financial status, and reproductive outcomes, while the latter asked about health. Results showed that spontaneous abortions occurred more frequently in women who had served in Vietnam than in comparable civilians, but not more frequently than in women veterans who did not serve in Vietnam. However, major demographic differences between the two veteran groups make it difficult to interpret the comparisons that were made.

Conclusions

Strength of Evidence in Epidemiologic Studies

There is inadequate or insufficient evidence to determine whether an association exists between exposure to herbicides (2,4-D, 2,4,5-T and its contaminant TCDD, cacodylic acid, and picloram) and spontaneous abortion.

Biologic Plausibility

Experimental animal evidence suggests that dioxin can alter hormones but does not provide direct clues about the reproductive significance of these hormonal changes and the risk of recognized pregnancy loss before 20 weeks of gestation.

A summary of the biologic plausibility for the reproductive effects of TCDD and the herbicides in general is presented in the conclusion to this chapter. A discussion of toxicological studies that concern biologic plausibility is contained in Chapter 3.

Increased Risk of Disease Among Vietnam Veterans

Few studies have addressed spontaneous abortion in Vietnam veterans. The recent doctoral dissertation examining female veterans provides weak evidence of an association between herbicides used in Vietnam and risk of spontaneous abortion among exposed women. Unfortunately, interpretation of the results is hampered by problems of comparability of the referent groups. Given the relatively weak data and the great uncertainties regarding the level of exposures experienced by servicepersons in Vietnam, it is not possible for the committee to quantify the degree of risk for spontaneous abortion likely to be or to have been experienced by Vietnam veterans because of their exposure to herbicides in Vietnam.

STILLBIRTH, NEONATAL DEATH, AND INFANT DEATH

Background

The term stillbirth or late fetal death is typically defined as the delivery of a fetus occurring at or after 28 weeks of gestation that shows no signs of life at birth, although a more recent definition includes deaths among all fetuses weighing more than 500 grams at birth, regardless of gestational age at delivery (Kline et al., 1989). Neonatal death refers to the death of a live-born infant within the first 28 days of life. Because the causes of stillbirths and early neonatal deaths overlap considerably, these are commonly analyzed as one group, referred to as perinatal mortality (Kallen, 1988). Stillbirths occur in less than 1 percent of all births (CDC, 2000). Among low-birthweight live- and stillborn infants (500–2,500 grams), placental and delivery complications such as abruptio placentae, placenta previa, malpresentation, and umbilical cord complications are the most common causes of perinatal mortality (Kallen, 1988). Among infants weighing more than 2,500 grams at birth, the most common causes of perinatal death are complications of the cord, placenta, and membranes and lethal congenital malformations (Kallen, 1988).

Summary of *VAO*, *Update 1996*, and *Update 1998*

The committee responsible for *VAO* found that there was inadequate or insufficient information to determine whether an association existed between exposure to the herbicides used in Vietnam or the contaminant dioxin and stillbirth, neonatal death, and infant death. Additional information available to the committees responsible for *Update 1996* and *Update 1998* did not change this finding. Reviews of the studies underlying these findings may be found in the earlier reports.

Update of the Scientific Literature

No new relevant data regarding stillbirths or infant mortality have come to the attention of the committee.

Conclusions

Strength of Evidence in Epidemiologic Studies

There is no information contained in the research reviewed for this report to change the conclusion that there is inadequate or insufficient evidence to determine whether an association exists between exposure to herbicides (2,4-D, 2,4,5-T and its contaminant TCDD, cacodylic acid, and picloram) and stillbirth, neonatal death, and infant death.

Biologic Plausibility

Laboratory studies of the potential male-mediated developmental toxicity of TCDD and herbicides as a result of exposure of adult male animals are too limited to permit conclusions.

A summary of the biologic plausibility for the reproductive effects of TCDD and the herbicides in general is presented in the conclusion to this chapter. A discussion of toxicological studies that concern biologic plausibility is contained in Chapter 3.

Increased Risk of Disease Among Vietnam Veterans

Given the large uncertainties that remain about the magnitude of potential risk of stillbirth, neonatal death, and infant death, it is not possible for the committee to quantify the degree of risk likely to be experienced by Vietnam veterans because of their exposure to herbicides in Vietnam. It is also possible that if such a risk exists, it would decline with time since service.

LOW BIRTHWEIGHT AND PRETERM BIRTH

Background

The World Health Organization (WHO) recommends a 2,500-gram cutpoint for the determination of low birthweight (Alberman, 1984). Reduced infant weight at birth is one of the most important causes of neonatal mortality and morbidity in the United States. Although often treated as a single entity, the concept of low birthweight actually encompasses two different causal pathways: (1) low birthweight secondary to intrauterine growth retardation (IUGR) or small for gestational age, and (2) low birthweight secondary to preterm delivery, which may have more long-term consequences. The concept of IUGR represents birthweight adjusted for gestational age. The currently used definition of preterm delivery (PTD) is delivery at less than 259 days, or 37 completed weeks of gestation, calculated on the basis of the date of the first day of the last menstrual period

(Bryce, 1991). Approximately 7 percent of live births have low birthweight. The incidence of IUGR is much more difficult to quantify since there are no universally applied standards for dividing the distribution of birthweight for gestational age. When no distinction is made between the causes of low birthweight (i.e., IUGR versus PTD), the factors most strongly associated with reduced birthweight are maternal smoking during pregnancy, multiple births, and race or ethnicity. Other potential risk factors for low birthweight include socioeconomic status (SES), maternal size, birth order, maternal complications during pregnancy (e.g., severe preeclampsia) and obstetric history, job stress, and cocaine or caffeine use during pregnancy (Kallen, 1988). Established risk factors for preterm birth include race (black); marital status (single); low SES; previous low birthweight or preterm birth; multiple gestations; cigarette smoking; and cervical, uterine, or placental abnormalities (Berkowitz and Papiernik, 1993).

Summary of *VAO*, *Update 1996*, and *Update 1998*

The committee responsible for *VAO* found that there was inadequate or insufficient information to determine whether an association existed between exposure to the herbicides used in Vietnam or the contaminant dioxin and low birthweight. Additional information available to the committees responsible for *Update 1996* and *Update 1998* did not change this finding. Reviews of the studies underlying these findings may be found in the earlier reports.

Update of Scientific Literature

A number of earlier studies found that mothers with high exposures to PCBs gave birth to infants that were lower in weight and remained smaller at later ages. These included the Yusho and Yucheng children, born to mothers in Japan and Taiwan, respectively, who were exposed accidentally when cooking oil with high concentrations of PCBs was sold commercially (Kuratsune et al., 1972; Chen et al., 1994). Infants born to women who consumed contaminated fish from Lake Michigan experienced a decrease in birthweight, a smaller head circumference, and a weight deficit at age 4 years (Fein et al., 1984; Jacobson et al., 1990). It was recognized that the cooking oil in Taiwan and Japan also was contaminated with dioxins; similarly, fish with PCBs are contaminated with dioxins.

More recently, Patandin et al. (1998) have been following a group of children with exposures to PCBs and dioxins beginning in utero. Cord and maternal plasma samples were used to estimate prenatal PCB exposures, and breast milk was collected for measurement of TCDD and other polychlorinated dibenzodioxin or dibenzofuran (PCDD/F) congeners, as well as three planar PCBs, three mono-ortho PCBs, two diortho PCBs, and eighteen nonplanar PCBs. A toxic equivalent (TEQ) was estimated according to the approach of Safe (1994), by applying the congener concentration in breast milk (nanograms per kilogram of milk fat) to the

TEQ factor and summing over all congeners. PCBs in cord plasma, expressed as the sum of the International Union of Pure and Applied Chemistry (IUPAC) numbers 118, 138, 153, and 180 (the four most abundant PCBs in human samples) were inversely associated with birthweight; findings were similar for maternal plasma. The authors also found that the rate of growth between birth and 3 months, among those who were not breast-fed, was negatively associated with prenatal PCB exposures. However, among breast-fed children, neither PCBs nor TEQs were associated with decreased rates of growth. No associations were found with the rate of growth after 3 months. Although no measurements of TCDD were made in the blood specimens collected at birth, dioxins are a contaminant of PCBs, and their presence in breast milk samples indicates clearly that these pregnant women also carried body burdens to which the fetus was exposed in utero. However, it is not possible to distinguish an effect of the dioxins from that of PCBs, some of which may operate by similar mechanisms. Planar PCBs and mono-ortho PCBs bind to the aryl hydrocarbon receptor (AhR) and may exert toxic effects through this same mechanism, believed to be a primary one for TCDD.

Rylander et al. (1998) conducted a study of low birthweight among children whose fathers were fishermen. The exposures were estimated by collecting blood samples in 1995 and extrapolating back to the time of pregnancies in 1973–1991. Cases of low birthweight (1,500–2,750 grams) were matched with controls on gender, parity, and calendar year of birth, and PCB 153 was used as a marker of exposure. In previous work, these authors had found that the correlation coefficient between PCB 153 and the total PCB toxic equivalent was 0.9 (Grimvall et al., 1997). Several extrapolation models were examined for the estimation of exposures during the pregnancies of interest. These were validated against a group of women for whom two blood samples in different years were available, although there were limitations to this validation. The analysis of low birthweight indicated an increase in risk with increasing exposure. The authors emphasized the strength of the association at the upper end of the exposure range and suggested that the effect might follow a threshold model. However there seemed to be an elevated risk (ORs of 1.8, 2.1, and 2.3) above several different cutpoints from different extrapolation models. The primary limitation of this study follows from uncertainties in the exposure assessment, which would likely have reduced the precision of this already small study.

Vartiainen et al. (1998) also analyzed PCBs, PCDDs, and PCDFs measured in breast milk samples in relation to birthweight. Their study was conducted in a Finnish population exposed primarily through consumption of contaminated fish in the Baltic Sea. Birthweight decreased slightly with increasing concentrations of PCDDs, PCDFs, and PCBs, including an index of the TEQ based on the WHO equivalencies; this difference was stronger in boys. When restricted to primiparous pregnancies, the association was not observed. This finding is difficult to interpret for several reasons. First, none of the analyses of birthweight and organochlorine compounds adjusted simultaneously for other factors. Second, fish consumption has been found in some studies to increase birthweight, probably because of the presence of omega-3 fatty acids (Olsen et al., 1992). Thus, any deficits in growth related to contaminants may have been offset by the benefits of fish consumption. This issue is further complicated by the fact that educated mothers consumed more fish (and hence had higher TEQs), which might partially explain the lack of association between education and birthweight among boys. There was an association of birthweight with education among girls; however, some data suggest that boys are more susceptible to the developmental effects of PCBs or dioxins. Finally, after the authors stratified on parity and sex of the child, the numbers of observations were small.

No studies appear to have examined the risk for preterm delivery associated with TCDD or related compounds.

Conclusions

Strength of Evidence in Epidemiologic Studies

There is no information contained in the research reviewed for this report to change the conclusion that there is inadequate or insufficient evidence to determine whether an association exists between exposure to herbicides (2,4-D, 2,4,5-T and its contaminant TCDD, cacodylic acid, and picloram) and either low birthweight or preterm birth. A handful of studies of populations with exposures to TCDD have observed some association with low birthweight, although these investigations are not fully consistent. All of the new studies addressing this outcome involved exposures to a variety of compounds other than dioxins, such as polychlorinated biphenyls and polychlorinated dibenzofurans. Additionally, for most of these studies, only maternal exposure was addressed. For these reasons, the evidence is weak regarding an association between herbicides used in Vietnam and low birthweight among offspring.

Biologic Plausibility

Laboratory studies of the potential male-mediated developmental toxicity of TCDD and herbicides as a result of exposure of adult male animals are too limited to permit conclusions. Regarding female-mediated developmental toxicity, TCDD and herbicides are found in follicular fluid (Tsutsumi et al., 1998), suggesting exposure of embryos, and are known to cross the placenta, leading to direct exposure of the fetus.

A summary of the biologic plausibility for the reproductive effects of TCDD and the herbicides in general is presented in the conclusion to this chapter. A discussion of toxicological studies that concern biologic plausibility is contained in Chapter 3.

Increased Risk of Disease Among Vietnam Veterans

Given the large uncertainties that remain about the exposure levels of Vietnam veterans and the magnitude of potential risk of low birthweight and preterm birth, it is not possible for the committee to quantify the degree of risk likely to be experienced by the offspring of Vietnam veterans because of exposure to herbicides in Vietnam.

CHILDHOOD CANCERS

Background

The American Cancer Society (ACS) estimates that approximately 8,600 children under the age of 15 will be diagnosed with cancer in the United States in 2001. Nearly half of these cases will be in children aged 0 to 4 years. Treatment and supportive care for children with cancer have greatly improved, leading to a decline in mortality rates by 50 percent over the last 3 decades. Despite these advances, cancer remains the leading cause of death from disease in children under the age of 15, with 1,500 deaths projected in 2001.

Leukemia is the most common cancer in children. It accounts for about one-third of all childhood cancer cases, with nearly 2,700 children projected to be diagnosed in 2001 (ACS, 2001). Of these children, nearly 2,000 will be diagnosed with acute lymphocytic leukemia (ALL) and most of the rest with acute myelogenous leukemia (AML).[1] The former is most common in early childhood, peaking between ages 2 and 3, while the latter is most common during the first two years of life. ALL incidence is consistently higher in males than females, while AML shows similar incidence for boys and girls (NCI, 2001). Through early adulthood, ALL rates are about twice as high in whites as in African Americans, whereas there is no consistent pattern for AML. Chapter 7 contains additional information on leukemia as part of the discussion of adult cancer outcomes.

The second most common group of cancers in children are those of the central nervous system—brain and spinal cord. Other cancers occurring in children include lymphomas, bone cancers, soft-tissue sarcomas, kidney cancers, eye cancers, and adrenal gland cancers. Compared with adult cancers, relatively little

---

[1] *Acute myelogenous leukemia* (ICD·9 205) is referred to by other names as well, including acute myeloid leukemia and acute nonlymphocytic leukemia. There are also numerous subtypes of the disease. For consistency, this report uses "acute myelogenous leukemia," or the abbreviation AML, no matter how the disease is referred to in the work being reviewed.

is known about the etiology of most childhood cancers and especially about potential environmental risk factors and the impact of parental exposures.

Summary of *VAO*, *Update 1996*, and *Update 1998*

The committee responsible for *VAO* found there to be inadequate or insufficient information to determine whether an association existed between exposure to herbicides used in Vietnam or the contaminant dioxin and childhood cancers. Additional information available to the committees responsible for *Update 1996* and *Update 1998* did not change this finding. Table 8-3 provides summaries of the results of the studies underlying these findings and a list of reports that contain details of the research.

Update of Scientific Literature

Occupational Studies

An earlier study, not previously summarized in *Veterans and Agent Orange* reports, examined occupational herbicide exposures in relation to acute myelogenous leukemia (Buckley et al., 1989). This study was assembled by the Children's Cancer Study Group and included cases diagnosed from 1980 to 1984. Initial analyses focused on self-reported job titles, with linkage to exposures based on a previously developed job–exposure matrix (Hoar et al., 1980). One hundred seventy-eight case-control pairs provided information regarding paternal occupational pesticide exposures, including weed killers. Using the job-title linkage, pesticide exposures were associated with a 2.3-fold increased risk. Using self-reported information on workplace exposure to specific types of products and on duration of exposure, a 2.7-fold increased risk of fathering a child who developed AML was found for men exposed more than 1,000 days. Results were comparable when interviews conducted with surrogates for the fathers were excluded from the analysis. An elevated risk was seen for exposure before, during, and after the pregnancy, but since these were highly correlated, it was not possible to determine which time period might have been most important.

A second study addressed childhood cancer in children born to male sawmill workers in British Columbia, Canada (Heacock et al., 2000). The primary exposures in these plants were to chlorophenate fungicides, which are contaminated with PCDDs and PCDFs formed during the production of these chemicals. Employees who worked at least 1 year at any of 11 such lumber mills in 1950–1985 formed the cohort of 23,829. Estimates of exposure were made from job title in each mill using information from mill records and interviews with persons knowledgeable about technology and formulation changes; a validation study that compared urinary chlorophenates with job-based estimates yielded a correlation of 0.5. The cohort was linked to birth files and also to marriage files that were linked to birth files (since the mother's name is on all birth certificates, whereas the father's name is not always), in order to identify the cohort of workers' children. The children's cohort was then linked to the British Columbia Cancer Registry to determine cancer diagnoses by age 20. Cancer cases in children born to sawmill plant workers from 1952 through 1988 and diagnosed in 1969–1993 were included. There were a total of 40 such cases, of which 22 were female and 18 male.

The initial analysis proceeded by calculation of a standardized incidence ratio (SIR), in which the cancer experience of these children was compared to that of the general population of the province of British Columbia, adjusted for age and sex of the children and calendar year. Results showed no elevation of risk for all cancers (SIR = 1.0, 0.7–1.4) or for leukemia (SIR = 1.0, 0.5–1.8); a slight but imprecise excess was observed for brain cancer (SIR = 1.3, 0.6–2.5). An internal comparison was conducted using a nested case-control design. For each case, five controls were selected from within the cohort matched on sex and year of birth. These results compared risks for differing cumulative exposure groups within four time windows: (1) more than 90 days prior to conception; (2) 90 days before conception to conception; (3) conception to birth; and (4) after birth. The risks for all cancers combined and for brain cancer were greater in the high-exposure groups than in the low-exposure groups for all windows except the first (more than 90 days before conception); however, these findings were not stable (i.e., all confidence intervals included values consistent with no effect or even a lowered risk in those with high exposures). The risk for leukemia was not elevated. The main limitations of the study were the small number of cases and the lack of quantitative data on chlorophenate or TCDD exposure.

Environmental Studies

Infante-Rivard et al. (1999) examined the risk of childhood acute lymphocytic leukemia associated with pesticide use: 491 cases in 0–9-year-old children were identified from tertiary care centers in the province of Quebec, Canada, over the years 1980–1993. These were age, gender, and location matched with controls. Interviewers administered questionnaires to the parents of all subjects to gather information on potential influencing and confounding variables, including home use of pesticides. Cases were significantly more likely than controls to be from households that used herbicides while the subject was in utero (OR = 1.8, 1.3–2.6) or during the subject's childhood (OR = 1.4, 1.1–1.9). Risk increased with frequency of use, although this observation was based on a very small number of cases in the higher of two use categories. The authors suggested that 2,4-D was probably the ingredient most frequently contained in the chlorophenoxy herbicides used at home. Because exposures were based entirely on self-reports after the diagnosis (and hence, for most cases, years after pregnancy), controls may have been less attuned to recalling events of the past than cases, producing recall bias. Additionally, specific products were not recorded (i.e., no analysis by chlorophenoxy herbicide use was possible).

A much larger population-based case-control interview study of several childhood cancers was conducted in West Germany by Meinert et al. (2000). The children were diagnosed at less than 15 years of age, and there were 1,184 cases of leukemia. Parental occupational exposures to herbicides, insecticides, or fungicides were found to be related to childhood cancer regardless of the time period of exposure and the type of cancer (lymphoma or leukemia) (see Table 8-3). Of particular note is the finding that there was a statistically significant association between paternal exposure in the year before pregnancy and leukemia (OR = 1.5, 1.1–2.2, based on 62 cases). Statistically significant associations were also found between leukemia and paternal exposure during pregnancy (1.6, 1.1–2.3) and "ever" (1.6, 1.1–2.3). However the strongest associations were in relation to maternal exposures during pregnancy (e.g., leukemia OR = 3.6, 1.5–8.8). No analyses of the separate types of leukemia were reported.

The data provide some evidence of an increased leukemia risk for children exposed in utero to herbicides, insecticides, or fungicides and also for children whose fathers were exposed preconceptionally. While this study may have been the largest ever to examine this hypothesis, the possibility of recall bias could not be ruled out, and there was some evidence suggesting that parents of cases consistently reported more occupational exposures than parents of controls. Neither study reported the effect of paternal preconception exposures independent of maternal exposures (or vice versa). The relevance of this study to exposures to the herbicides used in Vietnam and their contaminants is uncertain because the data did not permit analysis by specific herbicides.

Pearce and Parker (2000) compared children who died of kidney cancer with children who died of other causes with regard to paternal occupation in agriculture at the time of the child's birth. No association was found, although the relatively small number of deaths (21) from kidney cancer complicates the analysis. However, the analysis compared these children to children who died of other causes, rather than to the full cohort. If other children who died were more (or perhaps less) likely to have had fathers who worked in agriculture, the results could be biased.

Vietnam Veteran Studies

In a large case-control study, Wen et al. (2000) examined service in Vietnam or Cambodia as a risk factor for childhood leukemia. The study included 1,805 cases of ALL and 528 cases of AML, including cases diagnosed through 17 years of age. It combined data from three studies conducted by the Children's Cancer Group, which represents a consortium of hospitals and medical centers in the United States and Canada that pool their cases to enable large studies of rare childhood cancers to achieve sufficient statistical power. The cases were matched to controls on year of birth, location of residence, sex, and race. Controls were found through random-digit dialing, and cases were restricted to those with a telephone in the home. The overall response rates were 89 percent for cases and 77 percent for controls, and they were slightly lower for those with paternal interviews (83 percent for cases, 70 percent for controls). Analyses were conducted using conditional logistic regression for all leukemias combined, for ALL and AML separately, and stratified by age at diagnosis. Regression models adjusted for potential confounders, including education, race, family income, smoking, exposure to X-rays, and paternal marijuana use.

The results indicated no increased risk of either leukemia subtype associated with military service in general. However, for service in Vietnam or Cambodia, the risk of AML, but not ALL, was increased: OR = 1.7 (1.0–2.9). Analyses examining tours in Vietnam or Cambodia led to small numbers, although the highest risk was for those with two or more tours there; for those serving less than or equal to 1 year in these countries, the OR was 2.4 (1.1–5.4), whereas those with more than 1 year had an OR of 1.5 (0.7–3.2). When stratified by years between service and conception of the child, the association was strongest in those who had served more than 15 years earlier; however, the numbers in this stratum were small. Self-reported exposure to Agent Orange showed no association. The strongest association was for cases diagnosed under the age of 2 years. It is believed that childhood cancers at very young ages are more likely to be etiologically related to preconception or in utero exposures than those diagnosed at later ages. Limitations of the study include possible residual confounding from not having detailed exposure data on smoking and marijuana use; the unexplained stronger association with increasing interval between service and conception; and possible other factors associated with service in Vietnam or Cambodia, including postwar exposures. The authors point out that the inconsistency in results for number of tours of duty versus number of years in Vietnam or Cambodia could have been related to exposures being correlated with movement in and out of these areas, rather than with duration, or to other exposures in Southeast Asian countries. Longer duration in Vietnam or Cambodia does not necessarily mean higher exposure to herbicides, since no information is available on the nature of these veterans' activities during their service.

Close to 50,000 Australian Vietnam veterans were surveyed about their and their children's health, and an 80 percent response rate was achieved (Commonwealth Department of Veterans' Affairs [CDVA], 1998). A follow-up validation study of selected conditions was conducted that included children's cancers (AIHW, 1999); a later supplement (AIHW, 2000) had, as one of its aims, the collection and analysis of data on specific subtypes of leukemia among children of veterans. Validation sources included pathology reports, doctor certifications, or records from a disease or death registry. Australia has had, since 1982, a cancer registry. Nine cases of reported AML were confirmed through clinical records. The investigators used various assumptions to adjust for nonrespondents in the validation study and for circumstances in which it was not possible to validate a reported case (e.g., physician could not be located or medical records were incomplete). Depending on the specific assumptions, up to nine additional cases of AML were estimated for the full cohort (for a total of from 9 to 18 cases). The assumptions adopted by the study's authors estimated 4 additional cases (i.e., 13 validated cases where 3 [range 0–6] were expected) using community standards. This represents a statistically significant 4.3-fold increased risk. All of the alternative analyses, including those with the most restrictive assumptions (i.e., assuming zero cases among nonrespondents and no valid AML diagnoses among reported cases for which validation was not possible), also yielded large, precise, and hence statistically significant excesses of AML. These analyses did not adjust for any sociodemographic or life-style factors associated with increased risk of AML, although adjustment for age and gender was achieved through the methods used to derive expected numbers of cases in Australia's community standard. As in the study of Wen et al., no excess risk was observed for childhood ALL. The number of cases of chronic lymphocytic leukemia (CLL) and chronic myelocytic leukemia (CML) was well within the range of the expected number of cases.

The study also examined adrenal gland cancer in the children of veterans. It found a much higher-than-expected incidence of the disease, reporting 10 cases where 1 (range 0 to 3) was expected, using community standards.

Synthesis

No firm evidence links exposures to the herbicides used in Vietnam with most childhood cancers, including acute lymphocytic leukemia, chronic leukemias, non-Hodgkin's lymphoma, brain tumors, neuroblastoma, and cancers at other sites. A cohort study reports a slight elevation in risk to children of sawmill workers (Heacock et al., 2000), but the estimate of effect is very imprecise, and it is unclear how the exposures studied inform the question of the effect of exposure to the chemicals of concern in this report. One case-control study shows elevated risks for all leukemias with either maternal or paternal occupational use of herbicides, pesticides, or fungicides, specifically during the year prior to conception (Meinert et al., 2000). A similar association, but with much less precision, was seen for non-Hodgkin's lymphoma. Another case-control study showed elevated risks for ALL with household herbicide use during pregnancy (Infante-Rivard et al., 1999) but did not address exposures prior to pregnancy. Both of these studies relied on self-reports of exposure, which can entail biased reporting: for example, parents of children without cancer may be less likely to recall having used pesticides some years in the past, whereas parents of children with cancer might have thought about it more and therefore be likely to recall such activities. Self-report of use of herbicides, pesticides, or fungicides does not necessarily imply that exposures to dioxin or the herbicides used in Vietnam occurred. Overall, the literature lacks consistency for most types of cancer in children of exposed persons. The one study that separated herbicides from pesticides or fungicides did not examine exposures prior to conception, the time period most relevant for births to Vietnam veterans.

Three studies provide evidence regarding an association between exposure to the herbicides used in Vietnam and acute myelogenous leukemia in the children of veterans. The first is a case-control study of AML and parental occupational exposures conducted by the Children's Cancer Study Group (Buckley et al., 1989). Use of pesticides by either the mother or the father, as reported in detailed interviews, was associated with an elevated risk. However, because of a high correlation among exposures in the three periods studied (before, during, and after pregnancy), it was not possible to determine whether exposure uniquely prior to the pregnancy was associated with increased risk of AML in the children. The strongest associations were for children diagnosed before 5 years of age and for children with M4/M5 morphology.

In a second case-control study of AML conducted by the Children's Cancer Group (Wen et al., 2000), self-reported service in Vietnam or Cambodia was associated with an elevated risk (OR = 1.7, CI 1.0–2.9), after adjusting for potential confounders including education, race, income, smoking, X-ray exposure, and paternal marijuana use. Since service in Vietnam or Cambodia would be an extremely memorable event, underreporting by controls or overreporting by cases seems unlikely. Also arguing against recall bias was the lack of association with ALL in this study, as well as the lack of association of AML with general paternal military service. When stratified by time spent in Vietnam or Cambodia, those with 1 year or less of service there showed a greater risk than those with more than 1 year; additionally, self-reported exposure to Agent Orange was not associated with AML. However, these outcomes are not particularly convincing evidence against a causal association since neither length of service in Vietnam or Cambodia nor self-reported exposure is known to be strongly related to the actual level of herbicide exposure. Two or more tours of duty in Vietnam showed a stronger association than a single tour, although the numbers were small. This study showed the strongest association to be with childhood AML diagnosed before the age of 2 years (OR = 4.6, 1.3–16.1). One concern was the apparent lack of adjustment for maternal marijuana use, which has been shown to be related to AML (Robison et al., 1989). Additionally, the authors point out that an unexplained increase in risk with longer time since service in Vietnam or Cambodia might have been due to random fluctuations, but could also have been due to an unmeasured postwar exposure that was different from those who did not serve in the military or those who served elsewhere.

A third study on this topic is that of the Australian Vietnam veterans. Investigators surveyed veterans regarding their medical conditions and the health of their children (CDVA, 1998), with a follow-up validation of the self-reported conditions and a calculation of the expected number of cases based on Australian community standards (AIHW, 1999, 2000). The results were thereby adjusted for age and gender but not for other potential confounding factors. Among respondents, 9 cases of AML were successfully validated, where 3 (range 0–6) were expected based on the community standard. Taking into account possible additional cases among nonrespondents and cases that might have been validated had the information been obtainable, the authors estimated that there were 13 cases of AML among the veterans' children, representing a 4.3-fold increased risk. As in the study of Wen et al., no excess risk was observed for ALL among the children. Sensitivity analyses were conducted using a variety of strategies for assignment of nonrespondent cases. These analyses yielded relative risks, compared to a community standard, that varied from 3.0 to 6.0—in all cases, these were significant.

The relatively thorough control for confounders in the study by Wen et al. combined with the magnitude of association among Australian veterans diminishes the likelihood of explanations unrelated to service in Vietnam. The results of the Buckley et al. study suggest that exposure to the herbicides used in Vietnam is a credible candidate for producing the observed outcomes.

Conclusions

Strength of Evidence in Epidemiologic Studies

Based on the scientific evidence reviewed above, the committee finds **there is limited/suggestive evidence of an association between exposure to the herbicides of concern in this report and acute myelogenous leukemia (AML) in the children of veterans.** This is a change in classification from previous *Veterans and Agent Orange* reports, which found inadequate/insufficient evidence to determine whether an association existed for AML and other cancers.

When the whole of the literature was considered, the committee found that it met the definition established for limited/suggestive evidence—that is, *evidence is suggestive of an association between herbicides and the outcome, but limited because chance, bias, and confounding could not be ruled out with confidence.* Two studies, in particular, support this conclusion. One is a case-control study of AML conducted by the Children's Cancer Group (Wen et al., 2000) in which self-reported service in Vietnam or Cambodia was associated with an elevated risk after adjusting for numerous potentially confounding lifestyle and sociodemographic factors. The other, a study of the children of Australian Vietnam veterans (AIHW, 2000), found a greater than fourfold risk, although confounding factors other than age and gender were not controlled. While direct measures of exposure are lacking, the committee found the following characteristics of these studies to be particularly persuasive: (1) both studies were conducted in Vietnam veteran populations; (2) the association was specific for AML, with no excess risk for ALL; (3) one study adjusted for numerous confounders, while the other had an association of sufficiently large magnitude to reduce the likelihood of being completely due to confounding; and (4) the strongest association was seen in children diagnosed at the youngest ages—cases that are considered the strongest candidates for an etiology of parental origin. These characteristics of the studies and their findings reduce the likelihood of alternative explanations.

A 1989 case-control study of AML and parental occupational exposures by Buckley et al. reported a 2.7-fold increased risk in the children of fathers with self-reported exposure of more than 1,000 days to pesticides or weed killers. The study also found an association with maternal occupational exposures of more than 1,000 days and a high correlation among parental exposures in different time periods (before, during, and after pregnancy). It is thus not possible to determine whether paternal exposure uniquely prior to the pregnancy was associated with increased risk of AML in the children.

The Meinert et al. (2000) study finds a statistically significant excess of leukemia in children whose fathers were exposed to herbicides, insecticides, or fungicides in the year preceding the pregnancy, but does not separate the types of leukemia for analysis. It is therefore not possible to assess whether this study provides additional supportive evidence regarding AML. If the information is available, the committee encourages these researchers to conduct separate analyses of ALL and AML (the two most common forms of childhood leukemia) and publish the results.

None of the studies of childhood cancer outcomes reviewed in previous *Veterans and Agent Orange* reports provide specific information regarding AML. The Centers for Disease Control Vietnam Experience Study (CDC, 1989) found an elevated risk for childhood leukemia in its veterans' cohort (OR = 1.6, 0.6–4.0, based on 12 cases), but the types of leukemia found were not reported. A study reviewed in *Update 1996* of subjects aged 0–19 living in the area surrounding Seveso, Italy—site of a 1976 industrial accident that released dioxin into the environment—found 3 cases of myelogenous leukemia in the 10 years following the event where 1.1 was expected (RR = 2.7, 0.7–11.4) (Pesatori et al., 1993). However, all were in individuals born prior to the accident.

There is inadequate or insufficient evidence to determine whether an association exists between exposure to the herbicides considered in this report or the contaminant dioxin and most childhood cancers, including acute lymphocytic leukemia, chronic leukemias, non-Hodgkin's lymphoma, brain tumors, neuroblastoma, and cancers at other sites. Although two moderately sized investigations did observe associations with ALL, all leukemia, or non-Hodgkin's lymphoma in children, these studies were still problematic, because of reliance on self-reports for exposure assessment and/or a lack of information on exposures prior to the child's conception, the time period relevant for cancer among children of Vietnam veterans. Additionally, both Vietnam veterans' studies (AIHW, 2000; Wen et al., 2000) observed no association with ALL.

Biologic Plausibility

As noted in Chapter 3, the reproductive systems of adult male laboratory animals are considered to be relatively insensitive to TCDD because high doses are required to elicit effects. Two animal studies reviewed in *Update 1998* have investigated developmental effects following paternal exposure to the chemicals of interest. No paternally mediated effects were observed in the offspring of mice exposed to a mixture of 2,4-D, 2,4,5-T, and dioxin (Lamb et al., 1980). The offspring of mice exposed to a mixture of 2,4-D and picloram, however, showed some effects but at doses that also caused paternal toxicity (Blakley et al., 1989).

The mechanism by which herbicide or TCDD exposures could lead to childhood cancer in the offspring of persons exposed many years previously is unclear. One possible mechanism would involve germ cell mutations whereby damaged cells might later undergo spermatogenesis and result in fertilization, leading to the birth of a genetically susceptible child. However, assays do not indicate that the herbicides of interest or TCDD are genotoxic except at very high doses or concentrations. The link between Down's syndrome and AML appears to imply some genetic origin for at least a portion of AML cases. Leukemias in younger children, the period during which childhood AML cases are more common, are believed to have a different etiology from those of older children because the genetic abnormalities underlying them are more likely to have been present at birth.

Given the present lack of information, the committee believes that further research aimed at evaluating long-term effects of herbicide exposures on male reproductive organs would be useful.

Increased Risk of Disease Among Vietnam Veterans

Recently published studies reported an increased incidence of AML in the children of U.S. and Australian veterans of Vietnam. Although the committee's finding regarding the strength of evidence for AML derives primarily from this research, there remain large uncertainties about the exposure levels both of the subjects who participated in the cited studies and of Vietnam veterans generally. There are additional uncertainties regarding the magnitude of risk for AML in the children of Vietnam veterans. For these reasons, it is not possible for the committee to quantify the degree of risk for AML likely to be experienced by the children of Vietnam veterans because of their fathers' exposure to herbicides in Vietnam.

There remains insufficient information to quantify the degree of risk for other childhood cancers in the children of veterans resulting from their fathers' exposures to herbicides in Vietnam.

TABLE 8-3 Selected Epidemiologic Studies—Childhood Cancers

Reference	Study Population	Exposed Cases	RR, OR, or SIR (95% CI)
OCCUPATIONAL STUDIES			
Heacock et al., 2000	Cohort of sawmill workers' offspring; exposure via fungicides contaminated with PCDDs and PCDFs		
	Leukemia, all workers	11	SIR = 1.0 (0.5–1.8)
	Brain cancer, all workers	9	SIR = 1.3 (0.6–2.5)
	Leukemia, high chlorophenate exposure	5	OR = 0.8 (0.2–3.6)
	Brain cancer, high chlorophenate exposure	5	OR = 1.5 (0.4–6.9)
Buckley et al., 1989	Children's Cancer Study Group—case-control study of children of parents exposed to pesticides or weed killers		
	AML in children with any paternal exposure	27	OR = 2.3 ($p = .05$)
	AML in children with paternal exposure >1,000 days	17	OR = 2.7 (1.0–7.0)
	AML in children with maternal exposure >1,000 days	7	OR undefined (no cases in controls)
ENVIRONMENTAL STUDIES			
New Studies			
Meinert et al., 2000	Population-based case-control study of childhood cancer		
	Leukemias, paternal exposure, year before pregnancy	62	1.5 (1.1–2.2)
	Leukemias, paternal exposure, during pregnancy	57	1.6 (1.1–2.3)
	Lymphomas, paternal exposure, year before pregnancy	11	1.5 (0.7–3.1)
	Lymphomas, paternal exposure, during pregnancy	10	1.6 (0.7–3.6)
	Leukemias, maternal exposure, year before pregnancy	19	2.1 (1.1–4.2)
	Leukemias, maternal exposure, during pregnancy	15	3.6 (1.5–8.8)
	Lymphomas, maternal exposure, year before pregnancy	3	2.9 (0.7–13)
	Lymphomas, maternal exposure, during pregnancy	4	11.8 (2.2–64)

TABLE 8-3 *Continued*

Reference	Study Population	Exposed Cases	RR, OR, or SIR (95% CI)
Pearce and Parker, 2000	Cohort study examining paternal occupation on death certificate of children who died of kidney cancer Paternal agricultural occupation	(total cases = 21)	0.9 (0.2–3.8)
Infante-Rivard et al., 1999	Population-based case-control study of childhood ALL and household herbicide use during pregnancy	118	1.8 (1.3–2.6)
Studies Reviewed in *Update 1996*			
Pesatori et al., 1993	Seveso residents aged 0–19 years—10-year follow-up, morbidity		
	All cancers	17	1.2 (0.7–2.1)
	Ovary and uterine adnexa	2	— (0 expected)
	Brain	3	1.1 (0.3–4.1)
	Thyroid	2	4.6 (0.6–32.7)
	Hodgkin's lymphoma	3	2.0 (0.5–7.6)
	Lymphatic leukemia	2	1.3 (0.3–6.2)
	Myeloid leukemia	3	2.7 (0.7–11.4)
Bertazzi et al., 1992	Seveso residents aged 0–19 years—10-year follow-up, mortality		
	All cancers	10	7.9 (3.8–13.6)
	Leukemias	5	3.9 (1.2–1.8)
	Lymphatic leukemia	2	1.6 (0.1–4.5)
	Myeloid leukemia	1	0.8 (0.0–3.1)
	Leukemia, others	2	1.6 (0.1–4.6)
	Central nervous system tumors	2	1.6 (0.1–4.6)
VIETNAM VETERANS			
New Studies			
AIHW, 2000	Australian Vietnam veterans' children— Validation Study		
	AML	13 (estimated)	3 expected (0–6)
Wen et al., 2000	Case-control study of children's leukemia (AML and ALL)		
	Father ever served in Vietnam or Cambodia	117	1.2 (0.9–1.6)
	<1 year in Vietnam or Cambodia	61	1.4 (0.9–2.0)
	>1 year in Vietnam or Cambodia	49	1.2 (0.8–1.7)
	AML only		
	Father ever served in Vietnam or Cambodia	40	1.7 (1.0–2.9)
	<1 year in Vietnam or Cambodia	13	2.4 (1.1–5.4)
	>1 year in Vietnam or Cambodia	16	1.5 (0.7–3.2)

TABLE 8-3 *Continued*

Reference	Study Population	Exposed Cases	RR, OR, or SIR (95% CI)
Studies Reviewed in *VAO*			
CDC, 1989	Vietnam Experience Study		
	Cancer in children of veterans	25	1.5 (0.7–2.8)
	Leukemia in children of veterans	12	1.6 (0.6–4.0)
Field and Kerr, 1988	Cancer in children of Australian Vietnam veterans	4	—
Erikson et al, 1984b	CDC Birth Defects Study		
	"Other" neoplasms — children of Vietnam veterans	87	1.8 (1.0–3.3)

SEX RATIO

Background

Sex ratio (ratio of males to females at birth, about 105–107 males per 100 females, or 51.4 percent males among all births) has been used for a number of years as a potential marker of genetic damage. It has been hypothesized that the induction of lethal mutations prior to birth will alter the sex ratio at birth. In general, it was thought that with paternal exposure that there would be a reduction in the frequency of female offspring since sex-linked lethals on the paternal X chromosome would differentially affect female conceptuses. Investigators have evaluated the sex ratio among various species in relation to exposures such as radiation for a number of years. More recently, it has been suggested that the sex ratio is controlled by parental hormone levels at conception, and changes in gonadotropin and steroid levels may result in an altered sex ratio (James, 1996). The specific mechanisms involved (zygote formation, implantation, regulation of sex-determining factors, selective fetal loss) are uncertain, and direct experimental evidence for or against the hypothesis is lacking. James (1997) has suggested that a reduction in testosterone and high gonadotropin levels after dioxin exposure would result in an excess of female offspring. Potential confounding factors for altered sex ratio are uncertain, but parental age, social class, illness, race, smoking, and stress have been considered.

Summary of *VAO*, *Update 1996*, and *Update 1998*

The potential association between exposure to herbicides used in Vietnam or the contaminant dioxin and altered sex ratio was not explored in the *VAO* and *Update 1996* reports. The committee responsible for *Update 1998* reviewed papers addressing altered sex ratio as part of its examination of the literature on fertility. That committee found there to be inadequate or insufficient information to determine whether an association existed between exposure to herbicides used in Vietnam or the contaminant dioxin and health outcomes related to fertility.

Update of Scientific Literature

Mocarelli et al. (2000) have recently published new findings on the sex ratio of births to parents from Seveso, Italy, where an explosion of a chemical plant resulted in widespread environmental exposure in 1976. The study was based on a total of 674 births, to parents aged 3 to 45 at the time of the accident. Birth records for all persons in zones A and B and for a part of zone R were investigated, and all available serum samples from these parents or persons living outside these zones were analyzed for TCDD. Those who lived outside the three zones or whose TCDD measurement was less than 15 parts per trillion (ppt) were considered unexposed. Couples were analyzed according to whether the mother alone, the father alone, or both were exposed, based on the TCDD value in the 1976 serum specimen. The sex ratio was 0.6 if both parents were unexposed, 0.6 if only the mother was exposed, and 0.4 if only the father or if both parents were exposed. When only the father's exposure was considered, there was a decreasing trend ($p = .008$) for increasing concentration of TCDD in serum in 1976. When the authors stratified by age of the father in 1976, those who were younger than 19 years had a lower sex ratio than those older than 19, although for both groups the sex ratio was significantly different from that expected.

An interesting finding from this study is that the sex ratio within zone A was decreased not only from 1977 to 1984, but also in the period 1973–1976, the 4 years before the accident occurred. The authors argue that TCDD contamination of the environment surrounding the plant occurred even before the explosion. As evidence, they report that five men living in zone A from 1964 to 1967, who left before the accident and never returned, had TCDD levels in 1976 ranging from 138 to 352 ppt. In contrast, the sex ratio in a nearby comparison town with similar types of industrial and socioeconomic conditions was normal throughout 1966–1996.

In contrast to the Seveso findings, Michalek et al. (1998b) failed to find a reduction in male births among Ranch Hand personnel. This study included 2,157 live births, of whom 903 were to Ranch Hand servicemen and 1,254 to comparison servicemen. Ranch Hand veterans were divided into those having background, low, or high dioxin levels. The sex ratio was actually higher in those with high exposure than in the comparison group. This held true for births whose conception occurred in four different time periods: up to 1 month postservice, up to 1 year postservice, up to 5 years postservice, and during the entire postservice period.

The sex ratio results from the Seveso study have been compared with changes in wildlife sexual differentiation and mating behaviors hypothesized to be due to environmental contamination by hormonally active compounds such as DDT, dichlorodiphenyldichloroethylene (DDE), PCBs, and dioxin. In the case of the Seveso studies, only TCDD was present, rendering it less likely that the findings are due to other environmental contaminants. The discrepancy with the Ranch Hand study could be due to higher exposures in Seveso.

Conclusions

Strength of the Evidence in Epidemiologic Studies

Newly available information from the Seveso cohort, although interesting, does not change the committee's conclusion that there is inadequate or insufficient evidence to determine whether an association exists between exposure to the herbicides (2,4-D, 2,4,5-T and its contaminant TCDD, cacodylic acid, and picloram) and altered sex ratio.

Biologic Plausibility

Laboratory studies of the potential developmental toxicity of TCDD and herbicides using male animals are too limited to permit conclusions. A summary of the biologic plausibility for the reproductive effects of TCDD and the herbicides in general is presented in the conclusion to this chapter. A discussion of toxicological studies that concern biologic plausibility is contained in Chapter 3.

Increased Risk of Disease Among Vietnam Veterans

Given the large uncertainties that remain about the magnitude of potential risk of altered sex ratio, it is not possible for the committee to quantify the degree of risk likely to be experienced by Vietnam veterans because of their exposure to herbicides in Vietnam. Furthermore, giving birth to a higher-than-expected number of females is not in itself an adverse event. This outcome should be viewed as indicative of hormonal disruption with other potential adverse consequences, rather than as an outcome in itself.

SUMMARY

Strength of the Evidence in Epidemiologic Studies

The committee responsible for *Update 1996* found that there was limited/ suggestive evidence of an association between exposure to the herbicides considered in this report and spina bifida in the children of veterans. The Australian veterans Validation Study lends further support to this conclusion. The committee therefore upholds the designation reached in *Update 1996*. Also, as detailed earlier in the text, the committee concludes there is also limited/suggestive evidence of an association between exposure to these herbicides and AML in the children of veterans.

There is inadequate or insufficient evidence to determine whether an association exists between exposure to herbicides and altered hormone levels, semen quality, or infertility; spontaneous abortion; late-fetal, neonatal, or infant death; low birthweight or preterm delivery; birth defects other than spina bifida; childhood cancers other than AML; and altered sex ratio.

Biologic Plausibility

This section summarizes the general biologic plausibility of a connection between exposure to dioxin or herbicides and reproductive and developmental effects on the basis of data from animal and cellular studies. Details of the committee's evaluation of data from these studies are presented in Chapter 3. Some of the preceding discussions of reproductive and developmental outcomes include references to papers relevant to specific reproductive and developmental effects.

TCDD is reported to cause a number of reproductive and developmental effects in laboratory animals. In males, sperm count and production and seminal vesicle weight have been affected by TCDD. Effects have also been seen on female reproductive organs. The mechanism(s) of these effects is not known, but one hypothesis is that they are mediated through effects on hormones. The effects on both male and female reproductive organs, however, are not always accompanied by effects on reproductive outcomes. However, based on supporting animal data, there is a biologically plausible mechanism for male and female reproductive effects in humans. In animal studies, offspring from female hamsters dosed orally with TCDD on gestation day 15 had reduced body weight. Although body weights are not consistently reduced in mice and rats exposed in utero to TCDD, it is suggestive that exposure to TCDD in utero could affect the body weight of newborn humans.

In addition, there is some evidence in animals that TCDD can exacerbate or cause endometriosis. Although a recent study did not show any increase in surgically induced endometriosis with TCDD exposure, early studies have demonstrated an association between TCDD exposure and endometriosis. Recent evidence does demonstrate that TCDD inhibits progesterone-associated transforming growth factor–β_2 (TGFβ_2) expression and endometrial matrix metalloproteinase suppression, which the authors suggest could be a mechanism underlying an association between TCDD and endometriosis. Animal data, therefore, support a possible association between exposure to TCDD and endometriosis.

Experiments have examined the effects of TCDD on the adult female reproductive system. TCDD exposure did not increase egg mortality, nor did it affect time-to-hatching of newly fertilized zebrafish eggs. However, pericardial edema and craniofacial malformations were observed in zebrafish larvae. In ovo TCDD exposure adversely affected the body and skeletal growth and hatchability of the domestic pigeon but had no effect on the domestic chicken or great blue heron.

Administration of TCDD to male rats, mice, guinea pigs, marmosets, monkeys, and chickens elicits reproductive toxicity by affecting testicular function, decreasing fertility, and decreasing the rate of sperm production. Effects on the prostate have been seen following TCDD exposure. TCDD also decreased the levels of hormones such as gonadotropin and testosterone in rats. High doses of TCDD, however, are required to elicit many of these effects.

TCDD is teratogenic in mice, inducing cleft palate and hydronephrosis. Research indicates that coexposure with either of two other chemicals, hydrocortisone or retinoic acid, synergistically enhances expression of cleft palate. This synergy suggests that the pathways controlled by these agents converge at one or more points in cells of the developing palate. Several reports describe developmental deficits in the cardiovascular system of TCDD-treated animals. Evidence suggests that the endothelial lining of blood vessels is a primary target site of TCDD-induced cardiovascular toxicity, with evidence suggesting that cytochrome P450 1A1 (CYP1A1) induction in the endothelium might mediate the early lesions that result in TCDD-induced vascular derangements. Antioxidant treatment provides significant protection against TCDD-induced embryotoxicity, suggesting that reactive oxygen species might be involved in the teratogenic effects of TCDD.

Studies in female rats show that a single dose of TCDD results in malformations of the external genitalia and functional reproductive alterations in female progeny (e.g., decreased fertility rate, reduced fecundity, cystic endometrial hyperplasia, increased incidences of constant estrus). These effects were dependent on the timing of exposure.

Little research has been conducted on the offspring of male animals exposed to herbicides. A study of male mice fed varying concentrations of simulated Agent Orange mixtures concluded there were no adverse effects in offspring. A statistically significant excess of fused sternebrae in the offspring of the two most highly exposed groups was attributed to an anomalously low rate of this defect in the controls.

The effects of in utero and lactational exposure on the male reproductive system have also been investigated. In utero and lactational exposure to TCDD led to decreased daily sperm production and cauda epididymal sperm number in male rat and hamster offspring. Research suggests that in utero and lactational TCDD exposure selectively impairs rat prostate growth and development without inhibiting testicular androgen production or consistently decreasing prostate dihydrotestosterone concentrations. In utero exposure to TCDD also caused decreased seminal vesicle weight and branching, and decreased sperm production and sperm transit time in male offspring. Effects on the reproductive system of females have also been seen following in utero exposure.

Studies in female animals are limited but demonstrate that in utero and lactational exposure reduced fertility, decreased the ability to carry pregnancy to term, decreased litter size, increased fetal death, impaired ovary function, and decreased levels of hormones such as estradiol and progesterone. Most of these effects may have occurred as a result of TCDD's general toxicity to the pregnant animal, however, and not as a result of a TCDD-specific mechanism that acted directly on the reproductive system. TCDD also induced changes in serum concentrations of reproductive hormones in immature female rats administered TCDD by gastric intubation, partially because of the action of TCDD on the pituitary gland.

The mechanism by which TCDD could exert reproductive and developmental effects is not established. Extrapolating results to humans is not straightforward because the factors that determine susceptibility to reproductive and developmental effects vary among species. TCDD has a wide range of effects on growth regulation, hormone systems, and other factors associated with the regulation of activities in normal cells; these effects could in turn lead to reproductive or developmental toxicity.

Most studies are consistent with the hypothesis that the effects of TCDD are mediated by the AhR, a protein in animal and human cells to which TCDD can bind. Following the binding of TCDD, the TCDD–AhR complex has been shown to bind DNA, leading to changes in transcription (i.e., genes are differentially regulated). Modulation of these genes may alter cell function.

Although structural differences in the AhR have been identified among different species, this receptor operates in a similar manner in animals and humans. Therefore, a common mechanism is likely to underlie the toxic effects of TCDD in humans and animals, and data in animals support a biological basis for TCDD's toxic effects. Because of the many species and strain differences in TCDD responses, however, controversy remains regarding the TCDD exposure level that causes reproductive or developmental effects.

Limited information is available on reproductive and developmental effects of the herbicides discussed in this report. Studies indicate that 2,4-D does not affect male or female fertility and does not produce fetal abnormalities, but when pregnant rats or mice are exposed to 4-(2,4-dichlorophenoxy)buric acid (2,4-DB), of which 2,4-D is a major metabolite, the rate of growth of offspring is reduced and their rate of mortality increased (Charles et al., 1999). Very high doses of 2,4-D and its metabolite were required to elicit these effects. 2,4-D has also been shown to alter the concentration and function of reproductive hormones and prostaglandins. One study reported an increased incidence of malformed offspring of male mice exposed to a mixture of 2,4-D and picloram in drinking water. However, paternal toxicity was observed in the high-dose group, and there was no clear dose–response relationship, both of which are a concern in that study. Limited data suggested that picloram alone may produce fetal abnormalities in rabbits at doses that are also toxic to the pregnant animals. 2,4,5-trichlorophenoxyacetic acid (2,4,5-T) was toxic to fetuses when administered to pregnant rats, mice, and hamsters. The ability of 2,4,5-T to interfere with calcium homeostasis in vitro has been documented and linked to its teratogenic effects on the early development of sea urchin eggs. Cacodylic acid is toxic to rat, mouse, and hamster fetuses at high doses that are also toxic to the pregnant mother.

The foregoing evidence suggests that a connection between TCDD exposure and human reproductive and developmental effects is, in general, biologically plausible. However, differences in sensitivity and susceptibility across individual animals, strains, and species; the lack of strong evidence of organ-specific effects across species; and differences in route, dose, duration, and timing of exposure complicate any more definitive conclusions about the presence or absence of a mechanism for the induction of such toxicity by TCDD in humans. Experiments with 2,4-D and 2,4,5-T indicate that these chemicals can have effects on cells at the subcellular level that could provide a biologically plausible mechanism for reproductive and developmental effects. Evidence in animals, however, indicates that these chemicals do not have reproductive effects and have developmental effects only at very high doses. There is inadequate information on picloram and cacodylic acid to assess the biologic plausibility of these compounds' having reproductive or developmental effects.

Considerable uncertainty remains about how to apply this information to the evaluation of potential health effects of herbicides or dioxin exposure in Vietnam veterans. Scientists disagree over the extent to which information derived from animals and cellular studies predicts human health outcomes and the extent to which the health effects resulting from high-dose exposure can be extrapolated to low-dose exposure. Investigating the biological mechanisms underlying TCDD's toxic effects continues to be a very active area of research, and subsequent updates of this report might have more and better information on which to base conclusions, at least for that compound.

Increased Risk of Disease Among Vietnam Veterans

As discussed in *Update 1998*, there are some data suggesting that the highest risks for spina bifida occur in the children of those veterans estimated to have been exposed to Agent Orange (e.g., Ranch Hands). It therefore follows that there is limited/suggestive evidence for an increased risk of spina bifida among offspring of Vietnam veterans. Recently published studies reviewed in this report reported an increased incidence of AML in the children of U.S. and Australian veterans of Vietnam.

Given the large uncertainties that remain about the magnitude of potential risk of other reproductive and developmental outcomes from exposure to herbicides in the studies that have been reviewed, it is not possible for the committee to quantify the degree of risk likely to be experienced by Vietnam veterans because of their exposure to herbicides in Vietnam.

REFERENCES

Abell A, Juul S, Bonde JP. 2000. Time to pregnancy among female greenhouse workers. Scandinavian Journal of Work, Environment, and Health 26(2):131–136.

AIHW (Australian Institute of Health and Welfare). 1999. Morbidity of Vietnam Veterans: A Study of the Health of Australia's Vietnam Veteran Community: Volume 3, Validation Study. Canberra: AIHW.

AIHW. 2000. Morbidity of Vietnam veterans. Adrenal gland cancer, leukaemia and non-Hodgkin's lymphoma: Supplementary report no. 2. (AIHW cat. no. PHE 28). Canberra: AIHW.

Alberman E. 1984. Low birthweight. In: Bracken MB, ed. Perinatal Epidemiology. New York: Oxford University Press. Pp. 86–98.

ACS (American Cancer Society). Childhood Leukemia Resource Center. 2001. http://www3.cancer.org/cancerinfo (accessed March 19, 2001).

Australia Department of Veterans Affairs. 1983. Case-Control Study of Congenital Abnormalities and Vietnam Service. Canberra.

Axmon A, Rylander L, Stromberg U, Hagmar L. 2000. Miscarriages and stillbirths in women with a high intake of fish contaminated with persistent organochlorine compounds. International Archives of Occupational and Environmental Health 73:204–208.

Berkowitz GS, Papiernik E. 1993. Epidemiology of preterm delivery. Epidemiologic Reviews 15:414–443.

Bertazzi PA, Zocchetti C, Pesatori AC, Guercilena S, Consonni D, Tironi A, Landi MT. 1992. Mortality of a young population after accidental exposure to 2,3,7,8-tetrachlorodibenzodioxin. International Journal of Epidemiology 21(1):118–123.

Blakley PM, Kim ES, Firneisz GD. 1989. Effects of paternal subacute exposure to Tordon 202c on fetal growth and development in CD-1 mice. Teratology 39(3):237–241.

Blatter BM, Hermens R, Bakker M, Roeleveld N, Verbeek AL, Zielhuis GA. 1997. Paternal occupational exposure around conception and spina bifida in offspring. American Journal of Industrial Medicine 32(3):283–291.

Bloom AD, ed. 1981. Guidelines for Studies of Human Populations Exposed to Mutagenic and Reproductive Hazards. White Plains, NY: March of Dimes Foundation.

Bonde JP, Giwercman A. 1995. Occupational hazards to male fecundity. Reproductive Medicine Review 4:59–73.

Bryce R. 1991. The epidemiology of preterm birth. In: Kiely M, ed. Reproductive and Perinatal Epidemiology. Boca Raton, FL: CRC Press. Pp. 437–444.

Buckley JD, Robison LL, Swotinsky R, Garabrant DH, LeBeau M, Manchester P, Nesbit ME, Odom L, Peters JM, Woods WG, Hammond GD. 1989. Occupational exposures of parents of children with acute nonlymphocytic leukemia: a report from the Children's Cancer Study Group. Cancer Research 49:4030–4037.

CDC (Centers for Disease Control and Prevention) 1989. Health Status of Vietnam Veterans. Vietnam Experience Study, Vol.V, Reproductive Outcomes and Child Health. Atlanta: U.S. Department of Health and Human Services.

CDC. 2000. National Center for Health Statistics. National Vital Statistics System. Vital Statistics of the United States, Vol. II, Mortality, Part A, for Data Years 1950–1993. Washington, U.S. Government Printing Office. Data for 1994 to 1998, data are available on the NCHS Web site at www.cdc.gov/nchs/datawh/statab/unpubd/mortabs.htm.

CDVA (Commonwealth Department of Veterans' Affairs). 1998. Morbidity of Vietnam Veterans: A Study of the Health of Australia's Vietnam Veteran Community. Vol. 1: Male Vietnam Veterans Survey and Community Comparison Outcomes. Canberra: Department of Veterans' Affairs.

Charles JM, Henwood SM, Leeming NM. 1999. Developmental toxicity studies in rats and rabbits and two-generation reproduction study in rats on 4-(2,4-dichlorophenoxy)butyric acid. International Journal of Toxicology 18:177–189.

Chen Y-C J, Yu M-L M, Rogan WJ, Gladen BC, Hsu C-C. 1994. A 6-year follow-up of behavior and activity disorders in the Taiwan Yu-cheng children. American Journal of Public Health 84:415–421.

Dimich-Ward H, Hertzman C, Teschke K, Hershler R, Marion SA, Ostry A, Kelly S. 1996. Reproductive effects of paternal exposure to chlorophenate wood preservatives in the sawmill industry. Scandinavian Journal of Work, Environment and Health 22(4):267–273.

Driscoll R. 1998. Epidemiologic Study of Adverse Reproductive Outcomes Among Women in the U.S. Forest Service. Section 2, Health Hazard Evaluation Report No. 93-1035-2686. Washington DC: U.S. Department of Agriculture, U.S. Forest Service.

Erickson J, Mulinare J, Mcclain P, Fitch T, James L, McClearn A, Adams M. 1984a. Vietnam Veterans' Risks for Fathering Babies with Birth Defects. Atlanta: U.S. Department of Health and Human Services, Centers for Disease Control.

Erickson JD, Mulinare J, McClain PW, Fitch TG, James LM, McClearn AB, Adams MJ. 1984b. Vietnam veterans' risks for fathering babies with birth defects. Journal of the American Medical Association 252(7): 903–912.

Eskenazi B. 2000. Endometriosis and dioxin exposure in females of Seveso. Bethesda, MD: Crisp Data Base, National Institutes of Health.

Fear NT, Roman E, Reeves G, Pannett B. 1998. Childhood cancer and paternal employment in agriculture: the role of pesticides. British Journal of Cancer 77(5):825–829.

Fein GG, Jacobson JL, Jacobson SW, Schwartz PM, Dowler JK. 1984. Prenatal exposure to polychlorinated biphenyls: effects on birth size and gestational age. Journal of Pediatrics 105:315–320.

Field B, Kerr C. 1988. Reproductive behaviour and consistent patterns of abnormality in offspring of Vietnam veterans. Journal of Medical Genetics 25:819–826.

Garcia AM, Benavides FG, Fletcher T, Orts E. 1998. Paternal exposure to pesticides and congenital malformations. Scandinavian Journal of Work, Environment and Health 24(6):473–480.

Garry VF, Schreinemachers D, Harkins ME, Griffith J. 1996. Pesticide appliers, biocides, and birth defects in rural Minnesota. Environmental Health Perspectives 104(4):394–399.

Grimvall E, Rylander L, Nilsson-Ehle P, Nilsson U, Strömberg U, Hagmar L, Östman C. 1997. Monitoring of polychlorinated biphenyls in human blood plasma: methodological developments and influence of age, lactation, and fish consumption. Archives of Environmental Contamination and Toxicology 32(3):329–336.

Hanify JA, Metcalf P, Nobbs CL, Worsley KJ. 1981. Aerial spraying of 2,4,5-T and human birth malformations: an epidemiological investigation. Science 212:349–351.

Heacock H, Hogg R, Marion SA, Hershler R, Teschke K, Dimich-Ward H, Demers P, Kelly S, Ostry A, Hertzman C. 1998. Fertility among a cohort of male sawmill workers exposed to chlorophenate fungicides. Epidemiology 9(1):56–60.

Heacock H, Hertzman C, Demers PA, Gallagher R, Hogg RS, Teschke K, Hershler R, Bajdik CD, Dimich-Ward H, Marion SA, Ostry A, Kelly S. 2000. Childhood cancer in the offspring of male sawmill workers occupationally exposed to chlorophenate fungicides. Environmental Health Perspectives 108:499–503.

Henriksen GL, Michalek JE. 1996. Serum dioxin, testosterone, and gonadotropins in veterans of Operation Ranch Hand. Epidemiology 7(4):454–455.

Henriksen GL, Michalek JE, Swaby JA, Rahe AJ. 1996. Serum dioxin, testosterone, and gonadotropins in veterans of Operation Ranch Hand. Epidemiology 7(4):352–357.

Hertz-Picciotto I, Samuels SJ. 1988. Incidence of early loss of pregnancy. New England Journal of Medicine 319(22):483–484.

Hoar SK, Morrison AS, Cole P, Silverman DT. 1980. An occupation and exposure linkage system for the study of occupational carcinogenesis. Journal of Occupational Medicine 22:722–726.

Infante-Rivard C, Labuda D, Krajinovic M, Sinnett D. 1999. Risk of childhood leukemia associated with exposure to pesticides and with gene polymorphisms. Epidemiology 10:481–487.

IOM (Institute of Medicine). 1994. Veterans and Agent Orange: Health Effects of Herbicides Used in Vietnam. Washington, DC: National Academy Press.

IOM. 1996. Veterans and Agent Orange: Update 1996. Washington, DC: National Academy Press.

IOM. 1999. Veterans and Agent Orange: Update 1998. Washington, DC: National Academy Press.

Jacobson JL, Jacobson SW, Humphrey HEB. 1990. Effects of in utero exposure to polychlorinated biphenyls and related contaminants on cognitive functioning in young children. Journal of Pediatrics 116:38–45.

James WH. 1996. Evidence that mammalian sex ratios at birth are partially controlled by parental hormone levels at the time of conception. Journal of Theoretical Biology 180(4):271–286.

James WH. 1997. Reproductive effects of male dioxin exposure. The use of offspring sex ratios to detect reproductive effects of male exposure to dioxins. Environmental Health Perspectives 105(2):162–163.

Kallen B. 1988. Epidemiology of Human Reproduction. Boca Raton, FL: CRC Press.

Kalter H, Warkany J. 1983. Congenital malformations. Etiologic factors and their role in prevention (first of two parts). New England Journal of Medicine 308:424–491.

Kline J, Stein Z, Susser M. 1989. Conception to Birth: Epidemiology of Prenatal Development. New York: Oxford University Press.

Knobil E, Neill JD, Greenwald GS, Markert CL, Pfaff DW, eds. 1994. The Physiology of Reproduction. New York: Raven Press.

Kristensen P, Irgens LM, Andersen A, Bye AS, Sundheim L. 1997. Birth defects among offspring of Norwegian farmers, 1967–1991. Epidemiology 8(5):537–544.

Kuratsune M, Yoshimura T, Matsuzaka J, Yamaguchi A. 1972. Epidemiologic study on Yusho, a poisoning caused by ingestion of rice oil contaminated with a commercial brand of polychlorinated biphenyls. Environmental Health Perspectives 1:119–128.

Lamb JC, Moore JA, Marks TA. 1980. Evaluation of 2,4-dichlorophenoxyacetic acid (2,4-D), 2,4,5-trichlorophenoxyacetic acid (2,4,5-T), and 2,3,7,8-tetrachlorodibenzo-p-dioxin (TCDD) toxicity in C57BL/6 mice. Reproduction and Fertility in Treated Male Mice and Evaluation of Congenital Malformations in Their Offspring. National Toxicology Program.

Larsen SB, Joffe M, Bonde JP. 1998. Time to pregnancy and exposure to pesticides in Danish farmers. Occupational and Environmental Medicine 55(4):278–283.

Meinert R, Schüz J, Kaletsch U, Kaatsch P, Michaelis J. 2000. Leukemia and non-Hodgkin's lymphoma in childhood and exposure to pesticides: results of a register-based case-control study in Germany. American Journal of Epidemiology 151(7):639–646.

Michalek JE, Albanese RA, Wolfe WH. 1998a. Project Ranch Hand II: An Epidemiologic Investigation of Health Effects in Air Force Personnel Following Exposure to Herbicides—Reproductive Outcome Update. U.S. Department of Commerce: National Technical Information Service. Report number AFRL-HE-BR-TR-1998-0073.

Michalek JE, Rahe AJ, Boyle CA. 1998b. Paternal dioxin, preterm birth, intrauterine growth retardation, and infant death. Epidemiology 9(2):161–167.

Mocarelli P, Gerthoux PM, Ferrari E, Patterson DG Jr, Kieszak SM, Brambilla P, Vincoli N, Signorini S, Tramacere P, Carreri V, Sampson EJ, Turner WE, Needham LL. 2000. Paternal concentrations of dioxin and sex ratio of offspring. Lancet 355(9218):1858–1863.

NCI (National Cancer Institute). 2001. Surveillance, Epidemiology, and End Results (SEER) database. http://seer.cancer.gov/ScientificSystems/CanQues (accessed March 19, 2001).

Olsen SF. Sorensen JD. Secher NJ. Hedegaard M. Henriksen TB. Hansen HS. Grant A. 1992. Randomised controlled trial of effect of fish-oil supplementation on pregnancy duration. Lancet 339(8800):1003–1007.

Patandin S, Koopman-Esseboom C, de Ridder MA, Weisglas-Kuperus N, Sauer PJ. 1998. Effects of environmental exposure to polychlorinated biphenyls and dioxins on birth size and growth in Dutch children. Pediatric Research 44(4):538–545.

Pearce MS, Parker L. 2000. Paternal employment in agriculture and childhood kidney cancer. Pediatric Hematology and Oncology 17:223–230.

Pesatori AC, Consonni D, Tironi A, Zocchetti C, Fini A, Bertazzi PA. 1993. Cancer in a young population in a dioxin-contaminated area. International Journal of Epidemiology 22(6):1010–1013.

Petrelli G, Figa-Talamanca I, Tropeano R, Tangucci M, Cini C, Aquilini S, Gasperini L, Meli P. 2000. Reproductive male-mediated risk: spontaneous abortion among wives of pesticide applicators. European Journal of Epidemiology 16(4):391–393.

Robison LL, Buckley JD, Daigle AE, Wells R, Benjamin D, Arthur DC, Hammond GD. 1989. Maternal drug use and risk of childhood nonlymphoblastic leukemia among offspring. An epidemiologic investigation implicating marijuana (a report from the Childrens' Cancer Study Group). Cancer 63(10):1904–1911.

Rylander L, Stromberg U, Dyremark E, Ostman C, Nilsson-Ehle P, Hagmar L. 1998. Polychlorinated biphenyls in blood plasma among Swedish female fish consumers in relation to low birthweight. American Journal of Epidemiology 147:493–502.

Safe SH. 1994. Polychlorinated biphenyls (PCBs): environmental impact, biochemical and toxic responses and implications for risk assessment. Critical Reviews in Toxicology 24:87–169.

Sallmén M, Lindbohm ML, Nurminen M. 2000. Paternal exposure to lead and infertility. Epidemiology 11(2):148–152.

Schwartz LS. 1998. Health Problems of Women Veterans of the Vietnam War. Doctoral dissertation, Yale University.

Stellman SD, Stellman JM, Sommer JF Jr. 1988. Health and reproductive outcomes among American Legionnaires in relation to combat and herbicide exposure in Vietnam. Environmental Research 47:150–174.

9

Neurobehavioral Disorders

INTRODUCTION

Neurologic problems in clinical medicine cover a wide variety of disorders. The nervous system is anatomically and functionally divided into central and peripheral subsystems. The central nervous system (CNS) includes the brain and spinal cord, and CNS dysfunction can be subdivided into two general categories: neurobehavioral and motor/sensory. Neurobehavioral difficulties involve two primary categories: cognitive decline, including memory problems and dementia; and neuropsychiatric disorders, including neurasthenia (a collection of symptoms including difficulty concentrating, headache, insomnia, and fatigue), depression, posttraumatic stress disorder (PTSD), and suicide. Other CNS problems can be associated with motor difficulties, characterized by problems such as weakness, tremors, involuntary movements, incoordination, and gait/walking abnormalities. These are usually associated with subcortical or cerebellar system dysfunction. The anatomic elements of the peripheral nervous system (PNS) include the spinal rootlets that exit the spinal cord, the brachial and lumbar plexus, and the peripheral nerves that innervate the muscles of the body. PNS dysfunctions, involving either the somatic nerves or the autonomic system, are known as neuropathies.

Neurologic dysfunction can be further classified, based on anatomic distribution, as either global or focal; temporal onset, as acute, subacute, or chronic; or temporal course, as transient or persistent. For example, global cerebral dysfunction may lead to altered levels of consciousness, whereas focal lesions cause isolated signs of cortical dysfunction, such as aphasia. Acute onset of motor/coordination disturbances leads to symptoms that develop over minutes or hours, whereas subacute onset occurs over days or weeks and chronic onset over months or years. Finally, transient peripheral neuropathies resolve spontaneously, whereas persistent ones may lead to chronic deficits. In the original report, *VAO*, attention was deliberately focused on persistent neurobehavioral dysfunction. In later reports including the present one, all new data pertinent to clinical neurobehavioral dysfunction as well as transient acute and subacute peripheral neuropathy are reviewed.

Case identification in neurology is often difficult. Despite advances in neuroimaging, many types of neurologic alterations are biochemical and show no abnormalities on scanning tests. The nervous system is not usually accessible for biopsy, so pathologic confirmation is not feasible for many neurologic disorders. Behavioral and neurophysiologic changes can be partly or largely subjective and, even when objectively documented, may often be reversible. Timing is important in assessing the effect of chemical exposures on neurologic function. Some symptoms of neurologic importance will appear acutely but be short-lived, whereas others will appear slowly and be detectable for extended periods. These caveats must be considered in the design and critique of epidemiologic studies evaluating an association between exposure to any chemical agent and neurologic or neurobehavioral dysfunction.

Many reports have addressed the possible contribution of herbicides and pesticides to nervous system dysfunction, and reported abnormalities have ranged from mild and reversible to severe and long-standing. These assessments have been conducted in three general settings, related to occupational, environmental, and Vietnam veteran exposures. This chapter reviews reports of neurologic alterations associated with exposure to herbicides, TCDD (2,3,7,8-tetrachlorodibenzo-*p*-dioxin), or other compounds used in herbicides in Vietnam. The potential neurotoxicity of TCDD and herbicides in animal studies is discussed in Chapter 3.

COGNITIVE AND NEUROPSYCHIATRIC EFFECTS

Update of the Scientific Literature

On the basis of the data available at the time, it was concluded in *Veterans and Agent Orange: Health Effects of Herbicides Used in Vietnam* (hereafter referred to as *VAO*; IOM, 1994), *Veterans and Agent Orange: Update 1996* (hereafter, *Update 1996*; IOM, 1996), and *Veterans and Agent Orange: Update 1998* (hereafter, *Update 1998*; IOM, 1999) that there was inadequate or insufficient evidence to determine whether an association exists between exposure to the herbicides 2, 4-dichlorophenoxyacetic acid (2,4-D), 2,4,5-trichlorophenoxyacetic acid (2,4,5-T) and its contaminant 2,3,7,8-tetrachlorodibenzo-*p*-dioxin (TCDD); cacodylic acid, and picloram and cognitive or neuropsychiatric disorders. The majority of the data that formed the basis for these conclusions came from the Air Force Health Studies (AFHS, 1991, 1995). AFHS (1991), originally reviewed in *VAO*, found no association between serum TCDD concentrations (both baseline and current concentrations) and variables such as anxiety, depression, and hostility on a symptom checklist (the Symptom Checklist-90—Revised, SCL-90-R) and between TCDD concentrations and the presence of problems with sleep. By contrast some scales on the Millon Clinical Multiaxial Inventory (MCMI) had significant associations with TCDD across a variety of analyses. The findings from the SCL-90-R, the MCMI, and the reported medical information were thought to be inconsistent, leading to the conclusion of inadequate or insufficient evidence for an association between exposure and cognitive or neuropsychiatric disorders (IOM, 1994). Although in the follow-up study (AFHS, 1995), some checklist variables (anxiety, hostility, obsessive–compulsive behavior, paranoid ideation, somatization, and global severity index, along with other neuroses) were significantly elevated across all occupations in Ranch Hands, the association was not significant for some after adjustment for covariates. Therefore, the conclusion of inadequate or insufficient evidence of an association remained unchanged (IOM, 1996).

Since *Update 1998* (IOM, 1999), results of the AFHS 1997 follow-up examination have been published (AFHS, 2000). In that follow-up, 870 Ranch Hand veterans and 1,251 comparison subjects received a psychological assessment that consisted of the SCL-90-R and reported psychological disorders that were verified through a medical records review. The verified psychological disorders from the 1997 examination were combined with the verified psychological disorders obtained at baseline, and in 1985, 1987, and 1992. Comparisons were made between Ranch Hand veterans and the comparison group. Of five psychological diagnoses, only "other neuroses" (i.e., hysteria, phobic disorder, obsessive–compulsive disorder, somatization disorder, somatoform disorder, personality disorders, sexual deviations and disorders, nondependent abuse of drugs, acute reaction to stress, adjustment reaction, depressive disorder, sleep disorders, eating disorders, psychogenic pain, and tension headache) were significantly elevated in any of the Ranch Hand veterans, and even this end point was elevated only compared to corresponding controls in the enlisted ground crew (64.7 percent in ground crew; 57.1 percent in comparison group). The enlisted ground crew was the occupational classification with the highest dioxin concentrations. A dose–response pattern among 1987 dioxin concentrations and the prevalence of other neuroses was seen among low-, medium-, and high-dioxin categories (45.0, 53.5, and 64.9 percent, respectively). When the relationship between the 1987 lipid-adjusted dioxin levels from all Ranch Hands and the psychological end points was examined, however, no significant results were found. No differences were found for any of the scales for the checklist across Ranch Hand occupational groups and the comparison group. The 12 outcome variables from the checklist were also not associated with dioxin exposure.

Synthesis

When drawing conclusions about associations between exposures and diseases or disorders, the underlying reasonableness of such an association must be considered. The AFHS (2000) found an association between other neuroses and dioxin exposure, but the biological plausibility for such an association is lacking. It is improbable that herbicide or dioxin exposure could be associated with other neuroses, a category that includes more than 100 clinically dissimilar International Classification of Diseases, Ninth Edition, Clinical Modification (ICD·9-CM) codes.

Furthermore, interpretation of the results for this end point is hindered because the percentage of diagnoses verified in the medical records and a frequency table listing the diagnoses included in other neuroses category are not provided in AFHS (2000). In addition, in cases where verified psychological diagnoses from AFHS (2000) were combined with verified psychological diagnoses from previous AFHS studies, it is not clear whether the past diagnoses were active at the time of follow-up (AFHS, 2000).

Also, if these other neuroses were associated with dioxin exposure, the onset of symptoms of specific conditions would have occurred at a much earlier time, when they would be more closely related to actual exposure. Moreover, the lack of correlation of these other neuroses with the SCL-90-R—a standardized and validated questionnaire that includes scales for anxiety, depression, hostility, interpersonal sensitivity, obsessive–compulsive behavior, paranoid ideation, phobic anxiety, psychoticism, somatization, global severity index, positive symptom total and positive symptom, distress index—brings into question the criteria used for the psychological diagnoses.

VAO identified that the SCL-90-R, MCMI and related medical outcomes information reported for an earlier AFHS (1991) examination were inconsistent. Because of the above-mentioned problems, such inconsistencies are also present in the 1997 examination results.

Conclusion

There is still inadequate or insufficient evidence to determine whether an association exists between exposure to the herbicides 2,4-D, 2,4,5-T and its contaminant TCDD, cacodylic acid, and picloram, and cognitive or neuropsychiatric disorders.

MOTOR/COORDINATION DYSFUNCTION

Update of the Scientific Literature

Because of the increasing concern of a possible link between Parkinson's disease (PD) and various chemicals used as herbicides and pesticides, *VAO,*

Update 1996, and *Update 1998* suggested that as Vietnam veterans move into the decades when PD is more prevalent, attention be paid to the frequency and character of new cases in exposed versus nonexposed individuals.

Table 9-1 summarizes studies (some reviewed in *Update 1996* and *Update 1998*) from numerous countries that examined the association between PD and pesticide (herbicide and insecticide) exposure. In these studies, cases of PD were identified using strict guidelines, either neurological examination or review of medical data that required the presence of signs of PD (resting tremor, bradykinesia, cogwheel rigidity, and postural reflex impairment). Routine clinical diagnosis of PD has an accuracy of 75 percent by neuropathological criteria that can be improved to 80–90 percent when more strict diagnostic criteria are applied (Langston, 1998). Clinical features were not verified in the large population studies that relied on death certificates or hospital admission diagnoses (Schulte et al., 1996; Chaturvedi et al., 1995; Ritz and Yu, 2000; Tuschen and Jensen, 2000). Exclusion criteria included the presence of atypical features such as cerebellar involvement, gaze impairment, pronounced autonomic dysfunction, or all other causes of secondary parkinsonism such as drugs, infections, or toxins. In the studies reviewed, pesticide exposure was usually required to occur prior to disease onset, but knowledge of when it occurred in relation to disease onset was not presented.

In *Update 1998,* emphasis on the detection of early-onset parkinsonism was considered vital to test the hypothesis that the disease is related to a toxic exposure because, currently, aging is the only known definitive risk factor for PD. PD becomes clinically apparent when approximately 60 to 70 percent of the neurons in the substantia nigra have deteriorated. One possible reason for the early onset of PD is that neuronal loss is accelerated in individuals with pesticide exposure, causing expression of the disease at a younger age than usually found in the general population (see review in Weiss, 2000).

When attempting to address the issue of early-onset PD, study populations with an onset prior to age 40 or 50 years have been investigated. Butterfield et al. (1993) studied 63 persons, mean age 41 years, diagnosed with PD on or before age 50. Sixty-eight controls were used from the same area with comparable age and diagnosis of rheumatoid arthritis. Standard diagnostic criteria for PD were verified with the treating neurologist. Exposure history for herbicides, obtained by questionnaire, was positive if exposure occurred more than 10 times in any year. Time of exposure ranged from 1 to 46 years before the diagnosis of PD. The adjusted odds ratio (OR) for herbicide exposure and PD was 3.22 ($p < .034$). No herbicides were identified. By contrast, a case-control study of young-onset and late-onset Parkinson's disease found no association with pesticide exposure (Stern et al., 1991). In that study, cases with PD were divided into 69 young-onset individuals, with the first symptoms of PD before age 40, and 80 old-onset individuals, with the first symptoms after age 60. Cases were matched for age, sex, and race. Exposure to herbicides, obtained through interview, was a summary variable for any exposure in the home, yard, or garden. Fifty-four percent of cases and fifty-two percent of controls were exposed to herbicides; the OR for herbicides was not significant (0.9; 95 percent confidence interval [95% CI] 0.6–1.5). The relationship between herbicide exposure and PD, when comparing younger and older matched pairs, also showed no significant differences. As seen in Table 9-1, cases of early-onset Parkinson's disease are included in the study groups of many other studies but are not analyzed as a separate subset.

Although the presence of PD is carefully assessed in studies investigating an association between exposure to herbicides and PD, exposure assessment for herbicides (and TCDD) in these studies (see Table 9-1) is not well documented or quantified. Specific chemical agents or classes of compounds of interest are not identified, and virtually any pesticide exposure for any duration has been accepted for an individual to be classified as exposed. Even the use of the term pesticide changes between studies, from its general use to reflect both insecticides and herbicides, to its use only for insecticides. Some studies used occupations in agriculture as surrogates for pesticide exposure (Tanner et al., 1989; Hertzman et al., 1990; Schulte et al., 1996; Fall et al., 1999; Tuchsen and Jensen, 2000). Ritz and Yu (2000) performed a study of PD mortality and pesticide exposure in which the level of pesticide use by county in California was determined through a required pesticide registry and the amount of land in each county that was treated. They found a 2.5 fold increase in the risk of dying from Parkinson's disease if more than 37 percent of the county land was treated. If 5–37 percent of the county's land was treated, the risk of dying from PD was increased by 50 percent.

In a case-control study conducted in Parma, Italy, 68 cases with PD fulfilling the criteria established the UK Parkinson's Disease Society Brain Bank enrolled from the Institute of Neurology were compared for herbicide and pesticide exposure to 86 controls from other outpatient clinics (Smargiassi et al., 1998). Exposure required either occupational or residential contact for at least ten consecutive years prior to the onset of PD. Twenty five cases and 20 controls fulfilled this criteria for pesticide/herbicide exposure, giving an odds ratio of 1.2 (0.6–2.4).

Liou et al. (1997) conducted a case-control study in Taiwan in which subjects identified specific herbicides and pesticides that they had used. When PD cases were compared to a referent group with no exposure, the use of paraquat with or without other herbicides or pesticides had an OR of 4.7 (2.0–11.5). When the cases were exposed to herbicides or pesticides other than paraquat, however, the OR was 2.2 (0.9–5.6). Paraquat is of interest to PD researchers because of its structural similarity to a neurotoxic metabolite of 1-methyl-4-phenyl-1,2,3,6-tetrahydropyridine (MPTP), MPP+, that causes parkinsonism with similar pathology to idiopathic PD. Paraquat, however, is not structurally or mechanistically related to 2,4-D or 2,4,5-T and is not relevant to Agent Orange.

In a study by Seidler et al. (1996), an effort was made to obtain specific names of products used, but in the final exposure assessment, exposure was categorized by use of herbicides, insecticides, organochlorines, alkylated phosphates, and carbamates; "inhibitors of cellular metabolism"; and "other." Comparison of cases with regional controls for the alkylated phosphates and carbamates had an OR of 2.5 (1.3–4.6). The other analyses with use of specific classes of pesticides found no differences even though the broad categories of herbicide and insecticide use were significant. Herbicide use for 41–80 dose-years had an OR of 3.0 (1.5–6.0), and pesticide use for 41–80 dose-years had an OR of 2.5 (1.4–4.5).

In the occupational setting, Gorell et al. (1998) stratified by years of exposure and found that PD cases had more frequent use of herbicides and insecticides at work than the referent group (herbicide exposure OR, 4.1, 1.6–12.2; insecticide exposure OR, 3.6, 1.8–7.2). The association was stronger when insecticide exposure was 10 or more years (OR = 5.8, 2.0–17.0). For individuals with more than 20 years of herbicide exposure, however, the OR (3.0, 0.6–15.4) was not statistically significant. Examination of these last two groups for age of onset of PD showed no difference from that of individuals with fewer years of occupational exposure.

Koller et al. (1990) had access to pesticide questionnaire responses previously used in a study of lymphoma in Kansas. Herbicide or pesticide exposure included type of application (aerial, direct, sprayer), number of years exposed, number of acres to which herbicide was applied, type of crop (corn, wheat, sorghum, or pastureland), and type of herbicide/pesticide used. Examination of the differences between cases and controls found a weak association with herbicide or pesticide use on corn and PD. That association, however, was discounted for statistical reasons. The same exposure variables were collected by Wong et al. (1991) to examine the risk of PD from pesticide exposure in 19 families with two or more siblings who have PD and a matched comparison group, as well as a second comparison group of 19 sibling pairs with essential tremor. No differences in herbicide or pesticide use, farming, drinking of well water, or rural living were found between the PD group and the comparison group with essential tremor. The group with essential tremor, however, was significantly different from the control group for rural living and farming.

A new approach to establish a link between pesticide exposure and PD is to determine whether the presence of mutant alleles that alter the enzymes needed to detoxify chemicals are more prevalent in PD. The prevalence of a cytochrome P450 *CYP2D6* polymorphism, a gene involved with xenobiotic metabolism, was examined in 215 Chinese individuals with PD and 313 controls of similar age, sex, and locality (Chan et al., 1998). Of the 874 alleles examined, only three mutant alleles were found; two were control subjects and one PD. Although polymorphism of the *CYP2D6* gene is common among Caucasians, it is rare in the Chinese people and did not contribute to PD. In the Chinese with PD, however, years of pesticide exposure while farming were significantly related to PD in women (OR = 6.8, 1.9–24.7) but not in men (OR = 0.7, 0.3–1.8).

Another study that examined the interaction between pesticide exposure and altered genetic makeup in PD used cases of PD with dementia and, as the comparison group, cases of PD with no dementia (Hubble, 1998). One-fifth of patients with PD develop dementia. Researchers found that patients with PD, past pesticide exposure (>20 days per year in any year of life), and the presence of the *CYP 2D6 29B+* gene had 83 percent predicted probability of PD and dementia. Neither pesticide exposure nor the allele alone had predictive value, but the gene–toxicant interaction was significant (OR = 3.2, 1.1–9.1).

Menegon et al. (1998) investigated the presence of a glutathione *s*-transferase (GST) polymorphism in PD. This polymorphism was investigated because GST is necessary for the metabolism of pesticides. No association with GST polymorphism was found. In the group of PD and controls exposed to pesticides, however, the GSTP1 genotypes differed significantly. GSTP1 is involved in pesticide metabolism, and in humans, GSTP1-1 is located in the brain and blood–brain barrier. It was hypothesized that this could influence how neurotoxic pesticides are metabolized and therefore provide one explanation of why individuals with PD are more susceptible to the effects of pesticides.

A recent meta-analysis of 19 studies (see Table 9-1) examined the association between PD and exposure to pesticides (Priydarshi et al., 2000). These are all case-control studies, and therefore, the parameter calculated to estimate relative risk is an odds ratio. Of the 19 studies, 17 had a positive association between PD and exposure to pesticides and 8 had an estimated odds ratio that was significant. Of the remaining two studies, one showed a negative association (Stern et al., 1991), and the other no association (Wong et al., 1991), between PD and exposure to pesticides. Heterogeneity was significant among the studies ($p < .001$), and therefore, the random-effect model used generated a combined estimate for the 19 studies of 1.9 (1.5–2.5). The combined estimates for these studies by geographic location was United States, 2.1 (1.1–4.1); Asia, 2.5 (1.6–4.1); Europe, 1.8 (1.4–2.2); and Canada, 1.9 (1.4–2.8). The presence of a dose–response relationship was examined in six studies in which duration of exposure was included (Smargiassi et al., 1998; Chan et al., 1998; Morano et al., 1994; Seidler et al., 1996; Gorell et al., 1998; Semchuk et al., 1992); no increased incidence of PD was found with increasing dose. Gorell et al. (1998) showed an increased risk of PD with longer duration of exposure to pesticide (>10 years), with an OR of 5.8 (2.0–17.0).

Although the results are intriguing, an association of PD with exposure to 2,4-D, 2,4,5-T, and its contaminant dioxin is not reported in any of these studies.

Synthesis

Of the 30 studies summarized in Table 9-1, only eight provide an estimate of relative risk for herbicides; of these studies, five had a significant association (Butterfield et al., 1993; Gorell et al., 1998; Liou et al., 1997; Seidler et al., 1996;

Semchuk et al., 1992), one had no association (Taylor et al., 1999), and the remaining two had a negative association (Kuopio et al., 1999; Stern, 1991). When a specific herbicide was examined in Taiwan (Liou, 1997) the OR for paraquat was 3.2 (2.4–4.3). Paraquat is of interest to PD researchers because of its structural similarity to the active metabolite of the neurotoxin MPTP, MPP+, that is known to produce pathology identical to PD. The biological plausibility for PD and pesticide exposure is further supported by a recent study of rats exposed to the lipophilic insecticide, rotenone, a known inhibitor of complex 1, a mitochondrial enzyme involved in oxidative phosphorylation. After receiving 2–3 mg/kg of rotenone for 5 weeks, the rats developed features of parkinsonism with hypokinetic and unsteady movement and hunched posture. Neuropathological examination showed degeneration of dopaminergic neurons and cytoplasmic inclusions that possessed ultrastructural and chemical properties suggestive of Lewy bodies, a hallmark of PD in humans (Betarbet et al., 2000). It is believed that the underlying mechanism of PD in humans is related to oxidative damage from free radicals and mitochondrial impairment.

Conclusions

There remains inadequate or insufficient evidence of an association between exposure to the herbicides in this report and motor or coordination dysfunction or Parkinson's disease. In the future, however, as diagnostic accuracy for Parkinson's disease improves, herbicide exposure assessment is quantitated with specific biomarkers, and further research confirms the gene–toxicant interaction in larger prospective studies of PD, this evidence for association may change. This underscores the importance of a prospective study of Vietnam veterans for the development of PD.

TABLE 9-1 Epidemiologic Studies of Pesticide Exposure and Parkinson's Disease[a]

Reference and Country	Study Group	Comparison Group	Exposure Assessment	Significant Association with Pesticides	OR (95 % CI)	Neurological Dysfunction
Butterfield et al., 1993; USA[b,c]	63 young onset, (age < 50 years)	68	Questionnaire—pesticide or insecticide use 10 times in any year	+	Insecticides 5.8, herbicides 3.2 (2.5–4.1), past dwelling fumigated 5.3	Standard criteria for PD by history
Chan et al., 1998; Hong Kong[c]	215	313	Interview—exposure to pesticides during farming (years)	+	Pesticides in women 6.8 (1.9–24.7) Pesticides in men 0.7 (0.3–1.8)	Neurological exam
Chaturvedi et al., 1995; Canada[c]	87 (age > 64 years)	2,070	Survey—exposure positive if frequently used		Pesticides 1.8 (0.9–3.4)	History of PD
Fall et al., 1999; Sweden[c]	113	263	Questionnaire—any job handling pesticides		Pesticides 2.8 (0.9–8.7)	Neurological exam
Golbe et al., 1990; USA[b,c]	106	106	Telephone survey—Sprayed pesticides or insect spray once a year for a total of 5 years	+	Sprayed pesticide 7.0 (5.8–8.5)	Neurological exam
Gorrell et al., 1998; USA[c]	144 (age > 50 years)	464	Interview—Herbicide and insecticide use while working on a farm or gardening	+	Occupational herbicides 4.1 (1.4–12.2) Occupational insecticides 3.6 (1.8–7.2)	Standard criteria for PD by history
Hertzman et al., 1990; Canada	57	122	Questionnaire—ever worked in an orchard	+	Working in orchards 3.7 (1.3–10.3)	Neurological exam

continued

TABLE 9-1 Continued

Reference and Country	Study Group	Comparison Group	Exposure Assessment	Significant Association with Pesticides	OR (95 % CI)	Neurological Dysfunction
Hertzman et al., 1994; Canada[c]	127	245	Interview—occupation with probable pesticide exposure	+	Pesticides in men 2.3(1.1–4.9)	Neurological exam
Ho et al., 1989; Hong Kong[c]	35 (age >60 years)	105	Interview—use of insecticides or herbicides (Y/N), farming, eating raw vegetables	+	Herbicides and pesticides 3.6 (1.0–12.9)	Neurological exam
Hubble et al., 1993; USA[c]	63	76	Questionnaire—pesticide or herbicide use 20 days per year for >5 years	+	Pesticide or herbicide 3.4 (1.3–7.3)	Neurological exam
Hubble et al., 1998; USA	43 PD with dementia	51 PD without dementia	Interviews—pesticide exposure > 20 days in any year and presence of allele for poor drug metabolism	+	Pesticide exposure and genetic trait 3.17 (1.1–9.1)	Neurological exam
Jimenez-Jimenez et al., 1992: Spain[c]	128	256	Interview—exposure: applied pesticides, or lived and ate vegetables where pesticides used		Pesticide 1.3 (0.9–2.1)	Standard criteria for PD by history
Koller et al., 1990; USA[c]	150	150	Interview—acre-years= acres multiplied by years of herbicide or pesticide used		Herbicide or pesticide use 1.1 (0.9–1.3)	Neurological exam

450

Study	N	Exposure assessment		Result	Diagnosis
Kuopio et al., 1999; Finland	123 (onset of PD before 1984)	Interview—pesticides or herbicides regular or occasional use		Regular use herbicides 0.7 (0.3–1.3)	Neurological exam
Liou et al., 1997; Taiwan[b,c]	120	Interview—occupational exposures to herbicides or pesticides	+	Herbicides or pesticides, no paraquat 2.2 (0.9–5.6) Paraquat use 3.2 (2.4–4.3)	Neurological exam
McCann et al., 1998; Australia[c]	224	Questionnaire—daily or weekly exposure to industrial herbicides and pesticides > 6 months		Herbicides or pesticides 1.2 (0.8–1.5)	Neurological exam
Menegon et al., 1998; Australia	96	Interview—pesticide exposure = more than once weekly for > 6 months before onset of PD	+	Pesticide 2.3 (1.2–4.4)	Standard criteria for PD by history
Morano et al., 1994; Spain[c]	74	Interview—direct and indirect—exposure to pesticides		Pesticide 1.73 (1.0–3.0)	Neurological exam
Ritz and Yu, 2000; USA	7,516 (PD cause of death 1984–1994)	Counties ranked by pesticide use from pesticide registry and agricultural census data	+	Prevalence odds ratio Moderate pesticide 1.36 (1.3–1.5) High insecticide 1.45 (1.3–1.6)	ICD-9 332
498,461 (ischemic heart disease cause of death 1984–1994)					

continued

TABLE 9-1 Continued

Reference and Country	Study Group	Comparison Group	Exposure Assessment	Significant Association with Pesticides	OR (95 % CI)	Neurological Dysfunction
Schulte et al., 1996; USA[b]	43,425 PD cause of death in 27 states 1982–1991		Occupational exposure	+	PMR excess in male pesticide appliers, horticultural farmers, farm workers, and graders and sorters of agricultural products.	ICD-9 332
Seidler et al., 1996; Germany[b,c]	380 (age < 66 years with PD after 1987)	755	Interview—dose-years (years of application weighted by usage.)	+	Neighborhood controls for herbicide 1.7 (1.0–2.7) Regional controls for herbicide 1.7 (1.0–2.6)	Neurological exam
Semchuk et al., 1992; Canada[b,c]	130	260	Interview—occupational exposure for each job held > 1 month	+	Pesticide 2.25 (1.3–4.0) Herbicide 3.06 (1.3–7.0) Insecticide 2.05 (1.0–4.1)	Neurological exam
Stern et al., 1991; USA[c]	69 (onset before age 40 years) 80 (onset after age 59 years)	149	Interview—insecticides and pesticides measured by self-report of home or garden use		Herbicide—young onset 0.9 (0.5–1.7) Herbicide—old onset 1.3 (0.7–2.4) Insecticide—young onset 0.6 (0.2–1.7) Insecticide—old onset 0.8 (0.3–2.1)	Standard criteria for PD by history

Study	N	Exposure assessment		Pesticides or herbicides	PD diagnosis
Smargiassi et al., 1998; Italy[c]	86	Interview—occupational exposure for at least 10 consecutive years		1.15 (0.6–2.4)	Standard criteria for PD by history
Tanner et al., 1989; China	100	Interview—exposure for at least 1 year before onset of PD		Fruit growing 1.00 (1.0–1.0) Corn growing 0.54 (0.3–1.1) Rice growing 1.29 (0.7–2.3)	Neurological exam
Taylor et al., 1999; USA	140	Interview—exposure recorded as total days for lifetime		Pesticide 1.02 (0.9–1.2) Herbicide 1.06 (0.7–1.7)	Neurological exam
Tuchsen and Jensen, 2000; Denmark	134	Occupations in farming, horticulture, and landscape were expected to have exposure to pesticides	+	Age-standardized hospitalization ratio for all men in agriculture and horticulture 134 (109–162)	First-time hospitalization for PD
Wechsler et al., 1991; USA	34 (age >39 years)	Questionnaire—duration of occupational and home pesticide use		Home pesticides used more frequently by cases	Standard criteria for PD by history
Wong et al., 1991; USA[c]	38 (19 sibling pairs with PD)	Interview—acre-year (number of years exposed multiplied by the number of acres applied herbicides or pesticides)		Herbicides or pesticides 1.0 (0.7–1.4)	Neurological exam

Note: PMR = proportionate mortality ratio. [a]Modified from Le Couteur et al. (1999). [b]Previously quoted in *Update 1996* or *Update 1998*. [c]Studies used in meta-analysis (Priyadarshi et al., 2000).

Additional row note: Smargiassi et al. row; Wong row sibling pairs with essential tremor 38 age and sex matched and 19 sibling pairs with essential tremor.

453

CHRONIC PERSISTENT PERIPHERAL NEUROPATHY

Update of Scientific Literature

On the basis of data available at the time, it was concluded in *VAO, Update 1996,* and *Update 1998* that there was inadequate or insufficient evidence of an association between exposure to the herbicides considered in this report and chronic persistent peripheral neuropathy. Data from the Air Force Health Studies were a large part of the basis for these conclusions. In 1982 a baseline study of 1,208 Air Force Ranch Hands and a comparison group of 1,238 Air Force personnel found no differences between the groups in measures of peripheral nerve function, including neurological symptom evaluation, physical examination, and nerve conduction velocity tests (AFHS, 1984). A follow-up study was conducted in 1985 using the same protocol, except that nerve conduction velocity was not assessed, and once again no differences were seen between groups (AFHS, 1987). In a 1987 follow-up, Ranch Hands had significantly more hereditary and degenerative diseases, such as benign essential tremor (not found to be associated with dioxin), but the peripheral nerve status was not remarkable (AFHS, 1991). In 1992, the neurological assessment was comparable between the two groups and there was no consistent evidence of a dose–response relationship to either estimated initial dioxin levels or current dioxin levels.

The most recent AFHS follow-up (AFHS, 2000) studied 870 Air Force Ranch Hand veterans and 1,251 Air Force personnel in the comparison group. The neurological examination was based on physical examinations and verified histories of neurological diseases. Vibrotactile measurement with the Vibratron II complemented the peripheral nerve examination. A history of peripheral nerve disorders was significantly associated with the covariates age, insecticide exposure, and diabetic class. The percentage of participants with a confirmed polyneuropathy index was consistently higher in Ranch Hands than in the comparison group. After adjustment for the covariates, the results with dioxin exposure were marginally significant for the enlisted ground crew.

A decreased range of motion in the neck was found to be more prevalent in Ranch Hands than in the comparison group; this finding was associated with dioxin levels and a history of peripheral nerve disorders. Decreased range of motion in the neck is commonly a result of degenerative disease of the cervical vertebrae that can lead to cervical nerve root compression. Decreased range of motion in the neck is not caused by a peripheral neuropathy and is not an outcome related to any known toxic exposure.

Synthesis

The recent Air Force Health Study (2000) is the first time since the baseline examination in 1982 that a difference in measures of peripheral nerve function between the Ranch Hands and comparison group was found. In the Ranch Hand population, many risk factors for peripheral neuropathy, including age-related changes, diabetic class, alcohol use, occupation, and insecticide exposure, were significantly associated with measures of peripheral nerve function. Other uncontrolled confounders (related to life-style) also might have been involved in the increased incidence of peripheral neuropathy in the Ranch Hand ground crew. Five cases of peripheral neuropathy were seen in the Ranch Hand ground crew (1.4 percent of the crew). This prevalence is consistent with the expected prevalence for peripheral neuropathy in the general population (2–8 percent) and the prevalence increases with age. The development of a peripheral neuropathy associated with a toxic exposure begins when the exposure is occurring or shortly after cessation of exposure. Furthermore, the peripheral nervous system has the ability to repair itself when exposure ceases. Therefore, it is not biologically plausible that peripheral neuropathies found for the first time in the recent examination (AFHS, 2000) were caused by an exposure to dioxin or herbicides that occurred 30 years earlier.

In addition, the clinical relevance of the peripheral neuropathy findings is questionable because the neurological examination and its analyses cannot be understood from the perspective of a clinical or preclinical peripheral neuropathy. The various indices of peripheral nerve function, as reported by AFHS (2000), do not correspond to clinical neuropathy. For example, the presence of a Romberg sign may be caused by lesions in the nervous system that are not necessarily peripheral nervous system effects. Also, in the clinical setting, the severity of sensory loss in a peripheral neuropathy is determined by examining the distribution of diminished perception of vibration, pin, and light touch, which should be more severe distally than proximally. The results of such an examination were not included in the results for peripheral neuropathy. Important measures of sensory loss described in the methods—vibration at the ankle and vibrotactile threshold at the great toe—were also not included in the results, even though these were two of the four variables used to classify an individual as having a confirmed peripheral neuropathy. Measuring vibrotactile threshold with a Vibratron II provides a quantitative value for a sensory test, allowing examination of sensory impairment on a continuous scale. Individuals with abnormal vibration at the ankle should have higher vibrotactile thresholds of the great toe. As with sensory loss in peripheral neuropathy, motor weakness and altered reflexes, when present, should also be more pronounced in the distal part of an extremity, and therefore, ankle reflexes are diminished compared to the corresponding knee reflexes in many peripheral neuropathies. The only diagnostic criterion for ankle reflex used in the AFHS (2000) evaluation of peripheral neuropathy was absence of reflex. However, this is a poor marker for anything other than an advanced neuropathy. A more clinically relevant criterion would have been based on a comparison of ankle jerk to knee jerk or an evaluation of diminished ankle jerk with relation to knee jerk.

Diabetic neuropathy is a common cause of peripheral neuropathy, occurring in approximately 50 percent of individuals with Type 2 diabetes over time, and is present in less than 10 percent when the diagnosis is first made (Pirart, 1978). A recent study of non-insulin-dependent outpatients with Type 2 diabetes (mean age, 70.6 years; mean duration, 11.7 years) found polyneuropathy in 49 percent of the individuals when using the criteria of lower limb sensory and motor nerve conduction velocity or latency more than 2 standard deviations above or below the age-matched controls (de Wytt et al., 1999). In mild diabetic neuropathy, a median mononeuropathy was found in 23 percent of patients at a time when the lower extremities did not differ significantly from controls in electrodiagnostic studies (Albers et al., 1996).

The common neuropathy associated with Type 2 diabetes is a distal symmetric sensorimotor polyneuropathy that primarily affects the sensory nerves. Type 2 diabetes can also affect other parts of the peripheral nervous system to produce an autonomic neuropathy, a polyradiculopathy, cranial mononeuropathies, limb mononeuropathy, and mononeuropathy multiplex.

Intensive glycemic control (i.e., careful attention to blood sugar levels) appears to diminish the rate of progression of diabetic polyneuropathy. Persistent glycemia indirectly leads to an increased release of free radicals and oxidative damage to the nervous system. It is believed that these oxidative stressors lead to mitochondrial dysfunction and programmed cell death. This theory is supported by the fact that administration of antioxidants prevents the neuropathy (Feldman et al., 1999).

The clinical presentation of a diabetic neuropathy versus a neuropathy secondary to toxic exposure may be difficult to differentiate except by the presence of other unique features in the clinical history and presentation, such as gastrointestinal symptoms with lead or arsenic exposure or alopecia with thallium exposure. In addition, if caused by a toxic exposure, over time the neuropathy should improve after cessation of exposure, but a diabetic neuropathy will usually progress unless a dramatic change is made in glycemic control. Complaints of peripheral nerve pathology, however, often occur in isolation and are monotonously similar. In the clinical setting, approximately 30 percent of peripheral neuropathies are left with no etiology after a complete evaluation (McLeod, 1995). Examination of family members for evidence of mild or subclinical neuropathy can provide a hereditary etiology for a subset of this group (Dyck et al., 1981). Also the peripheral nervous system undergoes constant age-related changes that may increase its susceptibility to other metabolic and toxic exposures.

Conclusion

There remains inadequate or insufficient evidence of an association between exposure to dioxin or the herbicides studied in this report and chronic persistent peripheral neuropathy.

ACUTE AND SUBACUTE TRANSIENT PERIPHERAL NEUROPATHY

Update of the Scientific Literature

The committee is aware of no new publications that investigate the association between exposure to the compounds of interest and acute and subacute transient peripheral neuropathy. If TCDD were associated with the development of transient acute and subacute peripheral neuropathy, the disorder would become evident shortly after exposure. The committee knows of no evidence that new cases of acute or subacute transient peripheral neuropathy that develop long after service in Vietnam are associated with herbicide exposure.

CONCLUSIONS FOR NEUROBEHAVIORAL DISORDERS

Strength of Evidence in Epidemiologic Studies

As in the earlier reports, this committee finds that there is inadequate or insufficient evidence to determine whether an association exists between exposure to the herbicides used in Vietnam and disorders involving cognitive and neuropsychiatric dysfunction, motor or coordination deficits, and chronic persistent peripheral neuropathy. The evidence regarding association is drawn from occupational and other studies in which subjects were exposed to a variety of herbicides and herbicide components, as reviewed in previous reports.

In *Update 1996*, the committee found that there was limited/suggestive evidence of an association between exposure to the herbicides considered in this report and acute or subacute transient peripheral neuropathy. The evidence regarding association was drawn from occupational and other studies in which subjects were exposed to a variety of herbicides and herbicide components. Information available to the committees responsible for *Update 1998* and this report continues to support this conclusion.

Biologic Plausibility

This section summarizes the biologic plausibility of a connection between exposure to dioxin or herbicides and various neurobehavioral disorders on the basis of data from animal and cellular studies. The details of the committee's evaluation of data from these studies are presented in Chapter 3. Some of the preceding discussions of neurobehavioral outcomes include references to papers relevant to specific neurobehavioral effects.

Some information exists on the development of neurobehavioral disorders and TCDD exposure in laboratory animals. In vivo experiments have demonstrated that TCDD can affect biochemical processes, including having effects on calcium uptake and neurotransmission. Acute doses of TCDD administered to rats affect the metabolism of serotonin, a neurotransmitter in the brain that is able to modulate food intake. This biochemical change is consistent with observations of progressive weight loss and anorexia in experimental animals exposed to TCDD. A study in adult male Wistar rats suggests that a single low-dose intraperitoneal injection of TCDD could cause a toxic polyneuropathy (Grahmann et al., 1993; Grehl et al., 1993); no other studies in animals have reported such an effect. TCDD treatment has also been demonstrated to affect learning and memory in rats.

The mechanism by which TCDD could exert neurotoxic effects is not established. TCDD has a wide range of effects on growth regulation, hormone systems, and other factors associated with the regulation of activities in normal cells; these effects could in turn influence nerve cells. Furthermore, animal studies and in vitro mechanistic studies continue to emphasize the importance of alterations in neurotransmitter systems as underlying mechanisms of TCDD-induced behavioral dysfunction.

Most studies are consistent with the hypothesis that the effects of TCDD are mediated by the aryl hydrocarbon receptor (AhR), a protein in animal and human cells to which TCDD can bind. Following the binding of TCDD, the TCDD–AhR complex is known to bind DNA, leading to changes in transcription (i.e., genes are differentially regulated). Modulation of genes could cause altered cell function.

Although structural differences in the AhR have been identified among different species, this receptor operates in a similar manner in animals and humans. Therefore, a common mechanism is likely to underlie the neurotoxic effects of TCDD in humans and animals, and data in animals can support a biologic basis for TCDD's neurotoxicity. Because of the many species and strain differences in TCDD responses, however, controversy remains regarding the TCDD exposure level that is neurotoxic.

Limited information is available on neurotoxic effects of exposure to the herbicides discussed in this report. At the cellular level, 2,4-D inhibited neurite extension. This effect was accompanied by a decrease in intracellular microtubules, inhibition of the polymerization of tubulin, disorganization of the Golgi apparatus, and inhibition of ganglioside synthesis. Studies in rats indicate an impairment of motor function, central nervous system depression, and inhibition of myelination in the brain. Behavioral alterations have also been seen following treatment of rats with 2,4-D. Results from in vitro mechanistic studies suggest that 2,4,5-T may acutely affect neuronal and muscular function by altering cellular metabolism and cholinergic transmission.

There is evidence that other chemicals can induce a Parkinson-like syndrome in humans, possibly through the generation of free radicals in the target tissue. These results might be biologically relevant because it is suspected that TCDD and some of the herbicides used in Vietnam could indirectly generate free radicals or sensitize cells to free-radical injury; the exact relevance, however, has not been established.

The foregoing evidence suggests that a connection between TCDD exposure and human neurotoxic effects is, in general, biologically plausible. However, differences in sensitivity and susceptibility across individual animals, strains, and species; the lack of strong evidence of organ-specific effects across species; and differences in route, dose, duration, and timing of exposure complicate any more definitive conclusions about the presence or absence of a mechanism for the induction of neurotoxicity by TCDD in humans. Experiments with 2,4-D and 2,4,5-T indicate these chemicals can have effects on brain cells at the subcellular level that could provide a biologically plausible mechanism for neurotoxicity, if such toxicity is seen in animals or humans, but alone do not provide a basis to conclude these compounds are neurotoxic. The observation of behavioral alterations in rats following exposure to 2,4-D also would support the neurotoxicity of this compound, but the species, strain, and dose specificities of these effects remain unknown.

Considerable uncertainty remains about how to apply this information to the evaluation of potential health effects of herbicides or dioxin exposure in Vietnam veterans. Scientists disagree over the extent to which information derived from animal and cellular studies predicts human health outcomes and the extent to which the health effects resulting from high-dose exposure are comparable to those resulting from low-dose exposure. Investigating the biological mechanisms underlying TCDD's toxic effects continues to be a very active area of research, and subsequent updates of this report might have more and better information on which to base conclusions, at least for this compound.

Increased Risk of Disease Among Vietnam Veterans

The most recent Air Force Health Study (AFHS, 2000) reported differences in prevelance of peripheral neuropathy between the Ranch Hand and comparison group, but the clinical relevance is not clear. However, data do not support the notion that these differences are associated with exposure to herbicides or dioxin.

REFERENCES

AFHS (Air Force Health Study). 1984. An Epidemiologic Investigation of Health Effects in Air Force Personnel Following Exposure to Herbicides. Baseline Morbidity Study Results. Brooks AFB, TX: USAF School of Aerospace Medicine. NTIS AD-A138 340. 362 pp.

AFHS. 1987. An Epidemiologic Investigation of Health Effects in Air Force Personnel Following Exposure to Herbicides. First Follow-up Examination Results. 2 vols. Brooks AFB, TX: USAF School of Aerospace Medicine. USAFSAM-TR-87-27. 629 pp.

AFHS. 1991. An Epidemiologic Investigation of Health Effects in Air Force Personnel Following Exposure to Herbicides. Serum Dioxin Analysis of 1987 Examination Results. 9 vols. Brooks AFB, TX: USAF School of Aerospace Medicine.

AFHS. 1995. An Epidemiologic Investigation of Health Effects in Air Force Personnel Following Exposure to Herbicides. 1992 Follow-up Examination Results. 10 vols. Brooks AFB, TX: Epidemiologic Research Division. Armstrong Laboratory.

AFHS. 2000. An Epidemiologic Investigation of Health Effects in Air Force Personnel Following Exposure to Herbicides. 1997 Follow-up examination and results. Reston, VA: Science Application International Corporation. F41624–96–C1012.

Albers JW, Brown MB, Sima AAF, Greene DA. 1996. Frequency of median mononeuropathy in patients with mild diabetic neuropathy in the early diabetes intervention trial (EDIT). Muscle and Nerve 19:140–146.

Betarbet R, Sherer TB, MacKenzie G, Garcis-Osuna M, Panov AV, Greenamyre JT. 2000. Chronic systemic pesticide exposure reproduces features of Parkinson's disease. Nature Neuroscience 3(12):1301–1306.

Butterfield PG, Valanis BG, Spencer PS, Lindeman CA, Nutt JG. 1993. Environmental antecedents of young-onset Parkinson's disease. Neurology 43:1150–1158.

Chan DK, Woo J, Ho SC, Pang CP, Law LK, Ng PW, Hung WT, Kwok T, Hui E, Orr K, Leung MF, Kay R. 1998. Genetic and environmental risk factors for Parkinson's disease in a Chinese population. Journal of Neurology, Neurosurgery, and Psychiatry 65(5):781–784.

Chaturvedi S, Ostbye T, Stoessl AJ, Merskey H, Hachinski V. 1995. Environmental exposures in elderly Canadians with Parkinson's disease. Canadian Journal of Neurological Sciences 22:232–234.

de Wytt CN, Jackson RV, Hockings GI, Joyner JM, Strakosch CR. 1999. Polyneuropathy in Australian outpatients with type II diabetes mellitus. Journal of Diabetes and Its Complications 13:74–78.

Dyck PJ, Oviatt KF, Lambert EH. 1981. Intensive evaluation of referred unclassified neuropathies yields improved diagnosis. Annals of Neurology 10:222–226.

Fall PA, Fredrikson M, Axelson O, Granerus AK. 1999. Nutritional and occupational factors influencing the risk of Parkinson's disease: a case-control study in southern Sweden. Movement Disorders 4:28–37.

Feldman EL, Russell JW, Sullivan KA, Golovoy D. 1999. New insights into the pathogenesis of diabetic neuropathy. Current Opinion in Neurology 12:553–563.

Golbe LI, Farrell TM, Davis PH. 1990. Follow-up study of early-life protective and risk factors in Parkinson's disease. Movement Disorders 5:66–70.

Gorell JM, Johnson CC, Rybicki BA, Peterson EL, Richardson RJ. 1998. The risk of Parkinson's disease with exposure to pesticides, farming, well water, and rural living. Neurology 50:1346–1350.

Grahmann F, Claus D, Grehl H, Neundoerfer B. 1993. Electrophysiologic evidence for a toxic polyneuropathy in rats after exposure to 2,3,7,8-tertachlorodibenzo-p-dioxin (TCDD). Journal of Neurological Sciences 115(1):71–75.

Grehl H, Grahmann F, Claus D, Neundorfer B. 1993. Histologic evidence for a toxic polyneuropathy due to exposure to 2,3,7,8-tetrachlorodibenzo-p-dioxin (TCDD) in rats. Acta Neurologica Scandinavica 88(5):354–357.

Hertzman C, Wiens M, Bowering D, Snow B, Calne D. 1990. Parkinson's disease: a case-control study of occupational and environmental risk factors. American Journal of Industrial Medicine 17:349–355.

Hertzman C, Wiens M, Snow B, Kelly S, Calne D. 1994. A case-control study of Parkinson's disease in a horticultural region of British Columbia. Movement Disorders 9:69–75.

Ho SC, Woo J, Lee CM. 1989. Epidemiologic study of Parkinson's disease in Hong Kong. Neurology 39:1314–1318.

Hubble JP, Cao T, Hassanein RE, Neuberger JS, Koller WC. 1993. Risk factors for Parkinson's disease. Neurology 43:1693–1697.

Hubble JP, Kurth JH, Glatt SL, Kurth MC, Schellenberg GD, Hassanein RE, Lieberman A, Koller WC 1998. Gene–toxin interaction as a putative risk factor for Parkinson's disease with dementia. Neuroepidemiology 17:96–104.
IOM (Institute of Medicine). 1994. Veterans and Agent Orange: Health Effects of Herbicides Used in Vietnam. Washington, DC: National Academy Press.
IOM. 1996. Veterans and Agent Orange: Update 1996. Washington, DC: National Academy Press.
IOM. 1999. Veterans and Agent Orange: Update 1998. Washington, DC: National Academy Press.
Jimenez-Jimenez FJ, Mateo D, Gimenez-Roldan S. 1992. Exposure to well water and pesticides in Parkinson's disease: a case-control study in the Madrid area. Movement Disorders 7:149–152.
Koller W, Vetere-Overfield B, Gray C, Alexander C, Chin T, Dolezal J, Hassanein R, Tanner C. 1990. Environmental risk factors in Parkinson's disease. Neurology 40:1218–1221.
Kuopio A, Marttila RJ, Helenius H, Rinne UK. 1999. Environmental risk factors in Parkinson's disease. Movement Disorders 14:928–939.
Langston, JW. 1998. Epidemiology versus genetics in Parkinson's disease: progress in resolving an age-old debate. Annals of Neurology 44(Suppl 1):S45–S52.
Le Couteur DG, McLean AJ, Taylor MC, Woodham BL, Board PG. 1999. Pesticides and Parkinson's disease. Biomedicine and Pharmacotherapy 53:122–130.
Liou HH, Tsai MC, Chen CJ, Jeng JS, Chang YC, Chen SY, Chen RC. 1997. Environmental risk factors and Parkinson's disease: a case-control study in Taiwan. Neurology 48:1583–1588.
McCann SJ, LeCouteur DG, Green AC Brayne C, Johnson AG, Chan D, McManus ME, Pond SM. 1998. The epidemiology of Parkinson's disease in an Australian population. Neuroepidemiology 17:310–317.
McLeod JG. 1995. Investigation of peripheral neuropathy. Journal of Neurology, Neurosurgery and Psychiatry 58:274–283.
Menegon A, Board PG, Blackburn AC, Mellick GD, LeCouteur DG. 1998. Parkinson's disease, pesticides, and glutathione transferase polymorphisms. Lancet 352:1344–1346.
Morano A, Jimenez-Jimenez FJ, Molina JA, Antolin MA. 1994. Risk-factors for Parkinson's disease: case-control study in the province of Caceres, Spain. Acta Neurologica Scandinavica 89(3):164–170.
Pirart J. 1978. Diabetes mellitus and its degenerative complications: a prospective study of 4,400 patients observed between 1947 and 1973. Diabetes Care 1:168–188.
Priyadarshi A, Khuder SA, Schaub EA, Shrivastava S. 2000. A meta-analysis of Parkinson's disease and exposure to pesticides. Neurotoxicology 21(4):435–440.
Ritz B, Yu F. 2000. Parkinson's disease mortality and pesticide exposure in California 1984–1994. International Journal of Epidemiology 29:323–329.
Schulte PA, Burnett CA, Boeniger MF, Johnson J. 1996. Neurodegenerative diseases: occupational occurrence and potential risk factors, 1982 through 1991. American Journal of Public Health 86(9):1281–1288.
Seidler A, Hellenbrand W, Robra BP, Vieregge P, Nischan P, Joerg J, Oertel WH, Ulm G, Schneider E. 1996. Possible environmental, occupational, and other etiologic factors for Parkinson's disease: a case-control study in Germany. Neurology 46(5):1275–1284.
Semchuk KM, Love EJ, Lee RG. 1992. Parkinson's disease and exposure to agricultural work and pesticide chemicals. Neurology 42:1328–1335.
Smargiassi A, Mutti A, DeRosa A, DePalma G, Negrotti A, Calzetti S. 1998. A case-control study of occupational and environment risk factors for Parkinson's disease in the Emilia-Romagna region of Italy. Neurotoxicology 19:709–712.
Stern M, Dulaney E, Gruber SB, Golbe L, Bergen M, Hurtig H, Gollomp S, Stolley P. 1991. The epidemiology of Parkinson's disease. A case-control study of young-onset and old-onset patients. Archives of Neurology 48:903–907.

Tanner CM, Chen B, Wang W, Peng M, Liu Z, Liang X, Kao LC, Gilley DW, Goetz CG, Schoenberg BS. 1989. Environmental factors and Parkinson's disease: a case-control study in China. Neurology 39:660–664.

Taylor CA, Saint-Hilaire MH, Cupples LA, Thomas CA, Burchard AE, Feldman RG, Myers RH. 1999. Environmental, medical, and family history risk factors for Parkinson's disease: a New England-based case control study. American Journal of Medical Genetics (Neuropsychiatric Genetics) 88:742–749.

Tuchsen F, Jensen AA. 2000. Agricultural work and the risk of Parkinson's disease in Denmark, 1981–1993. Scandinavian Journal of Work, Environment, and Health 26:359–362.

Wechsler LS, Checkoway H, Franklin GM, Costa LG. 1991. A pilot study of occupational and environment risk factors for Parkinson's disease. NeuroToxicology 12:387–392.

Weiss B. 2000. Vulnerability to pesticide neurotoxicity is a lifetime issue. Neurotoxicology 21(1–2):67–73.

Wong GF, Gray CS, Hassanein RS, Koller WC. 1991. Environmental risk factors in siblings with Parkinson's disease. Archives of Neurology 48:287–289.

10

Other Health Effects

INTRODUCTION

This chapter addresses a variety of noncancer health outcomes: chloracne, porphyria cutanea tarda, respiratory disorders, immune system disorders, diabetes, lipid and lipoprotein disorders, gastrointestinal and digestive disease (including liver toxicity), and circulatory disorders. Additionally, in response to a request from the U.S. Department of Veterans Affairs (DVA), the scientific literature regarding AL-type primary amyloidosis and herbicide or dioxin exposure is evaluated.

The health outcomes reviewed in this chapter follow a common format. Each section begins by providing some background information about the outcome under discussion. A brief summary of the findings described in earlier Veterans and Agent Orange reports is then presented, followed by a discussion of the most recent scientific literature and a synthesis of the material reviewed. Where appropriate, reviews are separated by the type of exposure (occupational, environmental, Vietnam veteran) being addressed. Each section concludes with the committee's finding regarding the strength of the evidence in epidemiologic studies, biologic plausibility, and evidence regarding Vietnam veterans.

CHLORACNE

Background

Chloracne is recognized to be an outcome of exposure to 2,3,7,8-tetrachlorodibenzo-p-dioxin (TCDD) and other cyclic organochlorine compounds. It appears shortly after exposure and, although refractory to treatment, usually regresses over time and does not appear after a long latency. New cases of chloracne are therefore not a concern of this report.

Chloracne is a highly characteristic form of acne. It shares some pathological processes, such as occlusion of the orifice of the sebaceous follicle, with much more common forms of acne such as acne vulgaris. However, it is marked by a unique feature, the epidermoid inclusion cyst, which is caused by proliferation and hyperkeratinization (horn-like cornification) of the epidermis. Although typically appearing in a characteristic distribution over the eyes, ears, and neck, patterns of chloracne among exposed chemical industry workers may involve the trunk, genitalia, and buttocks (Neuberger et al., 1998).

Chloracne has been extensively studied and is used as a marker of exposure in studies of populations exposed to TCDD, as such residents involved in the 1976 industrial incident in Seveso, Italy, and to other organochlorine compounds such as polychlorinated biphenyls (PCBs) and pentachlorophenol. It is one of the few findings consistently associated with such exposure and is a well-validated indicator of high exposure to these compounds, particularly TCDD (Sweeney et al., 1997/98). The predictive value of chloracne as a biomarker is suggested by its strong association with other health outcomes, such as goiter, arthritis, and anemia in the Taiwanese population affected by the "Yucheng" (cooking oil disease) incident in 1979, in which there was exposure to high levels of PCBs (Guo et al., 1999).

Despite the utility of chloracne as a biomarker, and the general association with high blood levels of TCDD and related compounds, it has not been possible to identify a threshold level for the skin condition. Kimbrough (1998) suggests that this may be because blood levels do not necessarily reflect levels in skin. She also suggests that susceptibility due to different skin conditions may obscure the association or that direct dermal deposition may play a greater role in some situations. Kimbrough suggests that Ranch Hand veterans have too narrow and too low a range of blood levels from which to draw conclusions and also that the time elapsed after exposure until the studies were performed may have introduced confounding factors such as aging, obesity, and onset of diabetes, all of which change blood lipid levels in ways that may not affect skin changes and that may obscure relationships with chloracne.

One new study to shed light on the elusive threshold for development of chloracne was contributed by Coenraads et al. (1999), reporting on four groups of Chinese workers involved in industrial incidents that exposed them to polycyclic organochlorines, particularly TCDD. They reported their findings in terms of 2,3,7,8-TCDD toxicity equivalents (TEQs) in pooled blood, levels of exposure to these compounds weighted by their TCDD-like activity. They inferred a threshold for chloracne (per gram of blood lipid) between 650 and 1,200 pg/g TEQ. They also suggested that in this population, the contribution to the risk of developing chloracne from exposure to TCDD itself was small compared to the hexachlorinated dibenzodioxins and furans, a finding that may be specific to this population and the exposure conditions.

Summary of *VAO*, *Update 1996*, and *Update 1998*

The committee responsible for the *Veterans and Agent Orange: Health Effects of Herbicides used in Vietnam* (hereafter referred to as *VAO*; IOM, 1994) report found there to be sufficient information to determine that an association existed between exposure to herbicides used in Vietnam or the contaminant dioxin and chloracne. Additional information available to the committees responsible for Veterans and Agent Orange: *Update 1996* (IOM, 1996) and *Update 1998* (IOM, 1999) did not change this finding. Reviews of the studies underlying these findings may be found in the earlier reports.

Previous reports discuss chloracne extensively as a toxicological phenomenon but do not treat it extensively as a health outcome. New cases are not expected after the long latency, and new information on the mechanism of chloracne would not be expected to alter the interpretation of existing data from Vietnam veterans exposed to Agent Orange.

Update of the Scientific Literature

Vietnam veterans enrolled in the Ranch Hand study were not found to have chloracne. Burton et al. (1998) examined the same group for evidence of an increased risk for acne in general. Their working hypothesis was that levels of exposure insufficient to cause florid chloracne may increase the risk of other acneiform rashes because some of the mechanisms of comedone formation are similar. They also suggested that the florid appearance in-country of "tropical acne" among many troops, which was a major cause of morbidity during the conflict, may have been unrecognized chloracne. Despite the high frequency of skin disorders reported during service in Vietnam, the authors found no evidence for an increased risk of acne among Ranch Hand participants compared to other theater veterans, either during the Vietnam conflict or subsequently, and no cases of chloracne. The authors suggested that Ranch Hand participants may not have accumulated a sufficient dose to be at risk for chloracne. This study classified troops by serum dioxin levels and may be considered definitive.

Synthesis

Chloracne is clearly associated with exposure to high levels of cyclic organochlorine compounds. Blood levels that may reflect tissue threshold concentrations remain estimations. Estimates of the mean threshold of exposure, dose, blood level, or tissue level for induction of chloracne in human beings remain highly uncertain, and there is strong evidence of considerable variation among individuals. Ranch Hand veterans did not show evidence of chloracne, probably because the tissue concentrations required to induce this skin disorder were not reached. No new cases of chloracne from exposure in Vietnam will appear among Vietnam veterans at this late date.

Conclusions

Strength of Evidence in Epidemiologic Studies

There is no change in the previous conclusion that there is sufficient and abundant evidence to conclude that chloracne is associated with exposure to herbicides (2,4-D, 2,4,5-T and its contaminant TCDD, cacodylic acid, and picloram) and to TCDD in particular. The fact that Ranch Hand veterans did not experience this condition does not change the overall conclusion.

Biologic Plausibility

The formation of chloracne lesions after administration of TCDD is observed in some species of laboratory animals, supporting a biologic basis for these effects in humans. Similar observations have not been reported for the purified herbicides (i.e., without TCDD contamination). A discussion of toxicological studies that comprise the biologic basis for an association between exposure to TCDD or herbicides and toxicity end points is contained in Chapter 3; a general summary of the biologic basis for various end points is presented in the conclusion to this chapter.

Increased Risk of Disease Among Vietnam Veterans

Vietnam veterans in the AFHS study were not found to have chloracne. Because chloracne appears shortly after exposure, regresses over time, and does not appear after a long latency, no new cases from wartime exposures are expected.

PORPHYRIA CUTANEA TARDA

Background

Porphyria cutanea tarda (PCT) is only incompletely understood, and investigation into its mechanisms may provide useful insights into iron metabolism and the formation of hemoglobin. For this reason, more than for its clinical benefit, there has been further investigation into the mechanisms of PCT. Unpublished data by Sinclair (2000) reporting on investigations using liver cells in tissue culture suggest that uroporphyrin accumulation following exposure to TCDD and other presumable inducers may be reduced by ascorbate (vitamin C) acting to inhibit the activity of a cytochrome P450 1A2 (CYP1A2) that is induced by TCDD. Human subjects who had developed PCT were also found to be ascorbate deficient in almost 80 percent of cases, suggesting that poor diet may be a risk factor along with the known risk factors of high alcohol intake, estrogens (as in oral contraceptives), liver disease, hemodialysis, HIV infection, and diabetes.

Cigarette smoking also induces CYP1A2 and may be a risk factor, but this was not investigated. The results were interpreted to suggest that PCT is not more common because adequate ascorbate levels are present in the normal diet but that deficiencies may predispose to the disease (Sinclair, 2000). An adequate diet may be protective against manifestations of the disease following exposure to TCDD, at least in most people. This finding may explain why PCT was not observed among Ranch Hand participants and was not identified as a health problem among Vietnam veterans exposed to Agent Orange.

The genetic basis for PCT has also been further elucidated since *Update 1998* with the identification of at least three genes determining susceptibility to hexachlorophene-induced PCT in mice. If the human disorder is as complex, the observation would explain why susceptibility to PCT is as rare as it is in humans (Akhtar and Smith, 1998).

Summary of *VAO*, *Update 1996*, and *Update 1998*

The committee responsible for *VAO* found there to be sufficient information to determine that an association existed between exposure to herbicides used in Vietnam or the contaminant dioxin and PCT in genetically susceptible individuals. Additional information available to the committee responsible for *Update 1996* led it to conclude that there was limited or suggestive evidence of an association; *Update 1998* did not change this finding. Reviews of the studies underlying these findings may be found in the earlier reports.

PCT has been discussed extensively in both *VAO* and the two prior updates. *VAO* reviewed case reports of PCT among chemical workers who showed subsequent resolution following removal from the workplace. These reports are anecdotal and difficult to interpret because of multiple exposures. *Update 1998* hypothesized that the absence of detectable PCT may also have been explained by the fortuitous absence of genetically predisposed individuals among exposed Vietnam veterans. Contemporary research suggests that susceptibility to the disease is indeed a rare trait and that adequate diet may have been protective for those who were susceptible.

PCT is an early response to TCDD and is therefore no longer of current concern because new cases are not expected.

Update of the Scientific Literature

Neuberger et al. (1999), following a group of 159 Austrian chemical workers exposed to TCDD in herbicide production in the 1970s, reported that urinary porphyrins remained abnormal, although not clinically characteristic of PCT. Coproporphyrinogen levels were within the normal range, but there was a reversal in the normal ratio of isomers (I compared to III) in almost half of the subjects. The authors inferred that this indicated persistent liver injury and abnormal porphyrin metabolism due to TCDD and implied that exposed workers may be at risk for related conditions, including PCT, for much longer than had been assumed previously.

Conclusions

Strength of Evidence in Epidemiologic Studies

There is no basis for changing the previous conclusion that there is limited/suggestive evidence of an association between exposure to herbicides (2,4-D, 2,4,5-T and its contaminant TCDD, cacodylic acid, and picloram) and PCT.

Biologic Plausibility

There is some evidence that TCDD can be associated with porphyrin abnormalities in laboratory animals, although PCT has not been reported. Porphyria has not been reported in animals exposed to the other herbicides relevant to Agent Orange. A discussion of toxicological studies that comprise the biologic basis for an association between exposure to TCDD or herbicides and toxicity end points is contained in Chapter 3; a general summary of the biologic basis for various end points is presented in the conclusion to this chapter.

Increased Risk of Disease Among Vietnam Veterans

PCT is an early response to TCDD and therefore no new cases due to wartime exposure are expected among Vietnam veterans.

RESPIRATORY DISORDERS

Background

In *Update 1998*, only passing mention was made of inflammation and immune function in relation to respiratory disorders and their possible association with exposure to Agent Orange. Recent findings of a possible association with exposure to TCDD and related organochlorines among Seveso residents require closer attention to this issue.

The lung expresses injury resulting from inflammation in two general ways. Inflammation may result in changes in resistance to airflow in the conducting airways. Inflammation may also result in permanent scarring, or fibrosis, in the tissue of the air sacs (alveoli), which leads to stiffening of lung tissue and impairment of the capacity of the lung to fully expand. As described in *Update 1998*, airflow obstruction is measured primarily by the forced expiratory volume at 1 second (FEV_1) and secondarily by the ratio of FEV_1 to forced vital capacity (FVC) (i.e., FEV_1/FVC) and other forced expiratory flow rates. Lung capacity is measured primarily by the FVC and secondarily by measurements of total lung capacity.

Airflow obstruction is variable; it may be completely reversible in asthma, or it may be constant in whole or in part in emphysema. Chronic bronchitis is a less common condition characterized by sputum production, which often accompanies asthma, and may also progress to fixed airway obstruction. These three conditions are associated with varying degrees and sites of inflammation occurring on a prolonged basis.

Asthma is fundamentally a disorder of chronic inflammation of the larger airways, which may be a response to allergy, infection, or irritation and expresses itself as constriction of smooth muscle tissue and edema in the wall of the airway. These inflammatory processes reduce the caliber of the airway inside diameter, or lumen, and—following a physical law that resistance increases exponentially with reduced diameter of the passage—obstruct airflow. Asthma commonly occurs in persons with other expressions of allergy, especially children, but it can develop in adults without a clear connection to allergies. Mild degrees of airflow reduction may not be noticed by the person so affected. Moderate to severe airflow obstruction is perceived as wheezing and shortness of breath. Cough in response to the inflammatory process is common and may be the principal manifestation of asthma. Asthma is reversible because these inflammatory processes can get better or worse and are usually controlled on medication, so that individuals with asthma experience the disease as a series of episodes, often occurring in response to allergic reactions, infections, stress, or irritation. Severe asthma does occur, and the frequency of deaths from asthma has risen in many countries, at least in part associated with suboptimal treatment or inadequate access to medical care. The prevalence of asthma is also rising in most developed and affluent countries for reasons that are not clear but are suspected to reflect changes in immune response to common allergens in homes. Asthma is identified by a compatible history of episodic shortness of breath and wheezing and by pulmonary function tests showing obstruction to airflow that varies in response to drugs that dilate the airways. In surveys, asthma is difficult to identify reliably by symptoms alone in a self-administered questionnaire, and the subject is usually asked whether the diagnosis of asthma has ever been made.

Emphysema is a disorder of chronic inflammation and disintegration of lung tissue adjacent to smaller airways such that their supporting structure is lost and the thin-walled airways collapse at pressures within the chest that are required to expel air. When this happens, airflow is obstructed and more than normal amounts of air may be trapped in the lung after an exhaled breath. The inflammatory process of primary significance in emphysema is localized to the lung tissue immediately surrounding the airway, as opposed to the airway itself as in asthma and chronic bronchitis. Aside from rare hereditary disorders and occupational exposures, the cause of emphysema is overwhelmingly cigarette smoking. Emphysema is identified by pulmonary function studies and often by chest films.

Chronic bronchitis is a more gross and nonspecific process of airway inflammation often associated with either asthma or emphysema when it occurs. It is characterized by increasing production of sputum and frequent coughing. Chronic bronchitis has become much less common in recent years and, when it occurs today, is almost always associated with cigarette smoking, although it can accompany allergies, severe air pollution, and occupational exposures. Acute bronchitis is much more common, is usually self-limited, occurs in response to common illnesses such as influenza in addition to environmental irritants, and does not carry the same risk of permanent respiratory injury. Chronic bronchitis is diagnosed by a history of productive cough and can be reliably screened for by a questionnaire.

Because the three conditions causing airflow obstruction frequently occur together, they are often difficult to distinguish. They all have a common association with cigarette smoking and are interrelated by inflammatory processes. Because these conditions often occur together and are interrelated, they are usually aggregated into a collective category of chronic obstructive pulmonary disease (COPD), which is considered a distinct entity in treatment and coding for most epidemiologic purposes. For practical purposes, COPD should be understood to include all three disorders occurring together, any two of them if they occur together, and either chronic bronchitis or emphysema if it occurs separately. Further, there is some evidence to suggest that these conditions are associated biologically, through common hereditary predisposition, and may be associated with an increased risk of lung cancer for a given history of cigarette smoking.

Asthma requires separate consideration. Asthma is always coded separately in hospital discharge summaries and death certificates if it occurs in isolation from the other two because asthma in isolation has distinct risk factors and is considered a distinct disease. Asthma is a common disease, but fatal asthma is rare, notwithstanding the fact that mortality rates rose in many countries in the 1980s. There are usually insufficient numbers to report asthma deaths separately, and the mortality rate for asthma varies from year to year because of the small numbers. For this reason, asthma is usually aggregated for epidemiologic purposes with the other two disorders under COPD or a category of nonmalignant respiratory disorders when causes of death are considered. Asthma is counted separately in prevalence surveys or incidence studies of respiratory disease.

Fibrosis of lung tissue is a response to inflammation resulting in diffuse damage to the walls of the air sacs, or alveoli, and supporting structures. The scarring that occurs reduces the resilience, or compliance, of the lung and reduces its capacity to expand. This is called restrictive lung disease. The scarring also has secondary effects on the distribution of blood to various parts of the lung where oxygen is taken up more or less efficiently and, as it progresses, may cause reduction (desaturation) in oxygenation of blood. Pulmonary fibrosis may occur as a consequence of severe injury deep in the lung due to infection, inhalation of a toxic chemical that is poorly soluble in water (and therefore not cleared in the upper respiratory tract), inflammatory conditions caused by inhalation of particles to which there is an allergy, and a variety of immunological disorders.

Pneumonia and other lung infections generally run a much more acute course, and although they may occur more frequently in cigarette smokers, they usually have different and distinct risk factors not necessarily shared with chronic lung diseases. Their clinical course and risk of death may also be modified by changes in host defenses and especially by reductions in immune function. This is why pneumonia is a frequent cause of death following aggressive cancer chemotherapy and viral infections such as AIDS that depress the immune response to bacterial and parasitic infections.

These conditions may be modified in their frequency and their expression by modifications in the immune process and other protective mechanisms. These mechanisms often occur together and may be mechanical (cough), immunological, or inflammatory, with or without an associated immune response. Collectively, these protective responses are called host defense mechanisms. If TCDD affects host defense mechanisms of the lung, it is most likely to affect immune mechanisms, as it is known to do elsewhere in the body. The immune system in the lung is partly compartmentalized, with its own sites of lymphocyte and alveolar macrophage proliferation, and partly shared with the rest of the body. Circulating immunoglobulins, polymorphonuclear white cells, and lymphocytes play an especially important role in the initial response. Thus, TCDD-induced immunomodulation of these responses could occur in response to exposure whether or not concentrations in lung tissue reach a toxic level. TCDD is a potent immunotoxic agent and may be expected to have effects on the expression of immune function in the lung. However, the net effect of TCDD exposure is unpredictable. The effect of TCDD may be to reduce or vary the expression of immune response in the lung. There are no studies that have investigated the response of the immune system in the lung, either to systemic exposure to TCDD or to TCDD levels in the lung that reflect actual tissue levels observed in exposed individuals.

Iida et al. (1999) demonstrated that in human beings, levels of TCDD in lipids extracted from the lung correlated closely with concentrations in lipid extracted from blood and were greater by a factor of approximately 1.7, but did not correlate closely for other dioxins and furans (except the relatively nontoxic octochloro variety). The concentration of dioxins and furans in lipid derived from lung was higher than in lipid derived from liver, brain, spleen, muscle, kidney, and adipose tissue. This raises the possibility of local effects in the lung that may be stronger than the effects in other tissues for a given level of personal exposure.

Summary of *VAO*, *Update 1996*, and *Update 1998*

The committee responsible for *VAO* found there to be inadequate or insufficient information to determine whether an association existed between exposure to herbicides used in Vietnam or the contaminant dioxin and the respiratory disorders discussed above. Additional information available to the committees responsible for *Update 1996* and *Update 1998* did not change this finding. Reviews of the studies underlying these findings may be found in the earlier reports.

Cigarette smoking is a major, often overwhelming, confounding exposure that dominates as a risk factor for respiratory disorders and may obscure weaker associations. Vietnam veterans are reported to smoke more heavily than non-Vietnam veterans (McKinney et al., 1997), making any such association more difficult to discern.

Update of the Scientific Literature

Bertazzi and colleagues (Bertazzi et al., 1998; Pesatori et al., 1998) continued their follow-up of residents of the town of Seveso, Italy, site of the industrial incident in 1976 that exposed the local population to substantial amounts of relatively pure TCDD. This is one of the few nonoccupationally exposed populations that has been studied in detail, the largest such population studied, and certainly the nonoccupational population with the highest exposure and best exposure assessment. Until long-term follow-up data became available for 15 years following the incident, no evidence had been observed for respiratory impairment. An elevated mortality for respiratory disorders that achieves statistical significance has now been observed among exposed residents of Seveso compared to unexposed residents in surrounding communities. Residents of zone A, the area most heavily contaminated by TCDD showed a relative risk (RR) for males of 2.4 (5 deaths observed, 95 percent confidence interval [95%CI] 1.0–5.7) and for females of 1.3 (2 deaths observed, 0.3–5.3). Residents of zone B, the "medium" contaminated area, showed a relative risk for males of 0.7 (13 observed, 0.4–1.2) and for females of 1.0 (10 observed, 0.5–1.9). Residents of zone R, the least exposed area, showed a relative risk for males of 1.1 (133 observed, 0.9–1.3) and for females of 1.0 (84 observed, 0.8–1.2). This pattern is consistent with an effect, primarily among males, at the highest exposure levels but is not sufficient to conclude that there is an exposure–response relationship for respiratory disorders as a whole.

Mortality from respiratory disorders in the adult Seveso population, as in most populations in developed societies of the world, is driven by deaths from chronic obstructive pulmonary disease, which is overwhelmingly attributable to cigarette smoking. Mortality from COPD is usually higher among males than females because of increased smoking prevalence, frequency, and duration among men, although women are thought to be more susceptible to the effects of cigarette smoke. The residents of zone A showed a RR for males of 3.7 (4 deaths observed, 1.4–9.8) and for females of 2.1 (only 1 case observed, 0.3–14.9). Residents of zone B showed a relative risk for males of 1.0 (9 observed, 0.5–1.9) and for females of 2.5 (8 observed, 1.2–5.0). Residents of zone R showed a RR for males of 1.2 (74 observed, 0.9–1.5) and for females of 1.3 (37 observed, 0.9–1.9). This is a stronger and somewhat more consistent correlation suggesting, but not proving, an exposure–response relationship and the possibility of an effect on both sexes (Bertazzi et al., 1998; Pesatori et al., 1998).

These findings were essentially unchanged in the exposed groups after 20 years and did not show suggestive evidence of a latency effect overall, with one exception. Women in zone A did show highest mortality in two peaks, one at 0 to 4 years, no mortality at 5 to 9 years, and another at 10 to 20 years, but this pattern, which could be compatible with an immediate effect, exhaustion of susceptibles, and a latent effect, is the result of only 3 cases (Bertazzi et al., 2001).

It is possible that these findings are confounded by cigarette smoking, but this is judged to be highly unlikely. Bertazzi and colleagues (Bertazzi et al., 1998; Pesatori et al., 1998) offer the observation that their survey data do not demonstrate a higher prevalence of smoking by Seveso residents of the exposed zones compared to their unexposed neighbors. They correctly point out that the proportionate differences in cigarette smoking required to achieve such an elevation in risk of morbidity or mortality would be highly unlikely (Pesatori et al., 1998). Such a lopsided result would also be obvious in the survey data. They also point out that smoking-related lung cancers are not increased among exposed residents. They ruled out misclassification and coding as plausible sources of error (Pesatori et al., 1998). Bertazzi et al. (1998) suggest that a stress-related or host defense-related impairment may be responsible that is not mediated by behavioral changes resulting in increased smoking. They state that "early deaths among persons with impaired respiratory systems may have been caused by the social and emotional impact of the disaster" and imply that changes in the immune response as a result of TCDD exposure may have altered the inflammatory response to cigarette smoking in earlier stages of the habit, presumably enhancing the adverse effects, accelerating the loss of lung function, and hastening the onset of COPD (Bertazzi et al., 1998). This mechanism is speculative and not further defined. If this hypothesis is correct, it may be predicted that the elevation in risk is confined to cigarette smokers.

Occupational studies of exposed workers have not duplicated the finding in Seveso of increased mortality from nonmalignant respiratory disease.

The National Institute of Occupational Safety and Health (NIOSH) conducted a cohort mortality study of 5,132 chemical workers at 12 plants in the United States who were known to have been exposed to TCDD (Steenland et al., 1999). This synthetic population, consisting of four previously studied cohorts pooled together, showed an increased risk for all cancers combined (RR = 1.1, 1.0–1.3), an increased risk for lung cancer that did not achieve statistical significance, and exposure–response relationships with lung cancer and with all smoking-related cancers that were statistically significant (two-sided test for trend, $p < .03$ and $p < .02$, respectively). This suggests that if it were present, an effect reflecting TCDD exposure could be observed in this group, which is large enough to have the statistical power to demonstrate such a risk. However, the RR for nonmalignant respiratory diseases, such as COPD, was 0.9 (86 observed, 0.7–1.1).

NIOSH conducted a follow-up study of 586 workers from two plants involved in the production of sodium trichlorophenol and the ester of 2,4,5-trichlorophenoxyacetic acid 2,4,5-T (Sweeney et al., 1997/98). Exposure levels had been documented 15 years before, and the relative exposure levels were confirmed by serum lipid-adjusted levels of TCDD. There was no statistical difference in the prevalence of chronic bronchitis, chronic obstructive pulmonary disease, or reductions in lung function by several measures in the exposed workers compared to an unexposed comparison group with documented low blood levels of TCDD. These findings were available for *Update 1996* and *Update 1998* but were reviewed and reconfirmed by NIOSH in 1998 (Sweeney et al., 1997/98).

Among Ranch Hand participants, respiratory conditions were assessed by questionnaire, physical examination, chest film, and spirometry. There was no excess reported for asthma, bronchitis, pneumonia, abnormal chest film (with the exception of one model that did not show an exposure–response relationship), or pulmonary function. Had differences been observed, it would be difficult to separate any potential effect of herbicide exposure from cigarette smoking in the Ranch Hand population. The unique Ranch Hand population shows a lifetime prevalence of cigarette smoking of 72 percent, with a mean consumption among smokers of 17.3 pack-years; 46 percent of smokers have a history exceeding 10 pack-years. Confounding any association with herbicide exposure, cigarette smoking covaries with 1987 dioxin levels, as do insecticide exposure and exposure to ionizing radiation. This would tend to obscure associations for respiratory outcomes and herbicide exposure (AFHS, 2000).

No further data have become available on the prevalence of cigarette smoking among Vietnam veterans outside the AFHS cohort, either current or historical.

Synthesis

New evidence suggests that there may be an increased risk for nonmalignant respiratory disorders, particularly chronic obstructive pulmonary disease, among individuals exposed to TCDD. This association is based on small numbers, is not adjusted for smoking, and is not internally consistent. This elevation is not obviously the result of different patterns of cigarette smoking, although some degree of confounding is possible. Other studies of occupationally exposed subjects do not show this association, although some of them are clearly large enough to have revealed it if it were present. It is biologically plausible that exposure to TCDD would affect the progression of nonmalignant respiratory diseases, especially among cigarette smokers. Additional evidence from following the Seveso population for a longer period will be required to determine whether the finding in this population is an anomaly or remains elevated over time. Comparison with other populations over similar time periods is required to determine whether any consistent risk in the Seveso population might be shared by other TCDD-exposed populations.

Conclusions

Strength of Evidence in Epidemiologic Studies

There is no information contained in the research reviewed for this report to change the conclusion that there is inadequate or insufficient evidence to determine whether an association exists between exposure to herbicides (2,4-D, 2,4,5-T and its contaminant TCDD, cacodylic acid, and picloram) and nonmalignant respiratory disorders, including asthma in isolation, pleurisy, pneumonia, and tuberculosis, or associated or isolated measures of lung function, chest films, or abnormalities on physical examination. There is also inadequate or insufficient evidence to determine that an association exists between exposure to herbicides or TCDD and risk of death from chronic obstructive pulmonary disease, including emphysema, chronic bronchitis, and asthma in combination with these conditions. Notwithstanding the tentative evidence reviewed above, the committee concluded that the body of new evidence, taken as a whole, cannot be considered limited or suggestive of an association between exposure to TCDD and obstructive airways disorders. The tentative evidence mentioned above is drawn from small numbers in studies of residents of Seveso, who sustained exposure to relatively pure TCDD and represents an isolated finding that should be considered unconfirmed at this time, particularly given uncertainty about smoking patterns.

Biologic Plausibility

There is no evidence from animals that the respiratory system is a target of TCDD or the other herbicides. A discussion of toxicological studies that comprise the biologic basis for an association between exposure to TCDD or herbicides and toxicity end points is contained in Chapter 3; a general summary of the biologic basis for various end points is presented in the conclusion to this chapter.

Increased Risk of Disease Among Vietnam Veterans

There are insufficient data on nonmalignant respiratory disorders in Vietnam veterans to draw a specific conclusion as to whether or not they are at increased risk.

IMMUNE SYSTEM DISORDERS

Background

Immunotoxicology is the study of the effects of xenobiotics (chemical compounds that are foreign to the human body) on the immune system. The compounds may produce an impaired immune response (immunosuppression) or an enhanced immune response (immune-mediated disease). Although alterations in the immune system can be related to increases in the incidence of infection and neoplasm (immune suppression) and immune-mediated diseases (allergy and autoimmunity), there has been no observed increase in infectious or immune-mediated disease in the populations examined after exposure to herbicides. However, alterations have been observed in measures of immune function or populations of immune cells. The question of possible increases in neoplastic diseases is dealt with in Chapter 7.

Immune Suppression

The immune system helps defend the host against foreign invaders. It confers resistance to infection by bacteria, viruses, and parasites; it is involved in the rejection of allografts (tissue transplants); and it may eliminate spontaneously occurring tumors (Paul, 1993). Proper function of the immune system is exquisitely sensitive to disruptions in physiologic homeostasis. The immune response is highly redundant, and several different mechanisms may be employed to eliminate an antigen. Therefore, a toxicant can affect one facet of the immune system without altering the ability of the host to survive challenge by an infectious agent.

Suppression of the immune system leads to increased susceptibility to infection and neoplasia. However, the degree of immune suppression necessary to cause disease is unknown and is the subject of intense scientific interest. Immune deficiency may result from genetic abnormalities (e.g., a deficiency in the enzyme adenosine deaminase, leading to severe combined immune deficiency), congenital malformations, surgical accidents, pregnancy, stress, disease (e.g., HIV-1 can lead to AIDS), and exposure to immunosuppressive agents (Paul, 1993). Immune suppression can also occur in patients with autoimmune disease (discussed below); for example, in systemic lupus erythematosus, the suppression of complement levels and leukocyte function has been noted. Impaired host defenses can result in severe and recurrent infections with opportunistic microorganisms. As noted, the immune system may prevent or limit tumor growth, and a high incidence of tumors may follow immune suppression (Paul, 1993).

Allergy and Autoimmunity

A number of diseases involve hyperresponsiveness of the immune system to either foreign allergens (e.g., allergy) or self-antigens (autoimmunity). Allergic responses have been noted to numerous environmental agents, including plant pollens and epithelial products of domestic animals. Allergy is the result of the formation of allergen-specific immunoglobulin E (IgE) antibodies, which bind to the surface of mast cells and lead to mastcell degranulation on subsequent exposure to antigen. The mediators of allergic reactions, such as histamine, are then released. The alterations discussed below reflect only in vitro immune parameters, not disease incidence. In fact, no increase in allergic disease related to herbicide exposure has been reported in any of the studies reviewed.

In general, the immune response is directed against foreign antigens. However, in some instances antibodies can be demonstrated that react with endogenous antigens (i.e., autoantibodies). Autoimmune disease is the pathological consequence of an immune response to autologous antigen. Some autoimmune diseases result when autoantibodies activate the complement cascade or interact with "killer" mononuclear cells to induce antibody-dependent cell-mediated cytotoxicity. Others are caused by cytotoxic T cells acting directly on their targets or by injurious cytokines released by activated T cells.

It is important to distinguish the mere presence of an autoimmune response from autoimmune disease. Autoimmunity, as indicated by the presence of autoantibodies, is relatively common, whereas autoimmune disease is relatively rare. Detecting autoantibodies, particularly in high titers and with high affinity, is the first step in diagnosing autoimmune disease in humans. A definite diagnosis of autoimmune disease, however, depends on careful correlation of history and clinical findings with detailed immunological investigations.

Summary of *VAO*, *Update 1996*, and *Update 1998*

The committee responsible for *VAO* found that there was inadequate or insufficient information to determine whether an association existed between exposure to the herbicides used in Vietnam or the contaminant dioxin and immune system disorders. Additional information available to the committees responsible for *Update 1996* and *Update 1998* did not change this finding. Reviews of the studies underlying these findings may be found in the earlier reports.

Update of the Scientific Literature

Suppression of the immune system can result in increased susceptibility to infectious and/or carcinogenic agents, while stimulation can result in allergy and/or autoimmunity. TCDD exposure generally suppresses the immune response of laboratory animals. However, the immune effects described in humans exposed to TCDD have been marginal and have varied from study to study—some showing increases, others decreases, and others no effect. It has been suggested that perinatal exposure to chlorinated aromatic hydrocarbons may influence the human fetal and neonatal immune system, but the effects to date have not been correlated with increased susceptibility to infection. Further, workers exposed to high levels of TCDD for several years with body burdens at least 10 times higher than the general population had no significant differences in lymphocyte subpopulations or mitogen-induced lymphocyte proliferation compared to controls (IOM, 1994, 1999).

Several recent studies have evaluated the immunotoxic effects of polychlorinated dibenzodioxins and dibenzofurans (PCDD/PCDF) in human workers. In a study in which blood concentrations of PCDD and PCDF were available from

187 workers of a pesticide plant that closed in 1984, no significant correlation between blood PCDD concentration and clinical impairment of the immune system was noted and immunological parameters did not correlate with the concentrations (Jung et al., 1998). However, the chromate resistance of phytohemagglutinin (PHA) stimulated lymphocytes of workers with the highest exposure was significantly lower than that of the control group. In another study where workers had been employed more than 15 years earlier in production of sodium trichlorophenol and 2,4,5-T ester, a positive relationship between serum 2,3,7,8-TCDD levels and CD3/Ta1 cells (helper lymphocytes) was noted (Sweeney et al., 1997/98). A comparative analysis was also conducted of phenotypes of peripheral blood leukocytes in former industrial workers who had high exposures to dioxins (Ernst et al., 1998). The median TCDD burden of exposed workers was 116 ng/kg versus 4 ng/kg for the controls. There were no significant differences in the proportions of $CD3^+$, $CD4^+$, or $CD8^+$ T lymphocytes, $CD16^+$ natural killer cells, or $CD19^+$ B lymphocytes between the two groups. However, the proportion of $CD45Ro^+$ (CD^+ memory T cells) was significantly higher than the $CD45RA^+$ (naïve) phenotype in TCDD-exposed workers, while the monocytes expressing human leukocyte antigen-DR (HLA-DR) molecules on their surface were significantly lower than in the control group. When the peripheral blood mononuclear cells were cultured, polyclonal-stimulated cytokine release did not differ between the two cohorts. Significantly reduced interferon release was noted in diluted whole blood cultures but not in cultures of isolated PBMCs in the TCDD-exposed cohort when the T-cells were stimulated with tetanus toxoid. In another group of workers exposed in 1951–1984 in a plant that produced organochlorine herbicides, pesticides, and opioids, peripheral blood lymphocytes were obtained from several cohorts of control or TCDD-exposed individuals (Germolec, 1999). The lymphocytes were mitogen stimulated in culture alone or in the presence of TCDD. In vitro treatment with TCDD resulted in a significant decrease in mitogen-stimulated interleukin-2 (IL2) and interferon-δ (IFN-δ) in the TCDD-exposed workers. The authors considered this primarily an in vitro TCDD effect.

Blood from breast-fed babies of mothers exposed to a mixture of PCDDs, PCDFs, and coplanar polychlorinated biphenyls (co-PCBs) was evaluated for percent $CD4^+$ and $CD8^+$ T lymphocytes (Nagayama et al., 1998). The toxic equivalent quantity converted to 2,3,7,8-TCDD equivalents correlated positively with the babies' (1-year-old) $CD4^+$ lymphocytes and negatively with the $CD8^+$ lymphocytes. Thus, the $CD4^+/CD8^+$ ratio was increased.

Children born between 1978 and 1987 to women exposed to a high dose of PCBs and PCDFs through consumption of contaminated rice bran oil (1978–1979) had a higher frequency of bronchitis during their first 6 months of life and of respiratory tract and ear infections for the first 6 years. In 1995, blood was collected from 29 in utero exposed and 24 control children. Serum immunoglobulin levels were similar between the two groups, there were no significant differences in the $CD3^+$, $CD4^+$, and $CD8^+$ phenotypes, and the B-cell and natural killer (NK) cell markers did not differ between exposed and control children (Yu et al., 1998). A dose–response relationship was not observed between exposure and immune markers. The authors concluded that 16 years after exposure, children exposed to high doses of PCBs or PCDFs in utero did not show suppressed immunity of serum immunological biomarkers.

Workers who were exposed to dioxin while manufacturing 2,4,5-trichlorophenate between 1951 and 1972 had a lipid-adjusted mean serum TCDD concentration of 229 parts per trillion (ppt) compared with a mean of 6 ppt in unexposed referents (Halperin et al., 1998). Immune parameters examined were lymphocyte subsets ($CD3^+$, $CD3^+CD26$, $CD4^+$, $CD4^+CD29^+$, $CD4^+CD45RA^+$, $CD8^+$, $CD8^+CD116^{+/-}$, CD20, CD56, and CD4/CD8 ratio), immunoglobulin concentrations (IgA, IgM, and IgG), complement, mitogen background and proliferation (concanavalin A [Con A], PHA, and pokeweed), antigen background and proliferation (tetanus, *Candida*, and mumps), and NK cell activity as well as complete blood counts. An association was noted between serum TCDD levels and a decrease in both the number of CD26 cells and spontaneous background proliferation of T cells. However, increases in T-lymphocyte proliferation were observed in the highest-TCDD-exposed workers when the lymphocytes were stimulated with Con A or PHA. The authors indicated that these results are unlikely to be of clinical importance, and there was no evidence that TCDD caused meaningful immunological changes in the exposed cohort.

The plasma concentrations of immunoglobulins (IgM, IgG, IgA, IgD) and selected cytokines (IL-1alpha, IL-1beta, IL-6, tumor necrosis factor-α [TNF-α]) were evaluated in worker volunteers who had increased body burdens of PCDD (Neubert et al., 2000). Volunteers were "grouped" according to low, medium, or high body burdens, with a "clearly exposed group" identified by definitely increased body burdens of PCDD. Although there was a slight but significant decrease in plasma concentration of IgG1 in this clearly exposed group, no influence of dioxin exposure occurred when all groups were pooled and a multi-regression analysis against international TCDD toxicity equivalencies was performed. There were no effects of exposure on the plasma concentrations of other immunoglobulins or cytokines tested. The authors concluded that their results did not confirm any suspicion of a possible relationship between PCDD exposure and the production of immunoglobulins or cytokines that were measured in the plasma.

Immune parameters were measured in veterans of Operation Ranch Hand in 1992 (Michalek et al., 1999a; AFHS, 2000). Test groups included a comparison group (Air Force veterans who served in Southeast Asia during the same period as the Ranch Hand veterans but were not involved in spraying herbicides) and Ranch Hand background-, low-, and high-dioxin groups. The current median blood dioxin levels for the comparison and background categories were 4.0 and 5.7 ppt, respectively. The initial median blood dioxin levels for the low and high categories were 52.8 and 194.7 ppt, respectively. Immune assays performed were a composite skin test (*Canidida albicans*, mumps, *Trichophyton,* and *Staphylococcus aureus* antigens); lymphocyte and lymphocyte subset counts; serum IgA, IgM, and IgG isotype concentrations; M proteins (serum monoclonal immunoglobulins of clonal B cells); and the presence of serum autoantibodies (antinuclear autoantibodies [ANAs], thyroid microsomal, smooth muscle, mitochondrial, parietal, and rheumatoid factor [RF]). Ranch Hand veterans in the background group had an increased (odds ratio [OR] = 1.8) skin test, while the high group had a slight suppression (OR = 0.7) of the skin test. There were no notable differences in immunoglobulin isotypes or monoclonal immunoglobulins between the four categories. The only significant effect on lymphocyte phenotyping was an increase in the absolute numbers of $CD20^+$ cells in the background group and a decrease in the absolute count of $CD16^+CD56^+CD3^+$ in the higher category compared to the comparison group. No significant differences were noted in the other lymphocyte subpopulations including $CD3^+$, $CD5^+$, $CD4^+CD3^+$, $CD8^+CD3^+$, $CD16^+CD56^+CD3^-$, $CD25^+$, or $CD25^+CD3^+$. Out of the six autoantibodies evaluated, thyroid microsomal autoantibodies were increased in the three Ranch Hand categories with a significant increase in the low group. The other five autoantibodies tested were within the normal odds ratio compared to the comparison group. In fact, three of them in the high category had a low odds ratio (ANA, 0.8; parietal cell autoantibodies PCA, 0.7; RF, 0.6). The authors concluded that there was no evidence of a consistent relationship between dioxin exposure and immune system alteration in these studies.

A prevailing perception is that dioxins suppress the immune response of humans. This perception putatively arises from the fact that dioxins are extremely immunosuppressive in animals and that they are considered to cause cancer in humans, which is often a consequence of a suppressed immune system. However, literature during the past several years has failed to demonstrate a consistent positive association between TCDD exposure and immune effects in humans, via either in utero, perinatal, or postnatal exposure. Many of the immune procedures conducted in humans, however, have not measured immune function (e.g., "action" of immunocytes and/or their secretory products) (Koller, 1990). These nonfunctional procedures are often considered "biomarkers," which are indicators of events occurring in biological systems when a host is exposed to environmental substances. For instance, protein markers (CD) on the surface of immunocytes are usually specific for identifying and enumerating subpopulations of cells, but they do not test their functional capacity. Nevertheless, the available data indicate that the universal immunosuppressive effects observed in laboratory animals have not been confirmed in humans.

Conclusions

Strength of Evidence in Epidemiologic Studies

There is no information contained in the research reviewed for this report to change the conclusion that there is inadequate or insufficient evidence to determine whether an association exists between exposure to herbicides (2,4-D, 2,4,5-

T and its contaminant TCDD, cacodylic acid, and picloram) and immune suppression or autoimmunity.

Biologic Plausibility

There are a large number of studies in animals indicating that one of the most sensitive organ systems to TCDD toxicity is the immune system. TCDD can alter the number and function of immune cells. The effects seen are species and strain specific, but based on the sensitivity of this system in animals, effects on the immune system in humans might be expected. Studies of the effect of exposure to TCDD on immune response following infection with influenza A have been conducted in mice. These demonstrate that the humoral and cell-mediated response is suppressed while cytolytic activity is preserved. A discussion of toxicological studies that comprise the biologic basis for an association between exposure to TCDD or herbicides and toxicity end points is contained in Chapter 3; a general summary of the biologic basis for various end points is presented in the conclusion to this chapter.

Increased Risk of Disease Among Vietnam Veterans

No evidence is available to associate defects in the immune response with Agent Orange exposure. A more thorough discussion of the issue of increased risk of disease among Vietnam veterans is included in Chapter 1.

DIABETES

Background

Primary diabetes (i.e., not secondary to another known disease or condition, such as pancreatitis or pancreatic surgery) is a heterogeneous metabolic disorder characterized by hyperglycemia and quantitative and/or qualitative deficiency of insulin action (Orchard et al., 1992). Historically, two main types have been recognized: insulin-dependent diabetes mellitus (IDDM) and non-insulin-dependent diabetes mellitus (NIDDM). In June 1997, the American Diabetes Association (ADA, 1997) suggested a revised classification, with IDDM being termed Type 1 and NIDDM, Type 2. This new terminology is used in the remainder of this review, although the older diagnostic criteria are utilized as appropriate.

Type 2 diabetes accounts for the majority (approximately 90 percent) of cases of primary diabetes. It is rare before age 30, but increases steadily with age thereafter. The etiology of Type 2 is unclear, but three cardinal components have been proposed: (1) peripheral insulin resistance (thought by many to be primary) in target tissues (e.g., muscle, adipose, liver); (2) beta-cell insulin secretory defect; and (3) hepatic glucose overproduction. Although the relative contributions of these features are controversial, it is generally accepted that the main factors for increased risk of Type 2 diabetes include age (with older individuals at higher risk), obesity, central fat deposition, a history of gestational diabetes (if female), physical inactivity, ethnicity (prevalence is greater in African Americans and Hispanic Americans, for example), and perhaps most importantly, a positive family history of Type 2. Defects at many intracellular sites could account for the impaired insulin action and secretion seen in Type 2 diabetes (Kruszynska and Olefsky, 1996). The insulin receptor itself, insulin receptor tyrosine kinase activity, insulin receptor substrate proteins, insulin-regulated glucose transporters, enhanced protein kinase C (PKC) activity, TNF-α, rad (ras associated with diabetes), and PC1 have all been proposed as potential mediators of insulin resistance; impaired insulin secretion has been linked to hyperglycemia itself, to abnormalities of glucokinase and hexokinase activity, and to abnormal fatty acid metabolism. Finally, an increasing number of "other" types of diabetes have been described that are linked to specific genetic mutations, for example, maturity-onset diabetes of youth, which results from a variety of mutations of the beta cell glucokinase gene.

Pathogenetic diversity and diagnostic uncertainty are two of the more significant problems associated with the epidemiologic study of diabetes. Given the multiple likely pathogenetic mechanisms leading to diabetes—which include diverse genetic susceptibilities (ranging from autoimmunity to obesity) and a variety of potential environmental and health behavior factors (e.g., viruses, nutrition, activity)—it is probable that many agents or behaviors contribute to diabetes risk, especially in genetically susceptible individuals. These multiple mechanisms may also lead to heterogeneous responses to various exposures. Because up to half of the affected diabetic population is currently undiagnosed, the potential for ascertainment bias is high (i.e., more intensively followed groups or those with more frequent health care contact are more likely to be diagnosed), and the need for formal standardized testing (to detect undiagnosed cases) is great. Furthermore, it may be difficult to differentiate cases developing during young to middle age (i.e., 20–44 years) into Type 1 or Type 2.

Summary of *VAO, Update 1996,* and *Update 1998*

The committee responsible for *VAO* found that there was inadequate or insufficient information to determine whether an association existed between exposure to the herbicides used in Vietnam or the contaminant dioxin and diabetes. Additional information available to the committees responsible for *Update 1996* and *Update 1998* did not change this finding.

In 1999, in response to a request from the DVA, the IOM called together a committee to conduct an interim review of the scientific evidence regarding Type 2 diabetes. This review, which focused on information published since the deliberations of the *Update 1998* committee, resulted in the report *Veterans and Agent Orange: Herbicide/Dioxin Exposure and Type 2 Diabetes* (IOM, 2000). The committee responsible for that report found there was limited/suggestive evidence of an association between Type 2 diabetes and exposure to the herbicide used in Vietnam. While the committee convened for the DVA request and the committee responsible for *Update 2000* have worked concurrently, the committees functioned independently in reviewing, discussing, and summarizing the relevant literature on diabetes.

Reviews of the studies underlying these findings may be found in the earlier reports.

Update of the Scientific Literature

In the course of its evaluation of evidence, the committee responsible for the *Type 2 Diabetes* report reviewed scientific papers on this condition published since the release of *Update 1998*. The sections below briefly summarize those reviews; more complete information may be found in that report.

Occupational Studies

Two studies have combined information from multiple occupational cohorts with potential exposure to dioxin. The International Agency for Research on Cancer (IARC) mortality study included 36 cohorts with exposure to the production or spraying of phenoxy acid herbicides and chlorophenols (Vena et al., 1998). Data from each cohort were used to identify workers exposed to TCDD or higher-chlorinated dioxins, and analyses for diabetes contrasted the mortality experience of exposed ($N = 13,831$) and nonexposed ($N = 7,553$) workers. Exposure to dioxin was associated with a twofold increase in mortality from diabetes (RR = 2.3, 0.5–9.5), with the imprecision attributable to the relatively small number of deaths (33 exposed, 11 nonexposed). Additional assessments of exposure duration and latency effects were also markedly imprecise. A separate analysis was conducted on data from the 12 U.S. cohorts included in the IARC study (Steenland et al., 1999). A standardized mortality ratio (SMR) analysis of mortality for all 12 cohorts found a slight and statistically nonsignificant excess mortality from diabetes (28 deaths, SMR = 1.2, 0.8–1.7). Detailed information from 8 of the 12 cohorts enabled Steenland et al. to create a job–exposure matrix and assign a dioxin exposure score to the 3,538 workers from the 8 cohorts. Workers were divided into septiles of cumulative exposure to dioxin, and mortality was analyzed with an internal referent (the lowest septile of exposure). The analysis of diabetes mortality, based on deaths with diabetes as either the underlying or a contributing cause (55 deaths), found an unexpected inverse relationship between dioxin exposure and mortality, with $p = .02$ for the two-sided test of trend. A pattern of declining rate ratios was shown in the three highest septiles of exposure (1.0, 0.7, 0.5), although each estimate also had a broad confidence interval (e.g., 0.2–2.1 and 0.2–1.9 for the top two septiles).

The relationship between serum dioxin levels and diabetes morbidity in a NIOSH study of dioxin-exposed workers from chemical plants in New Jersey and

Missouri was summarized in *Update 1998* (Sweeney et al., 1997/98), but Calvert et al. (1999) provided a more detailed analysis of diabetes-related outcomes. Workers were recruited for the study 15 to 20 years after occupational exposure to dioxin, and a comparison group was formed by selecting neighbors matched to the workers on age, race, and gender. Examinations were conducted on 281 workers and 260 matched neighbors, and diabetes was defined by self-reported history of physician diagnosis (not verified) or elevated fasting glucose levels (≥ 7.8 mmol/l) on 2 consecutive days. All individuals in the neighborhood comparison group had current dioxin levels of less than 20 pg/g, while dioxin levels of the chemical workers ranged from nondetectable to 3,400 pg/g, with a median of 68 pg/g. Four subgroups of roughly equal size were defined among the chemical workers to represent levels of dioxin exposure for the analysis of data. Diabetes was found in 26 workers and 18 adults from the neighborhood comparison group. In the overall comparison of workers and their neighbors, the former were 50 percent more likely to have diabetes (OR = 1.5) after adjustment for body mass index, family history of diabetes, and the matching characteristics. However, this estimate was imprecise (0.8–2.9), and there was no support for a dose–response trend in risk of diabetes across the four levels of serum dioxin. The chemical workers also had a slight and statistically nonsignificant elevation in fasting serum glucose levels; in detailed analyses of current and half-life extrapolated dioxin levels, only the subgroup with the highest half-life extrapolated concentration (1,860–30,000 pg/g) demonstrated a statistically significant elevation in fasting glucose.

Environmental Studies

The 15-year follow-up for the Seveso study was reported by gender for three levels of exposure (Bertazzi et al., 1998; Pesatori et al., 1998). For men, no deaths were attributed to diabetes in zone A, the zone of highest exposure (with 0.6 death expected), and a small, statistically nonsignificant excess in deaths from diabetes was reported in the areas with medium (zone B, 6 deaths, SMR = 1.3) and low (zone R, 37 deaths, SMR = 1.1) exposure to dioxin. In women after 15 years of follow-up, the SMRs for diabetes were 1.8 (0.4–7.3; based on 2 deaths), 1.9 (1.1–3.2; 13 deaths), and 1.2 (1.0–1.6; 74 deaths) for zones A, B, and R respectively. The analysis of data on diabetes from the 20-year follow-up of the Seveso study became available after the publication of the Type 2 Diabetes report and was limited to zones A and B (Bertazzi et al., 2001). In these data there is no evidence of elevated mortality from diabetes in men, and there is a reduced excess for women in zone A (SMR = 1.3, 0.3–5.1; 2 deaths). The increased mortality from diabetes in women of zone B persisted (SMR = 1.8, 1.1–2.9; 18 deaths), and analyses for latency show a consistent excess across the follow-up period.

The only other study of environmental effects was an analysis of serum dioxin and insulin among nondiabetic adults in a larger population-based study of health effects from residing near the Vertac/Hercules Superfund site in Arkansas (Cranmer et al., 2000). Study subjects lived near the Superfund site or in a comparison community 25 miles away. A total of 69 individuals with no history of diabetes and a normal glucose response to an oral glucose tolerance test were divided into deciles of serum dioxin levels for the analysis of insulin at baseline (fasting) and 30, 60, and 120 minutes after the glucose challenge. Fasting insulin was elevated only among those in the top decile of exposure (dioxin > 15 ppt), and elevated insulin levels in this subgroup were sustained for 6 of these 7 individuals during the subsequent 2 hours (compared with 6 of 62 in the remaining nine deciles of exposure, $p < .05$ using Fisher's exact test). The seven subjects in the highest decile of dioxin exposure had slightly higher levels of lipids and body mass index, but the small numbers precluded mathematical adjustment for these differences.

Vietnam Veteran Studies

In a letter regarding the Ranch Hand publication by Henriksen et al. (1997), Slade (1998) suggested that the association observed between dioxin exposure categories and diabetes may have been attributable to the influence of triglycerides on the measurement of dioxin. In response to this letter, Michalek et al., (1998) presented analyses showing that adjustment (via stratification and logistic regression modeling) for serum triglyceride level at the time of the dioxin blood draw did not account for the association between dioxin and diabetes. In addition, there was no evidence in the logistic regression model for interaction between triglycerides and dioxin (i.e., the relationship between dioxin level and risk of diabetes did not vary by level of triglycerides).

Longnecker and Michalek (2000) published a study of serum dioxin and diabetes that focused exclusively on comparison veterans enrolled in the Ranch Hand study. These individuals were Air Force veterans who served in Southeast Asia between 1962 and 1971 but were not involved in the spraying of herbicides; in addition, all comparison veterans were required to have serum dioxin levels at or below 10 ng/kg in order to represent individuals with background levels of exposure. A total of 1,197 men were available for this analysis, and quartiles of serum dioxin levels were formed within the range of background exposure (between undetectable and 10 ng/kg) to evaluate the association between low-dose exposure to dioxin and diabetes, fasting and postchallenge glucose, and insulin. For most of these men, serum dioxin levels were measured in 1987, but others had measurements in 1992 or 1997. Glucose and insulin levels were measured in 1992, while diabetes was based on a verified physician diagnosis (at any time between the end of military service and 1995) or a postchallenge glucose level of 200 mg/dl in 1992. The number of men with diabetes by quartile of dioxin level was 26, 25, 57, and 61 for quartiles 1, 2, 3, and 4, respectively. In unadjusted analyses, the second quartile had no increase in diabetes, but men in the third (4–5.1 ng/kg) and fourth (5.2–10 ng/kg) quartiles were approximately 2.5 times more likely to have diabetes than men in the first quartile (below 2.8 ng/kg). The odds ratios for quartiles 3 and 4 were reduced to 1.8 (1.0–3.0) and 1.6 (0.9–2.7), respectively, after adjustment for age, race, military occupation, family history of diabetes, serum triglycerides, waist circumference, and body mass index. Fasting glucose and postchallenge glucose and insulin were directly related to quartile of dioxin in the simple analysis, while in the multivariate analysis, glucose and insulin levels in the top three quartiles were much closer to each other and only modestly above levels in the lowest quartile.

In February 2000, the Air Force Heath Study (AFHS) released a report based on data from the 1997 physical examination of Ranch Hand veterans and their comparison cohort (AFHS, 2000). The study included evaluations of Type 2 diabetes incidence, time to onset, and associated laboratory values using four statistical models based on a different approach to exposure measurement. All models were run both "unadjusted" and "adjusted" for a set of potential confounders: age, race, military occupation, personality type, body fat, and family history of diabetes. Individuals who were diagnosed with diabetes prior to their service in Southeast Asia were excluded from these analyses.

The composite diabetes indicator was coded "yes" if the participant had either a verified history of diabetes (a medical records measure) or a 2-hour postprandial glucose level of at least 200 mg/dl (a laboratory examination measure). Overall, approximately 17 percent of each cohort (16.9 percent of the Ranch Hands and 17.0 percent of the comparisons) were considered diabetic based on the indicator criteria. The unadjusted and adjusted comparisons of the groups did not yield statistically significant differences in the number of diabetic participants (RR = 1.0, 0.8–1.3; Model 1). However, the percentage of Ranch Hands with diabetes varied in a dose–response fashion among the dioxin-categorized subgroups: 9.8 percent in the background category, 20.9 percent in the low category, and 23.8 percent in the high category. This pattern of results is consistent with the report by Henriksen et al. (1997), which was based on data collected through June, 1995 and was summarized in *Update 1998*. The adjusted forms of Models 2, 3, and 4 all yielded statistically significant associations between the exposure measure and the composite diabetes indicator. There was a significant positive association between initial serum dioxin level and the percentage of diabetic participants among Ranch Hands (RR = 1.4, 1.1–1.7; Model 2). Ranch Hands in the low (RR = 1.2, 0.8–1.8), high (RR = 1.5, 1.0–2.2), and combined low and high (RR = 1.3, 1.0–1.8) dioxin categories were more likely to be diabetic than were comparisons (Model 3). Finally, there was a significant positive association between 1987 serum dioxin levels and diabetes (RR = 1.5, 1.2–1.7; Model 4). The unadjusted form of Model 4 also yielded a statistically significant positive relationship; the unadjusted forms of Models 2 and 3 did not.

The date on which a participant was first diagnosed with diabetes was used to measure a time to diabetes onset by determining the number of years between the date of diagnosis and the end date of the last tour of duty in Southeast Asia. Models adjusted for known confounders showed that time to onset was significantly shorter for Ranch Hand veterans with higher initial (Model 2, $p = .013$) and 1987 serum dioxin levels (Model 4, $p < .001$), compared to other Ranch Hand veterans. However, diabetic Ranch Hand and comparison subjects did not differ significantly in time to onset (Model 1), and only Ranch Hand veterans with background levels of dioxin showed a significantly shorter time to onset than the comparison groups (Model 3). It should be noted that for a condition like Type 2 diabetes, time to onset might be affected by characteristics associated with the utilization of medical care. The relationship between measures of exposure and potential variation in post-Vietnam utilization of medical care was not assessed in this analysis.

The government of Australia conducted mail surveys of males (CDVA, 1998a) and females (CDVA, 1998b) who served in Vietnam, comparing the self-report data with age-matched Australian national data. Questionnaires were mailed to 49,944 male veterans (80 percent response rate) and 278 female veterans (81 percent response rate). The authors found an excess of diabetes among male veterans and a deficit among female veterans when comparing the number of Vietnam veterans responding yes to the question, *Since your first day of service in Vietnam, have you been told by a doctor that you have diabetes?* compared to expected national rates: 6 percent (2,391) of the male veterans responded yes compared to the expected 4.5 percent (1,780; range 1,558–2,003) for an observed–expected ratio of 1.34. For female veterans 2 percent (5) responded yes, while 10 (9–11) were expected, for an observed–expected ratio of 0.5. The reports acknowledge that the questionnaire did not define diabetes and that misreporting was possible since respondents whose doctors had informed them of a single high blood sugar measure may have interpreted that as "having diabetes."

Synthesis

The new literature on mortality from diabetes is somewhat inconsistent. A general pattern of increased mortality from diabetes continued among women from zone B of Seveso but is not present for men. Elevated mortality was reported for exposed workers in the IARC analyses, but most of the estimates are very imprecise. Furthermore, a refined study of exposure effects in eight U.S. cohorts included in the IARC study documented an inverse relationship between exposure gradient and diabetes mortality. This inconsistency may be due in part to differences in the outcome studied; the Steenland et al. (1999) study used deaths with any mention of diabetes (underlying or contributing cause), while Vena et al. (1998) limited their analysis to underlying cause of death only. As mentioned in earlier *VAO* reports, mortality studies of diabetes are invariably problematic because of the uncertain validity of the assigned cause of death and the likely (but often unrecorded) contribution of diabetes to many deaths assigned to diabetes-related causes such as coronary heart disease, stroke, and renal failure.

Among the diabetes morbidity studies, the *Update 1998* summary of the NIOSH study of chemical workers from New Jersey and Missouri had been based on an abstract and review paper. More complete information is now available in the 1999 paper by Calvert and colleagues. This paper and the analysis of AFHS data by Henriksen et al. (1997) (with elaboration by Michalek et al., 1998 and AFHS, 2000) suggest that dioxin exposure may be associated with an increased risk of developing diabetes. The association in each study is modest and imprecise, but the rough consistency across studies compensates in part for the imprecision. Each study also provides some evidence that the association cannot be attributed to other factors (e.g., measures of obesity, family history of diabetes, lipid profile). Longnecker and Michalek's (2000) study of the Ranch Hand comparison cohort raises the possibility of low-dose effects of dioxin on risk for diabetes; if valid, a revised definition of the referent group employed by Calvert et al. and Henriksen et al. may reveal a clearer association between exposure and risk of diabetes.

In summary, positive associations are reported in multiple mortality studies, which may underestimate the incidence of diabetes, and in most of the morbidity studies identified by the committee. Taken together, these studies and the reports reviewed in *VAO*, *Update 1996*, and *Update 1998* meet the definition established for limited/suggestive evidence—that is, *evidence is suggestive of an association between herbicides and the outcome, but limited because chance, bias, and confounding could not be ruled out with confidence*. Although some of the risk estimates in the studies examined by the committee are not statistically significant and, individually, studies can be faulted for various methodological reasons, the accumulation of positive evidence is suggestive.

Conclusions

Strength of Evidence in Epidemiologic Studies

Based on its evaluation of the epidemiologic evidence reviewed in this and previous *Veterans and Agent Orange* reports, the committee finds there is limited/suggestive evidence of an association between exposure to herbicides (2,4-D, 2,4,5-T and its contaminant TCDD, cacodylic acid, and picloram) and diabetes. This change from previous *Update* report findings reflects the availability of multiple studies with direct measures of diabetes and adjustment for several important potential confounders. The report *Veterans and Agent Orange: Herbicide/Dioxin Exposure and Type 2 Diabetes* (IOM, 2000) provides additional detail for the reasoning underlying this conclusion.

Biologic Plausibility

Animal, laboratory, and human data provide reasonable evidence that TCDD exposure could affect Type 2 diabetes risk in humans. TCDD's association with triglyceride and high-density lipoprotein concentrations suggests a general consistency because these are the hallmarks of altered lipid metabolism in diabetes, since fatty acid metabolism, insulin resistance, and glucose metabolism are closely linked. Other observed effects include alteration of glucose transport in a variety of cells, modulation of protein kinase C activity, reduction in adipose tissue lipoprotein lipase in guinea pigs, hypertriglyceridemia in rabbits, and down-regulation of low-density lipoprotein receptors on the plasma membrane in guinea pig hepatocytes.

Recently published studies of humans report a compensatory metabolic relation between dioxin and insulin regulation in Air Force Health Study participants (Michalek et al., 1999b), an apparent association between serum dioxin levels and fasting glucose levels among nondiabetic AFHS comparison group members with less than 10 ppt serum dioxin (Longnecker and Michalek, 2000), and an elevated incidence of hyperinsulinemia among a nondiabetic cohort with serum TCDD levels greater than 15 ppt (Cranmer et al., 2000). These studies, however, have methodologic limitations—primarily, inadequate measures of individual characteristics such as percentage of body fat at the time of exposure—that prevent more definitive conclusions from being drawn.

Increased Risk of Disease Among Vietnam Veterans

Presently available data allow for the possibility of an increased risk of Type 2 diabetes in Vietnam veterans. It must be noted, however, that these studies indicate that the increased risk, if any, from herbicide or dioxin exposure appears to be small. The known predictors of diabetes risk—family history, physical inactivity, and obesity—continue to greatly outweigh any suggested increased risk from wartime exposure to herbicides.

TABLE 10-1 Selected Epidemiologic Studies—Diabetes

Reference	Study Population	Exposed Cases	Estimated Risk (95% CI)
OCCUPATIONAL			
New Studies			
Calvert et al., 1999	Workers exposed to 2,4,5-T and derivatives		
	All workers	26	1.49 (0.77–2.91)
	Serum TCDD <20 pg/g (ng/kg) lipid	7	2.11 (0.77–5.75)
	20<TCDD <75	6	1.51 (0.53–4.27)
	75<TCDD <238	3	0.67 (0.17–2.57)
	238<TCDD <3,400	10	1.97 (0.79–4.90)
Steenland et al., 1999	Highly exposed industrial cohorts ($N = 5,132$)		
	Diabetes as underlying cause	26	1.18 (0.77–1.73)
	Diabetes among multiple causes	89	1.08 (0.87–1.33)
	Chloracne subcohort ($N = 608$)	4	1.06 (0.29–2.71)

TABLE 10-1 *Continued*

Reference	Study Population	Exposed Cases	Estimated Risk (95% CI)
Vena et al., 1998	Exposed production workers and sprayers in 12 countries[a]	33	2.25 (0.53–9.5)
Calvert et al., 1996[c]	Workers (N = 273) exposed to 2,4,5-T and derivatives vs. matched referents (N = 259)		
	OR for abnormal total cholesterol concentration	95	Overall: 1.1(0.8–1.6)
		18	High TCDD: 1.0 (0.5–1.7)
	OR for abnormal HDL cholesterol concentration	46	Overall: 1.2(0.7–2.1)
		16	High TCDD: 2.2 (1.1–4.7)
	OR for abnormal mean total/HDL cholesterol ratio	131	Overall: 1.1(0.8–1.6)
		36	High TCDD: 1.5 (0.8–2.7)
	OR for abnormal mean triglyceride cholesterol ratio	20	Overall: 1.0(0.5–2.0)
		7	High TCDD: 1.7 (0.6–4.6)
Steenland et al., 1992[b]	Dioxin-exposed workers–mortality rates		
	Diabetes as underlying cause	16	1.07 (0.61–1.75)
	Diabetes among multiple causes	58	1.05 (0.80–1.36)
Studies Reviewed in *Update 1998*			
Sweeney et al., 1997/98	NIOSH production workers		
Ramlow et al., 1996	Pentachlorophenol production workers	4	SMR = 1.2 (0.3–3.0)
Studies Reviewed in *Update 1996*			
Ott et al., 1994	Trichlorophenol production workers		p = 0.06
Von Benner et al., 1994	West German chemical production workers	N/A	N/A
Zober et al., 1994	BASF production workers	10	0.5 (0.2–1.0)
Studies Reviewed in *VAO*			
Sweeney et al., 1992	NIOSH production workers	26	1.6 (0.9–3.0)
Henneberger et al., 1989	Paper and pulp workers	9	1.4 (0.7–2.7)
Cook et al., 1987	Production workers	4	SMR = 0.7 (0.2–1.9)
Moses et al., 1984	2,4,5-T and TCP production workers (chloracne)	22	2.3 (1.1–4.8)
May, 1982	TCP production workers	2	—
Pazderova-Vejlupkova et al., 1981	2,4,5-T and TCP production workers	11	—

TABLE 10-1 Continued

Reference	Study Population	Exposed Cases	Estimated Risk (95% CI)
ENVIRONMENTAL			
New Studies			
Bertazzi et al., 2001	Seveso residents—20-year follow-up		
	Zone A females	2	1.3 (0.3–5.1)
	Zone B males	6	0.9 (0.4–2.0)
	Zone B females	18	1.8 (1.1–2.9)
Cranmer et al., 2000	Vertac/Hercules Superfund site nondiabetic residents		
	OR for "high" fasting insulin–subjects 7: >15 ppt with serum TCDD>15 ppt vs. <15ppt 62: <15 ppt		8.5 (1.49–49.4)
	"high" 30-minute insulin…	"	7 (1.26–39.0)
	"high" 60-minute insulin…	"	12 (2.23–70.1)
	"high" 120-minute insulin…	"	56 (5.7–556)
Bertazzi et al., 1998	Seveso residents—15-year follow-up		
	Zone A females	2	1.8 (0.4–7.0)
	Zone B males	6	1.2 (0.5–2.7)
	Zone B females	13	1.8 (1.0–3.0)
Pesatori et al., 1998	Seveso residents—15-year follow-up		
	Zone A females	2	1.8 (0.4–7.3)
	Zone B males	6	1.3 (0.6–2.9)
	Zone B females	13	1.9 (1.1–3.2)
	Zone R males	37	1.1 (0.8–1.6)
	Zone R females	74	1.2 (1.0–1.6)
VIETNAM VETERANS			
New Studies			
AFHS, 2000	Air Force Ranch Hand veterans and comparisons		(Numerous analyses discussed in text)
Longnecker and Michalek, 2000	Ranch Hand unexposed referents only, OR by quartile and serum dioxin concentration		
	Quartile 1: <2.8 ng/kg (pg/g)	26	1.00—referent
	Quartile 2: 2.8–<4.0 ng/kg	25	0.91 (0.50–1.68)[c]
	Quartile 3: 4.0–<5.2 ng/kg	57	1.77 (1.04–3.02)[c]
	Quartile 4: ≥5.2 ng/kg	61	1.56 (0.91–2.67)[c]
CDVA, 1998a	Australian Vietnam veterans—male	2,391 reported[b] (6% of respondents)	1,780 expected (1,558–2,003)
CDVA, 1998b	Australian Vietnam veterans—female	5 reported[d] (2% of respondents)	10 expected (9–11)
Henriksen et al., 1997	Ranch Hands—high-exposure group		
	Glucose abnormalities		1.4 (1.1–1.8)
	Diabetes prevalence		1.5 (1.2–2.0)
	Use of oral medications for diabetes		2.3 (1.3–3.9)
	Serum insulin abnormalities		3.4 (1.9–6.1)

TABLE 10-1 Continued

Reference	Study Population	Exposed Cases	Estimated Risk (95% CI)
Studies reviewed in *Update 1998*			
Henriksen et al., 1997	Ranch Hands		
	High-exposure category	57	1.5 (1.2–2.0)
	All Ranch Hands	146	1.1 (0.9–1.4)
O'Toole et al., 1996	Australian Vietnam veterans	12	1.6 (0.4–2.7)[d]
Studies Reviewed in *VAO*			
AFHS, 1991	Air Force Ranch Hand veterans	85	$p = 0.001$, $p = 0.028$
AFHS, 1984	Air Force Ranch Hand veterans	158	$p = 0.234$

NOTE: N/A = not applicable; TCP = trichlorophenol, HDL=high-density lipoprotein; OR=Odds Ratio; 2,4,5-T=2,4,5-trichlorophenoxyacetic acid

[a] May include some of the same subjects covered in the NIOSH cohorts addressed in the other references cited in the Occupational cohorts category.

[b] Studies are not discussed in this report, but discussed as new studies in *Veterans and Agent Orange: Type 2 Diabetes* (IOM, 2000).

[c] Adjusted for age, race, body mass index, waist size, family history of diabetes, body mass index at the time dioxin was measured, serum triglycerides, and military occupation.

[d] Self-reported medical history; answer to question, Since your first day of service in Vietnam, have you been told by a doctor that you have diabetes?

LIPID AND LIPOPROTEIN DISORDERS

Background

Plasma lipid concentrations (notably cholesterol) have been shown to predict cardiovascular disease and are considered fundamental to the underlying atherosclerotic process (Kuller and Orchard, 1988). The two major lipids, cholesterol and triglycerides, are carried in the blood attached to proteins to form lipoproteins, which are classed according to their density: very low density lipoprotein (VLDL—the major "triglyceride" particle) produced in the liver and progressively catabolized (hydrolyzed) mainly by an insulin-mediated enzyme (lipoprotein lipase) to form intermediate-density lipoprotein (IDL) or VLDL remnants, most of which are rapidly cleared by the liver B/E receptors, with the rest going to form low-density lipoprotein (LDL), the major "bad" cholesterol particle. This is cleared by LDL receptors in the liver and other tissues. The "good" cholesterol particle, high-density lipoprotein (HDL), is produced in the small intestine and the liver and also results from the catabolism of VLDL. Although LDL is thought to be involved in the delivery of cholesterol to the tissues, HDL in contrast is involved in "reverse" transport and facilitates the return of cholesterol to the liver for biliary excretion (LaRosa, 1990).

Disorders of lipoprotein metabolism usually result from overproduction or decreased clearance of lipoproteins, or both. Common examples are hypercholesterolemia, which may be familial (due to an LDL receptor genetic defect) or polygenic (due to multiple minor genetic susceptibilities); familial hypertriglyceridemia (sometimes linked to susceptibility to diabetes); and mixed hyperlipidemias in which both cholesterol and triglycerides are elevated. This group includes familial combined hyperlipidemia, thought by many to result from hepatic overproduction of VLDL and apoprotein B, and type III dyslipidemia (defective clearance of IDL–VLDL remnants, leading to a buildup of these atherogenic particles). Although the bulk of blood lipid concentration is genetically determined, diet, activity, and other factors (concurrent illness, drugs, age, gender, hormones, etc.) do have major effects. In particular, the saturated fat content of the diet may raise LDL cholesterol concentrations via decreased LDL receptor activity, whereas obesity and a high-carbohydrate diet may increase VLDL triglycerides, possibly linked to insulin resistance and reduced lipoprotein lipase activity. Intercurrent illness may increase the triglyceride (and lower the cholesterol) concentration. Diabetes is also associated with increased triglycerides and decreased HDL cholesterol, whereas other diseases (e.g., thyroid, renal) often result in hypercholesterolemia. It is thus evident that multiple host and environmental factors influence lipid and lipoprotein concentrations and that these influences must be accounted for before the effect of a new factor can be assessed (LaRosa, 1990). In the current context, obesity as a primary determinant of both triglyceride and TCDD concentrations has to be fully controlled in any analysis. Furthermore, the ability of acute or chronic illness to raise triglyceride (and glucose) concentrations and lower HDL (and LDL) cholesterol must be recognized.

Summary of *VAO*, *Update 1996*, and *Update 1998*

The committee responsible for *VAO* found that there was inadequate or insufficient information to determine whether an association existed between exposure to the herbicides used in Vietnam or the contaminant dioxin and lipid and lipoprotein disorders. Additional information available to the committees responsible for *Update 1996* and *Update 1998* did not change this finding. Reviews of the studies underlying these findings may be found in the earlier reports.

Update of the Scientific Literature

Occupational and Environmental Studies

No new findings have appeared in occupational or environmental studies in the peer-reviewed epidemiologic literature regarding dioxin exposure and the occurrence of elevated lipids or lipoproteins since publication of the last *VAO* series report. Recently published results for triglyceride and HDL cholesterol levels of chemical plant workers in New Jersey and Missouri (Calvert et al., 1998; Sweeney et al., 1997/98) were identical to those given in *Update 1998*.

Vietnam Veteran Studies

The most recent report of the Air Force Health Study (AFHS, 2000) provided analyses of total cholesterol, HDL cholesterol, and triglyceride levels at the 1997 examination and across examinations between 1982 and 1997.[1] Regression analyses of lipids included adjustment for age, race, military occupation, current and lifetime alcohol use, and history of industrial or degreasing chemical exposure. Some analyses also adjusted for body fat at the time of blood measurement of dioxin. In regression analysis with body fat and the covariates listed above, the 238 Ranch Hands in the highest category of dioxin (initial level > 94 ppt, 1987 level > 10 ppt) had a small, statistically nonsignificant elevation in total cholesterol (217.3 mg/dl versus 212.9 mg/dl in comparison veterans, $p = .12$). Continuous and categorical measures of dioxin were not related to change in total cholesterol over time, and results by occupation were inconsistent (e.g., Ranch Hand veterans had slightly more favorable trends in cholesterol among officers but slightly less favorable trends among enlisted ground crew).

Level of HDL cholesterol in 1997 was inversely associated with level of dioxin in 1987 (49.2 mg/dl versus 46.3 mg/dl for low versus high tertiles of dioxin, $p = .04$). However, body fat was not included in regression models for the analysis of 1987 dioxin levels, and other potential predictors of HDL (e.g., change in body fat, distribution of body fat, smoking status, physical activity, medication use) were not assessed. In addition, HDL levels were not associated with occupational definitions of dioxin exposure or estimates of initial dioxin level. Longitudinal analyses of change in HDL cholesterol revealed no relationships to any measures of exposure to dioxin. The aforementioned Ranch Hand veterans with the highest combination of initial dioxin level (> 94 ppt) and 1987 dioxin level (> 10 ppt) had elevated triglyceride levels in 1997 (118.2 mg/dl versus 105.9 mg/dl in comparison veterans, $p = .01$). The longitudinal analysis also revealed that this category of Ranch Hand veterans experienced the largest increase in trigyceride levels over the 15-year follow-up (+13.1 mg/dl versus +1.3 mg/dl in comparison veterans, $p = .02$). No elevation in triglyceride level was evident in Ranch Hands with low or background levels of dioxin.

Synthesis

The new reports from the Air Force Health Study offer useful but incomplete evidence on the association between dioxin exposure and lipid abnormalities. The longitudinal analyses are particularly valuable in addressing alternative explanations for these associations (e.g., antecedent–consequent uncertainty and the effect of lipid level on dioxin level). The findings for total cholesterol and

---

[1] This material is also reviewed in *Veterans and Agent Orange: Herbicide/Dioxin Exposure and Type 2 Diabetes* (IOM, 2000).

HDL cholesterol, in aggregate, do not suggest a clear or consistent relationship with dioxin exposure. A stronger association was observed for serum triglyceride level, but the role of body fat and its distribution as a shared determinant of dioxin and lipid levels must be evaluated more rigorously. Unfortunately, there are no other new studies to add in order to evaluate any evolving direction in the body of evidence.

Conclusions

Strength of Evidence in Epidemiologic Studies

There is no information contained in the research reviewed for this report to change the conclusion that there is inadequate or insufficient evidence to determine whether an association exists between exposure to herbicides (2,4-D, 2,4,5-T and its contaminant TCDD, cacodylic acid, and picloram) and lipid and lipoprotein disorders. No peer-reviewed studies have been added to a literature of weak and inconsistent findings summarized in *Update 1998*, and more detailed analyses are needed from the Air Force Health Study on the role of obesity and other predictors of triglyceride and cholesterol levels.

Biologic Plausibility

Although animal studies suggest potential mechanisms whereby TCDD may cause lipid disturbances, human data (e.g., lipoprotein kinetic studies) are still needed to determine whether, and how, TCDD-exposed subjects have altered lipoprotein metabolism. A discussion of animal toxicological studies that could contribute to a biologic basis for an association between exposure to TCDD and herbicides and toxicity end points is contained in Chapter 3; a general summary of the biologic basis for various end points is presented in the conclusion to this chapter.

Increased Risk of Disease Among Vietnam Veterans

As indicated above, the most recent AFHS study (AFHS, 2000) reports an inconsistent association between dioxin exposure and lipid abnormalities in U.S. veterans of Vietnam. Data are at present insufficient to permit a conclusion about whether or not they are at increased risk for these disorders.

TABLE 10-2 Selected Epidemiologic Studies—Lipid and Lipoprotein Disorders

Reference	Study Population	Exposed Cases	Cholesterol	Triglycerides	HDL Cholesterol
OCCUPATIONAL					
Studies Reviewed in *Update 1998*					
Calvert et al., 1996[c]	Production workers	18, 16, 7	1.0 (0.5–1.7)	1.7 (0.6–4.6)	2.2 (1.1–4.7)
Ott and Zober, 1996[a]	Production workers	42	NS	NS	↑ $p = .05$
Studies Reviewed in *VAO*					
Martin, 1984[a]	Production workers	53 (some exposure)	↑ $p < .005$	↑ $p < .005$	NS
		39 (chloracne)	↑ $p < .05$	↑ $p < .01$	NS
Moses et al., 1984[b]	TCP and 2,4,5-T production workers	118 (chloracne)	NS	NS	No data
Suskind and Hertzberg, 1984[a]	TCP production workers	204	NS	NS	NS
May, 1982[a]	TCP production workers	94	NS	NS	No data
Pazderova-Vejlupkova et al., 1981[a]	TCP and 2,4,5-T production workers	55	NS	NS ↑ VLDL $p = .01$	No data
ENVIRONMENTAL					
Studies Reviewed in *VAO*					
Assennato et al., 1989[a]	Adults exposed near Seveso	193 (chloracne)	NS	NS	No data
Mocarelli et al., 1986[a]	Children exposed near Seveso	63	NS	NS	No data
VIETNAM VETERANS					
New Studies					
AFHS, 2000	Air Force Ranch Hand veterans	858	NS	NS	NS

Study		N			
Studies reviewed in *Update 1998*					
AFHS, 1996[i]	Longitudinal analysis (1992 exam data)	884	NS (cholesterol: HDL ratio)	NS	NS (cholesterol: HDL ratio)
O'Toole et al., 1996[d]	Australian Vietnam veterans	20	3.0 (1.3–4.7)	No data	No data
Studies reviewed in *VAO*					
AFHS, 1991[g]	Serum dioxin analysis (1987 exam data)	283–304[g]	$p = .175$	$p < .001^d$	$p < .001$
AFHS, 1990[f,j]	Original exposure group analysis (1987 exam data)	8–142[g]	1.2 (0.9–1.5)	1.3 (0.9–1.8)	1.0 (0.4–2.4)
AFHS, 1984;[e] Wolfe et al., 1990	Vietnam veterans exposed to herbicide spraying (1982 data)	1,027 total exposed	NS	NS	NS

NOTE: Estimated risk and 95% CI reported unless p-values are specified; NS = not significant; TCP = trichlorophenol.

[a] p-values comparing means to controls. Univariate analysis.
[b] p-values comparing means in production workers with subsequent chloracne to those without.
[c] OR for abnormal lipid in highest-exposure category.
[d] Compared to Australian population.
[e] Comparing means.
[f] Number of exposed Ranch Hand with "high" lipid values.
[g] Comparing mean dioxin across lipid groups.
[h] Continuous analysis.
[i] Comparing change over time between exposed and comparison groups.
[j] Model 1, Ranch Hands vs. Comparisons–Adjusted.

GASTROINTESTINAL AND DIGESTIVE DISEASE, INCLUDING LIVER TOXICITY

Background

The discussion in this section of gastrointestinal and digestive disease, including liver toxicity, encompasses a variety of conditions included under International Classification of Diseases, Ninth edition (ICD·9) codes 520–579. Conditions in this category include diseases of the esophagus, stomach, intestines, rectum, liver, and pancreas. Additional detail on peptic ulcer and liver disease—the two conditions most frequently discussed in the literature reviewed—is provided below. The symptoms and signs of gastrointestinal disease and liver toxicity are highly varied and often vague, depending on the specific condition involved.

The essential function of the gastrointestinal tract is to absorb nutrients and eliminate waste products. This complex task involves numerous chemical and molecular interactions at the mucosal surface, as well as complex local and distant neural and endocrine factors. One of the most common conditions affecting the gastrointestinal tract is motility disorder, which may be present in as many as 15 percent of adults. The range of diseases affecting the gastrointestinal system can most conveniently be categorized by the anatomic segment involved. These conditions include esophageal disorders that predominantly affect swallowing, gastric disorders related to acid secretion, and conditions affecting the small and large intestine and reflected by alterations in nutrition, mucosal integrity, and motility. Systemic disorders may also affect the gastrointestinal system; these include inflammatory, vascular, infectious, and neoplastic conditions.

Peptic Ulcer Disease

Peptic ulcer disease refers to ulcerative disorders of the gastrointestinal tract that are caused by the action of acid and pepsin on the stomach duodenal mucosa. Peptic ulcer disease is characterized as gastric ulcer or duodenal ulcer, depending on the anatomic site of origin. Peptic ulcer disease occurs when the corrosive action of gastric acid and pepsin exceeds the normal mucosal defense mechanisms protecting against ulceration. Approximately 10 percent of the population has clinical evidence of duodenal ulcer during their lifetime, with a similar percentage affected by gastric ulcer. The peak incidence for duodenal ulcer occurs in the fifth decade of life, whereas the peak for gastric ulcer occurs approximately 10 years later. The natural history of duodenal ulcer is one of spontaneous remission (healing) and recurrences. It is estimated that 60 percent of healed duodenal ulcers may recur in the first year and that 80–90 percent will recur within 2 years.

Increasing evidence indicates that the bacterium *Helicobacter pylori* (*H. pylori*) may be closely linked to both duodenal and gastric ulcer disease. This bacterium colonizes the gastric mucosa in 95–100 percent of patients with duodenal ulcer and 75–80 percent of patients with gastric ulcer. Healthy subjects in the United States under 30 years of age have gastric colonization rates of approximately 10 percent. Over age 60, colonization rates exceed 60 percent. Colonization alone, however, is not sufficient for the development of ulcer disease; only 15–20 percent of subjects with *H. pylori* colonization will develop ulcer disease in their lifetimes.

There are other risk factors for peptic ulcer disease. Genetic predisposition appears to be important; first-degree relatives of duodenal ulcer patients have approximately three times the risk of developing duodenal ulcer as the general population. Certain blood groups are associated with increased risk for duodenal ulcer, and HLA-B5 antigen appears to be increased among white males with duodenal ulcer. Cigarette smoking has also been linked to duodenal ulcer prevalence and mortality. Finally, psychological factors, particularly chronic anxiety and psychological stress, may act to exacerbate duodenal ulcer disease.

Liver Disease

Blood tests reflecting liver function are the mainstay of diagnosis for liver disease. Increases in serum bilirubin levels and in the serum activity of certain hepatic enzymes—including aspartate aminotransferase (AST or SGOT), alanine aminotransferase (ALT or SGPT), alkaline phosphatase, and γ-glutamyltransferase (GGT)—are commonly noted in many liver disorders. The relative sensitivity and specificity of these enzymes for liver disease vary, and several different tests may be required for diagnosis. The only regularly reported abnormality in liver function associated with TCDD exposure in humans is an elevation in GGT. Estimates of the serum activity of this enzyme provide a sensitive indicator of a variety of conditions, including alcohol and drug hepatotoxicity, infiltrative lesions of the liver, parenchymal liver disease, and biliary tract obstruction. Elevations are noted with many chemical and drug exposures without evidence of liver injury. The confounding effects of alcohol ingestion (frequently associated with increased GGT) make interpretation of changes in GGT in exposed individuals difficult (Calvert et al., 1992). Moreover, elevation in GGT may be considered a normal biologic adaptation to chemical, drug, or hormone exposure.

Cirrhosis of the liver is the most commonly reported liver disease outcome in epidemiologic studies of herbicide and/or TCDD exposure. Pathologically, cirrhosis reflects irreversible chronic injury of the liver, with extensive scarring and resultant loss of liver function. Clinical symptoms and signs include jaundice, edema, abnormalities in blood clotting, and metabolic disturbances. Ultimately, cirrhosis may lead to portal hypertension with associated gastroesophageal varices, enlarged spleen, abdominal swelling due to ascites, and ultimately hepatic encephalopathy, which may progress to coma. It is generally not possible to distinguish the various causes of cirrhosis by the clinical signs and symptoms or pathological characteristics. The most common cause of cirrhosis in North America and many parts of Western Europe and South America is excessive alcohol consumption. Other causes include chronic viral infections (hepatitis B or hepatitis C), a poorly understood condition called primary biliary cirrhosis, chronic right-sided heart failure, and a variety of less common metabolic and drug-related causes.

Summary of *VAO*, *Update 1996*, and *Update 1998*

The committee responsible for *VAO* found that there was inadequate or insufficient information to determine whether an association existed between exposure to the herbicides used in Vietnam or the contaminant dioxin and gastrointestinal and digestive disease, including liver toxicity. Additional information available to the committees responsible for *Update 1996* and *Update 1998* did not change this finding. Reviews of the studies underlying these findings may be found in the earlier reports.

Update of the Scientific Literature

Occupational Studies

Hooiveld et al. (1998) conducted a retrospective cohort study of Dutch production and contract workers exposed to phenoxy herbicides, chlorophenols, and contaminants between 1950 and 1976. Of the 1,129 workers identified in the original cohort, 562 exposed and 567 unexposed workers were included in this study. The standardized mortality ratio for "digestive system disorders" (ICD·9 520–579) was 0.6 (0.1–2.2), based on 2 deaths. Neither of these deaths was in a subcohort of 140 workers with presumed higher exposures due to an industrial accident. An analysis was also conducted of digestive system disease deaths among workers with medium and high TCDD levels compared to workers with low TCDD levels. Limited measurements of serum TCDD level were combined with information on occupation and duration of employment to form the TCDD level estimates. The relative risks were 1.0 (0.1–17.2) for workers with medium TCDD levels and 0.8 (0.1–14.4) for the high-TCDD group.

An Austrian cohort of 159 TCDD-exposed workers reporting chloracne between 1968 and 1975 was examined by Neuberger et al. (1999). The workers were involved in the production of 2,4,5-T and 2,4,5-trichlorophenol (TCP). In 1996, blood and urine samples were taken from 50 surviving exposed workers and matched controls. Liver disease, as evidenced by blood chemistry analyses and medical records data, was more frequent in exposed workers than in controls. Within the exposed cohort, the mean serum TCDD level was significantly higher in workers with a history of liver disease (801 pg/g; 7 cases) than those without (407 pg/g). Adjustment for smoking did not affect the statistical significance of the result. Analyses that controlled for age, alcohol, and TCDD concentration found the effects of TCDD and its interaction with age to be significant, suggesting chronic liver damage after high TCDD exposure at a young age. The authors raised the idea that liver disease might affect the toxicokinetics of dioxin but did not have the data that would allow this hypothesis to be tested empirically. They also acknowledged that other unmeasured occupational exposures could have influenced the results.

Vena et al. (1998) examined noncancer mortality among 21,863 phenoxy acid herbicide and chlorophenol production workers and sprayers included in the IARC study. This international study comprises 36 cohorts from 12 countries. An analysis of the 4,159 deaths occurring from 1939 to 1992 revealed 96 deaths from diseases of the digestive system (SMR = 0.7, 0.6–0.9) among 13,831 workers exposed to TCDD or higher chlorinated dioxins (TCDD/HCD) and 47 deaths (SMR = 1.0, 0.7–1.3) among 7,553 nonexposed workers. When liver cirrhosis (ICD·9 571) was treated as a separate category, 53 deaths (0.8, 0.6–1.1) were identified among exposed workers; and 19 (1.3, 0.8–2.0) among nonexposed.

Environmental Studies

Bertazzi et al. (1998) conducted a review of early and long-term effects of dioxin exposure following a 1976 industrial accident in Seveso, Italy, where a large population was exposed to a substantial amount of relatively pure 2,3,7,8-TCDD. Extensive monitoring of soil levels and measurements of a limited number of human blood samples allowed for classification of the exposed population into three categories: zone A—highest exposure, zone B—medium exposure, and zone R—lowest exposure. When the authors looked at digestive disease mortality in zone A males, 2 deaths were observed when 3.1 (RR = 0.7, 0.2–2.6) were expected. Among females, 2 deaths were observed when 1.6 were expected (RR = 1.2, 0.3–5.0). In zone B, 15 digestive disease deaths among males were observed when 20.8 were expected (RR = 0.7, 0.4–1.2), and there were 13 deaths among females when 10.3 were expected (RR = 1.3, 0.7–2.2). For males in zone R, there were 165 deaths from digestive diseases when 144.3 (RR = 1.1, 1.0–1.3) were expected. Among females in this zone, there were 89 deaths when 83.5 (RR = 1.1, 0.8–1.3) were expected.

A later study (Bertazzi et al., 2001) extends the mortality analysis to 20 years following the event for zones A and B only. For zone A, there were no additional deaths from digestive system ailments among males (0.5, 0.1–2.1) and one additional death among females (1.4, 0.4–4.3). In zone B, there were 7 additional deaths among males (RR = 0.9, 0.6–1.3; based on 22 deaths total) and 3 additional deaths among females (RR = 1.2, 0.7–1.9). An examination of these deaths as a function of years since first exposure did not indicate a time trend in the data. The analysis also separated data for cirrhosis of the liver from other gastrointestinal diseases. There were no deaths from the ailment among females in zone A; the number of deaths among zone A males (2) was slightly lower than expected (RR = 0.7, 0.2–3.0).

Liver cirrhosis deaths in zone B males (0.8, 0.5–1.4; 14 deaths) and females (0.7, 0.3–1.6; 5 deaths) were also slightly lower than expected.

Vietnam Veteran Studies

Michalek et al. (1998) conducted a 15–year follow-up study examining postservice mortality of U.S. Air Force veterans occupationally exposed to herbicides in Vietnam. Although cause-specific mortality did not differ from that expected regarding deaths from accidents, cancer, or circulatory system diseases, the authors found an increased number of deaths due to digestive diseases. When comparing 1,261 exposed Ranch Hands to a group of 19,080 veterans who were not involved in spraying operations, 9 deaths were observed when 5.1 were expected (SMR = 1.7, 0.9–3.2). Chronic liver disease and cirrhosis accounted for most of the increase in digestive disease deaths.

The latest in the series of Air Force Health Study reports describes the results of the 1997 physical examination of Ranch Hand veterans and their comparison cohort (AFHS, 2000). More details on this study series are contained in Chapter 3. An extensive assessment of liver disease outcomes was conducted: data were collected on eight medical conditions and 29 laboratory measurements or indices. Analyses were adjusted for age, race, military occupation, alcohol history, industrial chemical exposure, and degreasing chemical exposure. Participants with a pre-Southeast Asia diagnosis of a condition were excluded from the analysis of that condition.

The authors evaluated the incidence of uncharacterized hepatitis, jaundice, acute necrosis of the liver, chronic liver disease and cirrhosis (both alcohol and non-alcohol related), liver abscess and sequelae of chronic liver disease, enlarged liver (hepatomegaly), and what was termed "other liver disorders." There were too few cases of acute necrosis of the liver and of liver abscess and sequelae of chronic liver disease to draw conclusions about incidence. Uncharacterized hepatitis incidence was similar among Ranch Hand (17 of 863) and comparison (21 of 1,244) veterans (RR = 1.2, 0.6–2.4; Model 1, adjusted). Significantly more comparison (35 of 1,219) than Ranch Hand veterans (12 of 846) experienced unspecified jaundice (RR = 0.5, 0.3–1.0; Model 1, adjusted). Eleven of the twelve cases in the Ranch Hand cohort were among veterans with background levels of serum dioxin. Proportionately more Ranch Hand (14 of 870) than comparison (14 of 1,250) veterans experienced non-alcohol-related chronic liver disease and cirrhosis, but the difference did not achieve statistical significance in the various models employed by AFHS researchers (RR = 1.4, 0.7–3.0; Model 1, adjusted). There was no association between serum dioxin level and incidence among Ranch Hand veterans for this outcome. The incidence of alcohol-related liver disease and cirrhosis was similar in the two cohorts. More comparison (27 of 1,249) than Ranch Hand (14 of 869) veterans experienced an enlarged liver (0.7, 0.4–1.4;

Model 1, adjusted). While the authors note that diagnosis of this condition is problematic in obese individuals, they do not adjust for weight in their analysis.

There was a marginally significant excess of so-called other liver disorders (ICD·9 573.0–573.9, 790.4, 790.5, and 794.8) among Ranch Hand veterans. The 249 (of 866) Ranch Hand cases were proportionately greater than the 312 (of 1,240) cases found among comparison veterans (RR = 1.2, 1.0–1.5; Model 1, adjusted). Analyses that factored serum dioxin levels yielded a statistically significant excess among Ranch Hand veterans in the high dioxin category (1.5, 1.1–2.1; Model 3, adjusted) but not the background or low dioxin categories. The authors note that they are preparing a separate report that will examine the relationship between other liver disorders and herbicide exposure and dioxin levels in greater detail.

Laboratory indices included measurements of hepatic (liver) enzyme activity, hepatobiliary function, lipid and carbohydrate indices, a protein profile, and tests for the presence of hepatitis and fecal occult blood. Combinations of these tests are often used to inform the diagnosis of gastrointestinal ailments because physical examination results and reporting of symptoms are not always reliable indicators of problems or good health. However, the presence of altered levels does not by itself indicate an adverse health effect.

Analyses of discrete measures of three of the four hepatic enzymes—ALT, AST, and GGT—and serum triglycerides showed borderline or statistically significant associations between serum dioxin level and elevated enzyme levels. The authors noted that these results were consistent with a dose–response effect but could also be explained by the hyperlipidemia and fatty infiltration of the liver that occur in association with obesity. Analyses of other laboratory indices yielded inconsistent and generally nonsignificant results that depended on whether the measure was treated as a continuous or discrete variable, the particular model used, and whether confounding influences were factored.

The government of Australia conducted mail surveys of approximately 50,000 male and female nationals who served in Vietnam, including those involved in combat, medical teams, war correspondents, entertainers, and philanthropy workers (CDVA, 1998a,b). The self-report data that were gathered were compared with age-matched Australian national data. The authors examined three gastrointestinal conditions: stomach and duodenal ulcers, cirrhosis of the liver, and gastric reflux. There was an excess of male veterans reporting a doctor had told them that they had a stomach or duodenal ulcer since their first day of service in Vietnam compared to age-standardized expected rates: 4,732 cases of stomach ulcer and 3,114 cases of duodenal ulcer were reported (CDVA, 1998a), with many veterans reporting both types (K. Horsley, Commonwealth Department of Veterans Affairs, personal communication, December 10, 2000). In contrast, 3,089 total cases were expected (range 2,872–3,306). The authors noted that there was some uncertainty in the number of cases, given that veterans may or may not have reported ulcers that were identified and treated in the past. The number of reported cases of cirrhosis of the liver, 1,132, was within the bounds of the expected number (41–1,207). Because the expected range for this condition was derived from European rather than Australian data, doubt was expressed about its applicability to Australian veterans. Thirty percent of male veterans reported that a doctor had told them they had gastric reflux. No conclusion was drawn from this result because no baseline was available from which to calculate an expected number of cases.

The survey of female veterans (CDVA, 1998b) included estimates of the range of "observed" number of cases because problems in locating veterans limited the size of the sample cohort. Stomach ulcers were reported by 15 (range 8–22) female veterans and duodenal ulcers by 9 (3–15). A total of 22 (15–29) veterans reported one or both types of ulcers when 17 (15–18) were expected. As noted in the survey of male veterans, there was some uncertainty in the numbers of cases, given that veterans may or may not have reported ulcers that were identified and treated in the past. One case of cirrhosis of the liver was reported— no estimated range was given. Of the veterans surveyed 56 (46–66) reported that they had been told by a doctor that they had gastric reflux since their first day of service in Vietnam. This was higher than the two estimates of expected prevalence, 11 and 33 cases, although the authors stated that this finding should be interpreted with caution because of the lack of precision in defining this condition in both the survey population and the community comparison.

Synthesis

Evaluation of the impact of herbicide and dioxin exposure on noncancer gastrointestinal ailments is more difficult than some of the other outcomes examined in this report. Clinical experience suggests that medical history and physical examination are undependable diagnostic tools for some of these ailments, making incidence data more problematic. The strong interdependence between weight, laboratory indices of hepatic function, and health, and body burden of dioxin, complicate the already difficult task of assessing association.

Most of the analyses of occupational or environmental cohorts reviewed for the first time in this report had insufficient numbers of cases to draw confident conclusions. The one study with a relatively large number of observations (Vena et al., 1998) found lower digestive system disease and liver cirrhosis mortality among exposed workers than unexposed controls. A set of studies of Australian veterans suggested a higher incidence of stomach and duodenal ulcers in both men and women, but the information was self-reported and the analyses were not controlled for confounding influences. The latest AFHS (2000) report found a significantly higher percentage of other liver disorders among Ranch Hands in the high–dioxin category than among comparisons. Data were consistent with an interpretation of a dose–response relationship, but other explanations were also plausible. The committee will give careful scrutiny to a planned paper by AFHS researchers that specifically addresses the results concerning other liver disorders.

Conclusions

Strength of Evidence in Epidemiologic Studies

There is no information contained in the research reviewed for this report to change the conclusion that there is inadequate or insufficient evidence to determine whether an association exists between exposure to herbicides (2,4-D, 2,4,5-T and its contaminant TCDD, cacodylic acid, and picloram) and gastrointestinal and digestive diseases.

Biologic Plausibility

The liver is a primary target organ of TCDD exposure in animals. Therefore, TCDD would be expected to induce liver toxicity in humans at appropriate doses. Direct effects of TCDD and herbicides on other gastrointestinal and digestive diseases have not been seen. A discussion of toxicological studies that comprise the biologic basis for an association between exposure to TCDD or herbicides and toxicity end points is contained in Chapter 3; a general summary of the biologic basis for various end points is presented in the conclusion to this chapter.

Increased Risk of Disease Among Vietnam Veterans

The available data on Vietnam veterans do not permit a conclusion about whether they are at elevated risk for gastrointestinal and digestive diseases.

CIRCULATORY DISORDERS

Background

The circulatory diseases reviewed in this section cover a variety of conditions encompassed by ICD·9 codes 390–459, including hypertension, heart failure, arteriosclerotic heart disease, peripheral vascular disease, and cerebrovascular disease. In morbidity studies, a variety of methods were used to assess the circulatory system, including analysis of symptoms or history, physical examination of the heart and peripheral arteries, Doppler measurement of peripheral pulses, electrocardiograms (ECG), and chest radiograph. Doppler measurements and physical examinations of the pulses in the arms and legs are used to detect decreased strength of the pulses, which can be caused by thickening and hardening of the arteries. ECGs can be used to detect heart conditions and abnormalities such as arrhythmias (abnormal heart rhythms), heart enlargement, and previous heart attacks. Chest radiographs can be used to assess whether the heart is enlarged, which can result from heart failure and other heart conditions. Mortality studies attribute cause of death to one or more of the circulatory disorders, with varying degrees of diagnostic confirmation.

Summary of *VAO*, *Update 1996*, and *Update 1998*

The committee responsible for *VAO* found that there was inadequate or insufficient information to determine whether an association existed between exposure to the herbicides used in Vietnam or the contaminant dioxin and circulatory disorders. Additional information available to the committees responsible for *Update 1996* and *Update 1998* did not change this finding. Reviews of the studies underlying these findings may be found in the earlier reports.

Update of the Scientific Literature

Occupational Studies

The most recent report (Vena et al., 1998) of the IARC international cohort study of phenoxy herbicide and chlorophenol production workers stratified subjects by likely exposure to dioxins and assessed mortality for exposed ($N = 13{,}831$) and nonexposed ($N = 7{,}553$) workers in relation to each other and to the general population. Both exposed and nonexposed workers exhibited a "healthy worker effect" for circulatory diseases (i.e., both employed groups had an SMR <1.0 for circulatory diseases, ischemic heart disease and stroke, indicating lower levels of mortality than those found in the general population). However, an analysis conducted within the cohort of workers revealed that exposure to dioxins was associated with a 50 percent increase in death from all circulatory diseases (1,151 deaths in the exposed; 582 deaths in the nonexposed; RR = 1.5, 1.2–2.0). This estimate was adjusted for age, gender, country, and calendar period, and the increased risk was evident for both ischemic heart disease and stroke (RR = 1.7 and 1.5, respectively). No clear patterns were present in the additional analyses of latency and duration of exposure.

Separate reports have also been published on some of the individual cohorts included in the IARC study. The analysis of a Dutch cohort was based on 549 exposed and 482 nonexposed male workers and included adjustment for age, time since first exposure, and calendar year at end of follow-up (Hooiveld et al., 1998). Workers exposed to phenoxy herbicides, chlorophenols, and contaminants were at increased risk of death from all circulatory diseases (45 deaths in the exposed, 16 deaths in the nonexposed; RR = 1.4, 0.8–2.5), ischemic heart disease (33 deaths in the exposed, 10 deaths in the nonexposed; RR = 1.8, 0.9–3.6) and stroke (9 deaths in the exposed; 3 deaths in the nonexposed; RR = 1.4, 0.4–5.1). A dose–response analysis based on TCDD levels extrapolated from serum analyses of a subgroup found a dose–response pattern for ischemic heart disease but not for stroke or circulatory diseases in general. When a similar procedure was used to evaluate the presence of a dose–response relationship across quintiles of exposure in a German cohort of 1,189 workers (Flesch-Janys, 1997/98), the test for trend was statistically significant ($p < .05$) for all circulatory diseases and for ischemic heart disease, but this was influenced primarily by a protective effect in the lowest two quintiles of exposure (e.g., RR = 0.7 and 0.7 for circulatory diseases) and an elevated risk in the highest decile of exposure (e.g., RR = 1.7, 1.0–2.9). Steenland et al. (1999) created an ordinal exposure score based on a job–exposure matrix for eight American cohorts included in the IARC study. A total of 3,538 workers were included in this analysis, and 290 deaths from ischemic heart disease were ascertained. A direct relationship was observed between cumulative exposure to TCDD and ischemic heart disease mortality, with RR = 1.8 (1.1–2.9) for the highest septile of exposure (43 deaths) compared to the lowest septile of exposure (29 deaths).

Morbidity from circulatory diseases was assessed in a cross-sectional study of 281 chemical plant workers and a comparison group of 260 neighbors with matching on age, race, and gender (Calvert et al., 1998). In the simple analysis of myocardial infarction (defined by ECG evidence or self-report of a physician diagnosis), workers in the highest quartile of serum TCDD (>238 pg/g) had nearly a twofold increase (9 cases in the exposed, 20 cases in the nonexposed; OR = 1.9, 0.8–4.4). This association was eliminated (adjusted OR = 1.1, 0.2–5.1) in a logistic regression model that adjusted for age, smoking, alcohol consumption, and family history of heart disease. Dioxin level was not related to the prevalence of angina, cardiac arrhythmias, or hypertension in either the simple or the multivariate analysis.

Environmental Studies

Two papers presented results from the 15-year follow-up of mortality in Seveso, Italy, after the population-based exposure to dioxin (Bertazzi et al., 1998; Pesatori et al., 1998). In the report of the 10-year follow-up, Bertazzi et al. (1989) noted that both men and women in zone A (the most exposed region) had similarly elevated SMRs for circulatory diseases (men: SMR = 1.8, 1.0–3.2; women: SMR = 1.9, 0.8–4.2). These estimates were based on few deaths (11 male, 6 female) and represented different cardiovascular diagnoses. With 5 additional years of follow-up, the SMR for circulatory diseases in zone A remained modestly elevated for men (21 deaths; SMR = 1.6, 1.1–2.5) but was not elevated for women (12 deaths; SMR = 1.0, 0.6–1.7). Elevated SMRs for some specific cardiovascular diagnoses (e.g., chronic rheumatic heart disease and hypertension for women in zone A), are difficult to interpret in view of the small number of deaths (3 for each of these outcomes). There was no evidence of increased general cardiovascular or cerebrovascular mortality in the region with intermediate levels of exposure (zone B). In the area with the lowest level of exposure (zone R), modest increases in deaths due to hypertension and chronic ischemic heart disease led to SMRs of 1.1 (1.0–1.2; 719 deaths) and 1.2 (1.0–1.6; 759 deaths) for circulatory diseases in men and women, respectively. This pattern of results remained essentially unchanged with the extension of mortality follow-up to 20 years (Bertazzi et al., 2001). The SMR for circulatory diseases in men of zone A was 1.4 (1.0–2.2; 24 deaths), with the increased risk attributable to both ischemic heart disease and cerebrovascular disease during the first 9 years of follow-up. There was no clear evidence of elevated risk of mortality from circulatory diseases in residents of zone B (SMR = 0.9 and 1.0 for women and men, respectively) or women from zone A (SMR = 0.7). A small excess in mortality from hypertension (SMR = 1.3, 1.1–1.6; 130 deaths), and chronic ischemic heart disease (SMR = 1.2, 1.1–1.4; 328 deaths), was noted for men and women combined in zone R.

Vietnam Veteran Studies

Michalek et al. (1998) presented the results of the 15-year mortality follow-up of Ranch Hand veterans. These findings were included in *Update 1998* based on the AFHS (1996) report. Mortality was analyzed for 1,261 Ranch Hand veterans, with expected mortality based on data from 19,080 nonexposed Air Force veterans who also served in Southeast Asia. In general, Ranch Hand veterans and comparison veterans experienced similar mortality from all circulatory diseases (39 deaths in Ranch Hand veterans; SMR = 1.0, 0.7–1.3), but an analysis by military occupation showed that among enlisted ground personnel, Ranch Hand veterans were at somewhat increased risk (24 deaths in Ranch Hand veterans; SMR = 1.5, 1.0–2.2).

Data on morbidity were reported from the Air Force Health Study 1997 Follow-up Examination Results (AFHS, 2000). Multiple models were computed to contrast Ranch Hands with comparison veterans (overall and by rank) and to analyze health effects in Ranch Hands by dioxin level (in 1987 or extrapolated to initial exposure). Myocardial infarction, stroke, and transient ischemic attack were unrelated to dioxin levels or exposure categories in all models. Null findings were also reported for all analyses of systolic and diastolic blood pressure and most analyses of the prevalence of hypertension, although the latter was modestly associated with 1987 dioxin levels (OR = 1.2, 1.0–1.3 for a twofold increase in dioxin). A general measure of self-reported history of heart disease (excluding hypertension) was more common among Ranch Hand personnel than comparison veterans (66.1 percent versus 60.8 percent, $p = .01$), and this difference persisted following adjustment for covariates. However, the prevalence of self-reported heart disease was not consistently related to more detailed gradients of exposure as defined by specific occupation or dioxin level. While the investigators reported use of medical records to verify self-reports, the high frequency of heart disease (more than 60 percent among the study sample) raises questions about validity for this outcome.

The government of Australia conducted mail surveys of approximately 50,000 male and female nationals who served in Vietnam, including those involved in combat, medical teams, war correspondents, entertainers, and philanthropy workers (CDVA, 1998a,b). The self-report data that were gathered were compared with age-matched Australian national data. An excess of male veterans reported that a doctor had told them they had ischemic heart disease since their first day of service in Vietnam, compared to age-standardized expected rates: 5,965 cases were reported while 3,236 (range 2,732–3,739) were expected (CDVA, 1998a). The authors noted that although there was the possibility of other circulatory ailments being misreported as ischemic heart disease, elevated mortality rates (SMR = 1.1, 1.0–1.2) found in an earlier study of this population (Crane et al., 1997) lent support to this finding.

The survey of female veterans (CDVA, 1998b) included estimates of the range of "observed" number of cases because problems in locating veterans limited the size of the sample cohort. Ischemic heart disease was reported by 25 (16–34) female veterans. Expected rate estimates depended on the definition of the disease used, varying from 9 (8–10) to 15 (14–17). As noted in the survey of male veterans, there was some uncertainty in the numbers of cases due to possible misreporting.

Synthesis

Evidence of increased circulatory disease mortality persists in the extended follow-up of the Seveso population, but the pattern is somewhat inconsistent across levels of exposure and the statistical power remains limited, particularly for women. The new studies from occupational epidemiology offer additional insight by providing "internal" comparisons among employed populations, thereby reducing the potential for the healthy worker effect and exposure effects to offset each other. In the comparison among workers, there is evidence of an association between dioxin and mortality from circulatory diseases in three separate studies and one larger study incorporating these three studies and others. However, key limitations recognized in *Update 1998* still generally exist—the reliance on mortality as an outcome, the unassessed validity of assigned cause of death, and the inability to address potential confounding by other causes of cardiovascular and cerebrovascular disease. It is noteworthy that in the occupational study that examined morbidity and measured potential confounders, an initial association between exposure and myocardial infarction was eliminated with mathematical adjustment for confounding.

Findings on circulatory conditions in the Air Force Health Study also tend to be inconsistent and inconclusive. Excess mortality is reported for enlisted ground personnel from Operation Ranch Hand, but this pattern of findings is not supported in subsequent analyses of cardiovascular and cerebrovascular morbidity. More generally, the most current AFHS (2000) report shows no dioxin-related increased risk for myocardial infarction and the combination of stroke and transient ischemic attack. In the 20 multivariable analyses of blood pressure (four definitions of exposure; five definitions of outcome: hypertension, diastolic—continuous, diastolic—discrete, systolic—continuous, systolic—discrete), only one model identifies a statistically significant association (prevalence of hypertension in relation to 1987 dioxin level). The magnitude of association is modest (OR = 1.2), and no adjustment is possible for pre-exposure level of blood pressure. A general measure of heart disease is more prevalent among Ranch Hand veterans and some categories of increased dioxin levels, but the gradients of risk are inconsistent and more information is needed to determine the validity of the outcome measure. Elevated rates are reported in both male and female Australian veterans studies.

Conclusions

Strength of Evidence in Epidemiologic Studies

There is no information contained in the research reviewed for this report to change the conclusion that there is inadequate or insufficient evidence to determine whether an association exists between exposure to herbicides (2,4-D, 2,4,5-T and its contaminant TCDD, cacodylic acid, and picloram) and specific circulatory disorders (e.g., coronary artery disease, myocardial infarction, stroke, hypertension) or circulatory conditions in general. As noted in earlier reports, important sources of uncertainty include the quality of measurement for health outcomes, incomplete assessment of confounding, and inconsistency of findings across levels of exposure.

Biologic Plausibility

There have been reports of developmental defects in the cardiovascular system of TCDD-treated birds and fish. However, little information is available to suggest that TCDD is a cardiovascular toxin following postnatal exposure of mammals to TCDD. A discussion of toxicological studies that comprise the biologic basis for an association between exposure to TCDD or herbicides and toxicity end points is contained in Chapter 3; a general summary of the biologic basis for various end points is presented in the conclusion to this chapter.

Increased Risk of Disease Among Vietnam Veterans

The available data on Vietnam veterans do not permit a conclusion about whether they are at an elevated risk for circulatory disorders.

AMYLOIDOSIS

Background

Amyloidosis (ICD·9 code 277.3) is the name given to a poorly understood and relatively rare group of bone marrow diseases. The name derives from amyloid, an abnormal type of protein that can be produced by bone marrow cells. Amyloid cannot be broken down by the body—it builds up in the bloodstream and is deposited in various organs as it circulates throughout the body. Amyloidosis occurs when enough amyloid builds up in one or more organs of the body to cause the organ(s) to malfunction (Mayo Clinic, 2000). Most cases of amyloidosis affect the heart, kidneys, nervous system, or gastrointestinal tract. Amyloid deposits can also build up in the skin.

There are several different types of amyloidosis, which are distinguished by the type of amyloid protein produced, the organ(s) affected, and whether the disease occurs alone or as a complication of another disease. *AL-type primary amyloidosis* is the most common form of systemic (i.e., occurring throughout the body) amyloidosis. *AL* is a reference to the type of amyloid involved (amyloid light chain); *primary*, to the fact that it occurs in the absence of a discernible preceding disease.

Systemic amyloidosis is a complication that occurs in approximately 15–20 percent of patients with multiple myeloma, which is also a bone marrow disease. Differentiation of the amyloid associated with myeloma from that of primary amyloidosis is artificial because the amyloid is of similar genesis and tissue distribution, and the conditions are more appropriately considered as parts of the spectrum of the same basic disease process.

Amyloidosis, like multiple myeloma, occurs primarily in individuals between 50 and 70 years of age and in more males than females. Annual incidence is estimated to be approximately 1 per 100,000, or approximately 2,000 new cases per year in the United States (Solomon, 1996).

Summary of *VAO*, *Update 1996*, and *Update 1998*

The Department of Veterans Affairs asked the committee responsible for this report to address the possible association between exposure to the herbicides used in Vietnam or the contaminant dioxin and AL-type primary amyloidosis, a condition that has not been examined in previous *Veterans and Agent Orange* reports.

Update of the Scientific Literature

The committee identified a single report that addressed exposure to the herbicides used in Vietnam and amyloidosis. In a letter to the journal *Nature*, Tóth et al. (1979) described the results of carcinogenicity tests of the herbicide 2,4,5-

trichlorophenoxyethanol (TCPE) containing dioxin and of pure dioxin in outbred Swiss/H/Riop mice. TCPE, like 2,4,5-T, is a derivative of TCP.

Mice were dosed via gastric tube once a week for a year, beginning at 10 weeks of age, and followed for the remainder of their lives. The authors reported that "TCDD caused severe chronic, ulcerous skin lesions (probably similar to chloracne in humans) followed by generalized lethal amyloidosis, which can be regarded as a process secondary to chronic lesion." The lesions and amyloidosis both exhibited a dose–response relationship to TCDD. These results are consistent with a small literature reporting amyloidosis secondary to chronic chemical insults in humans (Jacob et al., 1978; Scholes et al., 1979).

The committee did not identify any literature addressing primary amyloidosis in animals or people exposed to the herbicides used in Vietnam or dioxin.

Synthesis

There is no direct evidence on which to base a finding concerning whether or not AL-type primary amyloidosis is associated with exposure to the herbicides used in Vietnam or dioxin. Although multiple myeloma and primary systemic amyloidosis are both clonal plasma cell proliferative disorders, there is no scientific reason to believe that available information regarding multiple myeloma and herbicide or dioxin exposure informs the question of an association with amyloidosis.

Conclusions

Strength of Evidence in Epidemiologic Studies

There is inadequate/insufficient evidence to determine whether an association exists between exposure to herbicides (2,4-D, 2,4,5-T and its contaminant TCDD, cacodylic acid, and picloram) and AL-type primary amyloidosis.

Biologic Plausibility

The single animal study (Tóth et al., 1979) reporting secondary amyloidosis in a strain of mice chronically exposed to TCDD suggests that the disease "should be considered a possible later complication of the most severe forms of human chloracne induced by TCDD." However, this study is only tangentially related to the issue of primary amyloidosis in humans. A discussion of toxicological studies that comprise the biologic basis for an association between exposure to TCDD or herbicides and toxicity end points is contained in Chapter 3; a general summary of the biologic basis for various end points is presented in the conclusion to this chapter.

Increased Risk of Disease Among Vietnam Veterans

There are no data on which to base a conclusion concerning whether Vietnam veterans may or may not be at increased risk for AL-type primary amyloidosis due to exposure to herbicides.

SUMMARY

Based on the occupational, environmental, and veterans studies reviewed, the committee reached one of four conclusions about the strength of the evidence regarding association between exposure to herbicides and/or TCDD and each of the other health effects under study. As explained in Chapter 4, these distinctions reflect the committee's judgment that if an association between exposure and an outcome were "real," it would be found in a large, well-designed epidemiologic study in which exposure to herbicides or dioxin was sufficiently high, well characterized, and appropriately measured on an individual basis. Consistent with the charge to the committee by the Secretary of Veterans Affairs in Public Law 102-4 and with accepted standards for scientific reviews, the distinctions between these standard conclusions are based on statistical association, not on causality. The committee used the same criteria to categorize diseases by the strength of the evidence as were used in *VAO*, *Update 1996*, and *Update 1998*.

Health Outcomes with Sufficient Evidence of an Association

In *VAO*, *Update 1996*, and *Update 1998*, the committee found sufficient evidence of an association between exposure to herbicides and/or TCDD and chloracne. The scientific literature continues to support the classification of chloracne in the category of sufficient evidence. Based on the literature, there are no additional health effects discussed in this chapter that satisfy the criteria necessary for this category.

For diseases in this category, a positive association between herbicides and the outcome must be observed in studies in which chance, bias, and confounding can be ruled out with reasonable confidence. The committee also regarded evidence from several small studies that are free from bias and confounding, and that show an association that is consistent in magnitude and direction, as sufficient evidence for an association.

Health Outcomes with Limited/Suggestive Evidence of Association

In *Update 1996* and *Update 1998*, the committee found limited/suggestive evidence of an association between herbicide or dioxin exposure and porphyria cutanea tarda. The scientific literature continues to support the classification of this disorder in the category of limited/suggestive evidence.

Based on its evaluation of newly available scientific evidence as well as the cumulative findings of research reviewed in the previous *Veterans and Agent Orange* reports, the committee responsible for the *Type 2 Diabetes* report found there was limited/suggestive evidence of an association between exposure to the herbicides used in Vietnam or the contaminant dioxin and Type 2 diabetes. Evidence reviewed in this report continues to support that finding. No other changes have been made to the list of health outcomes in the limited/suggestive evidence category.

For this category, the evidence must be suggestive of an association between herbicides and the outcome, but may be limited because chance, bias, or confounding could not be ruled out with confidence. Typically, at least one high-quality study indicates a positive association, but the results of other studies may be inconsistent.

Health Outcomes with Inadequate/Insufficient Evidence to Determine Whether an Association Exists

The scientific data for many of the health effects reviewed by the committee were inadequate or insufficient to determine whether an association exists. For the health effects discussed in this chapter, the available studies are of insufficient quality, consistency, or statistical power to permit a conclusion regarding the presence or absence of an association. For example, studies fail to control for confounding or have inadequate exposure assessment. This category includes nonmalignant respiratory disorders such as asthma in isolation, pleurisy, pneumonia, and tuberculosis; immune system disorders (immune suppression and autoimmunity); lipid and lipoprotein disorders; gastrointestinal diseases; digestive diseases; liver toxicity; and circulatory disorders. Since *Update 1998*, the committee responsible for this report has been asked to address the possible association between exposure to the herbicides used in Vietnam or the contaminant dioxin and AL-type primary amyloidosis. Based on the scientific literature reviewed, there is inadequate/insufficient evidence to determine whether an association exists between herbicide or dioxin exposure and AL-type primary amyloidosis.

Health Outcomes with Limited/Suggestive Evidence of *No* Association

In *VAO*, *Update 1996*, and *Update 1998*, the committee did not find any evidence to conclude that there is limited/suggestive evidence of *no* association between the health effects discussed in this chapter and exposure to TCDD or herbicides. The most recent scientific evidence continues to support this conclusion.

In order to classify outcomes in this category, several adequate studies covering the full range of levels of exposure that human beings are known to encounter must be mutually consistent in not showing a positive association between exposure to herbicides and the outcome at any level of exposure. These studies must also have relatively narrow confidence intervals. A conclusion of "no association" is inevitably limited to the conditions, level of exposure, and length of observation covered by the available studies. In addition, the possibility of a very small elevation in risk at the levels of exposure studied can never be excluded.

Biologic Plausibility

This section summarizes the biologic plausibility of a connection between exposure to dioxin or herbicides and various noncancer health effects on the basis of data from animal and cellular studies. Details of the committee's evaluation of data from those studies are presented in Chapter 3. Some of the preceding discussions of reproductive and developmental outcomes include references to papers relevant to specific effects.

TCDD has been shown to elicit a diverse spectrum of effects, including immunotoxicity, hepatotoxicity, chloracne, loss of body weight, and numerous biological responses, including the induction of phase I and phase II drug-metabolizing enzymes, the modulation of hormone systems, and factors associated with the regulation of cellular differentiation and proliferation. These effects are dependent upon sex, strain, age, and species.

Effects of TCDD on the liver include modulating of the rate at which liver cells multiply, increasing the rate of cell death for other types of cells, increasing fat levels in liver cells, decreasing bile flow, and increasing the levels of protein and of substances that are precursors to heme synthesis. TCDD also increases the levels of certain enzymes in the liver, but this effect in itself is not considered toxic. Liver toxicity is species specific; mice and rats are susceptible to TCDD-induced liver toxicity, but guinea pigs and hamsters are not. It is possible that liver toxicity is associated with susceptibility to liver cancer, but the extent to which TCDD effects mediate noncancer end points is not clear.

TCDD has been shown to inhibit hepatocyte DNA synthesis; decrease hepatic plasma membrane epidermal growth factor receptor; inhibit hepatic pyruvate carboxylase activity; induce porphyrin accumulation in fish and chick embryo hepatocyte cultures; and alter liver enzyme levels and activity. Hepatomegaly has occurred following high subchronic doses. The myocardium has also been shown to be a target of TCDD toxicity; impairment of a contraction modulated by adenosine $3',5'$-cyclic-monophosphate has been implicated.

The mechanism of TCDD hepatoxicity is not established, but most studies are consistent with the hypothesis that the effects of TCDD are mediated by the aryl hydrocarbon receptor (AhR), a protein in animal and human cells to which TCDD can bind. Following the binding of TCDD, the TCDD–AhR complex is thought to bind DNA, leading to changes in transcription (i.e., genes are differentially regulated), that alter cell function.

Although structural differences in the AhR have been identified among different species, this receptor operates in a similar manner in animals and humans. Data in animals support a biological basis for TCDD's toxic effects. Because of the many species and strain differences in TCDD responses, however, controversy remains regarding the extent to which animal data inform the evaluation of human health outcomes.

The immune system is one of the most sensitive organs to TCDD toxicity. Studies in mice, rats, guinea pigs, and monkeys indicate that TCDD suppresses the function of certain components of the immune system in a dose-related manner; that is, as the dose of TCDD increases, its ability to suppress immune function increases. TCDD suppresses cell-mediated immunity, primarily by affecting the T cell arm of the immune response, including a decrease in the number and response of certain types of T cells. It is not known whether TCDD directly affects T cells. TCDD may indirectly affect T cells and cell-mediated immunity by altering thymus gland function or cytokine production. The generation of antibodies by B cells, an indication of humoral immunity, may also be affected by TCDD. Effects of arachidonic acid have also been hypothesized to mediate TCDD's immunotoxicity, but recent evidence indicates that not all of TCDD's immunotoxic effects are mediated by arachidonic acid. As with other effects of TCDD, the immunotoxic effects are species and strain specific.

Increased susceptibility to infectious disease has been reported following TCDD administration. In addition, TCDD increased the number of tumors that formed in mice following injection of tumor cells. It should be emphasized, however, that very little change in the overall immune competence of the intact animal (i.e., animals not knowingly challenged with a pathogen or tumor cells) has been reported.

Despite considerable laboratory research, the mechanisms underlying the immunotoxic effects of TCDD are still unclear, but most studies are consistent with the hypothesis that these immunotoxic effects are mediated by the AhR. TCDD's wide range of effects on growth regulation, hormone systems, and other factors could also mediate its immunotoxicity. As with other TCDD-mediated effects, the similarity in function of the AhR among animals and humans suggests a possible common mechanism of immunotoxicity. Nevertheless, from the data available, the universal immunosuppressive effects observed in laboratory animals have not been confirmed in humans.

TCDD has been shown to induce differentiation in human keratinocytes. TCDD has been reported to decrease an acidic type I keratin involved in epidermal development, leading to keratinocyte hyperproliferation and skin irritations such as chloracne. These data provide a biologically plausible mechanism for the induction of chloracne by TCDD.

Although there is limited information on the health effects of the herbicides discussed in this report, they have been reported to elicit adverse effects in a number of organs in laboratory animals. The liver is a target organ for toxicity induced by 2,4-dichlorophenoxyacetic acid (2,4-D), 2,4,5-T, and picloram, with changes reportedly similar to those induced by TCDD. Some kidney toxicity was reported in animals exposed to 2,4-D and cacodylic acid. Exposure to 2,4-D has also been associated with effects on blood, such as reduced levels of heme and red blood cells. Cacodylic acid was reported to induce renal lesions in rats. Other studies provide evidence that 2,4-D binds covalently to hepatic proteins and lipids; the molecular basis of this interaction and its biologic consequences are unknown. 2,4,5-T has been shown to be a weak myelotoxin.

The potential immunotoxicity of the herbicides used in Vietnam other than TCDD has been studied to only a limited extent. Effects on the immune system of mice were reported for 2,4-D administered at doses that were high enough to produce clinical toxicity, but these effects did not occur at low doses. The potential for picloram to act as a contact sensitizer (i.e., to produce an allergic response on the skin) was tested, but other aspects of immunotoxicology were not examined.

The foregoing evidence suggests that a connection between TCDD or other herbicide exposure and human toxic effects is, in general, biologically plausible. However, differences in sensitivity and susceptibility across individual animals, strains, and species; the lack of strong evidence of organ-specific effects across species; and differences in route, dose, duration, and timing of exposure complicate definitive conclusions about the presence or absence of a mechanism for the induction of specific toxicity by these compounds in humans.

Considerable uncertainty remains about how to apply this information to the evaluation of potential health effects of herbicides or dioxin exposure in Vietnam veterans. Scientists disagree about the extent to which information derived from animals and cellular studies predicts human health outcomes and the extent to which the health effects resulting from high-dose exposure are comparable to those resulting from low-dose exposure. Investigating the biological mechanisms underlying TCDD's toxic effects continues to be a very active area of research, and subsequent updates of this report might have more and better information on which to base conclusions, at least for that compound.

Increased Risk of Disease Among Vietnam Veterans

Under the Agent Orange Act of 1991, the committee is asked to determine (to the extent that available scientific data permit meaningful determinations) the increased risk of the diseases it studies among those exposed to herbicides during their service in Vietnam. Where specific information about particular health outcomes is available, it is related in the preceding discussions of those diseases.

REFERENCES

ADA (American Diabetes Association). 1997. Report of the Expert Committee on the Diagnosis and Classification of Diabetes Mellitus. Diabetes Care 20(7):1183.

AFHS (Air Force Health Study). 1984. An Epidemiologic Investigation of Health Effects in Air Force Personnel Following Exposure to Herbicides. Baseline Morbidity Study Results. Brooks AFB, TX: USAF School of Aerospace Medicine. NTIS AD-A138 340.

AFHS. 1990. An Epidemiologic Investigation of Health Effects in Air Force Personnel Following Exposure to Herbicides. 2 vols. Brooks AFB, TX: USAF School of Aerospace Medicine. USAFSAM-TR-90-2.

AFHS. 1991. An Epidemiologic Investigation of Health Effects in Air Force Personnel Following Exposure to Herbicides. Serum Dioxin Analysis of 1987 Examination Results. 9 vols. Brooks AFB, TX: USAF School of Aerospace Medicine.

AFHS. 1996. An Epidemiologic Investigation of Health Effects in Air Force Personnel Following Exposure to Herbicides. Mortality Update 1996. Brooks AFB, TX: Epidemiologic Research Division. Armstrong Laboratory. AL/AO-TR-1996-0068.

AFHS. 2000. An Epidemiologic Investigation of Health Effects in Air Force Personnel Following Exposure to Herbicides. 1997 Follow-up Examination and Results. Reston, VA: Science Application International Corporation. F41624–96–C1012.

Akhtar RA, Smith AG. 1998. Chromosomal linkage analysis of porphyria in mice induced by hexachlorobenzene–iron synergism: a model of sporadic porphyria cutanea tarda. Pharmacogenetics 8(6):485–494.

Assennato G, Cervino D, Emmett E, Longo G, Merlo F. 1989. Follow-up of subjects who developed chloracne following TCDD exposure at Seveso. American Journal of Industrial Medicine 16:119–125.

Bertazzi PA, Zocchetti C, Pesatori AC, Guercilena S, Sanarico M, Radice L. 1989. Mortality in an area contaminated by TCDD following an industrial incident. Medicina Del Lavoro 80:316–329.

Bertazzi PA, Bernucci I, Brambilla G, Consonni D, Pesatori AC. 1998. The Seveso studies on early and long-term effects of dioxin exposure: a review. Environmental Health Perspectives 106 (Suppl 2):625–633.

Bertazzi PA, Consonni D, Bachetti S, Rubagotti M, Baccarelli A, Zocchetti C, Pesatori AC. 2001. Health effects of dioxin exposure: a 20-year mortality study. American Journal of Epidemiology 153(11):1031–1044.

Burton JE, Michalek JA, Rahe AJ. 1998. Serum dioxin, chloracne, and acne in veterans of Operation Ranch Hand. Archives of Environmental Health 53(3):199–204.

Calvert GM, Hornung RV, Sweeney MH, Fingerhut MA, Halperin WE. 1992. Hepatic and gastrointestinal effects in an occupational cohort exposed to 2,3,7,8-tetrachlorodibenzo-*para*-dioxin. Journal of the American Medical Association 267:2209–2214.

Calvert GM, Willie KK, Sweeney MH, Fingerhut MA, Halperin WE. 1996. Evaluation of serum lipid concentrations among U.S. workers exposed to 2,3,7,8-tetrachlorodibenzo-*p*-dioxin. Archives of Environmental Health 51(2):100–107.

Calvert GM, Wall DK, Sweeney MH, Fingerhut MA. 1998. Evaluation of cardiovascular outcomes among U.S. workers exposed to 2,3,7,8-tetrachlorodibenzo-*p*-dioxin. Environmental Health Perspectives 106(Suppl 2):635–643.

Calvert GM, Sweeney MH, Deddens J, Wall DK. 1999. Evaluation of diabetes mellitus, serum glucose, and thyroid function among United States workers exposed to 2,3,7,8-tetrachlorodibenzo-*p*-dioxin. Occupational and Environmental Medicine 56(4):270–276.

CDVA (Commonwealth Department of Veterans' Affairs). 1998a. Morbidity of Vietnam Veterans: A Study of the Health of Australia's Vietnam Veteran Community. Volume 1: Male Vietnam Veterans Survey and Community Comparison Outcomes. Canberra: Department of Veterans' Affairs.

CDVA. 1998b. Morbidity of Vietnam Veterans: A Study of the Health of Australia's Vietnam Veteran Community. Volume 2: Female Vietnam Veterans Survey and Community Comparison Outcomes. Canberra: Department of Veterans' Affairs.

Coenraads PJ, Olie K, Tang NJ. 1999. Blood lipid concentrations of dioxins and dibenzofurans causing chloracne. British Journal of Dermatology 141:694–697.

Cook RR, Bond GG, Olson RA, Ott MG. 1987. Update of the mortality experience of workers exposed to chlorinated dioxins. Chemosphere 16:2111–2116.

Crane PJ, Barnard DL, Horsley KW, Adena MA. 1997. Mortality of Vietnam veterans: the veteran cohort study. A report of the 1996 retrospective cohort study of Australian Vietnam veterans. Canberra: Department of Veterans' Affairs.

Cranmer M, Louie S, Kennedy RH, Kern PA, Fonseca VA. 2000. Exposure to 2,3,7,8-tetrachlorodibenzo-p-dioxin (TCDD) is associated with hyperinsulinemia and insulin resistance. Toxicological Sciences 56(2):431–436.

Ernst M, Flesch-Janys D, Morgenstern I, Manz A. 1998. Immunological findings in former industrial workers after high exposure to dioxins at the workplace. Arbeitsmedizin Sozialmedizin Umweltmedizin Supplement 24:14–47.

Flesch-Janys D. 1997/98. Analyses of exposure to polychlorinated dibenzo-p-dioxins, furans, and hexachlorocyclohexane and different health outcomes in a cohort of former herbicide-producing workers in Hamburg, Germany. Teratogenesis, Carcinogenesis, Mutagenesis 17(4-5):257–264.

Germolec DR. 1999. Expression of CytoKines and Immunoglobulius in Toxicant Exposed Human Lymphocytes. CRISP Data Base, Bethesda, MD: NIH.

Guo YL, Yu M-L, Hsu C-C, Rogan WJ. 1999. Chloracne, goiter, arthritis, and anemia after polychlorinated biphenyl poisoning: 14-year follow-up of the Taiwan Yucheng cohort. Environmental Health Perspectives 107(9):715–719.

Halperin W, Vogt R, Sweeney MH, Shopp G, Fingerhut M, Petersen M. 1998. Immunological markers among workers exposed to 2,3,7,8-tetrachlorodibenzo-p-dioxin. Occupational and Environmental Medicine 55(11):742–749.

Henneberger PK, Ferris BG Jr, Monson RR. 1989. Mortality among pulp and paper workers in Berlin, New Hampshire. British Journal of Industrial Medicine 46:658–664.

Henriksen GL, Ketchum NS, Michalek JE, Swaby JA. 1997. Serum dioxin and diabetes mellitus in veterans of Operation Ranch Hand. Epidemiology 8(3):252–258.

Hooiveld M, Heederik DJ, Kogevinas M, Boffetta P, Needham LL, Patterson DG Jr, Bueno de Mesquita HB. 1998. Second follow-up of a Dutch cohort occupationally exposed to phenoxy herbicides, chlorophenols, and contaminants. American Journal of Epidemiology 147(9):891–901.

Horsley K. 2000. Personal communication. Commonwealth Department of Veterans' Affairs, Canberra, Australia. December 10.

Iida T, Hirakawa H, Matsueda T, Nagayama J, Nagata Y. 1999. Polychlorinated dibenzo-p-dioxins and related compounds: correlations of levels in human tissues and in blood. Chemosphere 38(12):2767–2774.

IOM (Institute of Medicine). 1994. Veterans and Agent Orange: Health Effects of Herbicides Used in Vietnam. Washington, DC: National Academy Press.

IOM. 1996. Veterans and Agent Orange: Update 1996. Washington, DC: National Academy Press.

IOM. 1999. Veterans and Agent Orange: Update 1998. Washington, DC: National Academy Press.

IOM. 2000. Veterans and Agent Orange: Herbicide/Dioxin Exposure and Type 2 Diabetes. Washington, DC: National Academy Press.

Jacob H, Charytan C, Rascoff JH, Golden R, Janis R. 1978. Amyloidosis secondary to drug abuse and chronic skin suppuration. Archives of Internal Medicine 138(7):1150–1151.

Kimbrough R. 1997/98. Selected other effects and TEFs. Teratogenesis, Carcinogenesis, Mutagenesis 17:265–273.

Koller LD. 1990. In: Immunotoxicity of Metals and Immunotoxicolgy, A.D. Dayan et al. ed., Plenum Press, NY, Pp 233–239.

Kruszynska YT, Olefsky JM. 1996. Cellular and molecular mechanisms of non-insulin dependent diabetes mellitus. Journal of Investigative Medicine 44(8):413–428.

Kuller LH, Orchard TJ. 1988. The epidemiology of atherosclerosis in 1987: unraveling a common-source epidemic. Clinical Chemistry 34(8B):B40–B48.

LaRosa JC. 1990. Lipid Disorders. Endocrinology and Metabolism Clinics of North America. Philadelphia: W.B. Saunders Company.

Longnecker MP, Michalek JE. 2000. Serum dioxin level in relation to diabetes mellitus among Air Force veterans with background levels of exposure. Epidemiology 11(1):44–48.

Martin JV. 1984. Lipid abnormalities in workers exposed to dioxin. British Journal of Industrial Medicine 41:254–256.

May G. 1982. Tetrachlorodibenzodioxin: a survey of subjects ten years after exposure. British Journal of Industrial Medicine 39:128–135.

Mayo Clinic. 2000. Primary Amyloidosis MC0137/R894. http://www.mayo.edu/mmgrg/rst/aapamph.htm (accessed March 31).

McKinney WP, McIntire DD, Carmody TJ, Joseph A. 1997. Comparing the smoking behavior of veterans and nonveterans. Public Health Reports 112(3):212–217.

Michalek, JE. 2000. Letter to Dr. David A. Butler responding to questions and comments offered by the Committee to Review the Evidence Regarding a Link Between Exposure to Agent Orange and Diabetes. July 28.

Michalek JE, Ketchum NS, Akhtar FZ. 1998. Postservice mortality of US Air Force veterans occupationally exposed to herbicides in Vietnam: 15-year follow-up. American Journal of Epidemiology 148(8):786–792.

Michalek JE, Ketchum NS, Check IL. 1999a. Serum dioxin and immunologic response in veterans of Operation Ranch Hand. American Journal of Epidemiology 149:1038–1046.

Michalek JE, Akhtar FZ, Kiel JL. 1999b. Serum dioxin, insulin, fasting glucose, and sex hormone-binding globulin in veterans of Operation Ranch Hand. Journal of Clinical Endocrinology and Metabolism 84(5):1540–1543.

Mocarelli P, Marocchi A, Brambilla P, Gerthoux P, Young DS, Mantel N. 1986. Clinical laboratory manifestations of exposure to dioxin in children. A six-year study of the effects of an environmental disaster near Seveso, Italy. Journal of the American Medical Association 256:2687–2695.

Moses M, Lilis R, Crow KD, Thornton J, Fischbein A, Anderson HA, Selikoff IJ. 1984. Health status of workers with past exposure to 2,3,7,8-tetrachlorodibenzo-p-dioxin in the manufacture of 2,4,5-trichlorophenoxyacetic acid: comparison of findings with and without chloracne. American Journal of Industrial Medicine 5:161–182.

Nagayama J, Tsuji H, Iida T et al. 1998. Postnatal exposure to chlorinated dioxins and related chemicals in lymphocyte subsets in Japanese breast-fed infants. Chemosphere 37:1781–1787.

Neuberger M, Kundi M, Jäger R. 1998. Chloracne and morbidity after dioxin exposure (preliminary results). Toxicology Letters 96, 97:347–350.

Neuberger M, Rappe C, Cai H, Hansson M, Jäger R, Kundi M, Lim CK, Wingfors H, Smith AG. 1999. Persistent health effects of dioxin contamination in herbicide production. Environmental Research 81(A):206–214.

Neubert R, Maskow L, Triebig G, Broding HC, Jacob-Muller U, Helge H, Neubert D. 2000. Chlorinated dibenzo-p-dioxins and dibenzofurans and the human immune system: 3. Plasma immunoglobulins and cytokines of workers with quantified moderately-increased body burdens. Life Sciences 66(22):2123–2142.

Orchard TJ, LaPorte RE, Dorman JS. 1992. Diabetes. In: Last JM, Wallace RB, eds, Public Health and Preventive Medicine, 13th Edition., Norwalk, CT: Appleton and Lange. Chapter 51: Pp. 873–883.

O'Toole BI, Marshall RP, Grayson DA, Schureck RJ, Dobson M, Ffrench M, Pulvertaft B, Meldrum L, Bolton J, Vennard J. 1996. The Australian Vietnam Veterans Health Study: II. Self-reported health of veterans compared with the Australian population. International Journal of Epidemiology 25(2):319–330.

Ott MG, Zober A. 1996. Cause specific mortality and cancer incidence among employees exposed to 2,3,7,8-TCDD after a 1953 reactor accident. Occupational and Environmental Medicine 53(9): 606–612.

Ott MG, Zober A, Germann C. 1994. Laboratory results for selected target organs in 138 individuals occupationally exposed to TCDD. Chemosphere 29:2423–2437.

Paul W, ed. 1993. Fundamental Immunology, 3rd edition. New York: Raven Press.

Pazderova-Vejlupkova J, Lukas E, Nemcova M, Pickova J, Jirasek L. 1981. The development and prognosis of chronic intoxication by tetrachlorodibenzo-p-dioxin in men. Archives of Environmental Health 36:5–11.

Pesatori AC, Zocchetti C, Guercilena S, Consonni D, Turrini D, Bertazzi PA. 1998. Dioxin exposure and non-malignant health effects: a mortality study. Occupational and Environmental Medicine 55:126–131.

Ramlow JM, Spadacene NW, Hoag SR, Stafford BA, Cartmill JB, Lerner PJ. 1996. Mortality in a cohort of pentachlorophenol manufacturing workers, 1940–1989. American Journal of Industrial Medicine 30(2):180–194.

Scholes J, Derosena R, Appel GB, Jao W, Boyd MT, Pirani CL. 1979. Amyloidosis in chronic heroin addicts with the nephrotic syndrome. Annals of Internal Medicine 91(1):26–29.

Sinclair P. 2000. Mechanisms of porphyria caused by TCDD and other compounds. FEDRIP database.

Slade BA. 1998. Dioxin and diabetes mellitus. Epidemiology 9(3): 359–360.

Solomon A. 1999. What is amyloidosis? Myeloma Today 3(2). (accessed December 19, 2000). http://myeloma.org/MyelomaToday/Volume2/Number3/imf_asa.html.

Steenland K, Piacitelli L, Deddens J, Fingerhut M, Chang LI. 1999. Cancer, heart disease, and diabetes in workers exposed to 2,3,7,8-tetrachlorodibenzo-p-dioxin. Journal of the National Cancer Institute 91(9):779–786.

Suskind RR, Hertzberg VS. 1984. Human health effects of 2,4,5-T and its toxic contaminants. Journal of the American Medical Association 251:2372–2380.

Sweeney MH, Hornung RW, Wall DK, Fingerhut MA, Halperin WE. 1992. Diabetes and serum glucose levels in TCDD-exposed workers. Abstract of a paper presented at the 12th International Symposium on Chlorinated Dioxins (Dioxin '92), Tampere, Finland, August 24–28.

Sweeney MH, Calvert GM, Egeland GA, Fingerhut MA, Halperin WE, Piacitelli LA. 1997/98. Review and update of the results of the NIOSH medical study of workers exposed to chemicals contaminated with 2,3,7,8-tetrachlorodibenzodioxin. Teratogenesis, Carcinogenesis, and Mutagenesis 17(4–5):241–247.

Tóth K, Somfai-Relle S, Sugár J, Bence J. 1979. Carcinogenicity testing of herbicide 2,4,5-trichlorophenoxyethanol containing dioxin and of pure dioxin in Swiss mice. Nature 278(5704):548–549.

Vena J, Boffeta P, Becher H, Benn T, Bueno de Mesquita HB, Coggon D, Colin D, Flesch-Janys D, Green L, Kauppinen T, Littorin M, Lynge E, Mathews JD, Neuberger M, Pearce N, Pesatori AC, Saracci R, Steenland K, Kogevinas M. 1998. Exposure to dioxin and nonneoplastic mortality in the expanded IARC international cohort study of phenoxy herbicide and chlorophenol production workers and sprayers. Environmental Health Perspectives 106(Suppl 2):645–653.

Von Benner A, Edler L, Mayer K, Zober A. 1994. 'Dioxin' investigation program of the chemical industry professional association. Arbeitsmedizin Sozialmedizin Praventivmedizin 29:11–16.

Wolfe WH, Michalek JE, Miner JC, Rahe A, Silva J, Thomas WF, Grubbs WD, Lustik MB, Karrison TG, Roegner RH, Williams DE. 1990. Health status of Air Force veterans occupationally exposed to herbicides in Vietnam. I. Physical health. Journal of the American Medical Association 264:1824–1831.

Yu ML, Hsin JW, Hsu CC, Chan WC, Guo HL. 1998. The immunologic evaluation of the Yucheng children. Chemosphere 37(9–12):1855–1865.

Zober A, Ott MG, Messerer P. 1994. Morbidity follow up study of BASF employees exposed to 2,3,7,8-tetrachlorodibenzo-p-dioxin (TCDD) after a 1953 chemical reactor incident. Occupational and Environmental Medicine 51:479–486.

APPENDIX A

Summary of Workshop on the Review of Health Effects in Vietnam Veterans of Exposure to Herbicides

PUBLIC WORKSHOP

May 23, 2000
Room 2004, The Foundry Building
Washington, D.C.

Workshop Presentations and Speakers

- **Veterans' Perspective of IOM's Task**
Lisa Spahr, The American Legion, Washington, D.C.

- **Where We Are, Where We're Headed**
George Claxton, Vietnam Veterans of America, Silver Spring, Maryland

- **Health Problems of Women Veterans of the Vietnam War**
Linda Spoonster Schwartz, R.N., M.S.N., Dr.P.H., Associate Research Scientist, Office of Research and Policy, Yale University School of Nursing, New Haven, Connecticut

- **Diabetes Mellitus, Related to Agent Orange Handling During Service in Wartime Vietnam**
Turner Camp, M.D., Silver Spring, Maryland

- **Husband's Death and Agent Orange**
Jennie LeFevre, Shady Side, Maryland

- **Veterans' Health Problems: Heart Disease, Diabetes, Peripheral Neuropathy, Soft Knots Covering Body, Chloracne**
Shelia Winsett, Jasper, Alabama

APPENDIX B

ICD·9 Codes for Cancer Outcomes

The International Classification of Diseases, Ninth Edition (ICD·9) is a system used by physicians and researchers around the world to group related disease entities and procedures for the reporting of statistical information. It is used for the purposes of classifying morbidity and mortality information for statistical purposes, indexing hospital records by disease and operations, reporting diagnosis by physicians, data storage and retrieval, reporting national morbidity and mortality data, and reporting and compiling health care data. Many of the studies reviewed by the committee use ICD·9 classifications. Table B-1 lists the codes for the various forms of cancer.

TABLE B-1 Surveillance, Epidemiology, and End Results (SEER) Program Site Groupings for ICD·9 National Center for Health Statistics (NCHS) Data

Site	ICD·9 codes
Buccal cavity and pharynx	
Lip	140.0–140.9
Tongue	141.0–141.9
Salivary glands	142.0–142.9
Floor of mouth	144.0–144.9
Gum and other mouth	143.0–143.9, 145.0–145.6, 145.8–145.9
Nasopharynx	147.0–147.9
Tonsil	146.0–146.2
Oropharynx	146.3–146.9
Hypopharynx	148.0–148.9
Other buccal cavity and pharynx	149.0–149.9

TABLE B-1 *Continued*

Site	ICD·9 codes
Digestive system	
Esophagus	150.0–150.9
Stomach	151.0–151.9
Small intestine	152.0–152.9
Colon excluding rectum	153.0–153.9, 159.0
Rectum and rectosigmoid	154.0–154.1
Anus, anal canal, and anorectum	154.2–154.3, 154.8
Liver and intrahepatic bile duct	
Liver	155.0, 155.2
Intrahepatic bile duct	155.1
Gallbladder	156.0
Other biliary	156.1–156.9
Pancreas	157.0–157.9
Retroperitoneum	158.0
Peritoneum, omentum, and mesentery	158.8–158.9
Other digestive organs	159.8–159.9
Respiratory system	
Nasal cavity, middle ear,	
and accessory sinuses	160.0–160.9
Larynx	161.0–161.9
Lung and bronchus	162.2–162.9
Pleura	163.0–163.9
Trachea, mediastinum, and	
other respiratory organs	162.0, 164.2–165.9
Bones and joints	170.0–170.9
Soft tissue (including heart)	171.0–171.9, 164.1
Skin	
Melanomas—skin	172.0–172.9
Other nonepithelial skin	173.0–173.9
Breast	174.0–174.9, 175
Female genital system	
Cervix	180.0–180.9
Corpus	182.0–182.1, 182.8
Uterus, NOS	179
Ovary	183.0
Vagina	184.0
Vulva	184.1–184.4
Other female genital organs	181, 183.2–183.9, 184.8, 184.9
Male genital system	
Prostate	185
Testis	186.0–186.9
Penis	187.1–187.4
Other male genital organs	187.5–187.9

TABLE B-1 *Continued*

Site	ICD·9 codes
Urinary system	
Urinary bladder	188.0–188.9
Kidney and renal pelvis	189.0, 189.1
Ureter	189.2
Other urinary organs	189.3–189.4, 189.8–189.9
Eye and orbit	190.0–190.9
Brain and other nervous system	
Brain	191.0–191.9
Other nervous system	192.0–192.3, 192.8–192.9
Endocrine system	
Thyroid	193
Other endocrine (including thymus)	164.0, 194.0–194.9
Lymphomas	
Hodgkin's disease	201.0–201.9
Non-Hodgkin's lymphomas	200.0–200.8, 202.0–202.2, 202.8–202.9
Multiple myeloma	203.0, 203.2–203.8
Leukemias	
Lymphocytic	
Acute lymphocytic	204.0
Chronic lymphocytic	204.1
Other lymphocytic	204.2–204.9
Granulocytic (myeloid)	
Acute myeloid	205.0
Chronic myeloid	205.1
Other myeloid	205.2–205.9
Monocytic	
Acute monocytic	206.0
Chronic monocytic	206.1
Other monocytic	206.2–206.9
Other	
Other acute	207.0, 208.0
Other chronic	207.1, 208.1
Aleukemic, subleukemic and NOS	202.4, 203.1, 207.2, 207.8, 208.2–208.9
Ill-defined and unspecified sites	159.1, 195.0–195.8, 196.0–196.9, 199.0–199.1, 202.3, 202.5–202.6

NOTE: NOS = not otherwise specified.
Source: Ries LAG, Kosary CL, Hankey BF, Miller BA, Harras A, Edwards BK (eds) 1997. SEER Cancer Statistics Review, 1973–1994, National Cancer Institute. NIH Pub. No. 97 2789. Bethesda, MD. Table A-4.

APPENDIX C

Committee and Staff Biographies

COMMITTEE BIOGRAPHIES

Irva Hertz-Picciotto, Ph.D. *(Chair)*, is professor in the Department of Epidemiology, School of Public Health, at the University of North Carolina, Chapel Hill; director of the Reproductive Epidemiology Program; and a fellow at the Carolina Population Center. She has published extensively on risk assessment, occupationally related cancer, environmental exposures, reproductive outcomes, and methods for epidemiologic data analysis. Dr. Hertz-Picciotto serves on several editorial boards and is currently president-elect of the International Society for Environmental Epidemiology.

Margit L. Bleecker, M.D., Ph.D., is director of the Center for Occupational and Environmental Neurology in Baltimore. Her research interests are in the areas of clinical industrial neurotoxicology and occupational neurology. Dr. Bleecker recently served on the Institute of Medicine (IOM) Committee on the Safety of Silicone Breast Implants and has served on the IOM Committee on the Evaluation of the Department of Defense Comprehensive Clinical Evaluation Protocol and the IOM Committee on the Persian Gulf Syndrome Comprehensive Clinical Evaluation Program.

Thomas A. Gasiewicz, Ph.D., is professor of Environmental Medicine and deputy director of the Environmental Health Sciences Center in the Department of Environmental Medicine at the University of Rochester School of Medicine. He serves on the editorial board of *Biochemical Pharmacology* and is the associate editor of *Toxicology and Applied Pharmacology*. He also is a peer reviewer for several scientific journals including *Biochemical Pharmacology, Cancer Research, Fundamental and Applied Toxicology, Journal of Biological Chemistry, Science,* and *Toxicology and Applied Pharmacology.* Dr. Gasiewicz has published extensively on the toxicokinetics of dioxin, dioxin toxicity, and the role of the aryl hydrocarbon receptor in the molecular mechanism of dioxin toxicity.

Tee L. Guidotti, M.D., M.P.H., holds the position of department chair, Department of Environmental and Occupational Health in the School of Public Health and Health Services of the George Washington University. He is also director of the Division of Occupational Medicine in the Department of Medicine of George Washington University School of Medicine and is cross-appointed as professor of pulmonary medicine. Prior to accepting this position, he served as professor of occupational and environmental medicine and director of the Occupational Health Program in the Department of Public Health Sciences at the University of Alberta Faculty of Medicine, Edmonton. Dr. Guidotti is certified as a specialist in internal medicine, lung diseases, and occupational medicine. His primary research interests are air quality, inhalation toxicology, and occupational and environmental lung diseases. Dr. Guidotti is president-elect of the Association of Occupational and Environmental Clinics, sits on the Board of Directors of the American College of Occupational and Environmental Medicine, and serves as chair of the Scientific Committee on Respiratory Disorders of the International Commission on Occupational Health.

Robert F. Herrick, Sc.D., is lecturer on industrial hygiene at the Harvard School of Public Health, where he earned a doctor of science in industrial hygiene. Dr. Herrick is certified in the comprehensive practice of industrial hygiene. His research interests are centered on the assessment of exposure as a cause of occupational and environmental disease. Dr. Herrick is past chair of the American Conference of Governmental and Industrial Hygienists, and past president of the International Occupational Hygiene Association. Prior to joining the faculty at Harvard, Dr. Herrick spent 17 years at the National Institute for Occupational Safety and Health where he conducted occupational health research.

David G. Hoel, Ph.D., holds the position of distinguished university professor and associate director of the Hollings Oncology Center at the Medical University of South Carolina. Before joining the Medical University of South Carolina, he held the posts of director of the Division of Biometry and Risk Assessment and acting director of the National Institute of Environmental Health Sciences. Dr. Hoel has been a member of numerous working groups of the International Agency for Cancer Research of the World Health Organization. He also serves as chair of the IOM Committee on the Assessment of Wartime Exposure to Herbicides.

Loren D. Koller, D.V.M., Ph.D., is professor, College of Veterinary Medicine, Oregon State University, Corvallis; he formerly served as dean of the college. His research focuses on toxicological, pathological, and immunological effects of toxic substances and on the effects of environmental contaminants on tumor growth and immunity. Dr. Koller also serves on the IOM Committee on the Assessment of Wartime Exposure to Herbicides.

Howard Ozer, M.D., Ph.D., is Eason Chair and chief of the Hematology/Oncology Section, director of the Cancer Center, and professor of medicine at the University of Oklahoma. Dr. Ozer is a member of several professional societies and has served on the Board of the Society for Biologic Therapy and the Governor's Cancer Advisory Board for the State of Georgia. He serves on the editorial boards of the *Journal of Cancer Biotherapy*; *Cancer Research, Therapy and Control*; *Cancer Biotherapy and Radiopharmaceuticals*; and *Emedicine;* he is a reviewer for numerous journals including *Cancer Research, Journal of the National Cancer Institute,* and *New England Journal of Medicine.* Dr. Ozer has published extensively on the treatment of hematologic malignancies.

John J. Stegeman, Ph.D., is senior scientist and chair of the Department of Biology at the Redfield Lab of the Woods Hole Oceanographic Institution, in Woods Hole, Massachusetts. He received his Ph.D. in biochemistry, concentrating on enzymology, from Northwestern University, Evanston, Illinois. His research interests center on metabolism of foreign chemicals in animals and humans, and the structure, function, and regulation of the enzymes that accomplish this metabolism.

David S. Strogatz, Ph.D., M.S.P.H., is associate professor and chair, Department of Epidemiology, University at Albany, State University of New York, and adjunct professor, Department of Epidemiology, University of North Carolina, Chapel Hill. He received his M.S.P.H and Ph.D. in epidemiology from the University of North Carolina, Chapel Hill. Dr. Strogatz's research examines the epidemiology of diseases, including diabetes and cardiovascular disease, and the impact of socioeconomic status and race on health.

STAFF BIOGRAPHIES

ROSE MARIE MARTINEZ, Sc.D., is director of the IOM Board on Health Promotion and Disease Prevention. Prior to joining IOM, she was a senior health researcher at Mathematica Policy Research, where she conducted research on the impact of health system change on the public health infrastructure, access to care for vulnerable populations, managed care, and the health care work force. Dr. Martinez is a former assistant director for health financing and policy with the U.S. General Accounting Office, where she directed evaluations and policy analysis in the area of national and public health issues. Dr. Martinez received her doctorate from the Johns Hopkins School of Hygiene and Public Health.

KATHLEEN STRATTON, Ph.D., was acting director of the Division of Health Promotion and Disease Prevention of IOM from 1997 to 1999. She received a B.A. in natural sciences from Johns Hopkins University and a Ph.D. from the University of Maryland at Baltimore. After completing a postdoctoral fellowship in the neuropharmacology of phencyclidine compounds at the University of Maryland School of Medicine and in the neurophysiology of second-messenger systems at the Johns Hopkins University School of Medicine, she joined the staff of the IOM in 1990. Dr. Stratton has worked on projects in environmental risk assessment, neurotoxicology, the organization of research and services in the Public Health Service, vaccine safety, fetal alcohol syndrome, and vaccine development. She has had primary responsibility for the reports *Adverse Events Associated with Childhood Vaccines: Evidence Bearing on Causality; DPT Vaccine and Chronic Nervous System Dysfunction; Fetal Alcohol Syndrome: Diagnosis, Epidemiology, Prevention, and Treatment;* and *Vaccines for the 21st Century: An Analytic Tool for Prioritization.*

DAVID A. BUTLER, Ph.D., is a senior project officer in the Division of Health Promotion and Disease Prevention. He received B.S. and M.S. degrees in engineering from the University of Rochester and a Ph.D. in public policy analysis from Carnegie-Mellon University. Prior to joining IOM, Dr. Butler served as an analyst for the U.S. Congress Office of Technology Assessment and was a research associate in the Department of Environmental Health at the Harvard School of Public Health. He is on the editorial advisory board of the journal *Risk: Health, Safety and Environment.* His research interests include exposure assessment and risk analysis.

JAMES A. BOWERS is a research assistant in the Division of Health Promotion and Disease Prevention. He received his undergraduate degree in environmental studies from Binghamton University. He has also been involved with the IOM committees that produced *Characterizing Exposure of Veterans to Agent Orange and Other Herbicides Used in Vietnam, Adequacy of the Comprehensive Clinical Evaluation Program: Nerve Agents; Clearing the Air: Asthma and Indoor Air Exposures;* and *Veterans and Agent Orange: Herbicide/Dioxin Exposure and Type 2 Diabetes.*

JENNIFER A. COHEN is a research assistant in the Division of Health Promotion and Disease Prevention. She received her undergraduate degree in art history from the University of Maryland. She has also been involved with the IOM committees that produced *Organ Procurement and Transplantation, Clearing* *the Air: Asthma and Indoor Air Exposures,* and *Veterans and Agent Orange: Herbicide/Dioxin Exposure and Type 2 Diabetes.*

MARJAN NAJAFI, M.P.H., is a research associate in the Division of Health Promotion and Disease Prevention. She received her undergraduate degrees in chemical engineering and applied mathematics from the University of Rhode Island. She served as a public health engineer with the Maryland Department of Environment and later, Research Triangle Institute. After obtaining a master of public health degree from the Johns Hopkins School of Hygiene and Public Health, she managed a lead poisoning prevention program in Micronesia for the U.S. Department of Health and Human Services.

PATRICIA SPAULDING is a senior project assistant in the IOM Division of Health Promotion and Disease Prevention. She has also been involved with a number of previous IOM committees, including those that produced *Safety of Silicone Breast Implants*, *National Center for Military Deployment Health Research*, and *Gulf War Veterans: Measuring Health.*

ANNA STATON is a project assistant in the Division of Health Promotion and Disease Prevention. Ms. Staton joined the IOM in December 1999 and has also worked with the committee that produced *No Time to Lose: Getting More from HIV Prevention*. Prior to joining the IOM, she worked at the Baltimore Women's Health Study. Ms. Staton graduated from the University of Maryland Baltimore County with a bachelor of arts degree in visual arts (major) and women's studies (minor) degree. She is currently working toward a master of public administration at the George Washington University School of Business and Public Management.

Index

A

Acquired immune deficiency syndrome. *See* AIDS/HIV
ACTH. *See* Adrenocorticotropic hormone
Acute lymphocytic leukemia (ALL). *See* Leukemia
Acute myelogenous leukemia (AML) *See* Leukemia
Acute myeloid leukemia (AML). *See* Leukemia
ADA. *See* American Diabetes Association
Adipose tissue
    TCDD distribution, I: 130, 131, 168-169, 259, 269, 280; IV: 42, 43, 64, 116, 117
Adrenocorticotropic hormone (ACTH), IV: 59
Aerial spraying, I: 3, 24; III: 135, 137, 139; IV: 117, 120, 123, 150, 160, 303
    military early research, I: 25-26; III: 28; IV: 150
    records of, I: 84-85, 287
    See also Herbicide application methods; Herbicides
AFHS. *See* Air Force Health Study
Aflatoxin, I: 453; IV: 267
Africa, sub-Saharan, II: 181; III: 282; IV: 267
Age and aging
    acute lymphocytic leukemia incidence, data for selected age groups, III: 384; IV: 9, 378
    acute myeloid leukemia incidence, data for selected age groups, III: 384; IV: 378
    bone cancer incidence, data for selected age groups, III: 302; IV: 288
    brain cancer incidence, data for selected age groups, III: 356; IV: 351
    breast cancer incidence in US women, data for selected age groups, III: 324; IV: 314
    cancer age-specific incidence, I: 436-438
    chronic lymphocytic leukemia incidence, data for selected age groups, III: 384; IV: 378
    chronic myeloid leukemia incidence, data for selected age groups, III: 384; IV: 378
    diabetes prevalence, data by age, III: 492
    epidemiologic studies, control of aging effects, II: 261-262; III: 409; IV: 3, 13, 23
    female reproductive system cancer incidence, data by type, for selected age groups, III: 329, 330; IV: 321
    gastrointestinal tract cancer incidence, data by type for selected age groups, III: 267; IV: 250
    Hodgkin's disease incidence, data for selected age groups, III: 372; IV: 365

immune system, IV: 31, 79
laryngeal cancer incidence, data for selected age groups, III: 292; IV: 277
latency and, II: 261-262, 273, 275; III: 409, 414-415, 425, 428, 430; IV: 254, 256, 264, 265
leukemia incidence, data by type, for selected age groups, III: 384; IV: 378
liver/intrahepatic bile duct cancers incidence, data for selected age groups, III: 282; IV: 267
lung cancer incidence, data for selected age groups, III: 296; IV: 281
melanoma incidence, data for selected age groups, III: 313; IV: 300
multiple myeloma incidence, data for selected age groups, III: 377
nasal/nasopharyngeal cancer incidence, data for selected age groups, III: 289; IV: 273
non-Hodgkin's lymphoma age of onset, I: 436
non-Hodgkin's lymphoma incidence, data for selected age groups, III: 362; IV: 356
prostate cancer incidence, data for selected age groups, III: 334; IV: 10, 327
renal cancers incidence, data for selected age groups, III: 352; IV: 346
reproductive disorders, IV: 51-52, 59, 63, 66, 71, 80, 200
soft-tissue sarcoma age of onset, I: 436
soft-tissue sarcoma incidence, data for selected age groups, III: 306; IV: 292
TCDD half-life, IV: 24, 28, 45
testicular cancer incidence, data for selected age groups, III: 343; IV: 335
urinary bladder cancer incidence, data for selected age groups, III: 347; IV: 340
See also Demographic data, Vietnam veterans

Agent Blue, I: 27, 89-90, 93, 97, 100; III: 136, 137; IV: 118
volume used in Operation Ranch Hand, data, III: 136

Agent Green, I: 27, 90, 92, 114; III: 136, 137, 140, 146; IV: 118
volume used in Operation Ranch Hand, data, III: 136; IV: 123

Agent Orange, II: 308; III: 130, 159, 315, 344, 359, 389, 407, 444, 460, 462, 489, 491; IV: 117-118, 150, 156

Air Force research activities, II: 31-32; III: 28-29
birth defects association, II: 298, 300; III: 435; IV: 400
cancer latency issues, II: 260-276; III: 407-431; IV: 284
chemical composition, I: 27; II: 102; IV: 119
chloracne association, II: 317, 318; III: 479; IV: 138, 463
congressional hearings, II: 27-28; III: 25
defoliant effectiveness, I: 90
Department of Veterans Affairs activities, II: 29-31, 153, 156-157; III: 27-28; IV: 15
Environmental Protection Agency research activities, II: 32; III: 29-30
exposure opportunity index (EOI), II: 290-291; III: 146, 147, 148; IV: 124, 405
federal government action/research, I: 45-60; II: 27-32; III: 27-32; IV: 13
health effects of, concerns, I: 2; II: 19-23, 26-27; III: 19-20, 236, 237, 240, 242, 243
International Agency for Research on Cancer research activities, III: 30
legislation, I: 47-52; II: 28-29; III: 26-27; IV: 1, 15
Orange II formulation, I: 90; III: 137; IV: 119
product liability litigation, I: 34-35
spontaneous abortion, II: 283; IV: 399-400, 409-412
suspension of use, I: 92-93; II: 26
TCDD as contaminant of, I: 91, 114, 126-127; II: 102; III: 140; IV: 133-135
Vietnam amount used, I: 1, 27, 74, 90, 97-98, 106; II: 1, 26; III: 136; IV: 115, 118-119
Vietnam military application, I: 1, 3, 27, 74, 84-85, 90, 92-93, 97-107, 543-545; II: 1, 26-27; III: 1, 25, 136, 137, 138, 140; IV: 125-126
Vietnam surplus disposal, I: 93-94
Vietnam veterans' concerns, I: 32-34; II: 26-27
Vietnam veterans' increased disease risk, II: 22-23; III: 22-23, 272; IV: 8-9, 12, 256, 270, 275, 279, 284, 290, 296, 305, 311, 318, 323, 332, 338, 343, 348, 353, 359, 367, 374, 381, 388

INDEX 535

volume used in Operation Ranch Hand, data, II: 136; IV, 120, 123, 150
See also Herbicides; Incineration, of Agent Orange
Agent Orange, the Deadly Fog, I: 33
Agent Orange Act of 1991. *See* Public Law 102-104
Agent Orange Briefs, I: 56; II: 31; III: 28
Agent Orange Registry (AOR), I: 20, 53, 56, 729; II: 29, 31, 153, 228; III: 28, 344
See also Department of Veterans Affairs (DVA)
Agent Orange Review, I: 56; II: 31; III: 28
Agent Orange Scientific Task Force, I: 60-61
Agent Orange Study, I: 19, 57, 58-59, 63-64, 276-278; II: 102; III: 147, 148; IV: 124
Agent Orange Task Force, II: 24-26; III: 24-25, 148; IV: 124
See also Department of Veterans Affairs, U.S. (DVA)
Agent Orange Validation Study, III: 240; IV: 156, 159, 160, 162, 283, 304, 327, 403
Agent Orange Victims International, I: 34
Agent Orange Working Group, I: 19, 46, 58, 277, 743
research methodology, I: 728
Agent Orange II. *See* Agent Orange
Agent Pink, I: 27, 90, 92, 114; III: 136, 137, 140, 146; IV: 118, 122-123
volume used in Operation Ranch Hand, data, III: 136; IV: 123
Agent Purple, I: 27, 89, 92, 114; III: 136, 140, 146; IV: 118, 122-123
Operation Ranch Hand, IV: 123
TCDD in, I: 126; IV: 122
volume used in Operation Ranch Hand, data, III: 136
Agent White, I: 27, 90, 92-93, 97, 115, 189; III: 136, 137; IV: 118-119,
volume used in Operation Ranch Hand, data, III: 136
Agricultural/forestry workers
brain tumors, I: 320, 523; II: 136
Canadian Farmer Cohort, II: 135-136
cancers, I: 13, 37, 320-323, 443, 447, 454; II: 133-137, 179
case-control studies, I: 326-341, 486-488; II: 118-122, 138-140; III: 185-195, 228-232
cohort studies, I: 318-323; II: 118-120, 135-137, 197-198; III: 178-185, 224-228; IV: 197-202

epidemiologic studies, I: 37, 318-323; II: 118-120, 135-137, 232-234, 238-239, 241-243; III: 178-195, 224-232, 284-285, 335, 364-365, 379-380, 387-388; IV: 134, 141-142, 145, 257, 260, 263, 265, 271, 285, 290, 296, 306, 312, 318, 324, 333, 338, 349, 353, 360, 368, 374, 381, 401
female reproductive and breast cancers, I: 510-511; IV: 324-325
hepatobiliary cancer, I: 454; II: 183-184; III: 284-285; IV: 271
herbicide exposure assessment, I: 265-266; III: 154-157; IV: 202
Hodgkin's disease, I: 550-553; II: 135
Irish agricultural workers study, II: 136-137
kidney cancer, I: 515
leukemia, I: 332-335, 566-568; II: 136; III: 387-388
malignant lymphoma in, IV: 201
multiple myelomas, I: 11-12, 558-561; II: 138-139, 238-239, 241-243; III: 379-380
non-Hodgkin's lymphoma, I: 9, 256-257, 530-540; II: 138, 139, 232-234; III: 364-365; IV: 359-361
prostate cancer, I: 11, 518, 519, 575; II: 8-9; III: 335; IV: 327-329
reproductive outcomes, I: 510-511, 598
respiratory cancer, I: 11, 466; II: 197-198
soft-tissue sarcomas, I: 37, 326-328, 479-481, 486-488
sperm dysfunction, I: 632
suicide, I: 650
See also Forests; Professional pesticide/herbicide applicators
Agricultural Health Study, IV: 142
See also Iowa
Agricultural herbicides, I: 24, 35, 39, 174-175, 181; II: 137-139
See also Herbicides
Agriculture. *See* Agricultural/forestry workers; Agricultural herbicides; Food crops; Forests
Ah receptor (AhR), I: 3, 123, 134; II: 3-4, 51-53, 54-56, 57-62; III: 54-58, 129; IV: 25-26, 29-30, 42, 47, 50-58, 60, 68, 69, 70-73, 76, 80, 82, 84, 85, 86, 87, 90, 93, 94, 95, 99-100
animal studies and, I: 114, 123; II: 3-4, 51-53, 54-56, 57-62, 92-93; III: 33, 34, 35, 54-58, 62-63, 67-69, 129; IV: 48-49, 61-62, 64-67, 74-75

anti-estrogenicity and, II: 62; III: 67-69
biological consequences of activation, II: 57; III: 62; IV: 56-60, 323
blood abnormalities, I: 125
cacodylic acid acute toxicity, I: 188
cacodylic acid carcinogenicity, I: 118, 119, 187; IV: 5, 387
cacodylic acid chronic exposure, I: 188-189
cacodylic acid developmental toxicity, I: 189
cacodylic acid genotoxicity, I: 187-188
cacodylic acid mechanism of action, I: 188-189
cacodylic acid and mechanism of toxicity, II: 50-51; IV: 24
cacodylic acid pharmokinetics, I: 186-187
cacodylic acid renal toxicity, II: 50-51
cacodylic acid reproductive toxicity, I: 189
cacodylic acid toxicity summary, II: 50; III: 48; IV: 38
cacodylic acid toxicokinetics, I: 188-189; IV: 24, 27, 38
combinatorial interactions, II: 57-58
DNA binding capability and transcription, activation of, II: 56-57; III: 58-61
free radicals and, II: 60; III: 64-65
growth/differentiation signaling, III: 62-63
growth factor and, II: 59
inconsistencies in, II: 57-62
ligand-independent activation, II: 58
multiple forms of, II: 57
nervous system and, I: 161
protein kinases and, II: 60-62; III: 65-67; IV: 69-71
redox signaling, III: 64-65; IV: 67-69
signaling interactions, II: 59-62; III: 62-69; IV: 60-61, 64, 71-74
structural and functional aspects of, II: 54-56; III: 54-58; IV: 54-56
TCDD biologic plausibility and, I: 3, 133-138, 452-453; IV: 4, 25-26, 29, 42, 47-53, 322, 386
TCDD carcinogenicity and, I: 118, 439
TCDD hepatotoxicity and, I: 151, 152, 457; II: 3-4
TCDD immunotoxicity and, I: 122, 150
TCDD reproductive toxicity and, I: 123
TCDD teratogenicity and, I: 159-160
transcriptional-independent responses, II: 58-59
See also ARNT

AIDS/HIV, I: 338, 527, 541, 695; II: 326; IV: 144, 214, 356, 47, 476
Air Force. *See* U.S. Air Force
Air Force Health Study (AFHS), I: 62-63, 260, 272, 622; II: 284, 293-295, 336; III: 23, 25, 29, 239, 438-439, 495, 505, 514; IV: 13, 232, 233, 234, 235
appropriation for, I: 51
autoimmune disease in, I: 698
basal/squamous cell skin cancer in, III: 318, 321, 322; IV: 309
baseline mortality studies, II: 151
birth defects in offspring, II: 286, 293-295; III: 436, 438, 439; IV: 402
bone cancer in, III: 303; IV: 289
cancer and latency in, III: 423, 424, 425, 427
circulatory disease in, I: 703-705, 706; II: 336; III: 514, 517; IV: 508-509
data sources, I: 385-386; II: 150-151
diabetes mellitus in, I: 684; II: 330; III: 495, 498-500, 502; IV: 485-487
epidemiological studies, II: 31, 32, 149, 150-152, 154-156, 293-295; III: 28-29, 206-207, 218, 237-240, 303, 309-310, 313-314, 318, 321, 322, 339, 340, 385, 436, 438, 439, 446-447, 449, 452-453, 457-458, 481, 486, 495, 498-500, 502, 505, 506, 507, 510, 513, 514, 517; IV: 291, 294-295, 298, 301, 305-306, 308-311, 313, 327, 329, 331, 334-36, 342, 345, 347, 350, 352, 355, 357, 362, 366, 370, 373, 376, 380, 383
exposure assessment in, I: 279-280, 281, 386; II: 4-5, 101, 103, 109; III: 6, 146-147, 157-158, 162; IV: 123-124
gastrointestinal ulcers in, I: 691; III: 510, 513
immune system disorders in, I: 696
infertility in, II: 280; III: 446-447, 449
lipid abnormalities in, I: 689; II: 333; III: 505, 506, 507; IV: 494
liver toxicity in, II: 332; III: 510, 513; IV: 502
low birthweight in, I: 626, 627; III: 457-458
melanoma in, III: 313-314; IV: 303-304
methodology, I: 230-231, 385-386, 445, 757-762
multiple myelomas in, I: 562; II: 244, 245; IV: 373

INDEX 537

neurological disorders in, I: 659; IV: 441-443, 445, 454-455, 459
non-Hodgkin's lymphoma in, I: 541; IV: 362
participants, I: 722-723; II: 150-152
perinatal death in offspring, III: 452-453
peripheral nervous system disorders in, I: 665; IV: 454-455
porphyria cutanea tarda in, I: 681-682; II: 321-322; III: 481
recommendations for, I: 16-17, 722-724; II: 23, 24; IV: 13
reproductive outcomes in, I: 601, 612-613, 632, 633, 727; II: 293-295; III: 436, 438, 439, 446-447, 449, 452-453, 457-458; IV: 403
respiratory cancers in, I: 469; II: 201
respiratory disorders in, I: 711-712; III: 486
role of, I: 53
skin cancers in, II: 209; IV: 303
skin disorders in, I: 678
soft tissue sarcoma in, I: 492-493; III: 309-310; IV: 294-295
spina bifida in offspring, II: 9, 295-296; III: 7, 8, 9-10, 438
spontaneous abortions in, II: 283-284
status of, I: 53; II: 31-32
TCDD half-life estimates, I: 260-261; II: 104-105; III: 37, 50, 157-158
TCDD serum levels, I: 273, 281, 285, 656; II: 101, 103, 105, 109, 351, 356, 357; III: 146, 147
See also Operation Ranch Hand; U.S. Air Force; Vietnam veterans
Aktiengesellschaft, Germany, IV: 137
Alanine aminotransferase (ALT), II: 331, 332; III: 45, 509, 510; IV: 37
Alaskan natives
Inuit, III: 50-51
See also Race/ethnicity
Alberta, Canada, II: 135-136, 232, 242, 246; III: 234-235, 319-320; IV: 149, 198, 229, 312-313
Alberta Cancer Registry, III: 235
Alberta Health Care Insurance Plan, III: 235
Alcohol consumption, I: 507
ALL. *See* Leukemia
Allergies, II: 327, 329; III: 487-488; IV: 469-470
See also Immune system disorders
Alsea, Oregon, I: 42-43, 372-373, 598

ALT. *See* Alanine aminotransferase
AL-type primary amyloidosis *See* Amyloidosis
American Association for the Advancement of Science, I: 29, 92
  Herbicide Assessment Commission, I: 30-31
American Cancer Society, I: 334; II: 177, 181, 189, 191, 204, 205, 209, 211, 217, 223, 228, 231, 239, 245; III: 267, 282, 289, 292, 295, 296, 302, 304, 312, 322, 324, 329, 334, 343, 347, 351, 356, 362, 371, 377, 383; IV: 250, 267, 273, 277, 281, 287, 291, 299, 300, 314, 320, 326, 335, 339, 345, 350, 355, 364, 371, 377
  Cancer Prevention Study, II: 239; III: 229
American College of Epidemiology, II: 25
American Diabetes Association (ADA), III: 492, 493, 502
American Industrial Hygiene Association, II: 25
American Journal of Epidemiology, II: 281
American Legion, I: 60, 278-279, 399, 601-602, 626, 633; II: 113, 157; IV: 133, 158
  Vietnam veterans' epidemiological studies, III: 212-213, 243
American Public Health Association, II: 25
American Thoracic Society
  Epidemiology Standardization Questionnaire, II: 136
d-Aminolevulinic acid synthetase, I: 153-154
Amitrole, I: 323
AML. *See* Leukemia
Amyloidosis, IV: 2, 7, 11, 511-513
Anencephaly, IV: 404-405
Angina, I: 708; IV: 135
  See also Circulatory disorders
Animal studies; III: 394-396, 524; IV: 254, 256, 269, 275, 279, 290, 293-294, 296
  2,4-D carcinogenicity, I: 118-119, 176-178; II: 48; III: 47, 396; IV: 37
  2,4-D chronic exposure, I: 179-180; IV: 34
  2,4-D developmental toxicity, I: 124, 180-181; III: 46
  2,4-D disease outcomes and mechanisms of toxicity, II: 48-49; III: 38-39, 44-47; IV: 30-32, 35
  2,4-D genotoxicity, I: 178-179; IV: 28, 33
  2,4-D immunotoxicity, I: 122-123, 181; III: 46, 423; IV: 36
  2,4-D lethality, III: 44-45; IV: 35

2,4-D mechanism of action, II: 47-48; III: 44; IV: 33
2,4-D mechanism of toxicity, II: 48-49; IV: 28, 37
2,4-D neurotoxicity, II: 48; III: 45-46, 473; IV: 30, 35
2,4-D pharmacokinetics, I: 175
2,4-D reproductive toxicity, I: 124, 180, 181; III: 46; IV: 29, 36
2,4-D toxicity profile update summary, II: 46; IV: 33
2,4-D toxicokinetics, II: 46-47; III: 43-44; IV: 24, 27
2,4,5-T acute toxicity, I: 184
2,4,5-T carcinogenicity, I: 118, 119, 182-184; III: 396
2,4,5-T chronic exposure, I: 184
2,4,5-T developmental/reproductive toxicity, I: 124, 185; II: 49-50
2,4,5-T genotoxicity, I: 184
2,4,5-T immunotoxicity, I: 123
2,4,5-T mechanism of action, III: 47-48
2,4,5-T mechanism of toxicity, II: 49-50; IV: 37
2,4,5-T pharmacokinetics, I: 182
2,4,5-T toxicity profile update summary, II: 49; IV: 37
2,4,5-T toxicokinetics, II: 49; III: 47; IV: 37
Ah receptor, I: 3, 123, 134; II: 3-4, 51-53, 54-56, 57-62; III: 54-58, 129; IV: 4, 30, 386
amyloidosis, IV: 512
blood abnormalities, I: 125; IV: 496
breast cancer, IV: 29, 317-318
cacodylic acid acute toxicity, I: 188
cacodylic acid carcinogenicity, I: 118, 119, 187; IV: 5, 387
cacodylic acid chronic exposure, I: 188-189
cacodylic acid developmental toxicity, I: 189
cacodylic acid genotoxicity, I: 187-188
cacodylic acid mechanism of action, II: 50; III: 49-50
cacodylic acid mechanism of toxicity, II: 50-51; IV: 24
cacodylic acid pharmacokinetics, I: 186-187
cacodylic acid renal toxicity, II: 50-51
cacodylic acid reproductive toxicity, I: 189
cacodylic acid toxicity summary, II: 50; IV: 38
cacodylic acid toxicokinetics, II: 50; III: 48; IV: 24, 27, 38

characteristics of, I: 111-114; IV: 48
epidemiologic studies, IV: 359, 361, 369, 381
evidentiary role, I: 228; IV: 85, 106, 385, 515-516
generalizability, I: 112, 113, 114, 118, 122-123, 160; IV: 26, 85, 426, 459
hepatic abnormalities, I: 124-125, 688; IV: 25, 57, 59-60
human health relevance of toxicology, III: 35-36; IV: 26, 48
male-mediated disorders, I: 593-594
nonhuman primates, I: 151
picloram in, I: 118, 119, 125, 190-192; III: 51
squamous cell carcinomas, IV: 284
TCDD acute toxicity, II: 75-76
TCDD and bladder cancer in; IV: 342
TCDD and bone cancer in; IV: 290
TCDD and Hodgkin's disease in; IV: 367
TCDD and leukemia disease in; IV: 380
TCDD and multiple myeloma in; IV: 374
TCDD and nasal and nasopharyngeal cancer in; IV: 275
TCDD and non-Hodgkin's lymphoma in; IV: 358
TCDD and prostate cancer in; IV: 332
TCDD and soft-tissue sarcoma in; IV: 279
TCDD carcinogenicity, I: 3, 116, 138-142; II: 3, 65-68; IV: 26, 305, 311
TCDD cardiovascular toxicity, I: 171; II: 76; III: 74-75
TCDD dermal toxicity, I: 173-174; II: 76
TCDD developmental toxicity, I: 123-124, 156-157, 159-160; II: 3, 71, 72-73; III: 92-105; IV: 58
TCDD disease outcomes, II: 3; III: 39-43, 71-105; IV: 3, 23
TCDD endocrine effects, III: 83-84
TCDD gastrointestinal toxicity, I: 169-170; IV: 256
TCDD hepatotoxicity, I: 124-125, 151-156; II: 3, 73-75; III: 76-79
TCDD immunotoxicity, I: 119-122, 146-151; II: 3, 68-71; III: 85-92; IV: 3, 26
TCDD-induced diabetes, IV: 488
TCDD-induced wasting syndrome, I: 162-166; II: 76-77; III: 80-83; IV: 57, 76
TCDD lethality, III: 71-73; IV: 76
TCDD mechanism of action, II: 3, 54-65; III: 51-53, 54-58, 62-63, 67-69; IV: 3, 24

INDEX   539

TCDD mechanism of toxicity, II: 65-77
TCDD metabolic toxicity, I: 166-169
TCDD neurotoxicity, I: 160-166; II: 3, 75;
    III: 84-85; IV: 352, 458
TCDD pharmacokinetics, I: 127-133
TCDD renal toxicity, II: 77; III: 75-76; IV:
    348
TCDD reproductive toxicity, I: 123-124,
    156-159; II: 3, 71-72; III: 92-105; IV:
    26, 64, 323, 337, 411, 432, 434
TCDD respiratory tract toxicity, I: 170
TCDD toxicity update summary, II: 51-53
TCDD toxicokinetics, II: 3, 53-54; III: 4-5,
    33; IV: 3, 23, 41, 47
toxicity, potential health risks and
    contributing factors, III: 106, 107, 108
Anthropometry. *See* Body weight
AOR. *See* Agent Orange Registry
Apoptosis, TCDD and, II: 3, 67
Arctic, Inuit natives, III: 50-51
Argentina, III: 224
Arkansas, I: 373-374, 663; III: 234; IV: 149,
    231
Armed Forces Institute of Pathology, I: 494
Army. *See* U.S. Army
Army Chemical Corps. *See* U.S. Army
    Chemical Corps
Army Reserve Personnel Center, II: 152
ARNT, II: 4, 45, 55, 56, 57, 58, 66; III: 38, 54-
    58, 63; IV: 30, 47-56, 61, 67, 69-73, 86
    See also Ah receptor (AhR)
Arsenic
    cacodylic acid component, IV: 117-118
    respiratory cancer and latency, II: 268; III:
    420
Aryl hydrocarbon hydroxylase, I: 135, 153,
    155-156, 170
Aryl hydrocarbon receptor (AhR). *See* Ah
    receptor (AhR)
Asbestos, respiratory cancer and latency, II:
    268; III: 420
Asia, III: 471
Asian Americans, II: 188
    See also Race/ethnicity
Aspartate aminotransferase (AST), II: 331, 333;
    III: 45, 509; IV: 37
Assembly of Life Sciences (ALS), I: 62, 63
Association of Birth Defect Children, II: 292
AST. *See* Aspartate aminotransferase (AST)
Asthma, I: 708, 711, 713; IV: 199
    See also Respiratory disorders

Ataxia, I: 658
    See also Motor/coordination dysfunction;
    Neurobehavioral toxicity
Atlanta Congenital Defects Program, I: 387
Atlanta, Georgia, II: 241, 296; III: 229
    CDC Birth Defects Study, II: 9; III: 438;
    IV: 237
Atlantic Ocean, III: 108
Australia, I: 61, 91, 340, 406, 418, 444, 470,
    488-489, 537, 546, 614-615, 633, 702,
    710; II: 113, 132, 149, 160, 202, 293;
    III: 216-217, 218, 237, 244-245; IV: 8,
    10, 144, 150, 159, 210, 304
    Air Force veterans, III: 244
    Army veterans, III: 244, 245; IV: 159
    Australian National Service Vietnam
    veterans, III: 273, 286
    Bureau of Statistics Health Interview
    Survey, 1989-1990, III: 245, 485, 511,
    517
    Department of Defense, III: 244, 245
    Department of Veterans Affairs, III: 244,
    245
    Electoral Commission rolls, III: 245
    Health Insurance Medicare, III: 245
    herbicide use by forces, III: 137-138
    lung cancer mortality in Vietnam veterans,
    III: 424
    National Death Index, III: 245
    Navy veterans, III: 244
    Victorian Cancer Registry, III: 232; IV: 144
    Vietnam veterans epidemiologic studies,
    III: 9, 273, 285-286, 290, 294, 295, 298,
    299, 303, 310, 311, 314, 315, 327, 329,
    339, 340, 343, 346, 349, 353, 355, 359,
    365, 380, 389, 469, 486, 489, 500, 506,
    512-513, 517; IV: 244-247, 255, 259,
    262, 264, 266, 272, 276, 280, 283, 287,
    295, 298-299, 305-308, 310, 313, 319,
    323-326, 332, 334-335, 337, 339, 345,
    350, 355, 362-363, 371, 376, 380, 383,
    404-405
    See also Tasmania
Austria, IV: 138-139, 189, 467-468, 500
Autoimmune disease, I: 697-699; IV: 475-481
    See also Immune system disorders;
    Systemic autoimmune disease; Systemic
    lupus erythematosus
Autoimmunity, I: 693, 697-699; II: 7, 21, 327,
    329; III: 487-488; IV: 476-477
    See also Immune system disorders

B

B cell function, I: 147, 148
Baltic Sea, II: 329; III: 108, 236, 272, 285, 358, 484, 515
Basal/squamous cell skin cancer
  biologic plausibility, III: 322; IV: 311
  epidemiologic studies, III: 317-322, 323
  herbicide environmental exposure and, III: 323; IV: 229, 309
  herbicide occupational exposure and, III: 321, 323; IV: 309
  herbicides association with, III: 317-322, 323
  incidence, III: 319-320
  mortality studies, III: 319, 321
  scientific literature update, III: 319-320; IV: 309
  Vietnam veterans and, III: 323
  See also Melanoma; Skin cancer
BASF, I: 312-313, 444, 530, 550, 558; II: 130-131, 238, 318-319, 325, 330-331, 332-333, 334, 336; III: 153, 154, 174, 221-222, 269-270, 273, 297, 349, 484, 495, 506, 511; IV: 112, 188-189, 257, 260, 271, 285, 290, 301, 333, 343-344, 368, 382
  Aktiengesellschaft, III: 221; IV: 137
  Dioxin Investigation Programme, II: 131
  Occupational Safety and Employee Protection Department, II: 131
Basic helix-loop-helix (BHLH), II: 54, 55, 56; IV: 49
Bayer, III: 154; IV: 112
Beck's Depression Inventory, I: 650, 651
Benefits. *See* Compensation, veterans
BHLH. *See* Basic helix-loop-helix (BHLH)
Bias, methodological. *See* Methodological bias
Binghamton, New York, III: 234; IV: 149
Biochemical warfare, I: 29, 45
Biologic plausibility, II: 88, 92; III: 2, 124, 128; IV: 2-3, 16, 20-22, 26, 29, 106-107, 249, 385-388
  Ah receptor-TCDD interaction, I: 3, 133-137, 439, 452-453; III: 129; IV: 48, 86
  altered sperm parameters, I: 634; III: 451
  animal studies, I: 228; II: 176; III: 460-462, 474-475; IV: 431-435
  basal/squamous cell skin cancer, III: 322
  birth defects, II: 298; III: 444; IV: 403
  bladder cancer, III: 351; IV: 342-343

bone cancer, I: 474; III: 304; IV: 290
brain tumors, I: 525; III: 362; IV: 352
breast cancer, II: 217; III: 327, 329; IV: 317-318
carcinogenicity, I: 116-118, 119, 146, 176-178, 182-184, 187, 190-191, 439, 451; II: 176; III: 394-397; IV: 385-387
childhood cancer, I: 630; II: 300; IV: 426
chloracne, I: 678; II: 320-321; III: 480; IV: 466
circulatory disorders, I: 708; III: 518; IV: 510
diabetes mellitus, I: 692; II: 335; III: 502-503; IV: 488
endometrial cancer, IV: 322
evidentiary role of, I: 111, 114, 223-224, 240-241, 434; II: 88, 92, 176; III: 23, 106-107
female reproductive system cancers, I: 512; III: 334; IV: 323
fetal/neonatal/infant death, I: 624; III: 453
gastrointestinal tract cancers, III: 281-282; IV: 256
gastrointestinal ulcers, III: 513-514
genitourinary tract cancers, I: 521-522
genotoxicity, I: 178-179, 184, 187-188, 191
hepatobiliary cancer, I: 453, 457; III: 286, 288; IV: 270
Hodgkin's disease, I: 557; III: 377; IV: 367
hyperlipidemia, I: 692
immunotoxicity, I: 122, 146-151, 181, 192, 699; III: 491
infertility, I: 634; II: 282; III: 451
laryngeal cancer, III: 295; IV: 279
leukemia, I: 571; III: 390; IV: 380-381
liver disorders, I: 691-692; II: 335; III: 513-514; IV: 270
low birthweight outcomes, I: 628; III: 458
lung cancer, III: 302; IV: 284
male-mediated reproductive outcomes, I: 593-595; III: 451; IV: 413, 416-417, 426
melanoma, III: 317; IV: 305
motor/coordination dysfunction, I: 661; III: 475; IV: 448
multiple myeloma, I: 12, 563; III: 383; IV: 374
nasal/nasopharyngeal cancer, I: 460; III: 292; IV: 275
neurobehavioral disorders, II: 314; III: 474-475

neuropsychological disorders, I: 658; IV: 457-459
non-Hodgkin's lymphoma, I: 549; III: 366; IV: 358-359
peripheral nervous system disorders, I: 666
porphyria cutanea tarda, I: 679, 682; II: 323; III: 482; IV: 468
prostate cancer, III: 343; IV: 331-332
renal cancers, III: 356; IV: 348
renal toxicity, I: 179-180
reproductive outcomes, I: 123-124, 180-181, 185, 189, 192, 605, 618, 628; II: 300-301; III: 458, 460-462; IV: 411
respiratory cancers, I: 472
respiratory disorders, I: 713; III: 486
skin cancer, I: 503; IV: 305, 311
soft-tissue sarcoma, I: 500; III: 311; IV: 296
squamous cell carcinomas, IV: 284
testicular cancer, III: 347; IV: 337
See also TCDD biologic plausibility
Biological samples, I: 20-21, 729-730
Biomarkers
  chloracne as, I: 4, 10, 172-173, 262, 401, 672-674; II: 318
  exposure assessment and, I: 259-262, 280-284; II: 101-104; III: 146-147; IV: 111, 123, 479, 448
  research recommendations, I: 17, 725; II: 25
  sperm parameters as, I: 631
Bionetics Research Laboratory, I: 30
Birth defects
  biologic plausibility, III: 444; IV: 403
  definition of, I: 605-606; II: 286; III: 435; IV: 400
  epidemiologic studies, II: 140, 286-296; III: 436, 437-438, 443; IV: 247, 403
  epidemiology, I: 606; II: 286; III: 435-436
  evaluation of epidemiologic data, I: 615-618; IV: 144-145, 403
  herbicide association first reports, I: 1
  herbicide association in, I: 13-14, 618; II: 7, 11, 20, 286-296; III: 436-444; IV 400-405
  herbicide environmental exposure studies, I: 608-609; II: 140, 287-288, 297; III: 437
  herbicide occupational exposure studies, I: 607-608; II: 286-287, 297; III: 437; IV: 197
  Ranch Hand participants' children and, II: 293-296; III: 436, 438, 439; IV: 18

  risk factors of, I: 606-607; II: 298; III: 444
  scientific literature update, III: 437, 439-443; IV: 401-402
  Seveso, Italy, study, II: 287; III: 436
  summary, II: 295-296; IV: 400-401
  TCDD biologic plausibility in, I: 618; II: 298; III: 460-461
  Vietnam veterans' children and, I: 609-615, 618; II: 288-296, 297, 298; III: 435, 436, 437-438; IV: 403
  See also Cleft lip/palate; Neural tube defects; Reproductive disorders; Spina bifida; Teratogenicity
Birth Defects Study, II: 9, 290-291, 296; III: 147, 436, 438, 439; IV: 405, 429
  See also Centers for Disease Control and Prevention (CDC)
Births. *See* Birth defects; Low birthweight; Perinatal death; Preterm delivery (PTD)
Bladder cancer and disorders
  biologic plausibility, III: 351; IV: 342-343
  epidemiologic studies, I: 515-517; II: 225-227; III: 347-351; IV: 19, 339-347, 385, 387
  epidemiology; II: 223; III: 347
  herbicide association in, I: 12, 521, 576; II: 7, 12, 21, 225-227, 250; III: 3, 10, 21, 132, 347-351; IV: 19, 31, 40
  herbicide environmental exposure and, III: 349, 350-351; IV: 341
  herbicide occupational exposure and, III: 348, 350; IV: 340-341
  histopathology, I: 513
  incidence, I: 513
  incidence, data by age/gender/race, for selected age groups, III: 347; IV: 340
  risk factors, I: 513-514
  scientific literature update, II: 226-227; III: 348-349; IV: 340
  TCDD, association with, IV: 19, 24
  Vietnam veterans' risk, I: 513, 517, 522; II: 223, 226; III: 349, 351
  See also Genitourinary cancers
Body mass index (BMI), II: 281; III: 499, 502
Body weight, loss of and TCDD, II: 3
Boehringer-Ingelheim, I: 313; III: 153-154; IV: 111-112
Bone cancer
  biologic plausibility, III: 304
  children and, I: 628
  chondrosarcomas of the skull, III: 2, 10, 266, 304

epidemiologic studies, III: 303-305
epidemiology, I: 472-473; II: 204; III: 302
herbicide association in, I: 13, 473-474,
    577; II: 6, 11, 20, 204-205, 249-250; III:
    7, 10, 303-305
herbicide environmental exposure and, III:
    303, 305; IV: 289
herbicide occupational exposure and, III:
    303, 305; IV: 288
incidence of, data by gender/race, for
    selected age groups, III: 302; IV: 288
scientific literature update, II: 204-205; III:
    303; IV: 288
Vietnam veterans' risk, I: 473, 474; II: 204;
    IV: 290
Vietnam veterans' studies, III: 303, 305;
    IV: 289
Boston Hospital for Women, II: 291-292
Brain tumors, I: 339; IV: 350
2,4-D exposure and, I: 119, 176-177
agricultural workers and, I: 320; II: 136
biologic plausibility, III: 362; IV: 352
clinical features, I: 522
epidemiologic studies, II: 136, 229-230; III:
    356-361; IV: 198
epidemiology, I: 522-523; II: 228-229; III:
    356
herbicide association in, I: 12, 525, 576; II:
    7, 12, 21, 229-230, 250; III: 8, 12, 21,
    356-362; IV: 19
herbicide environmental exposure and, III:
    358, 361; IV: 351
herbicide occupational exposure and, III:
    357-358, 360; IV: 351
incidence, data by gender/race, for selected
    age groups, III: 356; IV: 351
scientific literature update, II: 229-230; III:
    357-359; IV: 351
TCDD, association with, IV: 19
Vietnam veterans' risk, I: 525; II: 228-229,
    230; IV: 353
Vietnam veterans' studies, III: 358-359,
    361; IV: 352
Breast cancer
agricultural workers and, I: 510; IV: 140
biologic plausibility, II: 217; III: 327, 329;
    IV: 318
epidemiologic studies, II: 214-216, 217; III:
    324-328; IV: 318-320
epidemiology, I: 505, 506-507; II: 213-214;
    III: 322, 324; IV: 144

herbicide association in, I: 13; II: 6, 11, 12,
    20, 89, 213-217, 249-250; III: 7, 10,
    324-329; IV: 24, 29, 38, 73
herbicide environmental exposure studies, I:
    511, 512; III: 328; IV: 315
herbicide occupational exposure studies, II:
    214-216; III: 324-326, 328; IV: 315
histopathology, I: 505-506
incidence in US women, data by race, for
    selected age groups, III: 324; IV: 314
risk, estimated, II: 218
risk factors, I: 507
scientific literature update, III: 326-327; IV:
    315
Vietnam veterans' risk, I: 213, 216-217,
    505, 511; III: 329; IV: 318
Vietnam veterans' studies, III: 326, 328;
    IV: 316
See also Reproductive system cancers,
    women
British Columbia, Canada, III: 10, 227-228,
    338, 439-440, 447-448, 449, 452, 453,
    457; IV: 419
Cancer Incidence File, III: 227
Death File, III: 227
Division of Vital Statistics, III: 452, 457
Health Surveillance Registry, III: 227, 439
Bronchitis, I: 708, 711, 713
See also Respiratory disorders
Bronchus cancer. See Lung cancer
Brown, Jesse, II: 24; III: 24, 25
Bureau of Census, III: 231
Bureau of Labor Statistics, I: 79, 80
n-Butyl esters, I: 27; IV: 117-119

C

Ca Mau peninsula, I: 100, 104
Cacodylic acid, I: 88-89; II: 4; III: 5, 19, 32,
    135, 136, 137, 218; IV: 22, 117-118,
    133
acute toxicity, I: 188
animal studies, I: 185-189; II: 50-51; III:
    34, 38, 48, 49-50, 396; IV: 5
carcinogenicity, I: 118, 119, 187; II: 40; III:
    396
chemical properties/structure, I: 111, 114,
    186; II: 38; III: 32
chronic exposure, I: 188-189
developmental toxicity, I: 124, 189

INDEX 543

dimethylarsenic radical formation and,
  II: 4
disease outcomes, III: 34, 50; IV: 25, 31
domestic use, I: 185-186
genotoxicity, I: 119, 187-188
kidney toxicity, I: 125; II: 42
mechanism of action, II: 50; III: 38, 49-50
mechanisms of toxicity, II: 50-51
metabolism, I: 115, 116
Operation Ranch Hand, use in, IV: 117
pharmacokinetics, I: 186-187
renal toxicity, II: 50-51
reproductive toxicity, I: 124, 189; II: 42;
  IV: 403
toxicity update summary, II: 50; IV: 23, 33,
  38
toxicokinetics, II: 50; III: 32-33, 48; IV: 24,
  27-29
Vietnam formulations, I: 186
volume used in Operation Ranch Hand,
  data, III: 136
Calcium, homeostasis of and 2,4,5-T, II: 4
California, I: 341; III: 232
  See also Irvine, California
Camp Drum, New York, I: 25-26, 89
Canada, I: 11, 319-320, 323, 374-375, 443,
  467-468, 537-539, 620, 650; II: 8, 132,
  135-136, 140, 219-220, 243, 248; III:
  226, 232, 303, 309, 335, 344, 348, 353;
  IV: 141, 199, 209, 257, 296, 333, 353,
  360, 374, 381
  Census of Agriculture, 1971, II: 135
  Census of Population, 1971, II: 135
  Central Farm Register, 1971, II: 135
  Central Farm Register, 1981, II: 135
  Mortality Data Base, II: 135; III: 227
  Mortality Study of Canadian Male Farm
    Operators, II: 135-136; III: 224; IV:
    140, 198-200
  Saskatchewan Cancer Foundation, II: 139
  Saskatchewan Hospital Services Plan, II:
    139
  Statistics Canada, III: 227
  See also Alberta, Canada; British Columbia,
    Canada; Manitoba, Canada; New
    Brunswick, Canada; Ontario, Canada;
    Saskatchewan, Canada
Cancer
  age-specific incidence, I: 436-438; IV: 250,
    267, 273, 277, 281, 288, 292, 300, 314,
    321, 327, 335, 346, 351, 356, 365, 372,
    378

agriculture workers and, I: 320-323, 443; II:
  136, 137-138
biologic plausibility, I: 116-118, 119, 434;
  II: 176; III: 394-397; IV: 249, 256, 270,
  275, 279, 284, 290, 296, 305, 311, 318,
  322, 323, 331, 332, 337, 342, 343, 348,
  352, 358, 359, 367, 374, 380, 381, 385
children and, I: 14, 594-595, 628-631; IV:
  345, 399, 400, 417-429
clinical features, I: 433-436
epidemiologic studies, I: 45, 317, 320-323,
  325-326, 367, 383-384, 391-393, 443-
  445; II: 133-138, 147-148; IV: 182,
  251-255, 268-269, 274-275, 277-278,
  282-283, 288-289, 292-295, 302-304,
  309-310, 315-316, 321-323, 327-329,
  336-337, 340-342, 346-347, 351-352,
  356-358, 365-367, 372-373, 379-380
epidemiology, I: 433, 435-438, 442, 525; II:
  175; III: 265-266
herbicide association, insufficient evidence
  for determining, I: 13-14, 577-578; II:
  249-250; III: 393; IV: 268, 270, 274,
  279, 286, 302, 305, 311, 314, 318, 321,
  323, 336, 337, 338, 340, 342, 346, 348,
  374, 378, 380, 384
herbicide association, limited/suggestive
  evidence of, I: 10-12, 574-576; II: 247-
  249; III: 393; IV: 256, 278, 279, 283,
  331, 373, 384, 385
herbicide association, no evidence of, I: 12-
  13, 576-577; II: 250; III: 393-394; IV:
  254, 256, 269, 289, 317
herbicide association, sufficient evidence
  of, I: 8-10, 572-574; II: 175, 176, 247;
  III: 390, 392; IV: 295, 358, 367, 384
herbicide environmental exposure
  epidemiologic studies, I: 444, 469; II:
  147-148; IV: 254, 269, 274, 278,
  282, 289, 293, 302, 309, 315, 321, 329,
  336, 341, 347, 351, 357, 366, 372, 379
herbicide exposure measures, II: 175, 176;
  III: 265-266
herbicide occupational exposure studies, I:
  443-444; II: 133, 134; IV: 251, 268,
  274, 282, 288, 292, 302, 309, 315, 321,
  327, 336, 340, 346, 351, 356, 365, 372,
  379
herbicide/pesticide applicators and, I: 320-
  321, 323, 325-326, 443, 447, 466-468,
  488, 491; II: 137-138; IV: 276

544

herbicides, categories of association in, I: 572
mortality studies, I: 442-445; II: 133, 134, 136, 137, 263; III: 410-411, 421, 422, 423, 424, 426, 427, 429; IV: 251-254, 268-270, 277, 282, 288, 289, 292, 293, 294, 299, 302, 303, 305, 327, 329, 330, 331, 332, 336, 341, 346, 347, 351, 352, 356, 357, 358, 365, 366, 367, 372, 373, 379, 380
multistage model, I: 142-143, 434, 439
P450 induction to, I: 144-145, 170
phenoxy herbicide association in, I: 483; III: 422, 423, 429
research priorities, I: 19, 727
research recommendations, I: 19, 727
risk assessment, I: 442-443, 578; II: 251, 276; III: 430-431
site groupings for ICD-9 cancer codes, III: 537-539
TCDD animal studies, I: 138-142; II: 176; III: 394, 396; IV: 306, 311, 317
TCDD genotoxicity, I: 143-144
TCDD in initiation/promotion, I: 116, 142-143, 434, 439
TCDD in P450 induction to, I: 144-145
Vietnam civilians, II: 148
Vietnam veterans, expected incidence, I: 439-440, 442, 452, 460-461, 473, 475, 501, 505, 513, 522, 526, 564; II: 176-177; III: 266-267
Vietnam veterans' risk, I: 391-393, 401, 402-403, 405, 436-438, 444-445, 578; II: 251, 276; III: 397, 430-431; IV: 256, 270, 275, 279, 284, 290, 296, 305, 311, 318, 323, 332, 338, 343, 348, 353, 359, 367, 374, 381, 388
See also Carcinogen(s); Latency effects in cancer studies; *specific cancers; specific cancer sites*
Carcinogen(s)
2,4-D as, I: 118-119, 176-178; II: 40, 48; III: 47, 396; IV: 5
2,4,5-T as, I: 118, 119, 182-184; II: 40; III: 396
cacodylic acid as, I: 118, 119, 187; II: 40; III: 396; IV: 29, 31
herbicides as, I: 3, 40; II: 273, 275; III: 426, 428, 430; IV: 10, 17, 267, 270, 341, 345, 511
mechanism of action, I: 434

INDEX

picloram as, I: 118, 119, 190-191; II: 40; III: 396
TCDD as, I: 3, 116-118, 434, 439; II: 3, 39-40, 65-68; III: 394, 396; IV: 3, 82-83, 134, 256, 274-275, 279, 284, 290, 296, 305, 311, 318, 330, 332, 337, 342, 348, 352, 358, 367, 374, 380, 385-387, 477
See also Cancer
Cardiovascular system disorders
cardiomegaly, I: 703
circulatory disorders, I: 699-709; IV: 182
lipid abnormalities in, I: 688
TCDD in, I: 171; II: 76; III: 74-75; IV: 76, 135, 156-157; IV: 23-26, 135, 156-157
See also Circulatory disorders; Myocardial infarction
Case-control studies
agriculture/forestry workers, I: 326-341; II: 138-140; III: 185-195, 228-232
evidentiary role of, I: 234-235, 727; II: 94-95, 178, 179, 180, 188; III: 130; IV: 105, 108
herbicide environmental exposure, II: 144-146, 148-149, 184, 186, 190, 193, 241; III: 201-204; IV: 227-231, 322
herbicide exposure assessment for, I: 256-257, 727; IV: 9, 137, 144-146, 207-221, 336, 369, 401, 418-420, 428, 444-445, 447
herbicide occupational exposure, II: 122-127, 138-140, 183, 184, 186, 188, 190, 193, 200, 222, 240; III: 173, 175, 185-196; IV: 133, 136, 187, 192, 207-221, 328
paper/pulp workers, II: 126-127, 200; IV: 147, 221-223
Vietnam veterans, II: 155-157, 159-160, 187, 223; III: 208-217; IV: 124, 236-245, 247, 420, 423-425, 427
Causality
statistical association vs., I: 7, 227, 239, 246; II: 5, 19, 97, 247; III: 6, 20, 132-133, 390; IV: 6
CDC. *See* Centers for Disease Control and Prevention
CDDs. *See* Chlorinated dibenzo-*p*-dioxins
Cell-mediated immunity (CMI)
TCDD and, II: 69-70
Cell proliferation
TCDD and, II: 3, 67; IV: 23, 60, 61, 63, 79, 82

INDEX

Cellular retinoic acid binding protein, type II (CRABP-II), II: 73
Census Bureau. *See* Bureau of Census
Centers for Disease Control and Prevention (CDC), I: 19, 40-41, 51; II: 9; III: 363, 517; IV: 115, 123, 133
  Agent Orange action/research, I: 57-62, 63-64; II: 28; III: 25; IV: 125-126
  Agent Orange Study, I: 276-278; II: 102; IV: 124
  birth defects research, I: 387-389, 609-612; II: 289; IV: 124
  epidemiological studies, II: 113, 155-156; III: 26, 207-209, 218, 240; IV: 156-157, 208, 235, 236, 237
  exposure opportunity index, I: 274-276, 611-612; II: 290-291; III: 147-148
  neural tube defects in children, studies by, IV: 18
  research methodology, I: 728
  TCDD half-life investigation, II: 104-105
  validation study, I: 59, 260-261, 281-284, 285, 387, 742-743; II: 103, 104; III: 240
  See also Birth Defects Study; Cerebrospinal Malformation (CSM) Study; General Birth Defects Study (GBDS); Selected Cancers Study; Vietnam Experience Study (VES)
Central nervous system (CNS). *See* Cognitive/neuropsychiatric disorders; Motor/coordination dysfunction; Neurologic disorders
Cerebrospinal Malformation (CSM) Study, I: 610; II: 289-290
Cerebrovascular disease, I: 702
  stroke, I: 658, 659, 660
Cervical cancer, I: 13, 505, 509, 510, 512; II: 6; III: 329, 330, 332; IV: 320-21, 324, 385
Chemical production. *See* Chemicals and chemical industry; Herbicides; Industrial accidents; Production workers
Chemicals and chemical industry
  Agent Orange product liability litigation, I: 34-35
  hexachlorophene production, I: 40; II: 128; IV: 134-135, 138, 148
  production workers exposure studies, I: 303-318; II: 114-118, 128-135, 171-175, 182-183, 191, 193-197, 206-207, 232, 237-238, 273-274, 275; III: 170-178, 218, 219-224, 284, 363-364, 378-379, 386-387, 420, 423, 426, 429; IV: 133-140, 194-197, 252, 257, 258, 260, 262, 263, 265, 266, 271, 276, 280, 285, 286, 293, 296, 297, 301, 306, 307, 318, 319, 325, 327, 333, 334, 338, 343, 344, 348, 349, 353, 354, 360, 368, 374, 381, 382
  TCDD contamination in production, I: 91, 126
  See also Herbicides; Industrial accidents
Chemoreception
  characteristics of, I: 133-134
  dioxin-responsive enhancers in, I: 135-136
  estrogen-mediated, I: 145
  TCDD dose-response linearity, I: 137-138
  TCDD hepatotoxicity and, I: 154-155
  TCDD-induced wasting syndrome and, I: 164
  See also Ah receptor
Child mortality studies, II: 147
  See also Deaths; Mortality studies
Children
  spina bifida in Vietnam veterans offspring, II: 9-10, 296, 298, 309; III: 7, 8, 9-10, 21, 24-25, 437-438
  See also Child mortality studies; Children, cancer in
Children, cancer in, I: 14, 594-595, 628-631; II: 7, 11, 20; IV: 399-400, 417-420, 422, 425-426, 427, 428, 432
  epidemiologic studies, II: 299
  epidemiology, II: 298; IV: 422-425
  herbicide association in, II: 299-300
  scientific literature update, II: 299-300; IV: 418-422
  Seveso, Italy, study, II: 299; IV: 428
  Vietnam veterans' offspring, II: 299; IV: 426, 429
  See also Wilm's tumor
China, I: 458; II: 188, 320; III: 159, 289; IV: 273
  See also Shanghai, China
Chloracne, I: 39
  animal studies, I: 173-174; III: 480
  biological plausibility, II: 320-321; III: 480; IV: 466
  chemical production workers and, I: 308, 310, 316; IV: 464, 466
  clinical features, I: 672-673
  diet and, I: 174; IV: 463-464
  epidemiologic studies, I: 674-678; II: 318-320; III: 479-480; IV: 135-136, 138-139, 147, 152, 186, 189, 194, 233
  epidemiology, II: 317-318; III: 478-479

herbicide association in, I: 10, 678; II: 5, 6, 20, 318-321; III: 6, 7, 20, 24, 479-480; IV: 185, 463-464
scientific literature update, II: 318-320; III: 480; IV: 465
Seveso, Italy, accident and, I: 366-367; IV: 464
skin cancer and, I: 502
TCDD biomarker for, I: 4, 10, 28, 172-173, 262, 401, 672-674; II: 3, 318
Vietnam veterans and, II: 317, 318, 321; III: 479, 480; IV: 233, 465-466
Vietnam veterans compensation for, I: 50, 51, 55, 56; II: 24, 28-29, 30, 31
See also Skin sensitivity
Chlordane, I: 91
Chlorinated dibenzo-p-dioxins (CDDs), II: 63-64, 65
Chlorodibenzodioxins, I: 28
4-Chloro-2-methylphenoxyacetic acid (MCPA), II: 113, 133, 188, 193, 195-196, 207; III: 218, 225; IV: 133, 197, 258, 259, 260, 262, 264, 265, 267, 276, 280, 286-287, 290, 291, 297, 299, 312, 334, 335, 338, 339, 344-345, 349, 350, 354, 355, 401
2-[4-Chloro-2-methylphenoxy]propanoic acid (MCPP), II: 133, 195-196
Chlorophenols, I: 9; III: 150, 151, 154, 218, 222, 223, 422, 423, 429; IV: 16
Chondrosarcomas of the skull. See Bone cancer
Chronic lymphocytic leukemia (CLL). See Leukemia
Chronic myeloid leukemia (CML). See Leukemia
Chronic obstructive pulmonary disease (COPD), II: 129; IV: 184, 470, 472, 474, 475
See also Respiratory disorders
Circulatory disorders
definition, II: 335, 337; III: 514; IV: 505
biologic plausibility, III: 518; IV: 510
epidemiologic studies, I: 700-707; II: 335-337; III: 514-518; IV: 506-509
epidemiology, III: 514
herbicide association in, I: 14, 708; II: 7, 11, 21, 335-337; III: 3, 8, 514-518
morbidity studies, II: 336
mortality studies, II: 335
research methodology, I: 699-700; II: 335

scientific literature update, II: 336-337; III: 515-518; IV: 506-509
Vietnam veterans and, II: 336; III: 514; IV: 510
See also Angina; Cardiovascular system disorders; Depressive disorders; Hypertension; Myocardial infarction
Cleanup efforts. See Hazardous materials disposal and cleanup
Cleft lip/palate, I: 373-374, 375, 611, 612; IV: 402, 433
See also Birth defects
Clinton, William J., III: 24
CLL. See Leukemia
CMI. See Cell-mediated immunity; Leukemia
CNS. See Cognitive/neuropsychiatric disorders; Motor/coordination dysfunction
Coast Guard. See U.S. Coast Guard
Cognitive/neuropsychiatric disorders
epidemiologic studies, II: 148, 307-308; III: 468-469
herbicide association in, I: 657-658; II: 7, 11, 20, 307-309; III: 468-469; IV: 441-443
herbicide environmental exposure studies, I: 651-653; II: 148
herbicide occupational exposure studies, I: 649-651
scientific literature update, II: 307-308; III: 469; IV: 441-442
Vietnam veterans' risk, I: 653-656; II: 308
See also Encephalopathy; Neurasthenia; Neurobehavioral toxicity; Neurological disorders; Posttraumatic stress disorder (PTSD)
Cohort studies
agriculture/forestry workers, I: 318-323; II: 118-122, 135-138; III: 178-182, 224-226; IV: 140-142, 197-206
definition, I: 229
herbicide environmental exposure, II: 141-147, 190, 218; III: 197-201; IV: 224-237
herbicide exposure assessment for, I: 254-256; II: 105-107, 178, 179, 180
herbicide occupational exposure, II: 107-108, 114-122, 130-133, 182-183, 186, 190, 192, 193, 218, 222, 240; III: 170-185, 196; IV: 134-140, 182-206, 222-230
methodology, I: 229-232

INDEX 547

Ranch Hand cohort, II: 109, 150-152, 154-156, 201; IV: 13, 18, 150-156
Vietnamese civilians cohort, II: 108-109
Vietnam veterans, II: 149-160, 187, 218; III: 206-217; IV: 232-247
Colon cancer
  agricultural workers and, I: 328-329
  epidemiologic studies, III: 276-278; IV: 250-252, 255-256, 262, 385
  herbicide association in, I: 12-13, 576-577; II: 7, 12; III: 8, 21
  See also Gastrointestinal (GI) tract cancers
Colorado, III: 47
Colorectal cancer, I: 446
  Vietnam veterans' risk, I: 447, 450, 451, 452; IV: 256
  See also Gastrointestinal (GI) tract cancers
Committee to Review the Health Effects in Vietnam Veterans of Exposure to Herbicides, II: 17, 18, 19, 22, 23, 264-266; III: 17, 18, 19, 23, 412; IV: 15
  epidemiologic studies of Vietnam Veterans, recommendations, II: 24-25
Compensation, veterans, I: 227
  congressional legislation, I: 47, 50-51; II: 28-29; III: 26-27
  Department of Veterans Affairs, I: 55-56; II: 24, 30-31; III: 28
  product liability litigation, I: 34-35
Confidence intervals, I: 244
Congress. *See* Congressional hearings; Legislation; U.S. Congress
Congressional hearings
  Agent Orange and, II: 27-28; III: 25
Connecticut, tumor registry, III: 235, 388
Con Thieu province, Vietnam, I: 96; III: 139; IV: 121
COPD. *See* Chronic obstructive pulmonary disease
Corticosterone, TCDD and, I: 168, 171-172
Cox Proportional Hazard, III: 499, 502
CRABP-II. *See* Cellular retinoic acid binding protein, type II
CSM. *See* Cerebrospinal Malformation (CSM) Study
Cytochrome P450. *See* P450
Cytogenetics
  non-Hodgkin's lymphoma studies, III: 365-366
Czechoslovakia, I: 317, 649, 675, 688; IV: 139
  See also Prague, Czechoslovakia

D

2,4-D. *See* 2,4-Dichlorophenoxyacetic acid
Data sources
  Agent Orange Registry, I: 20, 53, 56, 729; II: 153
  agricultural/forestry worker studies, I: 265-266, 318-341; IV: 140-142
  animal studies, I: 111-114, 228
  biological stored samples as, I: 20-21, 729-730
  Cancerlit, IV: 253
  case reports, I: 235-236
  Centers for Disease Control studies, I: 387-391; II: 113, 155-156; III: 207-209, 218, 240; IV: 133, 156-157
  chemical production workers, I: 303-318; IV: 134-140
  computerized data bases, I: 735-736; II: 24-25, 31
  Department of Veterans Affairs
    epidemiologic studies, I: 393-399; II: 152, 153; III: 209-212, 218, 240-243; IV: 151, 157-158
  epidemiologic controlled studies, I: 228-237; II: 150-153
  epidemiologic studies as, I: 737-738
  herbicide environmental exposure studies, I: 267-269, 372-375, 383-384; IV: 147-150
  herbicide exposure reconstruction model, I: 725-726
  herbicide non-military exposures, I: 4-5, 222-223, 241-242
  herbicide/pesticide applicators, I: 266-267, 323-326; IV: 142-143
  HERBS tapes, I: 20, 62, 85, 96-98, 273-279, 287, 291, 602, 725; III: 146, 148; IV: 123, 125
  International Register of Workers Exposed to Phenoxy Herbicides and Their Contaminants, I: 313-314; IV: 137
  mandated efforts, I: 20-21
  Medline, IV: 252
  organization of, I: 737
  paper/pulp mill workers, I: 341, 364; IV: 114, 134
  presentations/reports to committee, I: 739-756; II: 343-348; III: 533-536
  randomized controlled trials, I: 227-228
  reproductive outcomes, I: 593-595

research future recommendations, I: 287-289, 291, 722-725, 729-730; IV: 13
review of, I: 244-245
self-reports, I: 270-271
state government, I: 60
state-sponsored Vietnam veteran studies, I: 400-405, 495-496; III: 213-215, 243-244
TCDD production workers, I: 264-265; IV: 134-140
Toxline, IV: 252
troop location, I: 273-279, 287; IV: 121
Vietnam casualties, I: 82-83
Vietnam military herbicide use, I: 84-85
Vietnam veteran demographics, I: 79, 80-84
Vietnam veteran exposure assessment use, I: 270-287
Vietnam veteran reproductive outcomes, I: 601
Vietnamese civilian health outcomes, I: 371-372
women veterans, I: 83-84; II: 152-153
See also Death certificates; Epidemiologic studies; Military records; Questionnaires
DBCP. *See* Dibromochloropropane
DDT, I: 87, 91; IV: 141
Death certificates, I: 236-237; II: 128, 136, 137-138, 151; III: 470; IV: 112
See also Data sources
Deaths
2,4-D lethality, III: 44-45; IV: 35
Australian Vietnam veterans lung cancer deaths, III: 424
female reproductive system cancer deaths, by cancer site, III: 329
Finland male herbicide applicators respiratory cancer mortality, II: 271
Germany herbicide/chemical production workers cancer mortality, III: 423, 429
non-Hodgkin's lymphoma mortality, III: 429; IV: 355
prostate cancer mortality, III: 426, 427; IV: 326
respiratory cancer mortality, III: 421, 422, 423; IV: 273
Seveso, Italy, male cancer mortality, II: 271, 275; III: 422, 427; IV: 282
TCDD lethality, III: 71-73
See also Child mortality studies; Death certificates; Mortality studies; Perinatal death

Defense Manpower Data Center (DMDC), II: 24-25
See also Department of Defense, U.S. (DoD)
Defoliants
Agent Orange as, I: 90; IV: 38
military applications, I: 25, 26; III: 135, 137; IV: 117
Vietnam herbicide mission maps, I: 99-100
Vietnam tactical role of, I: 85
See also Herbicides
Dekonta Company, II: 329
Demilitarized Zone (DMZ), IV: 120
Demographic data, Vietnam veterans, I: 79, 80-84
DEN. *See* Diethylnitrosamine
Denmark, I: 317, 443, 444, 454, 463, 477, 480, 509, 510, 537, 553, 565, 567; II: 131-134, 139-140, 183, 194-195, 207, 209-210, 212, 215, 232, 238; III: 223, 224, 307, 313, 318, 325, 330-331; IV: 199-200, 209, 252, 406, 408
Cancer Registry, III: 232
Central Population Register, II: 133, 139, 224; III: 352
Danish National Institute for Social Research, II: 140
National Cancer Register, II: 133, 139, 215, 224; III: 325, 352; IV: 144
Deoxyribonucleic acid (DNA), II: 45, 48, 50, 51, 54, 55, 56, 57-58, 60, 61, 64, 74, 75; III: 34, 35, 39, 42, 43, 48, 49, 53, 54, 56, 57, 58-61, 65, 67, 69, 75, 77, 83, 90, 91, 98, 99, 103, 104, 109; IV: 29, 33, 40, 47, 48, 49, 53, 60, 64, 67, 68, 69, 70, 73, 75, 77, 85, 458
Department of Agriculture, U.S. (USDA), I: 35, 39, 443; II: 178, 219, 224, 229, 238-239, 248; III: 230, 335, 352; IV: 212, 213, 257, 259, 262, 264, 267, 301, 345, 350, 355, 364, 371, 376, 383
Agricultural Census, IV: 149
extension agents, IV: 144
Department of Air Force, U.S.
Vietnam herbicide use by military, response, II: 31-32; III: 28-29
Department of Defense, U.S. (DoD), I: 17, 27, 29, 31, 78; II: 24; III: 138, 139, 140; IV: 119, 121
Environmental Services Group, III: 148
herbicide spray mission records, I: 84-85

INDEX
549

herbicide use precautions, I: 95; IV: 121
military records, I: 78, 724-725
See also Defense Manpower Data Center (DMDC)
Department of Veterans Affairs, U.S. (DVA), I: 2, 8, 17, 18, 20, 50-51, 284; II: 2, 5, 8, 11, 13, 17, 18, 19, 26, 27, 89, 153, 176, 181, 187, 218, 249, 260, 278, 305, 312; III: 1, 2, 3, 6, 11, 12, 17, 18, 20, 24, 25, 26, 125, 132, 266, 303, 304, 390, 407, 434, 468, 478, 519; IV: 1, 2, 6, 15, 16, 18, 123, 133, 151, 158, 284, 463
  Agent Orange controversy and, I: 33, 53-54; II: 29-31; III: 28-29
  Agent Orange Coordinator, II: 31
  Death Beneficiary Identification and Record Location System (BIRLS), II: 151, 152, 153; III: 238, 241, 242; IV: 151, 157
  health care in, I: 54; II: 28; III: 27
  military records, I: 78-79, 724-725; II: 151, 152, 153
  mortality studies, II: 101, 152-153, 156-157; III: 146; IV: 151, 157-158
  outreach activities, I: 56; II: 31; III: 28
  Patient Treatment File (PTF), III: 242
  recommendations for, I: 724-725, 726-730; II: 24-25
  research efforts, I: 54-55; II: 29-30; III: 27-28
  veterans' advocacy groups and, I: 61
  Vietnam veteran compensation and benefits, II: 24, 30-31; III: 28
  Vietnam veteran epidemiologic studies, I: 50, 393-399, 445, 469-470, 493-495, 543-547, 562; II: 101, 113, 156-157, 201-202; III: 209-212, 218, 240-243
  women veterans epidemiological studies, II: 152-153; IV: 399
  See also Agent Orange Registry (AOR); Agent Orange Task Force; Environmental Agents Service (EAS); Environmental Epidemiology Service (EES)
Depressive disorders, I: 650, 651
  See also Cognitive/neuropsychiatric disorders; Neurobehavioral toxicity
Dermal toxicity
  TCDD and, II: 76; III: 73-74; IV: 76
Desiccant herbicides, I: 88-89; III: 136
  See also Herbicides
Detroit, Michigan, II: 241; III: 229

Developmental disorders
  2,4-D in, I: 180-181; II: 42; III: 46
  2,4,5-T in, I: 185; II: 42, 49-50
  cacodylic acid in, I: 189; II: 42
  neurological, I: 660
  picloram in, I: 192; II: 42
  TCDD in, I: 123-124, 149, 156-157, 159-160, 185; II: 3, 41-42, 71, 72-73; III: 92-105
  See also Low birthweight
Diabetes mellitus, I: 683-685, 691, 692, 698; II: 7; IV: 481
  biologic plausibility, III: 502-503; IV: 488
  diagnostic criteria, III: 493, 494
  epidemiologic concerns, III: 494
  epidemiologic studies, II: 330-331; III: 494-502; IV: 182, 232
  epidemiology, II: 330; III: 491-492, 493
  herbicide environmental exposure and, III: 497; IV: 484-485
  herbicide exposure and, II: 332-333; III: 2, 11-12, 125, 494-503; IV: 152
  herbicide occupational exposure and, III: 496; IV: 483-484
  pathogenetic diversity of, III: 494
  peripheral neuropathy and, relationship, III: 471-472
  prevalence, data by age/race/gender, III: 492
  scientific literature update, II: 330-331; III: 496, 497; IV: 483
  Type 2 (adult-onset), IV: 1, 8, 16-18, 21, 150-151, 182-183
  Vietnam veterans and, II: 330; III: 2, 11-12, 495, 497, 498, 500, 502; IV: 154-156, 485-487
Diamond Shamrock Corporation, I: 34, 35
Diazinon, I: 91
Dibenzofurans, I: 126; IV: 41, 64, 138
Dibromochloropropane (DBCP), II: 279
2,4-Dichlorophenoxyacetic acid (2,4-D); II: 4, 18; III: 5, 19, 135, 136, 137; IV: 4-5, 110-111, 122, 133
  acute toxicity, I: 179
  Agent Orange and, I: 27
  Agent White and, I: 90
  altered sperm parameters, I: 632
  animal studies, I: 174-181; II: 46-49; III: 34, 36-37, 38-39, 43-47, 396, 462, 475
  carcinogenicity, I: 118-119, 176-178, 439; II: 40, 48; III: 47, 396

chemical properties, I: 114, 175; II: 38; III: 32
chemical structure, I: 111, 114
chronic exposure, I: 179-180
development of, I: 24, 26, 35
developmental toxicity, I: 124, 180-181; II: 42; III: 46
disease outcomes, III: 34, 38-39, 44-47
domestic use, I: 174-175, 177-178
formulations, I: 175
genotoxicity, I: 119, 178-179
half-life of, II: 4
immunotoxicity, I: 122, 181; II: 41; III: 46, 524
infertility and, II: 280-282
ingestion of, I: 653
kidney toxicity, I: 125; II: 42
lethality, III: 44-45
liver toxicity, I: 125; II: 42; III: 524
mechanism of action, II: 47-48; III: 44
mechanisms of toxicity, II: 48-49
metabolism, I: 115, 116
military field tests, I: 26
neurobehavioral disorders and, II: 305; III: 475
neuropsychiatric outcomes and, I: 649, 650, 653
neurotoxicity, II: 48; III: 45-46
non-Hodgkin's lymphoma and, I: 256-257, 574
occupational exposure, I: 36, 37, 310-311, 321; III: 218, 224, 225, 226; IV: 117
peripheral neuropathy and, II: 312; III: 473
pharmacokinetics, Ì: 175
porphyria cutanea tarda and, II: 322
reproductive toxicity, I: 124, 180-181, 597-598; II: 41, 280-282; III: 46, 460, 461-462
role of, I: 88
teratogenic potential, I: 30, 92
therapeutic application, I: 659
toxicokinetics, II: 46-47; III: 32-33, 36-37, 43-44; IV: 27-28
toxicologic properties, IV: 22-25, 27-31, 33-37
volume used in Operation Ranch Hand, data, III: 136, IV: 117-119
See also Herbicides
2,4-Dichlorophenoxybutyric acid (2,4-DB)
differences with 2,4-Dichlorophenoxyacetic acid (2,4-D); IV: 5

Diet
breast cancer and, I: 507
cancer risk and, I: 442
chloracne and, I: 174
gastrointestinal cancers and, I: 446
TCDD interactions, II: 64
Diethylnitrosamine (DEN)
TCDD and, II: 67; IV: 71
Digestive disorders. *See* Metabolic and digestive disorders
Dimethylarsenic radical
bladder hyperplasia and tumors associated with, IV: 31, 40
cacodylic acid and formation of, II: 4
Dinoxol, I: 91; III: 137; IV: 119
Dioxin. *See* Dioxin congeners; Dioxin-responsive enhancers; Dioxin toxic equivalent factors (Teq factors); 2,3,7,8-Tetrachlorodibenzo-*p*-dioxin
Dioxin congeners, II: 105-107; III: 158-159
Dioxin Registry, I: 36-37
Dioxin-responsive enhancers, I: 135-136
Dioxin toxic equivalent factors (Teq factors), II: 106, 107; III: 99, 106, 107, 108, 158, 159; IV: 139
Diquat, I: 91; III: 137; IV: 119
Diseases and disorders. *See* Health outcomes of herbicide exposure; Military health care; specific cancers; *specific cancer sites; specific diseases and disorders*
DMA. *See* Cacodylic acid; Dimethylarsenic radical
DMDC. *See* Defense Manpower Data Center
DNA. *See* Deoxyribonucleic acid
DoD. *See* Department of Defense, U.S.
Domestic herbicide use
2,4-D, I: 174-175
2,4,5-T, I: 181-182
agricultural use, I: 24, 35, 39, 174-175, 181
pet cancers and, I: 119, 177-178
picloram, I: 189
TCDD contamination in, I: 91
See also Agricultural/forestry workers
Dopaminergic system, I: 163-164, 165
Dormagen, Germany, III: 154; IV: 112
Dose-response relationship
2,4-D pharmacokinetics, I: 175
animal fetal mortality, I: 159
animal studies, I: 111-114, 118
evidentiary role of, I: 239-230, 252
research recommendations, I: 19, 727

INDEX   551

TCDD-chloracne, I: 673; II: 318
TCDD dermal application, I: 128-129
TCDD-exposed workers and, I: 445
TCDD-immune system processes, I: 696
TCDD immunotoxicity, I: 122
TCDD threshold, I: 137-138
TCDD tissue distribution, I: 130
Doubs, France, IV: 116
Dow Chemical Company, I: 34, 35, 307-312, 461-462, 529, 558, 598, 607, 620, 674; II: 115-116, 130, 178, 191, 193, 207, 232, 238, 286; III: 152-153, 172-174, 220-221, 270-271, 357-358, 387, 484, 511, 516; IV: 136, 186-188
DVA. *See* Department of Veterans Affairs, U.S.
Dystonia, I: 658
See also Motor/coordination dysfunction

E

EAS. *See* Environmental Agents Service
East Germany. *See* German Democratic Republic
EES. *See* Environmental Epidemiology Service
EGF. *See* Epidermal growth factor
EGFR. *See* Epidermal growth factor receptor
Electrical transformers, I: 364-365, 444, 626, 675
Electrophoretic mobility shift gene (EMSA)
  TCDD and, II: 66
Emphysema, I: 708, 713
  See also Respiratory disorders
EMSA. *See* Electrophoretic mobility shift gene
Encephalopathy, I: 649
  See also Cognitive/neuropsychiatric disorders
Endocrine system, I: 150-151; IV: 156
  TCDD toxicity, III: 83-84; IV: 77, 331
Endometrial cancer, IV: 320-324, 385
England. *See* United Kingdom
Environmental Agents Service (EAS), II: 31; III: 28
  See also Department of Veterans Affairs (DVA)
Environmental Epidemiology Service (EES), II: 29
  See also Department of Veterans Affairs (DVA)

Environmental herbicide exposure
  accidental exposures, I: 364-365, 368-370; II: 141-143, 144, 148; IV: 114-116
  acute and subacute transient peripheral neuropathy and, II: 312-313
  agricultural areas exposure, I: 372-375
  Alsea, Oregon, I: 39, 42-43, 372-373, 598; II: 149
  assessment strategies, I: 262-263, 267-270; III: 144-145, 156-157
  basal/squamous cell skin cancer and, III: 323
  birth defects and, I: 608-609; II: 140, 287-288; III: 437
  birthweight, low, and, III: 459
  bladder cancer and, I: 516-517; III: 349, 350-351
  bone cancer and, III: 303, 305
  brain tumors and, I: 523; III: 358, 361
  breast cancer and, III: 328
  breast cancer estimated risk, II: 218
  cancer risk factor, I: 442
  cancer studies, I: 442, 444, 454-455, 469; II: 147-148, 179-180, 184
  chloracne and, I: 676-677
  circulatory disorders and, I: 701-702
  diabetes and, III: 497
  epidemiologic studies, I: 3, 301, 365-384, 469; II: 3, 6-7, 140-149; III: 197-205, 218, 232-236, 271-272, 275, 277, 279-281, 283, 285, 287-288, 290, 291, 297-298, 301, 303, 305, 309, 316, 323, 328, 333, 336, 338, 342, 344, 345, 349, 350-351, 353, 354, 358, 361, 365, 369, 373, 375, 380, 382, 388-389, 392, 437, 454, 455, 456, 459, 467, 497, 520; IV: 147-150, 224-231, 254
  evidentiary role of research on, I: 4-5, 222-223, 241-242
  female reproductive system cancers and, I: 511; III: 333
  gastrointestinal tract tumors and, II: 179-180; III: 271-272, 275, 277, 279-281; IV: 254
  hepatobiliary cancers and, I: 454-455; II: 184, 185, 186; III: 283, 285, 287-288; IV: 269
  Hodgkin's disease and, II: 236; III: 373, 375; IV: 366
  immune modulation and, I: 693-694
  infant death and, III: 456

leukemia and, I: 568-570; III: 388-389, 392; IV: 379
lipid/lipoprotein disorders and, III: 520; IV: 493
lung cancer and, III: 297-298, 301; IV: 282-283
melanoma and, III: 316; IV: 302-303
motor/coordination dysfunction and, I: 658-659
multiple myeloma and, I: 562; II: 243; III: 380, 382
nasal/nasopharyngeal cancer, II: 189; III: 290, 291; IV: 274-275
neonatal death and, I: 621; III: 455
neural tube defects, II: 297; III: 437; IV: 18
neurobehavioral disorders association studies, II: 306; III: 467
neuropsychiatric outcomes and, I: 651-653; II: 148
non-Hodgkin's lymphoma and, I: 540-541; II: 234; III: 365, 369; IV: 17
ovarian cancer and, III: 333; IV: 321-322
peripheral nervous system disorders and, I: 663-665
porphyria cutanea tarda and, I: 680-681
preterm birth and, III: 459
prostate cancer and, II: 221, 222; III: 336, 338, 342; IV: 329
renal cancers and, III: 353, 354; IV: 347
respiratory cancers and, I: 469; II: 190, 193, 200-201
soft-tissue sarcomas and, I: 491-492; II: 207-208; III: 319; IV: 116
spontaneous abortion and, I: 598-599
stillbirth and, I: 620; III: 454
testicular cancer and, III: 344, 345
uterine cancer and, III: 333
Vietnam exposure studies, III: 156-157
Washington residents, II: 149
See also Herbicide exposure assessment; Herbicides; Seveso, Italy; Times Beach, Missouri
Environmental Protection Agency (EPA), I: 39, 59-60, 93
  Alsea, Oregon, I: 42-43
  directives, IV: 117
  Science Advisory Board (SAB), II: 32; III: 29
  TCDD cancer potency estimate, I: 138
  Times Beach, Missouri, I: 41; III: 234; IV: 148
  Vietnam military use of herbicides, response, II: 32; III: 29-30, 136
Enzyme induction
  liver, I: 155-156
  lung, I: 170
  porphyria, I: 153-154
  TCDD and, II: 3, 66-67
EPA. *See* Environmental Protection Agency
Epidemiologic studies
  acute and subacute transient peripheral neuropathy, II: 312-314
  aging effects control, II: 261-262; III: 409
  agricultural/forestry workers, I: 318-323, 326-341; II: 118-120, 135-137, 183, 197-198, 232-234, 238-239, 241-243; III: 178-195, 224-232, 335, 364-365, 379-380, 387-388; IV: 134, 140, 144-145, 197-206
  Air Force personnel involved in herbicide spraying, II: 31-32; III: 28-29; IV: 232-235
  altered sperm parameters, I: 632; III: 445-449, 450
  amyloidosis, IV: 512
  autoimmunity, I: 697-698; II: 7; III: 488-491
  basal/squamous cell skin cancer, III: 317-322, 323
  birth defects, I: 607-618; II: 7, 140, 286-296; III: 436, 437-438, 443; IV: 400-405
  bladder cancer, I: 515-517; II: 7, 225-227; III: 7, 10, 347-351; IV: 340-342
  bone cancer, I: 472-473; II: 6, 204-205; III: 7, 10, 303-305; IV: 288-289
  brain tumors, I: 523; II: 7, 136, 229-230; III: 8, 12, 356-361; IV: 351-352
  breast cancer, II: 6, 176, 213-217, 218; III: 7, 10, 324-328; IV: 315-316
  cancer, I: 45, 59, 317, 320-323, 367, 383-384, 391-393, 401, 402-403, 435-445, 574; II: 133-138, 147-148, 175, 176; III: 265-266
  cancer latency issues, II: 260-276; III: 407-431
  case-control studies, I: 326-341; II: 94-95, 118-127, 138-140, 144-146, 148-149, 155, 157, 159-160, 183-184, 186-187, 188, 190, 193, 200, 222-223, 240-241; III: 173, 175, 185-195, 201-204, 208-217, 228-232; IV: 143-146, 207-220, 227-231, 236-245, 247

cervical cancer, III: 332
chemical industry production workers, I: 303-318; II: 114-118, 128-135, 191, 193-197, 206-207, 232, 237-238; III: 170-178, 218, 219-224, 363-364, 378-379, 386-387; IV: 134-140, 182-197
childhood cancer, I: 628-630; II: 7, 299-300
chloracne, I: 674-678; II: 5, 6, 318-320; III: 6, 7, 479-480
chronic persistent peripheral neuropathy, II: 310-311
circulatory disorders, I: 700-707; II: 7, 335-337; III: 8, 514-518; IV: 510
cleft lip/palate, I: 373-374, 375
cognitive/neuropsychiatric disorders, II: 7, 307-308; III: 468-469
cohort studies, I: 229-232; II: 105-109, 135-138, 141-147, 154-160, 178, 179, 180, 182-183, 186, 187, 190, 192-193, 204, 218, 222, 240; III: 170-185, 196, 197-200, 206-208, 217; IV: 140-143, 182-206, 222-230, 232-247
colon cancer, I: 12, 328-329, 576-577; II: 7; III: 8, 276-278
congressionally mandated, I: 50; II: 5
controlled observational, I: 228
cost of, I: 727
cross-sectional studies, IV: 187, 188, 196, 197, 199, 204, 226, 228, 229, 238, 242
cytogenetic studies, III: 365-366
developmental studies: 196, 227, 229, 231, 242
diabetes mellitus, I: 684-685; II: 7, 330-331; III: 494-502; IV: 482, 488-492
ecological design studies, IV: 231
evaluation of, I: 300-301, 591-592, 737-738; II: 5, 93-94; III: 129-130
evidentiary role of, I: 224-225, 228-237, 300, 305; II: 175, 176; III: 265, 266; IV: 104-105
female reproductive system/breast cancers, I: 508-511; II: 6, 211-213; III: 7, 10, 330-334
gastrointestinal tract cancers, I: 446-447; II: 7, 177-181; III: 8, 12, 268-281
gastrointestinal ulcers, I: 691; II: 334; III: 510-513; IV: 505
hepatic enzyme disorders, I: 686-688
hepatobiliary cancers, I: 453-455; II: 6, 176, 181-187; III: 7, 10, 282-288

herbicide environmental exposures, I: 365-384; II: 140-149, 189, 190, 193, 200-201, 207-208, 218, 221, 222, 234, 236, 241, 243, 287-288, 297, 306, 312-313; III: 197-205, 218, 232-236, 275, 277, 279-281, 283, 285, 287-288, 290, 291, 297-298, 301, 303, 305, 309, 316, 323, 328, 333, 336, 338, 342, 344, 345, 349, 350-351, 353, 354, 358, 361, 365, 369, 373, 375, 380, 382, 388-389, 392, 437, 454, 455, 456, 459, 467, 497, 520; IV: 147-149, 224-231, 255, 269, 274-275, 278, 282-283, 289, 293, 294, 302-303, 315-316, 321-322, 329, 336, 341, 347, 351-352, 357, 366, 372-373, 379
herbicide exposure assessment for, I: 251-259; II: 99-109; III: 142-146
herbicide exposure indices development, II: 107-109
herbicide exposure levels, II: 175
herbicide exposure reconstruction model and, I: 725, 726-728
herbicide occupational exposure studies, II: 107-108, 112, 113-140, 188-189, 190, 191-199, 206-207, 214-216, 218, 219-220, 222, 232-234, 235-236, 237-243, 286-287, 297, 306, 312; III: 170-196, 218, 219-232, 274-280, 282-283, 284, 287, 290, 291, 293-294, 296-297, 300-301, 303, 305, 308-309, 312, 316, 317, 321, 323, 324-326, 328, 332-333, 335-336, 337, 338, 341, 344, 345, 348, 350, 353, 354, 360, 363-365, 367-369, 372-373, 374-375, 378-380, 381-382, 386-388, 391-392, 437, 450, 454, 455, 456, 459, 467, 483-485, 489, 491, 496, 510-512, 515-516, 520; IV: 134-143, 182-223, 251-254, 268-269, 274, 277-278, 282, 288-289, 292-293, 302, 321, 327-329, 336, 340-341, 346, 351, 356, 365-366, 372, 379
herbicide/pesticide applicators, I: 323-326; II: 31-32, 120-122, 137-138, 198-200; III: 182-185, 226-228; IV: 202-206
Hodgkin's disease, I: 9, 329, 331, 335-336, 341, 384, 391, 393, 549-556, 574; II: 5, 6, 138, 235-236; III: 6, 7, 372-376
immune modulation, I: 693-696
immune system disorders, II: 7, 327-329; III: 488-491; IV: 480-481
infant death, III: 456

infertility, I: 632-633; II: 7, 280-282; III: 445-449, 450
kidney cancer, I: 515; II: 7, 139-140, 224-225; III: 352-355
laryngeal cancer, II: 202-203; III: 293-295
latency (cancer) issues, II: 260-276; III: 407-431
leukemia, I: 13, 332-333, 334-335, 564-571, 577-578; II: 7, 136, 245-247; III: 7, 10, 385-390, 391-392; IV: 379-380
limitations, I: 4, 223
lipid abnormalities, I: 688-690; II: 7, 333-334; III: 504-506, 520-521; IV: 493, 495
liver cancer, I: 13, 329, 391, 393
liver toxicity, II: 332-333; III: 510-513; IV: 499
low birthweight, I: 626-627; II: 7; III: 456-457, 459
lung cancer, III: 296-298, 300-301; IV: 282-283
melanoma, III: 313-317
meta-analysis, I: 225, 237-238, 242-243, 244
metabolic and digestive disorders, II: 7, 330-337
motor/coordination dysfunction, I: 658-661; II: 7, 309-310; III: 469-470
multiple myeloma, I: 11-12, 331, 334, 335, 336, 341, 557-563, 576; II: 6, 138-139, 176, 237-244; III: 7, 8, 9, 377-383
nasal/nasopharyngeal cancer, I: 459; II: 6, 176, 187-189; III: 7, 10, 290-291
neonatal death, III: 455
neural tube defects numbers, II: 297
neurobehavioral disorders, II: 305-308, 309-311, 312-314; III: 457
neurological disorders, I: 365-366, 642-648; II: 141
neuropsychiatric disorders, I: 649-657; II: 7, 148; III: 468-469
non-Hodgkin's lymphoma, I: 9, 328, 329, 330, 331, 333-334, 335-338, 383, 384, 391-393, 401, 528-548, 573-574; II: 5, 6, 134-135, 136, 138, 139, 231-234; III: 6, 7, 362-371, 428-430; IV: 356-358
NRC Commission on Life Sciences, I: 63
ovarian cancer, III: 333
pancreatic cancer, III: 280-281
paper/pulp workers, II: 126-127, 200, 243; III: 196, 232; IV: 134, 252

perinatal death, I: 620-624; II: 7, 285-286; III: 451-453, 454, 455, 456
peripheral nervous system disorders, I: 662-666; II: 6, 7, 310-311, 312-314; III: 7, 8, 470-471, 473
porphyria cutanea tarda, I: 680-682; II: 5, 6, 129, 321-323; III: 7, 8, 481-482
proportionate mortality studies, I: 232-233
prostate cancer, I: 11, 518-519, 575-576; II: 6, 176, 219-223; III: 7, 8, 9, 335-342, 426-428; IV: 327-329
Ranch Hand cohort, II: 31, 32, 109, 150-152, 154-156, 201, 209, 280, 283-284, 286, 293-295, 321-322, 330, 332, 336; III: 28-29, 218, 206-207, 237-240, 309-310, 313-314, 318, 321, 322, 339, 340, 385, 436, 438, 439, 446-447, 449, 452-453, 457-458, 481, 486, 495, 498, 502; IV: 13, 232-235
rare diseases in, I: 231, 499
recommendations, I: 15-20, 721-725, 731; II: 24-25; III: 23
rectal cancer, III: 278-279
reproductive outcomes, I: 41-42, 311-312, 321, 364-365, 368, 370, 371-375, 387-388, 389-390, 591-592; II: 280-282, 283-284, 285, 286-296; III: 436, 437-438, 443, 445-449, 450, 451-453, 454, 455, 456-457, 459; IV: 401-402, 406-407, 410-411
resolution in, I: 242-243; IV: 513
respiratory cancers, I: 10-11, 364, 461-472, 575; II: 6, 176, 189-203; III: 7, 8, 9, 418, 420-426; IV: 273, 278, 282, 284
respiratory disease, I: 709-713; II: 7, 324-326; III: 483-486; IV: 475
Seveso, Italy, population studies, I: 44-45, 365-368, 444, 454-455, 469, 491-492, 503, 511, 517, 523, 540, 568-570, 571, 598-599; II: 141-143, 148, 200-201, 206, 207-208, 209, 210, 211-212, 213, 216, 221, 225, 226-227, 228, 230, 234, 236, 243, 245, 246, 287, 299-300, 312-313; III: 197-200, 218, 232-233, 283, 285, 290, 296, 297-298, 299, 303, 307, 309, 314, 318, 324-326, 327, 330, 331, 332, 336, 338, 344, 348, 349, 352, 353, 356, 358, 363, 365, 372, 373, 380, 385, 386, 388-389, 390, 408, 414, 420, 422, 427, 436, 449, 495, 505; IV: 114-115, 464, 468, 472-475, 484, 487, 491, 501, 507, 509

INDEX 555

skin cancer, I: 502-503; II: 7, 209-211; III: 8, 10, 312-313; IV: 302-303
soft-tissue sarcoma, I: 8, 311, 326-328, 329-330, 335-336, 337, 339-340, 384, 391, 393, 395-396, 401, 403, 476, 477-500, 572-573, 574; II: 5, 6, 132, 134-135, 205-208; III: 6, 7, 306-311; IV: 116, 292-296
sperm abnormal parameters, II: 7; III: 445-449, 450
spina bifida, II: 6; III: 7, 8, 9-10, 437-438; IV: 404-405
spontaneous abortion, I: 42, 336-337, 372-373, 405-406, 596-605; II: 7, 283-284; IV: 410-411
state-sponsored, I: 399-405, 495-496, 546; II: 153, 158-159, 161, 202, 292; III: 213-215, 243-244
stillbirth, III: 454
stomach cancer, III: 274-275; IV: 251-255
strength of evidence in assessment of, I: 238-241
TCDD biomarkers, I: 259-262; II: 101-105, 318
testicular cancer, I: 405, 519; II: 7, 153, 227-228; III: 7, 10, 343-346; IV: 336
Times Beach, Missouri, I: 368-370; II: 144; III: 200-201, 218, 234, 283; IV: 115-116, 133, 148
usefulness of, IV: 103-108
uterine cancer, III: 333; IV: 321-324
Vietnam environmental herbicide exposure, II: 144-145; III: 201-202, 218, 234, 283
Vietnam veterans in, I: 50, 57-59, 62-63, 384-418; II: 149-161, 189, 190, 201-202, 204, 205, 208, 209, 212, 213, 216, 217, 218, 221, 223, 224, 226, 227, 228, 229, 230, 231, 234, 235, 236, 244, 245, 246, 278, 283, 285, 286, 288-296, 299, 300-301, 305, 306, 308, 309, 310, 311, 313, 314, 317, 318, 321-322, 323, 330, 332, 333, 336; III: 206-217, 236-245, 275, 277-278, 279, 281, 283, 285-286, 288, 290, 291, 294-295, 298, 301, 303, 305, 309-310, 312, 316, 317, 323, 326, 328, 333, 336, 338, 339, 340, 342, 343-344, 345-346, 349, 351, 353, 355, 358-359, 361, 363, 365, 370-371, 372, 373, 376, 380, 382, 385, 386, 389, 392, 435, 436, 437-438, 445, 446, 450, 454, 456, 457, 459, 467, 468, 469, 470, 473, 475, 479, 480, 481, 482, 485-486, 489, 491, 495, 497, 498, 500, 502, 505-506, 512-513, 516-518, 523; IV: 150-160, 232-247, 255, 269, 275, 278, 282-283, 289, 294-295, 303-304, 309-310, 316, 322-323, 329, 336-337, 342, 347, 352, 357-358, 366-367, 373, 380
Vietnamese in, I: 370-372, 599-601; II: 108-109, 144-145, 148, 287-288; III: 217, 245, 283; IV: 116-117, 227-228
See also Epidemiology; Exposure assessment

Epidemiology
acute lymphocytic leukemia, III: 383
acute myeloid leukemia, III: 383-384
birth defects, I: 606; II: 286; III: 435-436
bladder cancer, II: 223; III: 347
bone cancer, I: 472-473; II: 204; III: 302
brain tumors, I: 522-523; II: 228-229; III: 356
breast cancer, I: 505, 506-507; II: 213-214; III: 322, 324
cancer, I: 433, 435-438, 442, 525; II: 175; III: 265-266
children, cancer in, II: 298
chloracne, II: 317-318; III: 478-479
chronic lymphocytic leukemia, III: 384-385
chronic myeloid leukemia, III: 385
circulatory disorders, III: 514
diabetes mellitus, II: 330; III: 491-492, 493
female reproductive system cancers, I: 505, 506-508; II: 211; III: 329-330
gastrointestinal (GI) tract cancers, I: 445-447; II: 177; III: 267-268
gastrointestinal ulcers, II: 334; III: 508-509
hepatobiliary cancers, I: 452-455; II: 181-182; III: 282
Hodgkin's disease, I: 526, 527-528; II: 231; III: 371-372
immune system disorders, II: 326-327; III: 487-488
infertility, II: 279; III: 444-445
kidney cancer, I: 513, 514; II: 223; III: 351-352
laryngeal cancer, III: 292
leukemia, I: 564; II: 245; III: 383-385
lipid abnormalities, II: 333; III: 503-504
liver disorders, II: 331-332; III: 509-510
low birthweight, I: 625-626; III: 454, 455, 456
lung cancer, III: 295-296

malignant lymphomas, II: 231; IV: 137
multiple myeloma, I: 526, 528; II: 236-237; III: 377
nasal/nasopharyngeal cancer, I: 458-459; II: 187-188; III: 288-289
neurobehavioral toxicity, II: 304-305, 307; III: 466
non-Hodgkin's lymphoma, I: 526, 527; II: 231; III: 362
porphyria cutanea tarda (PCT), II: 321; III: 480-481; IV: 10
prostate cancer, I: 513, 514-515; II: 217, 219; III: 334
respiratory cancers, I: 460-461; II: 189-191
respiratory disorders, III: 482-483
skin cancer, I: 501-502; II: 209; III: 312, 313
soft-tissue sarcoma, I: 475; II: 205; III: 304, 306; IV: 116
spontaneous abortion, II: 282-283
stillbirth/neonatal deaths/infant death, III: 451
testicular cancer, I: 515; II: 223-224; III: 343
See also Epidemiologic studies
Epidermal growth factor (EGF), I: 145, 154; II: 59, 73-74; III: 77, 97; IV: 51, 64, 66
Epidermal growth factor receptor (EGFR), II: 67; III: 78, 80, 97; IV: 64, 67, 70
Epigenetic events. *See* Apoptosis; Cell proliferation; Enzyme induction; Intracellular communication
Epstein-Barr virus, I: 528; II: 188
Erbon, I: 309; II: 128; III: 219; IV: 134
EROD. *See* Ethoxyresorufin O-deethylase
Erythrocyte sedimentation, I: 696
Estrogen
  hepatic binding, I: 154
  receptor mediated responses, I: 145
  receptor signaling, III: 65-67
  transduction pathway, TCDD interaction, II: 4
Ethoxyresorufin O-deethylase (EROD), I: 153, 155; II: 52, 59, 60, 62, 63, 64, 65, 67, 69, 74; III: 40, 42, 51, 52, 53, 68, 69, 71, 72, 74, 75, 77, 91, 96; IV: 386
Europe, III: 108, 308, 471
European registry, II: 197
Evidence of herbicide association. *See* Herbicide association, insufficient evidence for determining; Herbicide association, limited/suggestive evidence; Herbicide association, limited/suggestive negative evidence; Herbicide association, sufficient evidence
Executive Order 11850, II: 27; III: 25
Experimental studies,
  evaluation of, II: 92-93
Exposure assessment. *See* Herbicide exposure assessment; Herbicide exposure reconstruction model
Exposure reconstruction model. *See* Herbicide exposure reconstruction model

F

Farmers. *See* Agricultural/forestry workers
Fecundity Ratio (FR), IV: 406
Federal government in herbicide management/research, I: 45-60; II: 27-32; III: 25-30; IV: 13
Federal Register, II: 30; III: 28
Federation of American Scientists, I: 29
Finland, I: 324, 364, 383-384, 443, 444, 467, 492, 541, 561; II: 134, 137, 140, 179, 183, 188-189, 198, 207, 220, 222, 226, 229-230, 233, 235, 243, 246, 269, 271; III: 226, 232, 234, 348, 372, 422, 472; IV: 142, 146, 149, 344, 353, 359, 361, 362, 368-369, 374-375, 381, 415
  Finnish Cancer Registry, II: 137
  Finnish Register of Congenital Malformations, II: 140
  Social Insurance Institution, II: 137
Florida, I: 324, 467; II: 199; III: 226; IV: 142, 258, 260, 263, 266, 286, 297, 327-328, 330, 333-334, 336, 338, 344, 349, 354
Follicle-stimulating hormone (FSH), II: 279, 280, 282; III: 41, 68, 72-73, 444, 445; IV: 399-400, 405, 408
Food crops, I: 89
  Agent Orange in destruction of, I: 62, 90
  as military target, I: 27, 31, 87, 97, 98-100, 106
Ford, Gerald, II: 27; III: 25
Foreign veterans, II: 113, 160, 202, 293; III: 9, 216-217, 218, 244-245, 273, 285-286, 290, 294, 295, 298, 299, 303, 310, 311, 314, 315, 327, 329, 339, 340, 343, 346, 349, 353, 355, 359, 365, 380, 389, 413, 423, 424, 469, 485, 486, 489, 500, 506, 512-513, 517

Forestry workers. See Agricultural/forestry workers
Forests
  2,4,5-T spraying, I: 42-43
  defoliant early field tests in, I: 26
  Vietnam forests, I: 31-32, 62, 90, 104; III: 137
  See also Agricultural/forestry workers; Lumber industry; Mangrove forests
Forest Service, U.S., I: 42; IV: 410
Fort Detrick, Maryland, I: 25
Free radicals, II: 4
  TCDD and, II: 60
Frierfjord, Norway, III: 236; IV: 149
FSH. See Follicle-stimulating hormone
Fungicides, I: 91

G

Gamma-glutamyltransferase (GGT), II: 331-332; III: 509, 510; IV: 499, 503
Gamma rays
  respiratory cancer and latency, II: 268; III: 418
Gastrointestinal (GI) disorders, III: 508-514; IV: 498-505
  cacodylic acid in, I: 188
  TCDD in, I: 169-170; IV: 19, 135, 156
  See also Gastrointestinal (GI) tract cancers; Ulcers, gastrointestinal
Gastrointestinal (GI) tract cancers
  biologic plausibility, I: 451; III: 281-282; IV: 256
  epidemiologic studies, III: 268-273, 274-281; IV: 251-255
  epidemiology, I: 445-447; II: 177; III: 267-268
  herbicide association in, I: 12, 447-451, 576-577; II: 7, 12, 21, 177-180, 250; III: 8, 12, 21, 268-282
  herbicide environmental exposure and, II: 179-180; III: 271-272, 275, 277-278, 279, 280-281; IV: 254
  herbicide occupational exposure and, II: 178-179; III: 268-271, 274-275, 276-277, 278-279, 280; IV: 251
  incidence, data by type/gender/race/selected age group, III: 267; IV: 250
  pancreatic cancer, epidemiologic studies, III: 280-281; IV: 250-254, 256, 385-386
  rectal cancer, epidemiologic studies, III: 278-279; IV: 250-251, 255-256, 262n, 264n, 385
  scientific literature update, II: 178-180; III: 268-273; IV 251-255
  Vietnam veterans and, I: 446, 452; II: 177, 180, 181; III: 272-273, 275, 277-278, 279, 281; IV: 255
  See also Colon cancer; Colorectal cancer; Gastrointestinal (GI) disorders
GBDS. See General Birth Defects Study
Gender
  acute lymphocytic leukemia incidence, data by gender, III: 384
  acute myeloid leukemia incidence, data by gender, III: 384
  bladder cancer incidence, data by gender, III: 347; IV: 339
  bone cancer incidence, data by gender, III: 302; IV: 387
  brain cancer incidence, data by gender, III: 356
  cancer studies and, II: 180, 181, 183, 190, 191, 204-205, 234, 242, 243, 246; IV: 199, 249
  chronic lymphocytic leukemia incidence, data by gender, III: 384
  chronic myeloid leukemia incidence, data by gender, III: 384
  diabetes prevalence, data by gender, III: 492
  gastrointestinal tract cancer incidence, data by type and gender, III: 267; IV: 145-146
  Hodgkin's disease incidence, data by gender, III: 372; IV: 356
  laryngeal cancer incidence, data by gender, III: 292; IV: 277
  leukemia incidence, data by type and gender, III: 384; IV: 378
  liver/intrahepatic bile duct cancers incidence, data by gender, III: 282; IV: 267
  lung cancer incidence, data by gender, III: 296; IV: 281
  melanoma incidence, data by gender, III: 313; IV: 300
  multiple myeloma incidence, data by gender, III: 377
  nasal/nasopharyngeal cancer incidence, data by gender, III: 289; IV: 273

non-Hodgkin's lymphoma incidence, data by gender, III: 362; IV: 356
renal cancers incidence, data by gender, III: 352
Seveso, Italy, in, IV: 148
soft-tissue sarcoma incidence, data by gender, III: 306; IV: 292
See also Demographic data, Vietnam veterans; Men; Women veterans
General Accounting Office, I: 52-53, 96; III: 139, 140; IV: 121
General Birth Defects Study (GBDS), I: 610, 626; II: 289, 290; III: 438, 439
See also Centers for Disease Control and Prevention (CDC)
General Services Administration, I: 77
Genetic alteration
 2,4-D in, I: 119, 178-179
 2,4,5-T in, I: 119, 184
 cacodylic acid in, I: 119, 187-188
 cancer mechanism, I: 433-434
 picloram in, I: 191
 reproductive outcomes, male-mediated, I: 593-594
 TCDD in, I: 118, 142, 143-144, 439
Genetic factors
 Ah receptor-mediated events and, I: 134
 cancer risk and, I: 10; IV: 249, 273, 300, 364, 386
 porphyria cutanea tarda and, I: 10, 679
Genetics. *See* Cytogenetics; Genetic alteration; Genetic factors
Geneva Protocol, I: 45; II: 27; III: 25
Genitourinary cancers, II: 223-224
 See also Bladder cancer; Kidney cancer; Prostate cancer; Testicular cancer
Georgia. *See* Atlanta, Georgia
German Democratic Republic, III: 226
Germany, I: 312-313, 326, 443, 477, 508-509, 530, 565, 675-676; II: 105, 108, 130-131, 149, 308, 319-320, 322, 323, 328, 331, 333; III: 221, 222, 223, 224, 232, 234, 235, 240, 269, 284, 308, 326, 332, 337, 357, 364, 365, 379, 386, 422, 423, 429, 470, 481, 483, 490, 506, 510-511, 515; IV: 137, 149, 156, 191, 195, 208, 420
German Cancer Research Center, III: 495, 506
 herbicide exposure assessment, III: 153-154, 158, 159-160; IV: 124, 257, 260, 263, 265, 271, 280, 285, 297, 301, 319, 333, 349, 353, 359, 368, 374, 381
 See also Aktiengesellschaft, Germany; Dormagen, Germany; Hamburg, Germany; Ludwigshafen, Germany; Uerdingen, Germany
GGT. *See* Gamma-glutamyltransferase
GI. *See* Gastrointestinal (GI) disorders; Gastrointestinal (GI) tract cancers
Givaudan Company, I: 43
Glucocorticoid receptor, I: 154
Great Britain. *See* United Kingdom
Ground/perimeter spraying, I: 20, 24, 74, 85, 90, 91, 94-96, 100, 272, 286, 287, 288-289; III: 138-140
 See also Herbicide application methods; Herbicides
Growth factors
 epidermal, I: 145, 154; II: 59
 TCDD induction of, I: 136-137; II: 4, 59; III: 62-63; IV: 66
 transforming, I: 145; II: 59
 tumor necrosis, II: 59
Guillain-Barre syndrome, II: 10, 312

H

Halogenated aromatic hydrocarbons, I: 125, 126, 151; IV: 41, 58, 68, 77
 hepatic enzyme induction and, I: 155
Hamburg, Germany, II: 195, 214-215, 329; III: 153, 223, 324-325, 515; IV: 191
Hamburg Boehringer Company, IV: 138
Hancock County, Ohio, III: 229; IV: 213
Hanoi, Vietnam, II: 148
Hawaii, I: 60, 400, 603; II: 292; III: 243
Hazardous materials disposal and cleanup
 Agent Orange surplus disposal, I: 93-94
 Nitro, West Virginia, accident efforts, I: 38; IV: 136
 Seveso, Italy, I: 43-44, 367-368
 See also Incineration, of Agent Orange
HBV_f. *See* Hepatitis B virus
HC. *See* Hydrocortisone
HD. *See* Hodgkin's disease
HDLP. *See* High-density lipoprotein (HDLP) receptors
Headaches, I: 650, 660
Health and Human Services, U.S., Department of, I: 57-59
Health care. *See* Military health care

INDEX 559

Health outcomes of herbicide exposure
    2,4-D outcomes, II: 48-49; III: 34, 38-39, 44-47
    2,4,5-T outcomes, II: 49; III: 48; IV: 185
    cacodylic acid outcomes, II: 50-51; III: 34, 50
    categories of evidence for assessing, I: 227-237
    categories of herbicide association in, I: 5-8, 221, 223-225, 246-247; II: 4-14, 19-22, 97; III: 6-15, 19-22, 132, 390, 392-394; IV: 6-12
    disease outcomes of, II: 37; III: 33-35, 38-43, 44-47, 48, 50, 71-105; IV: 22, 27, 110
    early herbicide research, I: 29-32, 35-36; II: 19-23; III: 19-23
    early TCDD research, I: 28-29
    evaluating exposure reconstruction model and, I: 289-290; IV: 85
    evidence insufficient for determining herbicide association in, I: 13-14, 19, 247, 457, 460, 473-474, 512, 521, 571, 577-578, 605, 618, 624, 627, 630, 634, 657, 666, 691, 699, 708, 713, 727; II: 6-7, 11-12, 20-21, 22, 97, 181-187, 249-250, 282, 284, 285-286, 298, 300, 325, 329, 334-335, 337; III: 7-8, 10-12, 21, 132, 133, 292, 304, 316, 322, 327, 332, 334, 346, 349, 351, 355, 390, 393, 444, 449, 453, 458, 459, 473-474, 486, 491, 503, 507, 513, 518, 522; IV: 11
    evidence limited/suggestive of herbicide association in, I: 10-12, 19, 247, 472, 519-521, 563, 574-576, 727; II: 6, 8-10, 20, 22, 97, 247-249, 298, 300, 323; III: 7, 8-10, 20-21, 133, 295, 299, 340, 342, 383, 393, 444, 458, 474, 482, 519; IV: 6, 7-11, 384
    evidence of no association of herbicides in, I: 12-13, 224, 247, 447-451, 503, 521, 525, 576-577; II: 7, 12-13, 21-22, 97, 177-181, 250-251; III: 8, 12, 21-22, 133, 359, 393-394, 522; IV: 7, 11, 384-385
    evidence sufficient for herbicide association in, I: 8-10, 246-247, 500, 548, 556-557, 572-574, 678, 682; II: 5, 6, 8, 19, 20, 21, 97, 247, 320; III: 6, 7, 8, 20, 132-133, 311, 366, 373, 374, 390, 392, 480, 519; IV: 8, 384

    research priorities, I: 19, 726-727
    research update, II: 37
    statistical association of herbicide exposure, II: 88, 90-91; III: 1-2, 6, 124, 126-127; IV: 6-12
    TCDD outcomes, III: 34-35, 71-105; IV: 20
    toxicity potential health risks, estimation of, III: 105-108; IV: 20
    Vietnam veterans' increased risk of disease, II: 14, 22-23, 88, 91, 218, 223, 251, 276, 283, 298, 300-301, 321, 323; III: 12-13, 14-15, 22-23, 124, 127-128, 329, 334, 343, 397, 430-431, 444, 462, 475-476, 491, 503, 507-508, 525; IV: 12, 403, 407, 411, 413, 417-418, 421-422, 424, 426, 431, 435, 459, 468, 475
    See also Epidemiologic studies; *specific cancers; specific cancer sites; specific diseases and disorders*
Healthy worker effect, I: 230
Hearing loss, I: 659-660
Heat shock protein (HSP90), IV: 30
Helicobacter pylori, II: 334; III: 268, 362, 509; IV: 145
Helicopters
    herbicide delivery use, I: 26, 86, 87, 93, 94; III: 135, 137, 138; IV: 117
Hematopoietic cancers, IV: 198
Hepatic phosphoenol pyruvate carboxy kinase (PEPCK), II: 63, 75-76, 77; III: 71, 72, 82
Hepatitis B infection, I: 453
Hepatitis B virus (HBV), II: 182, 183
Hepatitis C infection, I: 453
Hepatitis C virus, II: 182
Hepatobiliary cancers
    biologic plausibility, III: 286, 288
    epidemiologic studies, III: 282-288; IV: 268-269
    epidemiology, I: 452-455; II: 181-182; III: 282
    herbicide association and, I: 13, 577; II: 2, 6, 11, 12, 20, 89, 182-187, 249-250; III: 7, 10, 282-288
    herbicide environmental exposure and, II: 184; III: 283, 285, 287-288; IV: 269
    herbicide occupational exposure and, II: 182-184; III: 282-283, 284, 287; IV: 268-269
    incidence, data by gender/race, for selected age groups, III: 282; IV: 267

risk estimates, II: 186-187
scientific literature update, III: 284-286; IV: 268
TCDD and, IV: 77
Vietnam veterans and, II: 181, 185, 187; III: 283, 285-286, 288; IV: 269
See also Liver cancer
Hepatocellular carcinoma, II: 148; IV: 149
Hepatotoxicity
  TCDD and, II: 3, 73-75; III: 76-79; IV: 23, 71, 77
Herbicide application methods
  military early research, I: 25-26
  Operation Ranch Hand use, I: 85-87; III: 135, 136, 137, 138, 139
  Vietnam use, I: 1, 3, 24, 27, 74, 85-87, 94-96; III: 135-142
  See also Aerial spraying; Ground/perimeter spraying; Herbicides; Professional herbicide/pesticide applicators
Herbicide association, insufficient evidence for determining
  altered sperm parameters and, I: 14, 634; II: 7, 20; III: 449, 458; IV: 7
  amyloidosis, IV: 7
  basal/squamous cell skin cancer and, III: 322, 393; IV: 311
  basis for finding of, I: 13, 247, 577; II: 6-7, 11-12, 20-21, 22, 97, 249-250; III: 7-8, 10-12, 21, 133, 393
  birth defects and, I: 14, 605; II: 7, 20, 298, 300; III: 444, 458; IV: 7
  bladder cancer and, III: 7, 10, 132, 349, 351, 393; IV: 7, 19
  bone cancer and, I: 13, 473-474, 577; II: 6, 20, 205; III: 7, 10, 304, 393; IV: 7
  breast cancer and, II: 217; III: 7, 10, 327, 393; IV: 7
  chronic persistent peripheral neuropathy, II: 311, 314; IV: 7
  circulatory disorders and, I: 14, 708; II: 7, 21, 337; III: 518, 522; IV: 7
  cognitive and neuropsychiatric disorders and, I: 14, 657-658; II: 7, 20, 308-309, 314; III: 473-474; IV: 441
  diabetes mellitus and, I: 14, 691; II: 7, 21, 335; III: 503, 522
  female reproductive system/breast cancers and, I: 13, 14, 512, 577; II: 6, 20, 213; III: 7, 10, 332, 334, 393; IV: 7
  gastrointestinal tract ulcers and, I: 14, 691; II: 335; III: 513, 522
  genitourinary tract cancers and, I: 13, 521, 577
  hepatic enzyme abnormalities and, I: 14, 691
  hepatobiliary cancers and, I: 13, 577; II: 6, 20, 187; III: 7, 10, 286, 393; IV: 7
  immune system disorders and, I: 14, 699; II: 7, 21, 329; III: 491, 522; IV: 7
  infertility and, I: 14, 634; II: 7, 282, 300; III: 449, 458; IV: 7
  leukemia and, I: 13, 571, 577-578; II: 7, 20, 247; III: 7, 10, 390, 393; IV: 7, 198
  lipid abnormalities and, I: 14, 691; II: 7, 21, 335; III: 507, 522
  liver cancer and, I: 13, 457, 577
  liver toxicity and, II: 335; III: 513, 522
  low birthweight and, I: 14, 627; II: 7, 20; III: 458; IV: 7
  melanoma and, III: 316
  metabolic and digestive disorders and, II: 334-335; IV: 7
  motor/coordination dysfunction and, I: 14, 661; II: 7, 21, 310, 314; III: 474; IV: 7
  nasal/nasopharyngeal cancer and, I: 13, 460, 577; II: 6, 20, 189; III: 7, 10, 292, 393; IV: 7
  neonatal/infant deaths and stillbirths, IV: 7
  neurobehavioral disorders, II: 314; III: 473-474
  neuropsychiatric outcomes and, I: 14, 657, 666; II: 7, 20, 308-309, 314; III: 473-474; IV: 7
  perinatal death and, I: 14, 624; II: 7, 20, 285-286, 300; III: 453, 458
  peripheral nervous system disorders and, I: 14, 666; II: 21; III: 474
  renal cancer and, I: 13, 521, 577; II: 7, 20, 225; III: 7, 10, 355, 393; IV: 7
  research recommendations, I: 19, 727
  respiratory disorders and, I: 14, 713; II: 7, 21, 325; III: 486, 522; IV: 7
  skin cancers, II: 210-211; III: 8, 10, 21, 393; IV: 7, 19
  spontaneous abortions and, I: 14, 605; II : 7, 20, 284, 300; IV: 7
  testicular cancer and, I: 13, 521, 577; II: 7, 20, 228; III: 7, 10, 346, 393; IV: 7
  Vietnam veterans' children, cancer in, I: 14, 630; II: 7, 20, 300; IV: 7
Herbicide association, limited/suggestive evidence

INDEX

acute and subacute transient peripheral neuropathy, II: 314; III: 7, 8, 21, 474; IV: 6, 18-19
acute myelogenous leukemia (AML), IV: 7
    basis for finding of, I: 10-12, 247, 574-575; II: 6, 8-10, 20, 22, 97, 247-249; III: 7, 8-10, 20-21, 133, 393
    birth defects, IV: 6, 18-19
    cancer, I: 10-12, 519-521, 574-576; II: 247-249; III: 393
    diabetes, Type 2, IV: 6
    laryngeal cancer, III: 295, 393
    lung cancer, III: 299, 393
    multiple myeloma, I: 10, 11-12, 563, 574, 576; II: 6, 20, 244; III: 7, 8, 9, 20, 383, 393; IV: 6, 18-19
    neurobehavioral disorders, II: 314
    peripheral neuropathy, II: 6
    porphyria cutanea tarda, II: 6, 323; III: 7, 8, 20, 482, 519; IV: 6, 18-19
    prostate cancer, I: 11, 519-521, 575-576; II: 6, 20, 223; III: 7, 8, 9, 20, 340, 342, 393; IV: 6, 10, 18-19
    research recommendations, I: 19, 727
    respiratory cancers, I: 10-11, 472, 574, 575; II: 6, 20, 203; III: 7, 8, 9, 20; IV: 6, 18-19
    spina bifida, II: 6, 298, 300; III: 7, 8, 9-10, 21, 444, 458; IV: 7, 18-19
Herbicide association, limited/suggestive negative evidence
    basis for finding of, I: 12-13, 224, 247, 576-577; II: 7, 12-13, 21, 97, 250; III: 8, 12, 21-22, 133, 393-394, 522; IV: 7, 19-20
    brain tumors, I: 12, 525, 576; II: 7, 21, 230; III: 8, 12, 21, 359, 394; IV: 7
    gastrointestinal tract cancers, I: 12-13, 447-451, 576-577; II: 7, 21, 177-181; III: 8, 12, 21, 268, 273, 282, 394; IV: 7,19
    skin cancer, I: 12, 503, 576; III: 21
    urinary bladder cancer, I: 12, 521, 576; II: 7, 21, 227; III: 21
Herbicide association, sufficient evidence
    basis for finding of, I: 8-10, 246-247, 572; II: 5, 6, 8, 19, 20, 21, 97, 247; III: 6, 7, 8, 20, 132-133, 390, 392; IV: 6, 17-18
    cancer and, I: 8-10, 572-574; II: 247; III: 390, 392; IV: 6, 17-18
    chloracne and, I: 10, 678; II: 5, 6, 20, 320; III: 6, 7, 20, 480, 519; IV: 6, 17-18
    Hodgkin's disease and, I: 8, 9-10, 556-557, 573-574; II: 5, 6, 20, 236; III: 6, 7, 20, 373, 374, 390; IV: 6, 17-18
    non-Hodgkin's lymphoma and, I: 8-9, 10, 548, 573-574; II: 5, 6, 20, 234; III: 6, 7, 20, 366, 390; IV: 6, 17-18
    porphyria cutanea tarda and, I: 10, 682; II: 5, 6, 20; III: 20; IV: 6, 17-18
    soft-tissue sarcoma and, I: 8, 9-10, 500; II: 5, 6, 20, 208; III: 6, 7, 20, 311, 390; IV: 6, 17-18
Herbicide exposure assessment
    agricultural/forestry workers studies, III: 154-155; IV: 111-113
    biomarkers for, I: 17, 259-262, 280-284; II: 101-104; IV: 111
    cancer studies use, I: 436-439
    case-control studies use, I: 256-257; IV: 124
    Centers for Disease Control Agent Orange Study, I: 58; II: 102; IV: 124-125
    Centers for Disease Control exposure opportunity index, I: 274-276, 611-612; III: 147-148; IV: 124-125
    Centers for Disease Control validation study, I: 59, 260-261, 281-284, 387; II: 103, 104; IV: 125-126
    Centers for Disease Control Vietnam Experience Study, II: 101; III: 240; IV: 123
    cohort studies use, I: 254-256; II: 107-109
    cumulative exposure, III: 144
    current estimates, I: 284-287
    data sources (existing) limitations, I: 14-15, 290-291
    definition of, methodological issues, II: 4-5; III: 5-6; IV: 16, 20
    Department of Veterans Affairs mortality studies, II: 101; IV: 151, 157-58; IV: 123
    difficulties in, I: 14-15, 222, 247-248, 284, 286-287
    dioxin congeners, recent literature, II: 106-107; III: 158-159
    environmental studies use, I: 262-263, 267-270; III: 156-157; IV: 111, 114-116
    epidemiologic studies evaluation and, II: 99-101; III: 142-146
    evidentiary role of, I: 4, 15, 250-253
    exposure-dose relationship, I: 252-253
    ground spraying, I: 288-289; III: 138-140
    historic exposure reconstruction, I: 17-18, 19-20, 254, 255-256, 725-726, 728; III: 143

indices development, II: 107-109; III: 161-162
individual differences, I: 261, 286
job exposure matrix, I: 259-262
literature update, II: 104-109; III: 157-162
methodological issues, II: 4-5; III: 5-6
misclassification bias in, I: 17, 257-259, 724
non-military settings and, I: 4-5, 15, 222-223, 241-242
occupational studies use, I: 262-267, 269-270; II: 107-108; III: 150-156
paper/pulp mill workers, I: 266-267; III: 155-156; IV: 114, 134
process perspective, I: 252-253
Ranch Hand study use, I: 386; II: 109; III: 145-147
research recommendations, I: 16-18, 287-290, 291, 721-722, 724-725
risk assessment use, I: 14-15, 247-248, 250, 578; III: 14-15
sawmill workers, III; 10, 156, 227-228, 338, 439-440, 447-448, 449, 452, 453, 457; IV: 114
self-reports, I: 270-271; IV: 113
serum TCDD in, I: 19, 20-21, 261, 282-285, 289, 290, 725, 742-743; III: 159-161; IV: 135, 400
Seveso, Italy, accident, I: 267-268, 285, 598-599; III: 156; IV: 400
state-sponsored studies, I: 400, 401-402, 403-404
Stellmans' study, I: 278-279, 284
strategies for, I: 253-254; III: 144-145
TCDD exposure levels for epidemiological studies, II: 105-106; III: 159-161
TCDD half-life investigation, II: 104-105; III: 157-158; IV: 112, 115-116, 125-126
Times Beach, Missouri, case, I: 268, 368-369
Vietnam military records in, I: 271-280; IV: 125
Vietnam service as element of, I: 271, 284-287; II: 101-104; III: 146-150
Vietnam spray data, I: 273-279
Vietnam troop movement data in, I: 95-96, 273-279, 287
Vietnamese population, I: 108-109, 269, 731; III: 156-157; IV: 148-149
workshop on, I: 746-747
See also Environmental herbicide exposure; Herbicide exposure reconstruction model; Herbicides; Occupational herbicide exposure
Herbicide exposure reconstruction model
data sources, I: 725-726
epidemiologic research and, I: 726-728
evaluation of, I: 18, 289-290, 726; II: 25
recommendations, I: 15-16, 17-20, 287-290, 291, 721-722, 725-728; II: 25
Request for Proposals (RFP), II: 25-26; IV: 5
See also Herbicide exposure assessment; Herbicides
Herbicide/pesticide applicators. *See* Professional herbicide/pesticide applicators
Herbicides
action of, I: 88
acute and subacute transient peripheral neuropathy and, II: 2, 312-313; III: 7, 8, 473; IV: 441, 457
agricultural role of, I: 24, 35, 39, 174-175, 181
Air Force research activities, II: 31-32; III: 28-29
basal/squamous cell skin cancer association, III: 317-322, 323; IV: 311
biologic plausibility, II: 88, 92, 176, 217, 282, 298, 300; III: 2, 23, 124, 128, 281-282, 286, 288, 292, 295, 302, 304, 311, 317, 322, 327, 329, 334, 343, 347, 351, 356, 362, 366, 377, 383, 390, 444, 451, 453, 458, 460-462, 467, 480, 482, 486, 491, 502-503, 507, 513-514, 518, 522-525; IV: 22, 26, 29, 48, 85, 86, 249, 256, 270, 275, 279, 284, 290, 296, 306, 311, 318, 322, 323, 331, 332, 337, 342, 343, 348, 352, 358, 359, 367, 374, 380-381, 385
birth defects association, II: 286-298; III: 436-444; IV: 403
bladder cancer association, II: 225-227; III: 7, 10, 132, 347-351; IV: 342
bone cancer association, II: 204-205; III: 7, 10, 303-305; IV: 289
brain tumors association, II: 229-230; III: 8, 12, 356-362; IV: 352
breast cancer association, II: 213-217; III: 7, 10, 324-329; IV: 318
cancer latency issues, II: 2, 13-14, 175, 260-276; III: 3, 12-14, 407-431; IV: 289

INDEX

cancer risk and development, II: 13-14, 175; III: 12-14, 265-266
carcinogenicity, I: 118-119; II: 175; III: 265-266; IV: 256, 270, 275, 279, 284, 290, 296, 305, 311, 318, 323, 332, 337, 342, 348, 352, 358, 367, 374, 380, 387
cervical cancer association, III: 332; IV: 323
chemistry of, II: 38
childhood cancer association, II: 299-300; IV: 424-425
chloracne association, II: 318-320; III: 6, 7, 479-480; IV: 466
chronic persistent peripheral neuropathy and, II: 310-311
circulatory disorders association, II: 335-337; III: 3, 514-518; IV: 510
cognitive/neuropsychiatric disorders and, II: 307-309; III: 468-469; IV: 443
congressional hearings, II: 27-28; III: 25
congressional legislation on, II: 28-29; III: 26-27
Department of Veterans Affairs activities, II: 29-31; III: 27-28; IV: 151, 157-158
developmental toxicity, I: 124; IV: 403, 413, 416, 431, 434
diabetes mellitus association, II: 330-331, 334-335; III: 2, 11-12, 125, 494-503
disease outcomes of exposure, III: 6-15, 33-35, 38-43, 44-47, 48, 50, 71-105
early concerns about, I: 29-32, 35-36, 17-19; II: 26; III: 25
environmental exposure studies, I: 140-149, 184, 186, 189, 190, 193, 200-201, 221, 222, 234, 236, 241, 243, 287-288, 306, 312-313; II: 271-272, 275, 277, 279-281; III: 197-205, 218, 232-236, 283, 285, 287-288, 290, 291, 297-298, 301, 303, 305, 309, 316, 323, 328, 333, 336, 338, 342, 344, 345, 349, 350-351, 353, 354, 358, 361, 365, 369, 373, 375, 380, 382, 388-389, 392, 437, 454, 455, 456, 459, 467, 497, 520; IV: 249, 254-255, 258, 261, 263, 266, 269, 271, 274, 276, 278, 280, 282, 286, 289, 291, 293, 297, 302. 305-306, 309, 312, 314-316, 319, 321, 323, 325-326, 328-329, 334, 336, 338, 341, 344, 347, 349, 351, 354, 356-357, 361, 366, 369, 372, 375, 379, 382-383

Environmental Protection Agency research activities, II: 32; III: 29-30
evidence insufficient for determining association in health outcomes, I: 13-14, 19, 247, 457, 460, 473-474, 512, 521, 571, 577-578, 605, 618, 624, 627, 630, 634, 657, 666, 691, 699, 708, 713, 727; II: 7, 11-12, 20-21, 22, 97, 181-187, 189, 205, 210-211, 213, 217, 225, 228, 247, 282, 284, 285-286, 298, 300, 308-309, 310, 311, 314, 325, 329, 334-335, 337; III: 7-8, 10-12, 21, 132, 133, 286, 292, 304, 316, 322, 327, 332, 334, 346, 349, 351, 355, 390, 393, 444, 449, 453, 458, 473-474, 486, 491, 503, 507, 513, 518, 522; IV: 268, 270, 274, 275, 279, 288, 289, 302, 305, 308, 311, 314, 318, 321, 323, 329, 336, 337, 342, 348, 374, 380, 384, 400, 403, 406, 407, 410-414, 416, 418, 424, 425, 426, 430-432, 441-443, 448, 454-457, 475, 480, 495, 500, 505, 506, 510, 512, 514
evidence limited/suggestive of association in health outcomes, I: 10-12, 19, 247, 472, 519-521, 563, 574-576, 727; II: 6, 8-10, 20, 22, 97, 203, 223, 244, 298, 300, 314, 323; III: 7, 8-10, 20-21, 133, 295, 299, 340, 342, 383, 393, 444, 458, 474, 482, 519; IV: 7
evidence of no association in health outcomes, I: 12-13, 224, 247, 447-451, 503, 521, 525, 576-577; II: 7, 12-13, 21, 22, 97, 181, 227, 230; III: 8, 12, 21-22, 133, 268, 273, 282, 359, 393-394, 522; IV: 251, 256, 340, 351, 352, 385, 514
evidence sufficient of association in health outcomes, I: 8-10, 246-247, 500, 548, 556-557, 572-574, 678, 682; II: 5, 6, 8, 19, 20, 21, 97, 208, 234, 236, 320; III: 6, 7, 8, 20, 132-133, 311, 366, 373, 374, 390, 392, 480, 519; IV: 6
exposure assessment issues, II: 4-5, 99-109; III: 5-6, 135-162
federal government response to concerns over military use of in Vietnam, II: 27-32; III: 25-30
female reproductive cancers association, II: 211-213; III: 7, 10, 330-334
gastrointestinal tract cancers association, II: 177-181; III: 8, 12, 268-282; IV: 256

gastrointestinal ulcers association, II: 334-335; III: 510-514
hepatobiliary cancer and, II: 2, 176, 181-187; III: 7, 10, 282-288; IV: 270
Hodgkin's disease association, II: 235-236; III: 6, 7, 372-376; IV: 367
immune system disorders and, II: 327-329; III: 3, 488-491; IV: 480
immunotoxicity, I: 122-123
infertility association, II: 280-282; III: 445-451; IV: 407
International Agency for Research on Cancer research activities, III: 30; IV: 17, 133, 137-139, 252
laryngeal cancer and, II: 202-203; III: 292-295; IV: 279
latency and cancer risk, II: 13-14, 175, 260-276; III: 3, 12-14, 265, 407-431
leukemia association, II: 245-246; III: 7, 10, 385-390, 391-392; IV: 380
lipid abnormalities association, II: 333-335; III: 504-508, 520-521; IV: 495
liver toxicity association, II: 332-333, 334-335; III: 510-514; IV: 505
low birthweight and, III: 456-458, 459; IV: 416
lung cancer and, III: 296-302, 421, 422, 423, 424; IV: 284
mechanism of action, II: 36; III: 33, 38, 44, 47-48, 49-50, 53-71
mechanisms of toxicity, II: 37
melanoma association, III: 313-317; IV: 306
metabolic and digestive disorders association, II: 330-335; III: 3
military research and development, I: 25-26
military (U.S.) use ban, I: 32, 45
motor/coordination dysfunction and, II: 309-310; III: 469-470
multiple myeloma association, II: 237-244; III: 7, 8, 9, 377-383; IV: 512
nasal/nasopharyngeal cancer and, II: 2, 176, 187-189; III: 7, 10, 290-292; IV: 275
neural tube defects associated with herbicides, numbers, II: 297
neurobehavioral disorders and, II: 305, 306, 314; III: 3, 467, 468, 473-476; IV: 457
non-Hodgkin's lymphoma association, II: 231-234; III: 6, 7, 362-371, 428-430; IV: 358

occupational exposure settings, I: 36-38; III: 150-156
occupational exposure studies, II: 113-140, 182-184, 186, 188-189, 190, 191-200, 214-216, 219-220, 222, 232-234, 235-236, 237-243, 286-287, 306, 312; III: 170-196, 218, 219-232, 268-271, 274-281, 282-283, 284, 287, 290, 291, 293-294, 296-297, 300-301, 303, 305, 308-309, 312, 316, 317, 321, 323, 324-326, 328, 332-333, 335-336, 337, 338, 341, 344, 345, 348, 350, 353, 354, 357-358, 360, 363-365, 367-369, 372-373, 374-375, 378-380, 381-382, 386-388, 391-392, 437, 450, 454, 455, 456, 459, 467, 483-485, 489, 491, 496, 510-512, 515-516, 520; IV: 114, 249, 251, 253, 255-257, 259, 262, 265, 268, 270-271, 273-274, 276-282, 285, 288-290, 292, 296, 300-303, 305-307, 309, 312, 315, 317-318, 321, 324-325, 327-329, 331-333, 336, 338, 340-342, 346-348, 351, 353, 356, 358-361, 364-365, 368-369, 371-374, 377, 379, 381, 383
Operation Ranch Hand volume use, data by herbicide type, III: 136
ovarian cancer association, III: 333
perinatal death association, II: 285-286; III: 451-454, 455, 456; IV: 413
porphyria cutanea tarda association, II: 321-323; III: 7, 8, 481-482; IV: 468
preterm birth and, III: 456-458, 459
prostate cancer association, II: 2, 176, 217-223, 273-275; III: 7, 8, 9, 335-343, 426-428; IV, 10
renal cancer association, II: 224-225; III: 7, 10, 352-356; IV: 348
reproductive toxicity, I: 124; II: 278-301; III: 434-435
research recommendations, II: 23-24; III: 23; IV: 13
respiratory cancers and, II: 189-203, 268-273; III: 7, 8, 9, 418, 420-426
respiratory disorders association, II: 335-337; III: 3, 483-486
skin cancers association, II: 209-211; III: 8, 10, 312; IV: 305
soft-tissue sarcomas association, II: 205-208; III: 6, 7, 306-311; IV: 384
spontaneous abortions association, II: 283-284; IV: 411

statistical association with diseases, II: 88, 90-91; III: 1-2, 6, 124, 126-127
TCDD contamination of, I: 2, 3, 27, 91-92, 114, 126-127; II: 2, 3, 26; III: 3, 4, 5, 140-142
testicular cancer association, II: 227-228; III: 7, 10, 343-347; IV: 337
time-related factors and cancer risk, II: 263-264, 270, 271, 273, 274; III: 411-412, 421, 422, 423, 424, 426, 427, 429
toxicity profiles update, II: 45-77; III: 43-108
toxicokinetics, II: 35, 36, 38-39; III: 32-33, 36-37, 43-44, 47, 48, 50-53
toxicology, III: 3-5, 32-110
types of, I: 88
uterine cancer association, III: 333
Vietnam use by U.S. military, I: 1, 3, 24, 27, 74, 84-96, 98-107, 286; II: 1, 2, 26-27; III: 135-142
Vietnam veterans' cancer risk and latency, II: 276; III: 12-13, 430-431
Vietnam veterans' disease increased risk, II: 14, 22-23, 88, 91, 298, 300-301, 321, 323; III: 12-13, 14-15, 22-23, 124, 127-128, 329, 334, 343, 430-431, 444, 462, 475-476, 491, 503, 507-508, 525; IV: 2, 9, 12, 20, 103, 105-106, 124
Vietnam veterans' exposure concerns, II: 26-32
Vietnam veterans' exposure studies, II: 149-161, 185, 187, 189, 190, 201-202, 204, 205, 208, 209, 211, 212, 213, 216-217, 218, 221, 223, 224, 225, 226, 227, 228, 229, 230, 231, 234, 235, 236, 244, 245, 246, 278, 280, 283, 285, 286, 288-296, 306, 308, 309, 310, 311, 313, 314, 318-320, 321-323, 324-326, 327-329, 330-337; III: 206-217, 236-245, 272-273, 275, 277-278, 279, 281, 282-283, 287-288, 290, 291, 294-295, 298, 301, 303, 305, 309-310, 312, 316, 317, 323, 326, 328, 333, 336, 338, 339, 340, 342, 343-344, 345-346, 349, 351, 353, 355, 358-359, 361, 363, 365, 370-371, 372, 373, 376, 380, 382, 385, 386, 389, 392, 435, 436, 437-438, 445, 446, 450, 454, 455, 456, 457, 459, 467, 468, 469, 470, 473, 475, 479, 480, 481, 482, 485-486, 489, 491, 495, 497, 498, 500, 502, 505-506, 512-513, 516-518, 521; IV: 249-250, 255-256, 259, 262, 264, 266-267, 269-270, 272, 275-276, 278-281, 283-284, 287, 289-292, 294, 296, 298-299, 301, 303-311, 313-314, 316-320, 322-327, 329-332, 334-336, 338-340, 342-343, 345, 347-348, 350, 352-353, 355-359, 362-364, 366-367, 370-371, 373-374, 376-378, 380-381, 383, 387-388
See also Aerial spraying; Agent Orange; Agricultural herbicides; Chemicals and chemical industry; Defoliants; Desiccant herbicides; 2,4-Dichlorophenoxyacetic acid; Domestic herbicide use; Environmental herbicide exposure; Ground/perimeter spraying; Herbicide application methods; Herbicide exposure assessment; Herbicide exposure reconstruction model; Occupational herbicide exposure; Phenoxy herbicides; Professional herbicide/pesticide applicators; Selective herbicides; 2,3,7,8-Tetrachlorodibenzo-*p*-dioxin (TCCD); 2,4,5-Trichlorophenoxyacetic acid (2,4,5-T)
HERBS tapes, I: 20, 97-98, 602, 725; II: 108-109; IV: 123, 125
contents, I: 96-97, 273
deficiencies, I: 97, 104-105
exposure assessment use, I: 273-279, 287, 291; III: 146, 148
source of, I: 62, 85, 96
Hercules, Inc., I: 35
2,2′,4,4′,5,5′-Hexachlorobiphenyl (HxCB), II: 64, 65
1,2,3,6,7,8-Hexachloro-dibenzo-*p*-dioxin (HxCDD), II: 64, 65, 67
Hexachlorophene, I: 40; II: 128; III: 218, 219, 234; IV: 133-135, 138, 148
HI. *See* Humoral immunity (HI)
High-density lipoprotein (HDLP) receptors, II: 333, 334; III: 501, 503, 520-521
Highway workers, I: 326
Historic exposure reconstruction, I: 17-18, 19-20, 254, 255-256, 725-726, 728; III: 143; IV: 126-127
HIV-I. *See* AIDS/HIV
Ho Chi Minh City, Vietnam, II: 108; IV: 228
Hodgkin's disease (HD)
agricultural/forestry workers and, I: 328, 329, 331, 335-336, 341, 550-553; II: 138

biologic plausibility, I: 557; III: 377; IV: 367
chemical industry workers and, I: 549-550
epidemiologic studies, II: 138, 235-236; III: 372-376; IV: 199, 211, 212
epidemiology, I: 526, 527-528; II: 231; III: 371-372
herbicide association in, I: 8, 9-10, 556-557, 574; II: 5, 6, 20, 138, 235-236, 247; III: 6, 7, 20, 24, 372-376; IV: 17
herbicide environmental exposure studies, I: 384; II: 236; III: 373, 375; IV: 366
herbicide occupational exposure studies, II: 235-236; III: 372-373, 374-375; IV: 365
histopathology, I: 526-527
incidence, data by race/gender, for selected age groups, III: 372; IV: 365
research recommendations, I: 19, 727
scientific literature update, II: 235-236; III: 372-373; IV: 365
Vietnam veterans and, I: 258, 526, 554-556; II: 231, 236; III: 372, 373, 376; IV: 366
Vietnam veterans' compensation, II: 24, 30, 31
See also Malignant lymphomas
Hoffman-Taff, I: 40
Hormonal system
estrogen-mediated responses, I: 145, 154
TCDD carcinogenesis and, I: 116, 145
TCDD in, I: 156-159; IV: 71
TCDD-induced wasting syndrome and, I: 165
Hormones. *See* Follicle-stimulating hormone (FSH); Hormonal system; Luteinizing hormone (LH); Testosterone
Hourglass spray system, I: 25
House Committee on Veterans Affairs, II: 27; III: 25
H.R. 1565, II: 28
Human immunodeficiency virus (HIV-I). *See* AIDS/HIV
Humoral immunity (HI)
TCDD and, II: 69-70
HxCB. *See* 2,2',4,4',5,5'-Hexachlorobiphenyl
HxCDD. *See* 1,2,3,6,7,8-Hexachloro-dibenzo-*p*-dioxin
Hydatidiform mole, I: 30, 600-601
See also Reproductive disorders
Hydrocephalus, I: 609, 611
See also Reproductive disorders
Hydrocortisone (HC), II: 73

Hypercholesterolemia, I: 690
See also Lipid abnormalities
Hyperlipidemia, I: 152-153, 688, 692
See also Lipid abnormalities
Hypertension, I: 705, 706, 707, 708; IV: 135
See also Circulatory disorders
Hyperthyroidism
TCDD-induced, I: 168
See also Metabolic and digestive disorders
Hypoglycemia
TCDD-induced, I: 166-168
See also Metabolic and digestive disorders
Hypospadias, I: 609, 611
See also Reproductive disorders

I

IARC. *See* International Agency for Research on Cancer
ICD. *See* International Classification of Diseases
Iceland, III: 228, 319, 338, 339, 344, 353; IV: 142, 312, 333, 338
Association of Vegetable Farmers, III: 228
Cancer Registry, III: 228, 338
Committee on Toxic Substances, III: 228
Farmers' Association of Iceland, III: 228
Horticultural College, III: 228
Horticulturist's Association, III: 228
Market Gardeners Association Pension Fund, III: 228
National Registry, III: 228
Register of Deaths, III: 228
I Corps, I: 52, 96, 98, 394, 493-494, 542, 543, 546; II: 201; III: 139, 140, 241
mortality study, I: 233; IV: 121
II Corps, I: 542
III Corps, I: 59, 104, 276, 281-282, 542, 543; II: 228; III: 148, 344; IV: 125-126
IL. *See* Interleukin-1; Interleukin-4
ILO. *See* International Labor Organization
Immune system disorders
2,4-D toxicity, I: 181; II: 41; III: 46, 524; IV: 197
cell-mediated immunity, II: 69-70
cellular immunity, I: 147
endocrine system and, I: 150-151
epidemiologic studies, II: 327-329; III: 488-491; IV: 79, 195
epidemiology, II: 326-327; III: 487

herbicide toxicity, I: 122-123; II: 7, 11, 21, 327-329; III: 3, 488-491
humoral immunity, I: 147-148; II: 69-70
immune modulation in, I: 692-696, 698-699
macrophage function, I: 148
picloram toxicity, I: 192; II: 41; IV: 5
research methodology, I: 692
scientific literature update, II: 328-329; III: 489-491
suppression in, I: 693; II: 326, 329
TCDD toxicity, I: 119-122, 146-151, 338; II: 3, 40-41, 68-71, 328-329; III: 85-92, 488, 489, 490, 491; IV: 31-32
See also Allergies; Autoimmune disease; Autoimmunity; Systemic autoimmune disease; Systemic lupus erythematosus; Viral infection
Immunoglobulin antibodies, I: 693, 696, 697
2,4-D and, IV: 31
Immunotoxicity
TDCC and, IV: 26, 77-81
Incineration, of Agent Orange, I: 93-94; IV: 116
Indiana, III: 47
Industrial accidents, I: 316-317; III: 224, 232-233
BASF, I: 312-313, 444, 530, 550, 558; III: 153, 221; IV: 188-189
Nitro, West Virginia, I: 38-39, 305-307, 597, 607, 686, 700; III: 152-153, 220; IV: 136
Industrie Chimiche Meda Societa Anonima, I: 43
Infant deaths. *See* Perinatal death
Infertility, I: 631-634; II: 7, 11
biologic plausibility, II: 282; III: 451
epidemiological studies, II: 280; III: 445-449, 450
epidemiology, II: 279; III: 444-445
herbicide association in, II: 278, 280-282; III: 445-451; IV: 405-409
new studies summary, II: 280-281; III: 446-449, 450
Vietnam veterans and, III: 445, 446, 450
See also Reproductive disorders
Influenza, I: 713
See also Respiratory disorders
Insecticides, I: 87-88, 91
Institute of Medicine (IOM), I: 2, 20, 57, 62-64, 742, 743-744; II: 1, 2, 17, 24, 25, 27; III: 1, 2, 5-6, 17, 23, 24, 25, 125, 150; IV: 1, 15, 126

Interagency Working Group on the Long-Term Health Effects of Phenoxyherbicides and Contaminants, I: 46
Interleukin-1, I: 148; II: 59
Interleukin-4, II: 70-71
Internal Revenue Service (IRS), II: 152, 153
Social Security database, II: 151; III: 238; IV: 151
International Agency for Research on Cancer (IARC), I: 8, 12-13, 246, 264-265, 270, 313-314, 478, 479, 499, 565, 573, 577, 731; II: 101, 107, 131-135, 178-179, 196, 206, 212, 215, 220, 226, 232, 269; III: 20, 151, 175-177, 218, 222-223, 268, 269, 284, 290, 293, 296, 303, 306, 307, 308, 310, 311, 314, 319, 325, 326, 331, 337, 344, 348, 353, 357, 364, 378, 379, 386, 422-423, 424, 425, 429, 484, 511, 516; IV: 17
herbicide exposure assessment in occupational studies, III: 151-152, 154; IV: 111, 137-139; IV: 189-194, 252, 257, 259-260, 262-263, 265, 271, 276, 280, 290, 293, 296-297, 300, 306, 312, 318-319, 324-325, 333, 338, 341, 343, 348-349, 353, 359-360, 368, 374-375, 381
Vietnam military use of herbicides, response, III: 30
International Classification of Diseases (ICD), II: 325; III: 265; IV: 248, 249
ICD.9 cancer codes, SEER program site groupings for, III: 537-539; IV: 524-526
International Labor Organization (ILO), II: 324
International Register of Workers Exposed to Phenoxy Herbicides and Their Contaminants, I: 313-314; II: 131-135, 220, 232, 235, 238, 245; III: 175-177, 218, 222-223
International Society of Exposure Analysis, II: 25
Intracellular communication
TCDD and, II: 3, 67-68
Intrauterine growth retardation (IUGR), I: 625, 626; III: 455, 457; IV: 413-414
See also Reproductive disorders
IOM. *See* Institute of Medicine
Iowa, I: 11, 37, 60, 318-319, 332, 333, 334-335, 374, 400, 447, 495, 534, 550, 560, 567, 603, 660, 677; II: 8, 138-139, 219, 239, 248, 292; III: 224, 229, 234, 243,

335; IV: 140, 142, 143, 144, 149, 158, 210, 258, 261, 266, 290, 300, 334, 344, 349, 354, 361, 369, 375, 382
Iowa Health Registry, II: 138-139
See also Agricultural health Study
Ireland, Republic of, II: 136, 230, 233, 242, 246; III: 224-225, 363; IV: 198
Agricultural Institute, II: 136
Central Statistics Office of Ireland, II: 136
IRS. See Internal Revenue Service
Irvine, California, III: 533
Italy, I: 320-321, 338-340, 340-341, 384, 486-487, 492, 523, 537, 552, 553, 561, 566, 632; II: 183, 229; III: 9, 224, 230, 232, 234, 235, 271, 284-285, 294, 297, 299, 337, 358, 364, 373, 379-380, 387, 388, 516; IV: 133, 140, 144, 147-148, 149, 208, 212, 214, 230, 278, 282, 315, 325, 336, 341, 347, 351, 354, 357, 360, 368, 372, 375, 379 381, 425, 430, 445, 464, 472, 501, 507
Forli Province, III: 230
National Statistics Institute, II: 141
Novara Province, III: 225; IV: 197
Piedmont area, III: 224, 232
See also Lombardy, Italy; Milan, Italy; Seveso, Italy
IUGR. See Intrauterine growth retardation
IV Corps, I: 81, 98, 542

J

Japan, II: 237; IV: 414
Job exposure matrix, I: 256
Johnston Island, I: 93

K

Kansas, I: 9, 37, 335-336, 487, 490, 550; II: 231; III: 363; IV: 215, 260, 297, 361, 369, 446
Kaposi's sarcoma, I: 338, 487, 695; IV: 144, 214
See also Soft-tissue sarcoma
Khe Sanh-Thonh Son Lam area, I: 96; III: 140; IV: 121
Kidney cancer
biologic plausibility, III: 356; IV: 348
children and, I: 628; IV: 417, 420, 428

epidemiologic studies, I: 515; II: 224-225; III: 352-355; IV: 346-348
epidemiology, I: 513, 514; II: 223; III: 351-352; IV: 345-346
herbicide association in, I: 13, 521, 577; II: 7, 11, 20, 139-140, 224-225, 249-250; III: 7, 10, 352-356; IV: 342, 346-348, 385
herbicide environmental exposure and, III: 353, 354; IV: 347
herbicide occupational exposure and, III: 353, 354; IV: 346
histopathology, I: 513
incidence, data by race/gender, for selected age groups, III: 352; IV: 345-346
risk factors, I: 514; IV: 342, 345
scientific literature update, II: 224-225; III: 353, 355; IV: 346-347
Vietnam veterans' risk, I: 522; II: 223, 224, 225; III: 353, 355; IV: 348
See also Genitourinary cancers; Wilm's tumor
Kidneys
2,4-D toxicity in, I: 125, 179-180; II: 42; IV: 28, 37, 42, 43, 66, 68, 73, 76
arsenic toxicity in; IV: 39
cacolydic acid toxity in, II: 42; IV: 387
Korea, III: 240; IV: 156
Korean War, II; 150; III: 237; IV: 150

L

Laos, I: 106
Laryngeal cancer, I: 461, 470-471; II: 202-203; IV: 277-280
biologic plausibility, III: 295; IV: 279
epidemiologic studies, III: 293-295; IV: 277-278, 280-281
epidemiology, III: 292; IV: 277
herbicide exposure and, III: 293-295; IV: 9, 277-278
herbicide occupational exposure studies, III: 293-294; IV: 277-278
incidence, data by race/gender, for selected age groups, III: 292; IV: 277
larynx, IV: 6, 8, 9
scientific literature update, III: 293-294, 295; IV: 277-278
Vietnam veterans studies, III: 294-295; IV: 278
See also Respiratory cancers

INDEX 569

Latency effects in cancer studies, I: 231-232,
434, 435, 436-438, 494, 495, 727; II: 2,
13-14, 175; III: 3, 12-14, 266, 407-408
  aging effects control, II: 261-262; III: 409
  arsenic and, II: 268; III: 420
  asbestos and, II: 268; III: 420
  data limitations, III: 413, 414, 415, 416
  data requirements, II: 264, 265, 266; III:
    412, 414, 415, 416; IV: 283
  epidemiological studies, analysis of, II:
    261-266; III: 408-412
  epidemiological studies, new, III: 419; IV:
    148, 254, 256, 269, 293, 329, 473, 483,
    484, 506
  gamma rays and, II: 268; III: 418
  literature review results, II: 266-267; III:
    416-418, 420-424, 426-427, 429; IV:
    257, 260, 263, 265, 271, 280, 297, 333,
    343, 353, 368, 375
  measurement errors, II: 263-264; III: 411-
    412
  mortality and incidence studies for
    examining, II: 263; III: 410-411, 421,
    422, 423, 424, 426, 427, 429
  nickel and, II: 269; III: 420
  non-Hodgkin's lymphoma, III: 428-430
  potential problems with, II: 264, 265, 266;
    III: 413, 414, 415, 416
  prostate cancer, II: 273-275; III: 426-428
  radon daughters and, II: 268; III: 418
  random misclassification and, II: 263-264;
    III: 411-412
  relative risks, II: 264, 265, 266, 271, 275,
    351; III: 412, 413, 414, 415, 418, 420,
    422, 426-427, 428, 430-431
  respiratory cancer, II: 268-273; III: 418,
    420-426; IV: 284, 285
  smoking and, II: 268; III: 418; IV: 250, 273
  time-related factors, II: 262, 263-264; III:
    411-412, 421, 422, 423, 424, 426, 427,
    429; IV: 464, 465
  Vietnam veterans, relevancy for, II: 276,
    351; III: 12-13, 430-431; IV: 466
  See also Cancer
Lawn care, I: 119, 177-178; IV: 274
LDL. See Low-density lipoprotein (LDL)
  receptors
Leather tanners, I: 486, 514
Legal issues
  Agent Orange manufacturers' liability, I:
    34-35
  federal government liability, I: 34
  South Korean Vietnam veterans, I: 62
  Times Beach, Missouri, I: 41; IV: 133
Legislation
  epidemiologic studies on Agent Orange, II:
    28; III: 26
  federal, I: 45-60; III: 26-27
  health care associated with Agent Orange,
    II: 28
  Public Law 91-441, I: 47, 62
  Public Law 96-151, I: 50, 52, 57; II: 28; III:
    26, 240
  Public Law 97-72, I: 50; II: 28; III: 26
  Public Law 98-181, I: 51
  Public Law 98-542, I: 50-51; II: 28-29; III:
    26-27
  Public Law 99-272, I: 50; II: 28; III: 26
  Public Law 100-687, I: 51
  Public Law 101-239, I: 51
  Public Law 102-4, I: 2, 7, 20, 21, 51, 572,
    721, 728-730; II: 1, 5, 17, 19, 29, 97,
    247; III: 1, 6, 14, 17, 20, 124, 132, 390,
    397, 462, 475, 519, 525; IV: 1, 2, 6, 15,
    103, 132, 388
  Public Law 102-585, II: 28; III: 26
  Public Law 103-452, II: 28; III: 26
  Public Law 104-110, III: 26
  Public Law 104-204, III: 24, 26
  Public Law 104-262, III: 26
  Public Law 105-114, III: 25
  Veterans' Health Programs Extension and
    Improvement Act of 1979, III: 240
  Vietnam veterans' compensation, I: 47, 50-
    51, 55-56; II: 28-29; III: 26-27
Leiomyosarcomas, I: 475
  See also Soft-tissue sarcoma
Lethality. See Deaths
Leukemia
  acute lymphocytic leukemia, III: 383, 384;
    IV: 377
  acute myelogenous leukemia, IV: 417-429,
    432
  acute myeloid leukemia, III: 383-384; IV:
    9, 377
  agricultural workers and, I: 13, 332-333,
    334-335, 566-568; II: 136; III: 387-388;
    IV: 140, 143-144, 216
  children and, I: 628; IV: 18, 417-424
  chronic lymphocytic leukemia, III: 384-
    385; IV: 208, 211, 377, 417, 422

chronic myeloid leukemia, III: 384, 385; IV: 377-378, 417
epidemiologic studies, I: 564-572; II: 136, 245-247; III: 385-390, 391-392; IV: 149, 198; IV: 379-380, 381-383, 418-422, 427-429
epidemiology, I: 564; II: 245; III: 383-385; IV: 377-378
herbicide association in, I: 13, 571, 577-578; II: 7, 11, 20, 245-247, 249-250; III: 7, 10, 385-390, 391-392; IV: 379-380, 385, 418-422
herbicide environmental exposure and, III: 388-389, 392; IV: 379, 419-420
herbicide occupational exposure and, III: 386-388, 391-392; IV: 379, 418-419
incidence, data by type/race/gender, for selected age groups, III: 384; IV: 377-378
production workers and, I: 564-566; III: 386-387; IV: 379
pulp/paper workers and, I: 568; IV: 379
risk factors, I: 564
scientific literature update, II: 245-246; III: 386-389; IV: 379-380, 418-422
Seveso, Italy, studies, I: 13, 568-570, 571, 577; III: 385, 386, 388-389, 390; IV: 379
TCDD biologic plausibility in, I: 571; III: 390; IV: 380-381, 426
Vietnam veterans' risk, I: 564, 570, 571-572; II: 245, 246; IV: 381, 426
Vietnam veterans' studies, III: 385, 386, 389, 392; IV: 373, 380, 420-422
Leydig cells, II: 71, 279; III: 445; IV: 405
LH. *See* Luteinizing hormone
Lindane, I: 91
Lipid and Lipoprotein Disorders, I: 688-690, 692; IV: 492-497
biologic plausibility, III: 507; IV: 495
epidemiologic studies, I: 45; II: 333, 334; III: 504-506, 520-521; IV: 479, 493-494, 496-497
epidemiology, II: 333; III: 503-504; IV: 492-493
herbicide environmental exposure and, III: 520; IV: 493-494
herbicide exposure association with, II: 7, 21, 333-334; III: 504-508, 520-521; IV: 493-494

herbicide occupational exposure and, III: 520; IV: 493-494
scientific literature update, II: 334; III: 504-506, 520, 521; IV: 493-494
TCDD in, I: 152-153, 259-260; II: 333, 334; III: 505, 506, 507; IV: 471, 474, 493-495
Vietnam veterans and, II: 333; III: 505-506, 521; IV: 494
See also Hypercholesterolemia; Hyperlipidemia; Liver disorders; Metabolic and digestive disorders
Listeria
TCDD exposure and, II: 68
Liver cancer
background, IV: 267
biologic plausibility, IV: 270
children and, I: 628
epidemiologic studies, I: 453-455; IV: 268-270
herbicide association in, I: 13, 457, 577; IV: 143, 157, 385
picloram in, I: 190
research recommendations, I: 19, 727
risk factors, I: 453
Seveso, Italy, studies, I: 454-455; IV: 269
TCDD in, I: 116, 138-139, 142, 143; IV: 267, 386-387, 515
Vietnam veterans and, I: 391, 393, 455, 457; IV: 269
See also Hepatobiliary cancers
Liver disorders
2,4-D in, I: 179; III: 524; IV: 505
2,4,5-T in, II: 42; III: 524; IV: 500, 505
arsenic and, IV: 39-41
biologic plausibility, III: 513-514, 524; IV: 505
enzyme activity, I: 155-156, 685-687, 691-692
epidemiologic studies, I: 45; II: 332-333; III: 510-513; IV 500-504
epidemiology, II: 331-332; III: 509-510; IV: 498-500
herbicide occupational exposure and, III: 510-512; IV: 500-501
herbicides in, I: 125; II: 332-333; III: 510-514; IV: 135, 139, 141, 500-505
picloram chronic toxicity, I: 191-192; II: 42; III: 524
scientific literature update, II: 332-333; III: 510-513; IV: 500-504

Seveso, Italy, studies, I: 367; IV: 501-502
TCDD in, I: 115, 124, 129-130, 151-156, 165-166; II: 42, 331-333; III: 509; IV: 25-30, 34, 37, 41-44, 56-60, 66-73, 77, 83, 498-505
Vietnam veterans and, II: 332; III: 512-513; IV: 502-504
See also Lipid abnormalities; Metabolic and digestive disorders
Lombardy, Italy, II: 147, 299; IV: 329
Low birthweight
biologic plausibility, III: 458; IV: 416-417
definition, I: 625; IV: 413-414
epidemiologic studies, III: 456-457, 459; IV: 414-416
epidemiology, I: 625-626; III: 454, 455, 456; IV: 413-414
herbicide association in, I: 14, 627-628; II: 7, 11, 20; III: 456-458, 459; IV: 413-417
herbicide environmental exposure and, III: 459; IV: 414-416
herbicide occupational exposure and, III: 459; IV: 414-416
risk factors, I: 625-626; IV: 412
scientific literature update, III: 457, 459; IV: 414-416
Vietnam veterans exposure studies, III: 457, 459; IV: 417
See also Preterm delivery (PTD); Reproductive disorders
Low-density lipoprotein (LDL) receptors, I: 154-155; II: 333, 334; III: 503; IV: 489, 492
Ludwigshafen, Germany; III: 153, 154, 269, 297, 484, 511
Lumber industry
sawmill workers herbicide exposure, III: 10, 156, 227-228, 338, 439-440, 447-448, 449, 452, 453, 457; IV: 114, 142, 290, 296, 306, 307, 312, 333, 338, 343, 368, 404, 408, 418, 419, 422, 427
See also Forests
Lung cancer
2,4-D in, I: 177
agricultural/forestry workers and, I: 466; IV: 142
biologic plausibility, III: 302; IV: 284
cacodylic acid and, I: 187; IV: 24
environmental exposure studies, III: 297-298, 301; IV: 282-283

epidemiological studies, II: 139; III: 296-298, 300-301; IV: 157, 210, 278, 282-284, 285-287, 473
epidemiology, III: 295-296; IV: 281
herbicide association in, I: 472; II: 6; III: 296-302; IV: 282-284
herbicide/pesticide applicators and, I: 326, 466-468; II: 139; IV: 142
incidence, data by gender/race, for selected age groups, III: 296; IV: 281
latency and, III: 421, 422, 423, 424
occupational exposure studies, III: 296-297, 300-301, 421, 423; IV: 142, 144, 282
paper/pulp mill workers and, I: 364, 468
production workers and, I: 461-466; III: 421, 423; IV: 282
Ranch Hands, IV: 9, 283
scientific literature update, III: 296-298; IV: 282-284
Seveso, Italy, studies, I: 469; III: 296, 297-298, 299, 422; IV: 278, 282-283
Vietnam veterans and, I: 469-470, 472; III: 298, 301, 424; IV: 283, 284
See also Respiratory cancers
Luteinizing hormone (LH), II: 182, 279, 280, 281; III: 41, 72-73, 444-445; IV: 34, 399, 405
Lymphocytic leukemia. *See* Leukemia

M

Maine, I: 60, 400, 603; II: 292; III: 243; IV: 158
Malathion, I: 87, 88, 91
Malignant lymphomas
2,4-D exposure and, I: 119, 177-178
epidemiology, II: 231; IV: 137, 140, 143
See also Hodgkin's disease (HD); Multiple myeloma; Non-Hodgkin's lymphoma (NHL)
Mangrove forests, I: 31, 62, 90, 104
See also Forests
Manitoba, Canada, II: 135-136, 232, 242, 246; IV: 198
March of Dimes, II: 286; III: 435; IV: 400
Marine Corps. *See* U.S. Marine Corps
Maryland. *See* Fort Detrick, Maryland
Massachusetts, I: 60, 400-401, 405-406, 445, 470, 496, 602-603, 613, 620, 621, 622; II: 202, 291; III: 243, 244, 303, 310,

315, 339, 346, 349, 353; IV: 158, 291, 298, 299, 308, 334, 339, 345, 350, 363
Cancer Registry, III: 244
Mast cells, I: 693
MC-1 spray system, I: 25
MCPA. *See* 4-Chloro-2-methylphenoxyacetic acid
MCPP. *See* 2-[4-chloro-2-methylphenoxy]-propanoic acid
Medical Literature Analysis and Retrieval System, I: 735
Mekong Delta, II: 104
Melanoma
  biologic plausibility, III: 317; IV: 305
  epidemiologic studies, III: 313-317; IV: 299-302, 306-308
  herbicide association with, III: 313-317; IV: 302-308
  herbicide environmental exposure and, III: 316; IV: 302, 303
  herbicide occupational exposure and, III: 316, 317; IV: 302
  incidence of, III: 313, 315; IV: 299-300
  mortality studies, III: 314-315, 316; IV: 306-307
  scientific literature update, III: 314-315; IV: 302-304
  Vietnam veterans studies, III: 316, 317; IV: 303-306
  See also Basal/squamous cell skin cancer; Skin cancer
Melatonin, TCDD-induced wasting syndrome and, I: 165
Meta-analysis, I: 243, 244
Meta risk ratio (MRR), IV: 253, 265, 267n
Metabolic and digestive disorders
  biological plausibility, II: 335; III: 513-514; IV: 505
  epidemiological studies, II: 330-331, 332-335; III: 510-513; IV: 500-504
  epidemiology, III: 508; IV: 498-500
  herbicides association in, II: 7, 11, 21, 330-331, 332-335; III: 3, 510-514; IV: 500-505
  herbicides occupational exposure and, III: 510-512; IV: 500-501
  scientific literature update, III: 510-513; IV: 500-504
  Vietnam veterans and, III: 510, 512-513; IV: 502-504

See also Diabetes mellitus; Hyperthyroidism; Hypoglycemia; Lipid abnormalities; Liver toxicity; Ulcers, gastrointestinal
Methodological bias
  biological stored samples, analysis, I: 20-21, 729-730
  cancer studies, I: 436
  controlling for, I: 33, 226-227, 234-235, 242-246; IV: 105, 108-09
  healthy worker effect, I: 230
  herbicide exposure assessment, I: 17, 257-259, 286-287, 291, 724
  latency studies, II: 263-264; III: 408-412
  proportionate mortality studies, I: 233
  recall bias, I: 256, 601
  reproductive outcome studies, I: 591-592, 601
  self-reports, I: 270-271; II: 109, 150
  See also Methodology
Methodology
  Agent Orange Study, I: 58-59, 63-64; II: 2
  Agent Orange Working Group, I: 19, 728
  Alsea, Oregon, investigation, I: 372-373, 598
  American Legion Agent Orange study, I: 602
  assessment of strength of evidence, I: 238-241; II: 88-97; III: 124-133
  BASF study, I: 312-313
  biologic plausibility, II: 88, 92; III: 124, 128
  burden of proof approach, I: 226-227, 245
  cancer expected incidence, I: 439-440
  cancer studies, I: 435-440, 442-443, 445; II: 175, 176; III: 265-266
  case-control studies, I: 234-235, 256-257, 326-341; II: 94-95; III: 130; VI: 9
  case reports, I: 235-236
  Centers for Disease Control Birth Defects Study, I: 611-612
  Centers for Disease Control epidemiologic studies, I: 19, 387-393, 498, 728
  circulatory disease studies, I: 699-700, 705-706, 707; II: 335; IV: 11, 463, 502, 506
  cohort studies, I: 229-232, 254-256, 318-323; IV: 8-13, 28, 43, 46, 111, 114, 123-161 *passim*, 182-247 *passim*, 251-253, 256-388 *passim*, 402, 409, 418-422, 425-431, 473-474, 478-479, 483, 486-492, 500-509

INDEX 573

confidence intervals, I: 244; IV: 19, 43, 251, 278, 342, 385, 419, 445, 472, 483, 515
controlled observational studies, I: 228
Department of Veterans Affairs studies, I: 393-399, 494-495; IV: 1, 15, 133, 151, 157-158, 255, 284, 399, 421
disease latency effects, I: 231-232, 434, 436-438, 494, 495, 727; II: 351-357
dose-response relationship, I: 239-230, 252; II: 89; IV: 40
Dow studies, I: 307-312
epidemiologic studies evaluation, I: 300-301; II: 93-94; III: 129-130; IV: 103-109, 132-161, 182-247
evidence categories, I: 227-237; III: 132; IV: 103-109 *passim*
experimental studies evaluation, II: 92-93
health outcome categories for herbicide association, I: 5-8, 223-225, 246-247; II: 97; III: 132; IV: 6-12
herbicide environmental exposure assessment, I: 262-263, 269-270; III: 156-157
herbicide exposure assessment strategies, I: 251-259, 270-287; III: 144-145
herbicide exposure reconstruction model evaluation, I: 18, 289-290, 726; II: 25
herbicide exposure, statistical association with diseases, II: 88, 90-91; III: 1-2, 6, 126-127; IV: 103
herbicide occupational exposure assessment, I: 262-264, 269-270; III: 150-156
immune system research, I: 692
indirect adjustment, I: 229
information management, I: 735-738
judgment in, I: 245-246; II: 96; III: 131-132
latency and cancer studies, II: 261-266, 351; III: 407-416
meta-analysis, I: 225, 237-238, 242-243
neurological assessment, I: 14, 641-642, 649
neuropsychiatric studies, I: 657
new evidence integration, II: 96; III: 132
NIOSH studies, I: 303-305; II: 350-351, 356, 357; IV: 111, 136
Nitro, West Virginia, industrial accident studies, I: 305-307
NRC Commission on Life Sciences, I: 63

odds ratio determination, I: 234, 239; II: 90; III: 126-127; IV: 105
Office of Technology Assessment, I: 19, 728
paper/pulp mill worker studies, I: 341, 364
publication bias, II: 95-96; III: 131; IV: 108
Ranch Hand study, I: 230-231, 385-386, 498, 757-762
random misclassification and latency, II: 263-264; III: 411-412
relative risk assessment, I: 229, 239, 258; II: 90, 351, 356; III: 126, 127; IV: 105
reproductive outcome studies, I: 591-592
respiratory disease studies, I: 708-709, 712-713; II: 324
risk assessment, I: 225-226; II: 89; III: 127-128
sample size and disease frequency, I: 231, 242-243, 440, 499
Selected Cancers Study, I: 234-235, 498
self-reports, I: 270-271; II: 109; IV: 9, 113, 122, 125-126, 135, 141, 154-157, 159, 255, 262, 287, 297, 299, 304, 308, 310, 313, 320, 324, 325, 326, 335, 336-337, 339, 364, 380, 383, 402, 406, 418-419, 421-425, 484, 487, 492, 503-504, 507-509
soft-tissue sarcoma studies, I: 482-490, 497-500
standardized mortality ratio, I: 229-230
statistical significance/power, I: 226-227, 243
TCDD biomarkers, I: 259-262
Times Beach studies, I: 368-370
toxicologic studies evaluation, III: 128-129
type I error, I: 243
type II error, I: 243
Vietnam veterans disease risk estimation and latency, II: 349-357
Vietnam veterans serum TCDD mean maximum estimation, II: 349-350
See also Data sources; Literature review; Methodological bias; Research needs; Risk assessment methodology
2-Methyl-4-chlorophenoxyacetic acid, I: 700
6-Methyl-1,3,8-trichlorodibenzofuran, I: 153
Michigan, I: 374, 375, 383; II: 113, 153, 161, 202, 308; III: 159, 160, 218, 221, 234, 235, 243, 270, 357-358, 363, 373, 387, 388, 484, 511, 516; IV: 133, 136, 149, 158, 231, 266, 335, 350, 355, 363, 368, 370, 381, 383, 414

Department of Management and Budget's Vietnam-era Bonus List, II: 153, 161, 202, 208, 221, 225, 230, 234, 236, 246; III: 308, 336, 353, 489
Department of Public Health, II: 161
 See also Detroit, Michigan; Midland, Michigan; Tecumseh, Michigan
Midland, Michigan, III: 152, 221, 234; IV: 149
Midwest Research Institute, I: 29-30
Milan, Italy, II: 243; III: 232; IV: 144
Military health care
 Agent Orange legislation, II: 28; III: 26, 27
 Department of Veterans Affairs activities, II: 29; III: 27
Military occupation specialty code (MOS), II: 153; III: 242
Military operations
 Agent Orange surplus disposal, I: 93-94
 herbicide early research, I: 25-26; II: 27-32; III: 25-30
 herbicide (strategic) use ban, I: 32, 45
 herbicide use precautions, I: 95
 South Vietnam tactical zones, I: 98
 Vietnam distribution of personnel, I: 81, 82
 Vietnam herbicide applications, I: 1, 3, 24, 27, 74, 84-96, 98-107, 286; II: 26-27; III: 135-142
 Vietnam herbicides aerial spraying, I: 27, 85-91; II: 26; III: 135, 137, 138
 Vietnam herbicides ground spraying, I: 94-96; II: 26; III: 138-140
 Vietnam herbicides use early objections, I: 29, 31-32; II: 26-27
 Vietnam troop movements, I: 52-53, 96, 273-279, 287
 Vietnam U.S. involvement, I: 75-76, 84
 See also Military records; Operation Ranch Hand
Military personnel. *See* Demographic data, Vietnam veterans; Foreign veterans; Military health care; Military occupation specialty code (MOS); Military operations; Military records; Operation Ranch Hand; U.S. Air Force; U.S. Army; U.S. Army Chemical Corps; U.S. Coast Guard; U.S. Marine Corps; U.S. Navy; U.S. Special Forces; Vietnam veterans; Women veterans
Military records, I: 742-743
 herbicide exposure assessment use, I: 271-280, 287-288; II: 101; III: 138, 140; IV: 125
 herbicide spray missions records, I: 27, 62, 84-85, 104-106
 HERBS tapes, I: 62, 96-98; III: 146, 148; IV: 123-125
 research recommendations, I: 17, 724-725
 Vietnam casualties, I: 82-83
 Vietnam herbicide ground spraying, I: 94, 95; IV: 110-111, 113-114
 Vietnam service identification in, II: 24-25, 175
 Vietnam veterans in, I: 75-80, 106; II: 150-153
Minnesota, I: 37, 326, 332, 333, 468; II: 47, 137-138, 178, 199, 325; III: 226-227, 229, 440-441; IV: 144, 210, 286, 306, 344, 349, 354, 362, 369, 375, 382
 Department of Agriculture, II: 137; III: 226, 440; IV: 149
Minnesota Multiphasic Personality Inventory, I: 641
Miscarriages. *See* Spontaneous abortion
Missouri, I: 621, 626, 664-665, 681; II: 280; III: 500; IV: 133, 135, 148, 227, 272, 404, 484, 487, 493
 See also Times Beach, Missouri; Verona, Missouri
Mixed-function oxidase activity, I: 131, 155, 156
Models and modeling. *See* Herbicide exposure reconstruction model; Quantitative structure-activity relationship (QSAR) models
Monsanto Company, I: 34, 35, 38, 305-307, 444, 674, 700; II: 114-115, 179, 182, 193, 204, 207, 220, 236; III: 152, 171-172, 220, 348; IV; 136, 185-186, 257, 260, 271, 371, 290, 301, 333, 343
Montagnards, I: 31, 371, 599
Montana, II: 268; III: 420; IV: 149, 344, 349, 354, 362, 369, 375, 382
Mortality. *See* Child mortality studies; Deaths; Mortality studies; Perinatal deaths
Mortality of Vietnam Veterans: The Veteran Cohort Study, III: 273, 285-286
Mortality studies, II: 130; IV: 140, 141, 144, 146, 149, 156, 157, 159, 184-194, 252, 253
 basal/squamous cell skin cancer, III: 319, 321
 cancer, I: 442-445; II: 133, 134, 136, 137, 185; IV: 137, 140, 142, 143, 150, 199-200-206

INDEX 575

circulatory disorders, II: 335
death certificate data, I: 236-237; II: 136, 137-138
female reproductive cancers statistics, II: 211
Finland respiratory cancer mortality and latency, II: 271; III: 422
Germany, in, IV: 137, 138
latency results, II: 263; III: 410-411, 421, 422, 423
melanoma, III: 314-315, 316
methodology, I: 229-233, 435
National Institute for Occupational Safety and Health (NIOSH) conducted by, IV: 105, 136, 251
non-Hodgkin's lymphoma and latency, III: 429
prostate cancer and latency, II: 273, 274, 275, 276; III: 426, 427
Ranch Hand baseline mortality studies, II: 151; IV: 151-153
respiratory cancer mortality and latency, II: 270, 271; III: 421, 422, 423, 424
Seveso, Italy, children study, II: 147; IV: 148
Seveso, Italy, males cancer mortality and latency, II: 271, 275; III: 422, 427; IV: 148
standardized mortality ratio, I: 229-230
women veterans, II: 152-153, 201
See also Child mortality studies; Deaths; Perinatal deaths
MOS. See Military occupation specialty code
Motor/coordination dysfunction
epidemiological studies, II: 309-310; III: 469-470; IV: 445-447
herbicide association in, I: 661-662; II: 4, 7, 11, 21, 309-310; III: 469-470; IV: 443-447
herbicide environmental exposure studies, I: 658-659; IV: 445-447
herbicide occupational exposure studies, I: 658; IV: 445-447
scientific literature update, II: 309-310; III: 470; IV: 445-447
Vietnam veterans' risk, I: 662; II: 309, 310
See also Ataxia; Dystonia; Neurobehavioral toxicity; Neurological disorders; Parkinsonism; Stroke
Motor/sensory/coordination problems, I: 14, 658-662

MPTP, I: 661; IV: 445, 448
MRR. See Meta risk ratio
Multiple myeloma, I: 331, 334, 335, 336, 341; IV: 6, 8, 10, 144, 149
agricultural/forestry workers and, I: 558-561; II: 138-139, 238-239, 241-243, III: 379-380; IV: 140
biologic plausibility, I: 563; III: 383; IV: 374
epidemiologic studies, I: 331, 334, 335, 336, 341, 557-563; II: 138-139, 237-244; III: 377-383; IV: 199, 209, 211, 212, 215, 372-373, 374-376
epidemiology, I: 526, 528; II: 236-237; III: 377; IV: 371-372
herbicide association in, I: 10, 11-12, 563, 574, 576; II: 6, 8, 20, 89, 236-244, 247; III: 7, 8, 9, 20, 24, 377-383, IV: 18, 143
herbicide environmental exposure and, II: 241, 243; III: 380, 382; IV: 372-373
herbicide occupational exposure and, II: 237-243; III: 378-380, 381-382; IV: 372
histopathology, I: 527
incidence, data by race/gender, for selected age groups, III: 377; IV: 371-372
paper/pulp workers and, II: 143
production workers and, II: 237-238; III: 378-379; IV: 373
risk estimates, II: 240-241
scientific literature update, III: 378-380; IV: 372-373
Vietnam veterans' compensation, II: 24, 30, 31
Vietnam veterans' risk, I: 563; II: 231, 244; IV: 374
Vietnam veterans' studies, III: 380, 382; IV: 373
See also Malignant lymphomas
Myeloid leukemia. See Leukemia
Myocardial infarction, I: 708; IV: 135, 507-510
See also Cardiovascular disorders; Circulatory disorders

N

NAS. See National Academy of Sciences
Nasal/nasopharyngeal cancer
biologic plausibility, III: 292; IV: 275
clinical description, I: 457-458
epidemiologic studies, II: 6, 187-189; III: 290-291; IV: 143, 274-276

epidemiology, I: 458-459; II: 187-188; III: 288-289; IV: 273
herbicide association in, I: 13, 19, 460, 577; II: 2, 6, 11, 12, 20, 89, 187-189, 249-250; III: 7, 10, 290-292; IV: 7, 11
herbicide environmental exposure and, II: 189; III: 290, 291; IV: 274-275
herbicide occupational exposure and, II: 188-189; III: 290, 291; IV: 274
incidence, data by race/gender, for selected age groups, III: 289; IV: 273
scientific literature update, III: 290; IV: 274-275
treatment, I: 458
Vietnam veterans' risk, I: 460; IV: 275
Vietnam veterans' studies, II: 189; III: 290, 291; IV: 275
Nasal olfactory mucosa, I: 130
National Academy of Sciences (NAS), I: 2, 28-29, 31, 43, 47, 51, 55, 57; II: 1, 17, 25, 29, 30, 63; III: 1, 23, 28, 146; IV: 1, 15
National Cancer Institute (NCI), I: 9, 30, 37, 439; II: 231; III: 218, 363
National Center for Health Statistics (NCHS), III: 266; IV: 249
  ICD-9 cancer codes, SEER program site groupings for, III: 537-539; IV: 524-526
National Death Index, II: 130, 152, 153
National Diabetes Data Group (NDDG), III: 492, 493
National Health and Nutrition Evaluation Survey III (NHANES III), III: 498
National Health Interview Survey (NHIS), III: 499; IV: 411
National Institute for Occupational Safety and Health (NIOSH), I: 8, 12, 36-37, 260, 264, 270, 285, 303-305, 443, 478, 479, 499, 564, 573, 577, 650-651, 686, 731; II: 13, 95, 101, 103, 105, 114-115, 128-129, 132, 178, 196, 206, 221, 229, 269, 270, 272, 273, 274, 275, 280, 309, 322, 350-351, 356, 357; III: 11, 12, 131, 144, 162, 170-171, 218, 219-220, 306, 310, 420, 421, 424, 425, 426, 428, 445, 449, 469, 481, 500, 502; IV: 10, 111, 133-134, 136, 182-184, 251, 257, 260, 263, 265, 268, 270-271, 277, 280, 282-283, 288, 290, 292, 295, 297, 300, 327, 331, 333, 341, 343, 346, 349, 351, 353, 356, 358, 366, 368, 372, 375, 379
National Institutes of Health (NIH), I: 92

National Library of Medicine, I: 735
National Medical Expenditures Survey (NMES), III: 243; IV: 238
National Occupational Mortality Surveillance System, III: 231, 470
National Personnel Records Center, I: 17, 77, 385, 724; II: 150, 152; III: 237, 242
National Research Council, I: 20, 62-64
National Survey of the Vietnam Generation, IV: 411
National Technical Information Service, III: 29
National Toxicology Program, I: 139-141; IV: 284
National Veterans Legal Services Project, I: 60
National Vietnam Veterans Birth Defects/Learning Disabilities Registry and Data Base, I: 741-742; II: 292-293
National Vietnam Veterans Readjustment Study, I: 79, 83, 655
Nature, IV: 511
Navy. *See* U.S. Navy
NCHS. *See* National Center for Health Statistics
NCI. *See* National Cancer Institute
NDDG. *See* National Diabetes Data Group
Nebraska, I: 9, 37, 332, 333-334, 535; II: 139, 231, 233-234, 241; III: 229, 363; IV: 143-144, 211, 216, 360, 375, 382
Nebraska Lymphoma Study, II: 139
Neonatal death. *See* Perinatal death
Netherlands, I: 316-317, 323, 325-326, 443, 464, 468, 477, 558; II: 132-133, 179, 196, 199, 220, 226, 232, 238, 243, 269; III: 10, 223, 226, 230, 236, 348, 441-442, 490; IV: 252-253, 256-257, 259-260, 262, 265, 293, 295-296, 302, 306, 333, 340, 343, 346, 348, 351, 353, 356, 358-360, 365, 368, 372, 374-375, 379, 381, 404-405
  Central Bureau of Statistics, II: 133
  herbicide exposure assessment, III: 150-151
  National Institute of Public Health and Environmental Protection, II: 132-133
  See also Rotterdam, Netherlands
Neural tube defects, II: 297; III: 437-438; IV, 18, 400-405
  See also Birth defects; Reproductive disorders; Spina bifida
Neurasthenia, I: 649; IV: 440
  See also Cognitive/neuropsychiatric disorders

Neurobehavioral toxicity
  2,4-D, I: 180; II: 305; III: 473, 474
  biological plausibility, II: 314; III: 474-475
  definition, II: 304
  epidemiological studies, II: 306, 307-308, 309-310, 311, 312-313, 314; III: 467-473
  epidemiology, II: 304-305, 307; III: 466, 468
  evidence in epidemiological studies, II: 314; III: 473-474
  herbicide association, II: 305-314; III: 3, 467-475
  herbicide environmental exposure studies, II: 306; III: 467
  herbicide occupational exposure studies, II: 306; III: 467
  TCDD, II: 305, 307-308, 309, 310-311, 314; III: 469, 470-471, 474, 475; IV: 25-26
  Vietnam veterans increased risk, II: 305, 306, 314; III: 475-476
  See also Ataxia; Cognitive/neuropsychiatric disorders; Depressive disorders; Motor/coordination dysfunction; Neurological disorders; Peripheral nervous system (PNS) disorders; Posttraumatic stress disorder (PTSD); Stroke
Neuroblastoma, I: 594
  children and, I: 628; IV: 422, 425
Neurologic disorders
  2,4-D in, I: 179; II: 48; III: 45-46, 473, 474
  assessment issues, I: 14, 641-642; IV: 440-441
  biologic plausibility, III: 474-475; IV: 457-459
  childhood cancer, I: 628
  classification of, I: 640; II: 304-305
  cognitive and neuropsychiatric effects, I: 649-658; III: 468-469; IV: 441-443
  epidemiologic studies, I: 44-45, 643-648; II: 141, 305, 307, 309; III: 467-473; IV: 441-459
  herbicide association in, I: 14, 657, 661, 666; III: 467-476; IV: 441-459
  herbicide occupational exposure studies and, I: 649-651, 658, 662-663; III: 467
  motor/coordination dysfunction, I: 14, 658-662; III: 469-470; IV: 443-448
  peripheral nervous system disorders, I: 662-666; III: 470-473; IV: 454-459
  Seveso, Italy, studies, I: 365-366, 523; II: 141; IV: 227
  TCDD in, I: 160-166; II: 3, 75; III: 84-85, 469, 470-471, 474, 475; IV: 441-443, 445
  Vietnam veterans' compensation, I: 55
  Vietnam veterans' offspring and, I: 609, 660
  Vietnam veterans' risk, I: 658, 662, 666; III: 475-476; IV: 459
  See also Cognitive/neuropsychiatric disorders; Motor/coordination dysfunction; Neurobehavioral toxicity; Peripheral nervous system (PNS) disorders
Newark, New Jersey, II: 128-129; III: 219, 220; IV: 134-135
New Brunswick, Canada, III: 234; IV: 149
New Hampshire, I: 341, 364; III: 232; IV: 146, 222
New Jersey, I: 656, 695; II: 280; III: 243, 500; IV: 158, 483, 487, 493
  Agent Orange Commission, I: 60, 280-281, 401-402, 741; II: 292
  See also Newark, New Jersey
New Mexico, I: 60, 402; III: 243; IV: 159
New York, I: 60, 364-365, 402-403, 444, 470, 495, 626; II: 202; IV: 149, 159, 230, 291, 298, 355, 364, 371
  See also Binghamton, New York; Camp Drum, New York
New Zealand, I: 329-331, 373, 486, 490, 535-536, 552, 560-561; II: 132, 134, 242; III: 226, 229; IV: 113, 142, 143, 149, 206, 215, 216, 297, 361, 369, 375, 404
  See also Northland, New Zealand
NHANES III. *See* National Health and Nutrition Evaluation Survey III
NHIS. *See* National Health Interview Survey
NHL. *See* Non-Hodgkin's lymphoma
Nickel, respiratory cancer and latency, II: 269; III: 420
NIH. *See* National Institutes of Health
NIOSH. *See* National Institute for Occupational Safety and Health
Nitro, West Virginia
  industrial accident, I: 38-39, 305-307, 597, 607, 686, 700; II: 287; III: 152, 220, 318; IV: 136
NMES. *See* National Medical Expenditures Survey

Non-Hodgkin's lymphoma (NHL)
  2,4-D in, I: 256-257
  age of onset, I: 436
  agricultural/forestry workers and, I: 530-540; II: 135, 138, 139, 232-234; III: 364-365; IV: 140
  biologic plausibility, III: 366; IV: 358-359
  cytogenetic studies, III: 365-366
  epidemiologic studies, I: 328, 329, 330, 331, 333-334, 335-338, 383, 384, 391-393, 401, 528-540, 573-574; II: 134-135, 138, 139, 231-234; III: 362-371; IV: 116, 137, 199, 211, 212, 213, 214, 215, 216, 294, 356-358, 359-364
  epidemiology, I: 526, 527; II: 231; III: 362; IV: 355-356
  herbicide association in, I: 8-10, 548, 573-574; II: 5, 6, 20, 102, 108, 231-234, 247; III: 6, 7, 20, 24, 362-371; IV: 6, 8, 17, 384, 422, 425
  herbicide environmental exposure studies, I: 540-541; II: 234; III: 365, 369; IV: 149, 357
  herbicide occupational exposure and, II: 232-234; III: 363-365, 367-369; IV: 142, 143-144, 146, 356
  histopathology, I: 526
  incidence, data by race/gender, for selected age groups, III: 362; IV: 355-356
  latency issues, III: 428-430
  paper/pulp workers and, I: 540
  production workers and, I: 9, 529-530, 548; II: 232; III: 363-364, 429
  research recommendations, I: 19, 727
  scientific literature update, II: 232-234; III: 363-366; IV: 356-358
  Selected Cancers Study and, I: 234-235
  Vietnam veterans and, I: 9, 401, 526, 541-548, 549; II: 231, 234; III: 363, 365, 370-371; IV: 156-157, 357-358, 359
  Vietnam veterans compensation, I: 51, 55-56; II: 24, 29, 30, 31
  See also Malignant lymphomas
Nonmelanoma skin cancer. *See* Basal/squamous cell skin cancer; Skin cancer
North America, II: 197; III: 510
North Carolina, IV: 202
  See also Agricultureal Health Study
North Dakota, IV: 149, 344, 349, 354, 362, 369, 375, 382

Northeast Pharmaceutical and Chemical Corporation, I: 40
Northland, New Zealand, III: 234; IV: 149
Norway, III: 10, 225, 442-443; IV:197, 209, 404
  Central Population Register, III: 225, 442
  Medical Birth Registry, III: 225, 442
  Population Registry, III: 236
  See also Frierfjord, Norway
Null hypothesis, I: 225

O

Occupational herbicide exposure, I: 5, 303
  acute and subacute transient peripheral neuropathy and, II: 312; IV: 10
  agricultural/forestry workers, II: 183-184, 197-198, 232-234, 238-239, 241-243; III: 178-195, 224-232, 284-285, 335, 364-365, 379-380, 387-388; IV: 112-113, 140-142
  basal/squamous cell skin cancer and, III: 321, 323; IV: 309
  birth defects and, II: 286-287; III: 437; IV: 404
  bladder cancer and, III: 348, 350; IV: 341-342
  bone cancer and, III: 303, 305; IV: 288-289
  brain tumors and, III: 357-358, 360; IV: 351
  breast cancer and, II: 214-216; III: 324-326, 328; IV: 317
  breast cancer estimated risk, II: 218
  cancer mortality, I: 443-444; II: 133, 134, 136, 137
  cancer risk factor, I: 442; II: 133-135
  cervical cancer and, III: 332
  childhood cancer, IV: 418-419, 427
  circulatory disorders and, III: 515-516; IV: 506-507
  diabetes mellitus and, III: 496; IV: 483-484
  epidemiologic studies, I: 303-365; II: 3, 6-7, 113-140; III: 170-196, 218, 219-232, 268-271, 274-280, 282-283, 284, 287, 290, 291, 293-294, 296-297, 300-301, 303, 305, 308-309, 312, 316, 317, 321, 323, 324-326, 328, 332-333, 335-336, 337, 338, 341, 344, 345, 348, 350, 353, 354, 357-378, 360, 363-365, 367-369, 372-373, 374-375, 378-380, 381-382, 386-388, 391-392, 437, 450, 454, 455, 456, 459, 467, 483-485, 489, 491, 496,

510-512, 515-516, 520; IV: 134-147, 251-254, 257-258, 259-260, 262-263, 265-266, 268-269, 276, 277-278, 280, 285-286, 290, 292-293, 306, 307, 312, 318-319, 324, 325, 333-334, 338, 343-344, 348-349, 353-354, 359-361, 368-369, 374-375, 381-382, 404, 408, 418-419, 427, 445, 446, 473-474, 483-484, 489-490, 500-501, 506-507
exposure assessment strategies, I: 253-256, 258-259, 262-267, 269-270; II: 5, 99-101, 107-108; III: 144-145, 150-156
exposure indices development, II: 107-108; III: 161-162
female reproductive system cancers and, III: 332-333; IV: 321
gastrointestinal/digestive disorders and, III: 510-512; IV: 500-501
gastrointestinal tract tumors and, II: 178-179; III: 268-271, 274-280; IV: 251-254
hepatobiliary cancer and, II: 182-184, 185, 186; III: 282-283, 284, 287; IV: 268-269
Hodgkin's disease and, II: 235-236; III: 372-373, 374-375; IV: 365-366
immune system disorders and, III: 489, 491
infant death and, III: 456
infertility and, III: 450; IV: 406-407
laryngeal cancer and, III: 293-294; IV: 277-278
leukemia and, III: 386-388, 391-392; IV: 198, 379
lipid abnormalities and, III: 520; IV: 114-15, 117, 493
low birthweight and, III: 459; IV: 414-416
lung cancer and, III: 296-297, 300-301, 421, 422, 423, 424; IV: 282
melanoma and, III: 316, 317; IV: 302
multiple myeloma and, II: 237-243; III: 378-380, 381-382; IV: 372
nasal/nasopharyngeal cancer and, II: 188-189; III: 290, 291; IV: 274
neonatal death and, III: 455
neural tube defects numbers, II: 297
neurobehavioral disorders association studies, II: 306; III: 467
non-Hodgkin's disease and, II: 232-234; III: 363-365, 367-369, 429; IV: 356
ovarian cancer and, III: 333
production workers, II: 182-183, 191, 193-197, 206-207, 232, 237-238; III: 170-

178, 219-224, 284, 363-364, 378-379, 386-387, 420, 423, 426, 429; IV: 111-112, 134-140, 251-254, 271, 282, 288-289, 296-297, 302, 321, 327-329, 336, 340-341, 346-347, 351, 356, 365-366, 372, 379
professional herbicide/pesticide applicators, II: 198-200; III: 182-185, 226-228; IV: 113-114, 142-143, 404
prostate cancer and, II: 219-220, 222; III: 335-336, 337, 338, 341, 426, 427; IV: 327-329
pulp/paper workers, I: 37-38, 267, 341, 364, 443, 447, 454, 468, 516, 523, 540, 561-562, 568; II: 126-127, 184, 200, 243; III: 196, 232; IV: 114, 134, 252, 268
renal cancers and, III: 353, 354; IV: 346-347
research recommendations, I: 15-16, 731
respiratory cancers and, II: 190, 191-200; IV: 282
respiratory disorders and, III: 483-485; IV: 473-474
sawmill workers, III: 10, 156, 227-228, 338, 439-440, 447-448, 449, 452, 453, 457; IV: 114
skin cancer and, III: 312; IV: 300, 301
soft-tissue sarcomas, II: 206-207; III: 308-309; IV: 292-293
stillbirths and, III: 454
testicular cancer and, III: 344, 345; IV: 336
uterine cancer and, III: 333
Vietnam veteran exposure vs., I: 4, 285, 290
See also Herbicide exposure assessment; Herbicides
Occupations. *See* Agricultural/forestry workers; Highway workers; Leather tanners; Paper/pulp industry workers; Production workers; Professional herbicide/pesticide applicators; Railroad workers; Tannery workers
Odds ratio, I: 224, 234; II: 90; III: 126-127; IV: 105
Office of Technology Assessment, I: 19, 50, 52, 57, 728; II: 28; III: 26
OGTT. *See* Oral glucose tolerance test
Ohio, I: 336, 550
See also Hancock County, Ohio
Olshan, Andrew, III: 25
Ontario, Canada, II: 199

Operation Ranch Hand, I: 3, 4, 15, 16-17, 24, 74; II: 5, 14, 18, 23, 54, 251, 293; III: 6, 11, 12, 22, 23, 37, 50, 135, 136, 137, 138, 139; IV: 13, 18, 117-119, 150-156, 160-161
  application techniques, I: 25, 85-86, 87-88; IV: 120-122
  Army Chemical Corps and, IV: 123-124
  birth defects in offspring of, IV: 18, 403-404, 408, 430
  chloracne and, IV: 8, 464-466
  continuation of, IV: 21, 160-161
  epidemiological studies, II: 31, 32, 150-152, 154-156; III: 28-29, 237, 438-439, 498; IV: 9, 10, 150-156, 255, 262, 269, 272, 275-276, 278, 280, 283-284, 287, 291, 295, 298-299, 301, 303-305, 308-310, 313, 327, 329, 331-332, 334-336, 339, 342-343, 345, 347, 350, 352, 355, 357, 359, 362-363, 366, 370, 373, 376, 380, 383, 430-431, 435, 474, 479, 480, 485-488, 494, 502-504, 508-510
  herbicide formulations, I: 88-91
  herbicide surplus disposal, I: 93-94
  herbicide volume used, data by type, III: 136
  neurological disorders in, IV: 442, 454-455, 459
  number of military personnel in, I: 94, 273
  objectives, I: 85
  operations data, I: 86, 87, 92, 106-107
  porphyria cutanea tarde (PCT), IV: 466-467
  questionnaires, self-administered, II: 109, 151; IV: 124
  start of, I: 84, 85
  suspension of, I: 27, 31, 32, 92-93; II: 109
  targeting procedures, I: 86
  TCDD half-life in, IV: 24, 28, 43
  See also Air Force Health Study (AFHS)
Operational Report Lessons Learned, IV: 125
Oral glucose tolerance test (OGTT), III: 498, 500
Oregon, I: 336-337, 341; II: 149; III: 230, 232, 234; IV: 149, 231
  See also Alsea, Oregon
Outreach activities
  Vietnam Veterans and, II: 31; III: 28
Ovarian cancer, I: 338-339, 506, 510-511; III: 333
  herbicide association in, I: 13, 512; II: 6; III: 333; IV: 320-323, 326, 385
  See also Reproductive system cancers, women

P

P450, I: 130, 144-145, 170, 709; II: 56, 70, 72, 74, 76; III: 220; IV: 27, 41-42, 47-48, 50-52, 54-55, 58-60, 63, 65, 67-69, 72-76, 78
PACER HO, I: 93
PAI-2. *See* Plasminogen activator inhibitor
Pancreatic cancer. *See* Gastrointestinal (GI) tract cancers
Paper/pulp industry workers
  cancers in, I: 443, 454, 468, 516, 523, 540, 568; II: 200; IV: 114, 134, 252, 268
  chemical exposures in, I: 37-38, 267; III: 155-156; IV: 134, 252
  epidemiologic studies, I: 38, 341, 364; II: 126-127, 184, 200, 243; III: 196, 232; IV: 134, 221-223, 252, 268
  hepatobiliary cancer, II: 184
  multiple myeloma and, II: 243
Parkinsonism, I: 661; II: 140, 149, 309-310; III: 469-470, 475; IV: 144, 443-445, 448, 458
  See also Motor/coordination dysfunction
Parma, Italy, IV: 445
  See Also Italy
PCBs. *See* Polychlorinated bephenyls
PCDDs. *See* Polychlorinated dibenzodioxins
PCDFs. *See* Polychlorinated dibensofurans
PCMR. *See* Proportionate cancer mortality ratio
PCP. *See* Pentachlorophenol
PCT. *See* Porphyria cutanea tarda
Pennsylvania, I: 60, 403, 562; II: 244; III: 243; IV: 186
1,2,3,7,8-Pentachlorodibenzo-*p*-dioxin (PnCDD), II: 64, 65
2,3,4,7,8-Pentachlorodibenzofuran (PnCDF), II: 64, 65
Pentachlorophenol (PCP), II: 320; III: 221, 511, 516; IV: 257, 260, 263, 265, 271, 280, 285, 290, 296, 338, 353, 359, 368, 381
Pentoxyresorufin-O-dealkylase (PROD)
  TCDD and, II: 64
PEPCK. *See* Hepatic phosphoenol pyruvate carboxy kinase
Perimeter spraying. *See* Ground/perimeter spraying
Perinatal death
  biologic plausibility, III: 453, 458; IV: 413
  definitions, I: 618-619; II: 284; III: 451; IV: 412

INDEX   581

descriptive epidemiology, I: 619-620; II: 284-285; III: 451
epidemiological studies, I: 620-624; II: 285-286; III: 451-453, 454, 455, 456
herbicide association in, I: 14, 624; II: 7, 11, 20, 278, 285-286; III: 451-454, 455, 456; IV: 413
herbicide environmental exposure and, III: 454, 455, 456
herbicide occupational exposure and, III: 454, 455, 456
risk factors, I: 619-620
scientific literature update, II: 285; III: 452-453, 454, 456
TCDD biologic plausibility in, I: 624
Vietnam veterans and, II: 285; III: 454, 455, 456; IV: 413
Peripheral nervous system (PNS) disorders, I: 55, 662-666; II: 304, 312; IV: 440
acute and subacute transient peripheral neuropathy, II: 2, 6, 89, 311-314; III: 7, 8, 473; IV: 10, 18, 457-459
chronic persistent peripheral neuropathy, II: 89, 310-311; III: 470-472; 454-456
epidemiological studies, II: 310-311, 312-314; III: 470-473; IV: 135, 454-455, 457
herbicide association with, I: 666; II: 2, 6, 10, 11, 21, 89, 310-314; III: 7, 8, 21, 470-473; 454-457
herbicide environmental exposure studies, I: 663-665; II: 312-313
herbicide occupational exposure studies, I: 662-663; II: 312
methodology, II: 311-312
scientific literature update, II: 310-311; III: 471, 473; IV: 454-455, 457
Seveso, Italy, residents and, II: 312-313
Vietnam veterans' risk, I: 666; II: 311, 313; IV: 457, 459
See also Neurobehavioral toxicity; Neurological disorders
Pesticide/herbicide applicators. *See* Professional herbicide/pesticide applicators
Pesticides. *See* Agricultural herbicides; Desiccant herbicides; Fungicides; Herbicides; Insecticides; Phenoxy herbicides; Selective herbicides
Pharmacokinetics
2,4-D, I: 175

2,4,5-T, I: 182
cacodylic acid, I: 186-187
picloram, I: 190
TCDD, I: 127-133, 260-261, 284; II: 53-54; III: 161; IV: 41, 42, 47
TCDD-induced wasting syndrome, I: 162-166
Phenoxy herbicides, I: 8, 9, 10, 11, 27; III: 150, 151, 154, 222, 223, 422, 423, 429
action of, I: 27; IV: 16
IARC registry and, IV: 137
See also Herbicides
Phenoxyenolpyruvate carboxykinase, I: 172
Phenoxypropionic acids, I: 327
Phytar 560-G, I: 89
Picloram, I: 88, 90, 91; II: 4; III: 5, 19, 135, 136, 137, 218; IV: 5, 117-119, 133
acute toxicity, I: 191
animal studies, I: 189-192; III: 50, 396, 460
biologic plausibility, III: 460, 524; IV: 426
carcinogenicity, I: 118, 119, 190-191; II: 40; III: 396
chemical properties/structure, I: 111, 114-115, 189; II: 38; III: 32
chronic exposure, I: 191-192
developmental/reproductive toxicity, I: 192; II: 42; III: 460; IV: 416, 426, 431, 434-435
domestic use, I: 189
genotoxicity, I: 191
immunotoxicity, I: 122-123, 192; II: 41
liver toxicity, I: 125; II: 42; III: 524
metabolism, I: 115, 116
pharmacokinetics, I: 190; IV: 27-28
toxicity profile update, II: 51; III: 50; IV: 22-24, 31, 33-34, 40-41
volume used in Operation Ranch Hand, data, III: 136; IV: 117
PKC. *See* Protein kinase C
Plasminogen activator inhibitor (PAI-2), II: 74
Plasmodium, TCDD exposure and, II: 68
Plausibility. *See* Biologic plausibility
Pleurisy, I: 711, 713
See also Respiratory disorders
PMRs. *See* Proportional mortality ratios
PnCDD. *See* 1,2,3,7,8-Pentachlorodibenzo-*p*-dioxin (PnCDD)
PnCDF. *See* 2,3,4,7,8-Pentachlorodibenzo-furan
Pneumoconiosis, I: 713
See also Respiratory disorders

Pneumonia, I: 710, 713
  See also Respiratory disorders
PNS. *See* Peripheral nervous system (PNS) disorders
Pointman Project, I: 60, 280, 401-402, 656
Polychlorinated biphenyls (PCBs), II: 64, 67, 68, 182, 329; III: 236, 515; IV: 138, 399
Polychlorinated dibenzodioxins (PCDDs), I: 126, 327; II: 53, 64, 133, 149, 320, 329; III: 153, 154, 156, 160, 221, 223, 236, 511, 515, 516; IV: 111-112, 114
Polychlorinated diensofurans (PCDFs), II: 53, 64, 68, 149, 320, 329; III: 153, 154, 160, 223, 236
Polymorphonuclear neutrophils, I: 148
Population characteristics. *See* Age and aging; Gender; Deaths; Demographic data, Vietnam veterans; Perinatal death; Race/ethnicity
Porphyria, I: 153-154
Porphyria cutanea tarda (PCT)
  biological plausibility, II: 323; III: 482; IV: 468
  clinical features, I: 679, IV: 466-467
  epidemiologic studies, I: 680-682; II: 6, 129, 321-323; III: 481-482; IV: 194, 467-468
  epidemiology, II: 321; III: 480-481; IV: 10, 466-467
  herbicide association in, I: 10, 682; II: 5, 6, 10, 20, 129, 321-323; III: 7, 8, 20, 24, 481-482; IV: 17, 18, 135, 183, 467, 468
  scientific literature update, II: 322-323; III: 482; IV: 467-468
  Vietnam veterans' compensation, I: 50, 55; II: 24, 28-29, 30, 31
  Vietnam veterans' risk, I: 682-683; II: 321, 322, 323; III: 481, 482; IV: 468
  See also Skin sensitivity
Posttraumatic stress disorder (PTSD), I: 397-398, 653-656, 658; II: 304, 308; IV: 440
  See also Cognitive/neuropsychiatric disorders
Prague, Czechoslovakia, III: 224
Preterm delivery (PTD), III: 454, 455, 456-458, 459; IV: 400, 413, 416, 432
  See also Low birthweight
PROD. *See* Pentoxyresorufin-O-dealkylase
Production workers
  bladder cancer, I: 513-517; IV: 341-342
  brain cancer, I: 523; IV: 351

cancer mortality, I: 443-444; II: 133, 134, 270, 273, 274; III: 423, 426, 429; IV: 251, 268
chemical industry production workers studies, I: 303-318; II: 114-118, 128-135, 171-175, 182-183, 191, 193-197, 206-207, 232, 237-238, 273-274, 275; III: 170-178, 219-224, 363-364, 378-379, 386-387, 422, 423, 426, 429; IV: 270, 292
chloracne, I: 674-676
circulatory disorders, I: 700-701; IV: 506-507
diabetes mellitus, I: 684 ; IV: 483-484
epidemiologic studies, I: 36-37, 303-318; II: 113, 114-118, 128-135, 182-183, 191, 193-197, 232, 237-238; III: 170-178, 219-224, 284, 363-364, 378-379, 386-387; IV: 182-197, 300, 312
female reproductive/breast cancer, I: 508-510; IV: 317, 321
gastrointestinal tract cancers, I: 447; IV: 251-254
gastrointestinal ulcers, I: 691
German herbicide employees, exposure assessment, II: 4-5, 105, 108; III: 423, 429
hepatic enzyme dysfunction, I: 686, 687
hepatobiliary cancers, I: 453-454, 455; II: 182-183; III: 284; IV: 268-269
herbicide exposure assessment, I: 264-265; II: 103, 105, 107-108; III: 150-154
Hodgkin's disease, I: 9; IV: 365-366
immune system disorders, I: 697-698
international register of workers exposed to phenoxy herbicides, II: 131-135; III: 175-177, 222-223
latency and cancer, II: 269, 270, 272, 273-274, 275; III: 422, 423, 426, 429; IV: 284, 293,
leukemia, I: 564-566, 570-571; III: 386-387; IV: 379
lipid abnormalities, I: 688-689; IV: 493
multiple myeloma, I: 557-578; II: 237-238; III: 378-379; IV: 372
nasal/nasopharyngeal cancers, I: 458, 459; IV: 274
neurologic/neuropsychiatric disorders, I: 649, 650-651, 662-663
non-Hodgkin's lymphoma, I: 9, 529-530, 548; II: 134, 135, 232; III: 363-364, 429; IV: 356

porphyria cutanea tarda, I: 680; II: 129
prostate cancer, I: 518; II: 273-274, 275;
   III: 426, 427; IV: 327-329
renal cancer, I: 515; IV: 346-347
reproductive outcomes, I: 596-598, 607,
   620, 621
respiratory cancer, I: 10, 461-466, 471; II:
   191, 193-197, 269, 270, 272; III: 423;
   IV: 282
respiratory disorders, I: 709-710; IV: 273-274
skin cancer, I: 502; IV: 300, 301
soft-tissue sarcoma, I: 8, 477-479, 499; II:
   132, 134-135, 206-207; IV: 292-293
testicular cancer, I: 519; IV: 336
See also Indutrial accidents
Professional herbicide/pesticide applicators
   cancer in, I: 320-321, 323, 325-326, 443,
      447, 466-468, 488, 491; II: 137-138,
      198-200; III: 422; IV: 321, 327-328,
      330, 336
   cohort studies, IV: 202-206
   epidemiologic studies, I: 323-326, 447,
      466-468; II: 120-126, 137-140; III: 182-
      185, 226-228; IV: 142-143, 144-145
   Finland respiratory cancer mortality and
      latency, II: 271; III: 422
   herbicide exposure assessment, I: 266-267;
      II: 107-108; III: 155; IV: 113-114
   reproductive outcomes, I: 324-325; IV: 410
   See also Herbicide application methods;
      Herbicides
Prolactin, I: 165
Proportionate cancer mortality ratio (PCMR),
   II: 179, 183, 197-198, 203, 204-205,
   207, 210, 212, 216, 219, 224, 226, 227,
   229, 233, 235, 246
Proportionate mortality ratio (PMR), I: 232-
   233; II: 161, 180, 185, 208, 225, 230,
   234, 236, 242, 246; III: 417-418, 428;
   IV: 253, 369
Prostate cancer
   biologic plausibility, III: 343; IV: 332
   epidemiologic studies, I: 518-519; II: 6,
      219-223; III: 335-342; IV: 202, 327-
      329, 330-331, 333-335
   epidemiology, I: 513, 514-515; II: 217, 219;
      III: 334; IV: 326-327
   evidence of association for, IV: 18
   herbicide association in, I: 10, 11, 519-521,
      575-576; II: 2, 6, 8-9, 20, 89, 217-223,
      247; III: 7, 8, 9, 20, 335-343; IV: 6, 8,
      10

herbicide environmental exposure studies,
   II: 221, 222; III: 336, 338, 342; IV: 329
herbicide occupational exposure studies, II:
   219-220, 222; III: 335-336, 337, 338,
   341; IV: 202, 327-329
histopathology, I: 513
incidence, data by race, for selected age
   groups, III: 334; IV: 249, 326-327
latency issues, II: 13, 14; III: 426-428
mortality and latency, II: 273, 274, 275; III:
   426, 427
research recommendations, I: 19, 727
risk, estimated, II: 222-223
scientific literature update, III: 336-339; IV:
   74, 327-331
Seveso, Italy, male mortality and latency,
   II: 275, III: 336, 338, 427; IV: 329
Vietnam veterans' risk, I: 11, 518, 519,
   522; II: 221, 223; III: 343, 431; IV: 332
Vietnam veterans' studies, III: 336, 338,
   339, 340, 342; IV: 329
See also Genitourinary cancers
Protein kinase C (PKC), II: 4, 52, 59, 60, 61,
   62; III: 65-67, 105; IV: 69-71, 72
Psychiatric disorders
   assessment for, I: 641
   epidemiological studies, I: 649-657
   herbicide association in, I: 14, 657; IV: 135,
      151
   posttraumatic stress disorder, I: 397-398,
      653-656, 658; IV: 440
PTD. *See* Preterm delivery
PTSD. *See* Posttraumatic stress disorder
Public concern, I: 1, 2, 23-24, 29-32, 35-36, 39
   federal government response to, I: 45-60; II:
      27-32; III: 25-30
Public Law 91-441, I: 47, 62
Public Law 96-151, I: 50, 52, 57; II: 28; III: 26,
   240
Public Law 97-72, I: 50; II: 28; III: 26, 240
Public Law 98-181, I: 51
Public Law 98-542, I: 50-51; II: 28-29; III: 26-
   27
Public Law 99-272, I: 50; II: 28; III: 26
Public Law 100-687, I: 51
Public Law 101-239, I: 51
Public Law 102-4, I: 2, 7, 20, 21, 51, 572, 721,
   728-730; II: 1, 5, 17, 19, 29, 97, 247;
   III: 1, 6, 14, 17, 20, 124, 132, 390, 397,
   462, 475, 519, 525; IV: 1, 2, 6, 15, 103,
   388
Public Law 102-585, II: 28; III: 26

Public Law 103-452, II: 28; III: 26
Public Law 104-110, III: 26
Public Law 104-204, III: 24, 26
Public Law 104-262, III: 26
Public Law 105-114, III: 25
Pulmonary system
  TCDD absorption, I: 129; IV: 135, 156
  Vietnam veterans disorders, I: 402
  See also Chronic obstructive pulmonary disease (COPD); Respiratory cancers; Respiratory disorders

Q

QSAR models. *See* Quantitative structure-activity relationship (QSAR) models
Quail Run mobile home park, I: 268, 369-370, 455, 665, 681, 687, 694; II: 144, 184; III: 200-201, 234, 283; IV: 115, 148
Quantitative structure-activity relationship (QSAR) models, III: 106; VI: 84
Questionnaires, II: 109, 136, 150, 292; IV: 111, 124

R

RA. *See* Retinoic acid
Race/ethnicity
  acute lymphocytic leukemia incidence, data by race, III: 384; IV: 378
  acute myeloid leukemia incidence, data by race, III: 384; IV: 378
  bladder cancer incidence, data by race, III: 347; IV: 340
  bone cancer incidence, data by race, III: 302; IV: 288
  brain tumor incidence, data by race, III: 356; IV: 351
  breast cancer incidence, data by race, III: 324; IV: 314
  cancer studies and, II: 179, 180, 181, 183, 214, 219, 227, 237; IV: 249-250
  cardiovascular disorders, adjusted by, IV: 494, 507
  chronic lymphocytic leukemia incidence, data by race, III: 384; IV: 378
  chronic myeloid leukemia incidence, data by race, III: 384; IV: 378
  diabetes prevalence, data by race, III: 492; IV: 484-486, 492
  female reproductive system cancer incidence and other effects, data by race, III: 330; IV: 321, 414, 421, 423, 429
  gastrointestinal tract cancer incidence, data by race and cancer type, III: 267; IV: 250
  Hodgkin's disease incidence, data by race, III: 372; IV: 365
  laryngeal cancer incidence, data by race, III: 292; IV: 273
  leukemia incidence, data by type and race, III: 384; IV: 378
  liver/intrahepatic bile duct cancer incidence, by race, III: 282; IV: 267, 502
  lung cancer incidence, data by race, III: 296; IV: 281
  melanoma incidence, data by race, III: 313; IV: 300
  motor dysfunction, adjusted by, IV: 444
  multiple myeloma incidence, data by race, III: 377; IV: 372
  nasal/nasopharyngeal cancer incidence, data by race, III: 289; V: 273
  non-Hodgkin's lymphoma incidence, data by race, III: 362; IV: 356
  prostate cancer incidence, data by race, III: 334; IV: 326-327
  renal cancers incidence, data by race, III: 352; IV: 346
  risk adjusted by, IV: 135, 150-152, 154-156
  soft-tissue sarcoma incidence, data by race, III: 306; IV: 292
  testicular cancer incidence, data by race, III: 343; IV: 335
  Vietnam veterans, I: 81, 82, 83, 84; II: 180
  See also Alaskan natives; Asian Americans; Demographic data, Vietnam veterans
Radiation exposure, I: 564, 595
Radon daughters
  respiratory cancer and latency, II: 268; III: 418
Railroad workers, I: 323-324, 467, 486, 649-650, 658; IV: 206
Ranch Hand study. *See* Air Force Health Study (AFHS)
RARb. *See* Retinoic acid receptor b
Reagan, Ronald, III: 26
Rectal cancer. *See* Gastrointestinal (GI) tract cancers

INDEX 585

Registries. *See* Agent Orange Registry (AOR); Dioxin Registry; European registry; National Vietnam Veterans Birth Defects/Learning Disabilities Registry and Data Base
Regression analysis, II: 281
Relative risk, I: 224, 229, 230, 239, 258; II: 90, 178, 264, 265, 266, 271, 275, 297, 351, 356; III: 126-127, 412, 413, 414, 415, 418, 420, 422, 426-427, 428, 430-431; IV: 83, 105, 138, 142, 153, 254, 277, 278, 282, 284, 303, 310, 315, 321, 322, 329, 331, 332, 366, 373, 379, 424, 447, 472, 500
Renal cancer
  See Kidney cancer
Renal toxicity
  cacodylic acid and, II: 50-51
  TCDD and, II: 77; III: 75-76; IV: 76-77
Reproductive disorders
  2,4-D in, I: 180-181; II: 42, 280-282; III: 46, 460, 461-462; IV: 416
  2,4,5-T in, I: 185; II: 42, 280-282, 287; III: 462; IV: 404; IV: 416
  animal studies, I: 123-124; III: 460-462; IV: 426, 431-435
  biologic plausibility, II: 300; III: 444, 451, 453, 458, 460-462; IV: 416, 426
  cacodylic acid in, I: 189; II: 42; IV: 403, 407, 411, 413, 416, 431, 435
  epidemiologic studies, III: 436, 437-438, 443, 445-449, 450, 451-453, 454, 455, 456-457, 459; IV: 135, 153, 209, 227, 228, 233, 431; IV: 416, 426
  herbicide association in, I: 13-14, 605, 634; II: 6, 7, 278-279, 300-301; III: 3, 434-435, 436-444, 445-454, 455, 456-458, 459; IV: 135
  male-mediated, I: 593-595; III: 444-451; IV: 413
  methodological approach to study of, I: 591-592
  occupational risk factors, I: 594-595; IV: 399-400, 402, 404, 408, 418-419
  picloram in, I: 192; II: 42; III: 462; IV: 403, 413, 416, 431
  Ranch Hand study, I: 758-762; II: 293-295; III: 436, 438, 439, 446-447, 449, 452-453, 457-458; IV: 233
  research recommendations, I: 727

  TCDD in, I: 123-124, 156-159; II: 3, 41-42, 71-72, 282, 285-286; III: 92-105, 446-449, 460-461, 462; IV: 26, 81-82, 416
  Vietnam veterans' increased disease risk, II: 278, 298, 300-301; III: 444, 462; IV: 417, 426, 431
  See also Birth defects; Cervical cancer; Endometrial cancer; Hydatidiform mole; Hydrocephalus; Hypospadias; Infertility; Intrauterine growth retardation (IUGR); Low birthweight; Neural tube defects; Ovarian cancer; Perinatal death; Preterm delivery (PTD); Reproductive system cancers, women; Sperm parameter disorders; Spontaneous abortion
Reproductive system cancers, women, I: 13, 14, 505-512, 577; II: 6; IV: 320-326
  biologic plausibility, III: 334; IV: 323
  epidemiologic studies, I: 508-512; II: 211-213; III: 330-334; IV: 321-326
  epidemiology, I: 505, 506-508; II: 211; III: 329-330; IV: 320-321
  herbicide association in, I: 13, 14, 512, 577; II: 6, 11, 20, 211-213, 249-250; III: 7, 10, 330-334; IV: 7, 11, 323, 385
  herbicide environmental exposure and, III: 333; IV: 321-322, 325, 326-329, 334
  herbicide occupational exposure and, III: 332-333; IV: 321
  histopathology, I: 506
  incidence and mortality statistics, II: 211; III: 329-330; IV; 321
  scientific literature update, II: 212; III: 331-332; IV: 321-324
  Vietnam veterans' risk, I: 512; II: 211, 213; III: 334; IV: 323-324
  Vietnam veterans' studies, III: 333; IV: 322-323
  See also Breast cancer; Ovarian cancer; Reproductive disorders; Uterine cancer
Request for Proposals (RFP), II: 25, 26; III: 6, 126, 150; IV: 5, 126-127
Research
  Department of Veterans Affairs efforts, II: 29-30; III: 27-28; IV: 151, 157-58
  experimental studies update, II: 43-45
  herbicide exposure and cancer latency, literature review, II: 266-275; III: 416-431

herbicide exposure assessment strategies, recent literature, II: 104-109; III: 157-162; IV: 5
publication bias, II: 95-96; III: 131; IV: 108
See also Research needs
Research needs
biomarkers, I: 17, 725; II: 25
cost of, I: 727
health outcome priorities, I: 19, 726-727
herbicide exposure assessment, I: 4, 15, 16-17, 287-290, 291, 721-722, 724-728
herbicide occupational exposure data, I: 731
Hodgkin's disease, I: 19, 727
military records, I: 17, 724-725; II: 24-25
motor/coordination dysfunction, I: 660-661
neurobehavioral functioning, I: 657
recommendations, I: 15-21, 721-731; II: 23-24; III: 23; IV: 13
research management, I: 16, 17-18, 723-724, 726
risk assessment, I: 731
serum mandated testing, I: 21, 730
Vietnamese population studies, I: 731
Respiratory cancers
agricultural/forestry workers and, I: 466; II: 197-198
arsenic and, latency, II: 268; III: 420
asbestos and, latency, II: 268; III: 420
epidemiologic studies, I: 461-472; II: 189-203; IV: 274-275, 276, 277-278, 280, 285-287
epidemiology, I: 460-461; II: 189-191; IV: 273-274, 277, 281
evidence of association for, IV: 6, 8, 18
Finland male herbicide/pesticide applicators mortality and latency, II: 271; III: 422
gamma rays and, latency, II: 268; III: 418
herbicide association in, I: 10-11, 19, 574-575; II: 6, 8, 20, 89; II: 189-203, 247, 269-273; III: 7, 8, 9, 20, 24; IV: 6, 8, 275, 279, 284,
herbicide environmental exposure and, II: 190, 193, 200-201; IV: 274-275, 278, 282-283
herbicide occupational exposure and, II: 190, 191-200; IV: 274, 277, 282
latency issues, II: 13-14, 268-273; III: 418, 420-426
literature review, II: 269-272; III: 420-424
nickel and, latency, II: 269; III: 420
paper/pulp workers and, I: 468-469; II: 200

production workers and, I: 461-466; II: 191, 193-197; III: 420, 422, 423, 429; IV: 277, 282
professional herbicide/pesticide applicators, II: 198-199
radon daughters and, latency, II: 268; III: 418
relative mortality and latency, II: 270; III: 421, 422, 423, 424
risk estimates, II: 190, 192-193
risk factors, I: 461
Seveso, Italy, men lung cancer mortality, II: 271; III: 422, 424; IV: 278
Seveso, Italy, outcomes, I: 469; IV: 275, 278, 282-283
smoking and, latency, II: 268; III: 418
Vietnam veterans' compensation, I: 55; II: 24, 30, 31
Vietnam veterans' risk, I: 460-461, 469-470, 472; II: 190, 201-202, 203; III: 430-431; IV: 275-276, 279, 283, 284
See also Laryngeal cancer; Lung cancer; Respiratory disorders
Respiratory disorders
biologic plausibility, III: 486; IV: 475
epidemiologic studies, II: 324-326; III: 483-486; IV: 272-274
epidemiology, III: 482-483; IV: 468-471
herbicide association in, I: 14, 713; II: 7, 11, 21, 324-336; III: 3, 483-486; IV: 275
herbicide occupational exposure and, III: 483-485; IV: 273-274
paper/pulp mill workers and, I: 341, 364
production workers and, I: 709-710; IV: 273-274
research methodology, I: 708-709, 712-713; II: 324
scientific literature update, II: 325; III: 483-486; IV: 272-274
TCDD in, I: 170, 472, 709-710, 712, 713-714; III: 484; IV: 468, 471-475
Vietnam veterans' risk, I: 713-714; III: 485-486; IV: 275
See also Asthma; Bronchitis; Chronic obstructive pulmonary disease (COPD); Emphysema; Influenza; Pleurisy; Pneumoconiosis; Pneumonia; Respiratory cancers; Tuberculosis
Retinoic acid (RA), II: 73; III: 53, 73, 98
Retinoic acid receptor b (RARb), II: 73

INDEX

RFP. *See* Request for Proposals
Ribonucleic acid (RNA), II: 55, 58, 59, 62, 74, 75; III: 80, 82, 99, 101, 102, 103, 104
Risk assessment methodology, I: 5, 221, 246
   EPA dioxin research, I: 59-60
   predisposing factors, I: 731
   relative risk determination, I: 224, 229, 258; II: 351, 356; IV: 105
   standardized mortality ratio in, I: 229-230
   strength of association in, I: 239
   terminology, I: 224
   Vietnam veterans' disease risk estimation, II: 349-357; IV: 17
   Vietnam veterans' TCDD concentrations with time after exposure, II: 356-357
   Vietnam veterans' TCDD serum levels back-extrapolated to measure dose, II: 357
   Vietnam veterans' TCDD serum levels linear extrapolation, II: 356
   Vietnam veterans' TCDD serum levels use to estimate disease risk, II: 350-357; IV: 182
Risk assessment, Vietnam veterans, I: 5, 14-15, 221, 225-226, 246, 247-248, 578; II: 14, 22-23, 91; III: 14-15, 22-23, 127-128, 475-476, 525; IV: 388, 517
   amyloidosis, IV: 513
   birth defects, I: 618; II: 298, 300-301
   bone cancer, I: 474-475; IV: 290
   breast cancer risk, II: 218; III: 329; IV: 318
   cancer, I: 440, 442-443, 578; II: 251, 276; III: 397, 430-431
   cancer in offspring, I: 630-631; IV: 426
   chloracne, I: 678-679; II: 321; IV: 466
   circulatory disorders, I: 708; IV: 510
   diabetes mellitus, I: 692; III: 503; IV: 489
   disease risk methodology, II: 349-357
   female reproductive system cancers, I: 512; III: 334; IV: 323
   fetal/infant death, I: 625; IV: 413
   gastrointestinal cancers, I: 452; IV: 356
   genitourinary tract cancers, I: 522
   hepatic enzyme disorders, I: 692; IV: 505
   hepatobiliary cancers, I: 457; II: 187; IV: 270
   Hodgkin's disease, I: 557; IV: 367
   immune system disorders, I: 699; III: 491; IV: 481
   leukemia, I: 571-572; IV: 381
   linear extrapolation of exposure and risk, II: 356
   lipid abnormalities, I: 692; III: 507-508; IV: 495
   low birthweight outcomes, I: 628; IV: 417
   motor/coordination dysfunction, I: 662
   multiple myeloma, I: 563; IV: 374
   nasal/nasopharyngeal, I: 460; IV: 275
   neuropsychiatric outcomes, I: 658
   non-Hodgkin's lymphoma, I: 549; IV: 359
   peripheral nervous system disorders, I: 666; II: 314; IV: 459
   porphyria cutanea tarda, I: 682-683; II: 323; IV: 468
   prostate cancer risk, II: 223; III: 343; IV: 332
   reproductive outcomes, I: 634; II: 300-301; IV: 407, 431
   respiratory cancer, I: 472; II: 190, 192-193; IV: 279, 284
   respiratory disorders, I: 713-714; IV: 475
   skin cancer, I: 505; IV: 305-306, 311
   soft-tissue sarcoma, I: 500; IV: 17, 296
   spina bifida in offspring, II: 298, 301; IV: 403
   spontaneous abortion, I: 605; IV: 411
   TCDD concentrations with time after exposure, II: 356-357
   TCDD serum levels back-extrapolated to measure dose, II: 357
   TCDD serum levels linear extrapolation, II: 356
   TCDD serum levels use to estimate disease risk, II: 350-357
RNA. *See* Ribonucleic acid
Ronnel, II: 128; III: 219; IV: 134
Rotterdam, Netherlands, III: 236
Rung Sat Special Zone, I: 100, 104, 105, 106
Russia, II: 319
   See also USSR

S

Salmonella, TCDD exposure and, II: 68
Saskatchewan, Canada, II: 135-136, 200, 232, 242, 246, 325; III: 232
Sawmills. *See* Lumber industry
Schistosoma haematobium, III: 347
Scientific literature update, IV: 27-32, 104-105, 108, 248-388 *passim,* 399-435 *passim*
Seasonal factors
   herbicide distribution and, I: 26, 87

SEER program. *See* Surveillance, Epidemiology, and End Results (SEER) program
Selected Cancers Study
  exposure assessment use, II: 101; III: 146, 231, 240
  goals, I: 59, 387, 391
  hepatobiliary cancers, II: 185; III: 283
  Hodgkin's disease in, I: 554-556
  liver cancer in, I: 455
  methodology, I: 57, 234-235, 243, 258, 391-393, 440, 527
  nasal/nasopharyngeal cancer, I: 459; II: 189
  non-Hodgkin's lymphoma in, I: 9, 541-543, 573; II: 231; IV: 17
  soft-tissue sarcoma in, I: 493, 498
Selective herbicides, I: 24, 88
  See also Herbicides
Self-Report Symptom Inventory, I: 641
Senate Committee on Veterans Affairs, II: 24, 27-28; III: 23-24, 25
Serontonergic system, I: 166
Serum levels, TCDD, I: 4, 19, 21, 261, 281-285, 289, 290, 725, 728, 729, 742-743; II: 4-5, 104-106; III: 140-142, 146-147; IV: 37, 46, 112, 114, 125-126, 252, 293, 331
  back-extrapolated serum TCDD as measure of dose, II: 357; IV: 154
  Centers for Disease Control validation study, I: 281-284; II: 103, 104
  concentrations of TCDD with time after exposure, II: 356-357; III: 159-161
  estimated mean maximum levels, II: 252-255
  latency results, linear extrapolation from long exposure, II: 356
  measurement technique, I: 260; II: 349-350
  pharmocokinetics, I: 259-261
  recommendations, I: 20-21
  significance of, I: 4, 19, 261, 284-285, 289, 290, 725, 742-743; II: 4-5, 102-106, 108-109
  testing, mandated, I: 728, 729
  Vietnam veterans disease risk estimation, use for, II: 350-357
Services HERBS tapes. *See* HERBS tapes
Seveso, Italy; III: 9; IV: 8-9, 147-148
  accidental contamination in, I: 43; II: 140-141; III: 232-233; IV: 147
  birth defects, II: 287; III: 436

bladder cancer, I: 517; II: 226-227; III: 348, 349; IV: 341
bone cancer, III: 303; IV: 289
brain tumors, I: 523; II: 230; III: 356, 358; IV: 351-352
breast cancer, II: 216; III: 324-326, 327; IV: 315
cancer incidence, II: 141, 148
cancer mortality, I: 444; III: 422, 424
childhood cancer, II: 299-300; IV: 425
child mortality study, II: 147
chloracne, I: 267, 676-677; IV: 464
circulatory disorders, I: 701-702; IV: 507-509
diabetes mellitus, III: 495; IV: 11, 484
epidemiologic studies, I: 44-45, 63, 365-368; II: 113, 141-143, 148; III: 130, 197-200, 232-233, 283, 285, 290, 296, 297-298, 303, 307, 309, 314, 318, 325-326, 327, 330, 331, 332, 336, 338, 344, 348, 349, 352, 353, 356, 358, 363, 365, 372, 373, 380, 385, 386, 388-389, 390, 436, 449, 495, 505; IV: 224, 225, 226, 227, 258-259, 261, 263-264, 266, 271-272, 276, 280, 286-287, 291, 297-298, 306-307, 313, 319, 325-326, 334, 338, 344, 349, 354-355, 361-362, 369-370, 375-376, 382-383, 428, 430-431, 491
exposure assessment, I: 267-268, 285, 598-599; II: 4-5, 103, 105-106; III: 150, 156, 158, 160-161, 162; IV: 111, 114-115, 126
female reproductive cancers, I: 511; II: 211-212, 213; III: 330, 331, 332; IV: 321-322
gastrointestinal tract tumors, II: 177, 180; III: 271, 273; IV: 254
gastrointestinal ulcers, I: 691; IV: 501-502
hepatic enzyme disorders, I: 686-687
hepatobiliary cancers, II: 184; III: 283, 285; IV: 269
Hodgkin's disease, II: 236; III: 372, 373
immune modulation, I: 695
infertility, III: 449
latency and cancer risk, II: 271, 272, 273, 274, 275; III: 13, 408, 414, 420, 422, 424, 425, 426, 427, 428, 430
leukemia, I: 13, 569-570, 571; II: 245-246; III: 385, 386, 388-389, 390; IV: 379, 425
lipid abnormalities, I: 689; III: 505

INDEX 589

liver cancer, I: 454-455
liver disorders, I: 367; IV: 501-502
lung cancer, I: 469; II: 271; III: 296, 297-298, 299, 422, 424; IV: 282-283
  mortality studies, I: 652; II: 141, 271, 272-273, 275; III: 422, 424, 426, 427
multiple myeloma, I: 562; II: 243; III: 380; IV: 372-373
nasal/nasopharyngeal cancer, II: 189; III: 290; IV: 275
neurological disorders, II: 141
neuropsychiatric outcomes, I: 651-652
non-Hodgkin's lymphoma, I: 540-541; II: 234; III: 363, 365; IV: 357
peripheral nervous system disorders, I: 663-664; II: 10, 312-313
porphyria cutanea tarda, I: 680-681
prostate cancer, I: 11; II: 9, 221, 248, 274, 275; III: 336, 338, 426, 427; IV: 329
renal cancer, II: 225; III: 352, 353; IV: 347
reproductive outcomes/toxicity, I: 598-599; II: 72; III: 436, 449; IV: 400, 430-431
respiratory cancer, II: 200-201, 269, 272; III: 422, 424; IV: 278, 279, 282-283, 284
respiratory outcomes, I: 710; IV: 472-473, 474, 475
response to accident, I: 43-44
skin cancer, I: 503; II: 12, 209, 210; III: 314, 318; IV: 302
soft-tissue sarcoma, I: 491-492; II: 206, 207, 208; III: 307, 309; IV: 293-294, 295
testicular cancer, II: 228; III: 344; IV: 336
SFR. *See* Standardized fertility ratio
SGOT. *See* Aspartate aminotransferase (AST)
SGPT. *See* Alanine aminotransferase (ALT)
Shanghai, China, II: 188
Silvex, I: 309, 324; II: 128; III: 219; IV: 134
Skaraborg, Sweden, III: 234; IV: 149
Skin cancer
  animal studies, I: 141, 142-143; IV: 5, 24, 31, 40
  biologic plausibility for TCDD, I: 503; IV: 305, 311
  clinical features, I: 501, 502
  epidemiologic studies, I: 502-503; II: 209-211; III: 312-313; IV: 19, 149, 154, 232, 302-305, 306-308, 312-313
  epidemiology, I: 501-502; II: 209; III: 312, 313; IV: 299-300

  herbicide association in, I: 12, 576; II: 7, 11-12, 21, 209-211, 249-250; III: 8, 10, 21, 312; IV: 7, 11
  herbicide occupational exposure and, III: 312; IV: 302
  TCDD in, I: 141, 142-143, 502-503; II: 209-211; III: 313-316, 317, 319, 320, 322; IV: 19
  Vietnam veterans and, II: 209; III: 312; IV: 303-304, 305, 309-311
  See also Basal/squamous cell skin cancer; Melanoma
Skin sensitivity
  2,4-D and, I: 181
  picloram and, I: 192
  Ranch hands, IV: 8
  TCDD and, I: 172-174
  See also Chloracne; Porphyria cutanea tarda
Sleep disorders, I: 650; IV: 442
SMRs. *See* Standardized mortality ratios
Social Security Administration, II: 130, 152, 153
Society for Epidemiologic Research, II: 25
Soft-tissue sarcoma (STS), I: 311, 314
  age of onset, I: 436
  agricultural/forestry workers and, I: 322, 326-328, 329-330, 335-336, 337, 339-340; IV: 140, 149
  biologic plausibility of TCDD in, I: 500; III: 311; IV: 296
  case-control studies, I: 481-491; IV: 143-44
  CDC Selected Cancers Study and, IV: 157
  children and, I: 628
  clinical features, I: 475, 476
  cohort studies, I: 231, 243
  epidemiologic studies, I: 231, 476, 477-500; II: 132, 134-135, 205-208; III: 306-310, 311; IV: 149, 187, 216, 292-295, 296-299
  epidemiology, I: 475; II: 205; III: 304, 306; IV: 116, 136-137, 140, 143-144, 149, 157
  herbicide association in, I: 8, 9-10, 500, 572-573; II: 5, 6, 20, 205-208, 247; III: 6, 7, 20, 24, 306-310, 311; IV: 6, 8, 17
  herbicide environmental exposure studies, I: 375, 383, 384; II: 207-208; III: 309; IV: 293-294
  herbicide occupational exposure studies, III: 308-309; IV: 292-293
  IARC registry and, IV: 137, 293

incidence, data by race/gender, for selected age groups, III: 306; IV: 292
Midland, Michigan cohort, IV: 136
pesticide applicators and, I: 491
production workers and, I: 8, 477-479, 499; II: 132, 134-135, 206-207; IV: 136, 292-293
research recommendations, I: 19, 727
risk factors, I: 10, 477
scientific literature update, II: 206-208; III: 308-310; 292-295
Vietnam veterans and, I: 395-396, 401, 475, 492-498, 500; II: 205, 208; III: 309-310; IV: 157, 294-295
Vietnam veterans compensation, I: 51, 55, 56; II: 24, 29, 30, 31
See also Kaposi's sarcoma; Leiomyosarcomas
Somatostatin, I: 168, 169
South America, III: 510
South Dakota, IV: 149, 344, 349, 354, 362, 369, 375, 382
Southeast Asia, II: 181, 188, 294, 295; III: 29, 237, 239, 241, 243, 282, 289, 318, 321, 452; IV: 267
South Korea, I: 61-62; II: 108-109
Soviet Union. *See* Russia; USSR
Spain, IV: 144-145, 207, 401
Special Forces. *See* U.S. Special Forces
Sperm parameter disorders
altered sperm parameters, I: 631, 632, 633-634; II: 7, 11, 20; III: 444-451; IV: 200, 405-406, 433
See also Reproductive disorders
Spina bifida, I: 609, 611, 612; II: 6, 295-296
Vietnam veterans offspring, II: 9-10, 296, 298, 309; III: 7, 8, 9-10, 21, 24-25, 437-438; IV: 7, 10, 18, 404-405
See also Birth defects; Neural tube defects
Spontaneous abortion, I: 592
agricultural/forestry workers and, I: 336-337; IV: 197, 410-411
Alsea, Oregon, case, I: 42-43, 372-373, 598
definition, I: 595-596; II: 282; IV: 409
epidemiologic data, quality of, I: 603-605
epidemiologic studies, II: 283; IV: 410-411
epidemiology, II: 282-283
herbicide association in, I: 14, 605; II: 7, 20, 278, 283-284; 411-412
herbicide environmental exposure and, I: 598-599; IV: 410-411

herbicide occupational exposure and, I: 596-598; IV: 410
maternal risk factors, I: 596
Ranch Hand participants, II: 283-284
risk factors, I: 594; IV: 409
scientific literature update, II: 283-284; IV: 410-411
Vietnamese civilians and, I: 599-601
Vietnam veterans' increased risk, II: 283; IV: 411
Vietnam veterans' wives and, I: 405-406, 601-603
See also Reproductive disorders
Standardized fertility ratio (SFR), III: 448
Standardized incidence ratio (SIR), IV: 252-253, 269, 289, 293-294, 328-329, 336, 357, 365-366, 379
Standardized mortality ratios (SMRs)
cancer studies, II: 134, 136, 137, 178, 182, 183, 191, 193, 194, 195, 198, 199, 200, 201, 202, 204, 206, 269, 270, 271, 273, 274; III: 420, 421, 422, 423, 424, 425, 426, 429; IV: 138, 142, 153; IV: 251-253, 268, 292, 302, 327, 332, 341, 346-347, 351-352, 365-366, 372, 379
role of, I: 229-230
State governments, I: 60
Vietnam veterans epidemiologic studies by, I: 399-405, 495-496; II: 153, 158-159, 161, 202, 292; III: 213-215, 243-244
See also specific state
Statistics Sweden, IV: 145
Umea Department of Oncology, II: 138; III: 228
University Hospital, Linkoping, II: 138; III: 228, 229
University Hospital, Umea, III: 228
See also Skaraborg, Sweden; Umea, Sweden; Uppsala, Sweden
Stillbirth. *See* Perinatal death
Stomach
cancer, I: 446, 447; II: 7, 12; III: 274-275; IV, 250-254, 256, 259n, 385
TCDD effects in, I: 169
See also Gastrointestinal (GI) tract cancers
Streptococcus pneumoniae
TCDD exposure and, II: 68
Stroke
herbicide exposure risk, I: 658, 659, 660
See also Motor/coordination dysfunction; Neurobehavioral toxicity

STS. *See* Soft-tissue sarcoma
Subcommittee on Hospitals and Health Care, III: 25
Substance abuse, I: 655
Suicide, I: 398, 650, 655-656; IV: 440
Surveillance, Epidemiology, and End Results (SEER) program, I: 336, 439-440, 506; II: 205, 213; III: 229, 266, 313; IV: 215, 249
 ICD-9 cancer codes, site groupings for, III: 537-539; IV: 524-526
Sweden, I: 8, 9, 13, 37, 322-323, 326-329, 375, 443, 444, 447, 467, 479, 480, 481, 482-486, 490, 510, 528-529, 530-533, 539, 548, 551-553, 561, 572-573; II: 138, 183-184, 185, 197, 198, 199, 209, 215, 231, 233, 235-236, 242-243; III: 226, 228-229, 236, 271-272, 285, 297, 306, 308, 309, 310, 314, 315, 317, 319, 325, 338, 340, 349, 353, 358, 363, 372, 484, 515; IV: 201, 202, 206, 207, 208, 209, 210, 212, 213, 214, 322, 328, 330, 367
 Cancer Environment Register, III: 224; IV: 140
 Cancer Registry, III: 224, 228, 229; IV: 142
 Lund University Hospital, III: 229
 National Register of Causes of Death IV: 141
 Orebro Medical Center Hospital, III: 229
 Regional Cancer Registry, II: 138; III: 228, 229
Switzerland, II: 134
Systemic autoimmune disease, I: 697-699
 See also Autoimmune disease; Immune system disorders
Systemic lupus erythematosus, I: 697
 See also Autoimmune disease; Immune system disorders

T

2,4,5-T. *See* 2,4,5-Trichlorophenoxyacetic acid
T cell function, I: 147-148, 151; II: 3; IV: 62, 80
 autoimmunity and, I: 697
 immune modulation and, I: 694, 695
 TCDD and, II: 68-70; IV: 61, 62, 78
 Vietnam veterans and, I: 698
Taiwan, III: 231, 470
 chloracne as a biomarker in, IV: 464
 Movement Disorders Clinic, National Taiwan University Hospital, III: 231
Tannery workers, I: 486, 514
Tasmania, I: 418, 603; II: 293; III: 244; IV: 246
TCDD. *See* TCDD biologic plausibiltiy;
 Serum levels, TCDD; 2,3,7,8-Tetrachlorodibenzo-*p*-dioxin
TCDD biologic plausibility, IV: 2, 3, 11-12, 107, 110, 385-387, 432-435, 515-517
 Ah receptor in, I: 133-138; IV: 25-27, 29-30, 42, 47-58, 85-86, 458
 animal carcinogenicity studies, I: 138-146, 439; III: 394, 396
 brain tumors and, I: 525; IV: 352
 cancer, II: 176; IV: 248-388 *passim*
 carcinogenesis, I: 116-118, 434, 439; III: 394, 396; IV: 279, 385
 cardiovascular toxicity, I: 171; IV: 510
 childhood cancer and, I: 630; IV: 426
 chloracne and, I: 172-174, 678; II: 320-321; III: 480; IV: 8, 17-18, 135; IV: 466
 cognitive/neuropsychiatric disorders and, II: 314
 diabetes mellitus, III: 502-503; IV: 488
 fetal/infant death and, I: 624; IV: 413
 gastrointestinal toxicity, I: 169-170, 451; III: 513-514
 genitourinary tract cancers and, I: 521-522
 hepatobiliary cancers and, I: 457; IV: 270
 Hodgkin's disease and, I: 557; IV: 8, 367
 immune system disorders and, I: 122, 146-151, 699; III: 523-524; IV: 481
 lethality, IV: 76, 137
 leukemia and, I: 571; IV: 380
 lipid abnormalities, III: 507; IV: 495
 liver disease, III: 522-524; IV: 10, 505
 motor/coordination dysfunction and, I: 661; II: 314
 multiple myeloma and, I: 563; IV: 374
 nasal/nasopharyngeal cancer and, I: 460; IV: 275
 neurological disorders and, I: 160-166; III: 474, 475; IV: 441-443, 445, 457-459
 non-Hodgkin's lymphoma and, I: 549; IV: 8, 116, 358
 peripheral neuropathy and, II: 314; IV: 457-459
 porphyria cutanea tarda and, I: 682; II: 323; IV: 468
 reproductive disorders and, I: 123-124, 156-159, 605, 618, 634; II: 282; III: 460-461, 462; IV: 323, 403, 407, 411, 431

respiratory toxicity, I: 170; IV: 475
skin cancer and, I: 503; IV: 305-311
soft-tissue sarcoma and, I: 500; IV: 8, 116, 296
See also Ah receptor (AhR); Biologic plausibility; 2,3,7,8-Tetrachlorodibenzo-*p*-dioxin (TCDD)
TCP. See 2,4,5-Trichlorophenol
TEC. See Toxic equivalent concentration
Tecumseh, Michigan, III: 235, 388
TEFs. See Toxic equivalency factors
Teq factors. See Dioxin toxic equivalent factors
Teratogenicity, I: 57, 62, 606-607
 2,4-D, I: 180-181
 2,4,5-T, I: 185, 373-374; II: 4
 cacodylic acid, I: 189
 picloram, I: 192
 TCDD, I: 28, 30, 123, 159-160, 185, 368, 370, 372; III: 461; IV: 29, 53
 viral potential, I: 607
 See also Birth defects
Testicular cancer, I: 405
 biologic plausibility, III: 347; IV: 337
 epidemiologic studies, I: 519; II: 153, 227-228; III: 343-346; IV: 336-337, 338-339
 epidemiology, I: 515; II: 223-224; III: 343; IV: 335
 herbicide association in, I: 13, 521; II: 7, 11, 20, 227-228, 249-250; III: 7, 10, 343-347; IV: 7, 11
 herbicide environmental exposure and, III: 344, 345; IV: 336
 herbicide occupational exposure and, III: 344, 345; IV: 336
 histopathology, I: 513
 incidence, data by race, for selected age groups, III: 343; IV: 335
 scientific literature update, II: 227-228; III: 344, 346; IV: 159, 336-337
 Vietnam veterans' risk, I: 519, 522; II: 153, 223-224, 227, 228; IV: 338
 Vietnam veterans' studies, III: 343-344, 345-346; IV: 157, 159, 336-337
 See also Genitourinary cancers
Testimony, I: 739-756; II: 343-348; III: 533-536
Testosterone, I: 123, 157-158; II: 280, 281, 282; IV: 183, 399-400, 405, 407-408, 429, 433
Tetrachlorobenzene, I: 28

2,3,7,8-Tetrachlorodibenzo-*p*-dioxin (TCDD), III: 5, 19; IV: 16, 132
 acute toxicity, II: 75-76
 Ah receptor interaction, I: 3, 114, 118, 122, 123, 133-138, 150, 151, 152, 159-160, 439, 452-453, 457; II: 3-4, 51-53, 54-56, 57-62, 176; III: 33, 34, 35, 53, 54, 58-61, 62-69, 129; IV: 25, 26, 30, 32, 47-53, 58, 60
 animal studies, I: 111-114, 138-142, 477; II: 3-4, 12, 51-77; III: 4-5, 33, 34-36, 37, 40-43, 54-58, 62-63, 67-69, 74-105, 128, 129, 130, 394, 396, 460-461, 474, 475, 482, 501, 522-523; IV: 26, 53-57, 59, 270, 284, 305, 311, 416, 426, 432-435, 458-459, 512
 anti-estrogenicity and, I: 512; II: 62; III: 67-69
 apoptosis of, II: 3, 67
 autoimmunity and, I: 697-699
 bioavailability, I: 128-129
 biological consequences of activation, II: 57; III: 61-62
 biomarkers, I: 4, 17, 259-262, 725; II: 101-104; III: 146-147
 bladder cancer association, II: 225-227; III: 347-348; IV: 341-342
 body burdens, III: 107-108; IV: 478
 body temperature regulation and, I: 169
 bone cancer association, II: 204-205; III: 303; IV: 289
 brain distribution, I: 160-161
 brain tumors association, II: 229, 230; III: 357, 358; IV: 351
 breast cancer association, II: 215-217; III: 327, 329; IV: 316-317
 carcinogenesis promoter capability, I: 116, 142-143, 434, 439
 carcinogenicity, I: 28-29, 116-118, 138-146, 439, 451; II: 3, 39-40, 65-68, 175, 176; III: 265, 394, 396, 430-431; IV: 60-66, 270, 279
 cardiovascular toxicity, I: 171; II: 76; III: 74-75
 cell proliferation capability of, I: 145; II: 3, 67; IV: 60
 chemical properties, I: 28, 114, 127
 chemical significant interactions, II: 64-65; III: 69-71
 chemical structure, I: 125-126; II: 38
 chloracne and, I: 4, 10, 28, 172-173, 262;

II: 3, 5, 6, 317-321; III: 479-480; IV: 135, 464
circulatory disorders and, I: 701-708; II: 336-337; III: 514, 515-516, 518; IV: 506-507
cognitive/neuropsychiatric disorders and, II: 308
concerns about, I: 1, 2, 23-24, 28-32, 35-36; II: 2, 17, 18, 19, 26-27; III: 3-5, 12, 13, 14
corticosteroids and, I: 168, 171-172;
cytochrome P4501A2 and, I: 130, 144-145, 170, 709; IV: 274, 386
dermal toxicity, II: 76; III: 73-74
developmental toxicity, I: 123-124, 149, 156-157, 159-160, 185; II: 3, 41-42, 71, 72-73; III: 92-105
diabetes mellitus and, I: 683; II: 330-331; III: 494, 495, 500-501, 502; IV: 483, 489
dietary significant interactions, II: 64
dioxin categorization, I: 23n, 125
DNA binding capability and transcription activation and, II: 56-57; III: 58-61
dose-response relationships, I: 111-114, 122, 128-129, 130, 137-138, 445, 673, 696; II: 318
endocrine effects, III: 83-84
environmental exposure assessment, I: 262-263, 267-270; II: 140-149, 179-180, 184, 186, 190, 193, 200-201, 221, 222, 234, 236, 243; III: 156-157, 232-233, 234, 235-236, 297-298, 303; IV: 114-116, 147-150, 254, 269, 274-275, 278, 293, 296, 336, 347, 351, 357, 379
environmental persistence, I: 288
enzyme induction of, II: 3, 66-67
estrogen-mediation of carcinogenesis, I: 144-145
excretion, I: 132-133
exposure assessment issues, II: 4-5, 104-106; III: 140-142, 144, 157-158, 159-161; IV: 122-127, 132
exposure sources, I: 127
fatty acid biosynthesis and, I: 168-169
female reproductive system/breast cancers and, I: 512; II: 211-213; III: 331, 332; IV: 315, 316, 322
free radicals, II: 59; III: 64-65
gastrointestinal toxicity, I: 169-170, 447-452, 690-692; II: 177-181; III: 268-272, 511; IV: 251-254, 499-501

gastrointestinal ulcers and, II: 334-335; III: 510
genotoxicity, I: 118, 143-144; II: 3
growth factor and, II: 59
H4IIE-luc cells and, III: 107
half-life, I: 129, 260-261; II: 104-105; III: 157-158; IV: 24, 27
hepatic enzyme disorders and, I: 155-156, 685-688, 691-692
hepatobiliary cancers and, I: 457; II: 181-187; III: 283-285
hepatotoxicity, II: 3, 73-75; III: 76-79
herbicide contaminant capacity, I: 2, 3, 27, 91-92, 114, 126-127; II: 2, 3, 26; III: 1, 3, 5, 6, 140-142
hexachlorophene manufacture and, I: 40; IV: 134-135, 138, 148
Hodgkin's lymphoma and, II: 5, 6, 235, 236; III: 372-373; IV: 366
hypoglycemia and, I: 166-168
immune modulation and, I: 694-696; II: 328-329; III: 488, 489, 490, 491; IV: 26
immunotoxicity, I: 119-122, 146-151, 338, 477; II: 3, 40-41, 68-71; III: 85-92; IV: 478-480
infertility association, II: 282
inflammatory responses and, I: 148
interactions, significant, III: 69-71
intracellular communication of, II: 3, 67-68
latency issues, II: 13-14, 269, 270, 272; III: 420, 421, 423, 424, 425, 426, 429, 431
lethality, III: 71-73
leukemia association, II: 246; III: 386-388, 390; IV: 379, 426
lipid abnormalities and, I: 688-690; II: 333-334; III: 505, 506, 507
liver toxicity, I: 115-116, 124, 138-139, 142, 143, 151-156, 165-166; II: 42, 331-333; III: 509; IV: 27, 268, 269, 499
lung cancer and, III: 297-298, 299, 421, 423; IV: 282-283
mechanism of action, animal studies, II: 3, 54-65; III: 54-58, 62-63, 67-69; IV: 28-30
mechanisms of toxicity, II: 65-77; IV: 67-76, 426
metabolism, I: 115-116, 131-133, 155
multiple myeloma association, II: 237-238, 243, 244; III: 378-380, 383; IV: 372-373

nasal/nasopharyngeal cancer and, I: 460;
    IV: 274-275
neuropsychiatric outcomes and, I: 649-650,
    651-652, 656, 657-658; II: 308
neurotoxicity, I: 160-166, 642; II: 3, 75; III:
    84-85, 469, 470-471; IV: 31
non-Ah-mediated toxicity, I: 138
non-Hodgkin's lymphoma and, I: 8, 9, 528-
    529, 574; II: 5, 6, 231-234; III: 364,
    429; IV: 357
occupational exposure, I: 36-39, 262-267,
    269-270, 303; II: 108-109, 113-140,
    178-179, 190, 191-200, 219-220, 222,
    232-234, 237-238; III: 153, 154, 155,
    219, 220, 221-222, 223, 224 284-285,
    293, 296-297, 303; IV: 111-114, 134-
    147, 187-190, 195-196, 251, 257, 259-
    260, 262, 265, 268, 271, 277, 280, 282,
    284, 289, 290, 292, 306, 312, 318, 341,
    343, 346, 348, 353, 359, 374
opioid antagonist capacity, I: 164
oral administration, I: 128
perinatal death association, II: 285-286
peripheral neuropathy and, II: 310-311,
    314; III: 470-471; IV: 184
pharmacokinetics, I: 127-133, 160, 259-
    261, 284
porphyria cutanea tarda and, II: 5, 6, 321-
    323; III: 481-482; IV: 466-468
potential health risk estimating, II: 63-65;
    III: 105-108
production of, I: 28, 114
prostate cancer association, II: 220-223,
    273, 274, 275; III: 336-337, 425, 426;
    IV: 327-328, 329-331
protein kinases and, II: 60-62; III: 65-67
Qsar model approach, III: 106
Ranch Hand study, II: 109; III: 50, 146-
    147; IV: 18
renal cancer association, II: 225; III: 353;
    IV: 346-347
renal toxicity, II: 77; III: 75-76
reproductive toxicity, I: 123-124, 156-159,
    368, 371-372, 597, 599, 605; II: 3, 41-
    42, 71-72; III: 92-105, 446, 449; IV:
    398-438 *passim*
respiratory cancers and, II: 13-14, 189-203,
    269, 270, 272; IV: 282-283
respiratory disorders and, I: 170, 472, 709-
    710, 712-714; III: 484; IV: 471-474
sensitivity interspecies and interindividual
    differences, II: 63-64; III: 108

skin cancer and, I: 141, 142-143, 502-503;
    II: 209-211; III: 313-316, 317, 319, 320,
    322
soft-tissue sarcoma and, I: 477, 478, 490,
    498-500; II: 5, 6, 205-208; III: 307, 308;
    IV: 292-293
solubility, I: 114, 115-116, 127
teratogenicity, I: 28-29, 30, 31, 123, 159-
    160, 185, 368, 370, 372; III: 461
testicular cancer association, II: 228; III:
    346; IV: 336
tissue specificity, II: 64
toxic equivalency factors approach, II: 63;
    III: 106, 158, 159
toxic equivalent concentration approach,
    III: 107
toxicity, factors influencing, II: 63-65; III:
    105-108; IV: 83-84
toxicity profile, III: 50-108; 33-84
toxicity update summary, II: 51-53; IV: 3-5,
    22, 26, 44, 62, 64, 83-86
toxicokinetics, animal studies, II: 3, 53-54;
    III: 4-5, 48; IV: 41-46
Vietnam amount used, I: 27, 106; II: 26;
    IV: 122
Vietnam military exposure, I: 17, 26, 149-
    161; II: 21, 22, 181, 185, 187, 190, 201-
    202, 204, 205, 208, 209, 211, 212, 226,
    276, 308; III: 146, 147, 237, 239, 240,
    430-431; IV: 150-160
Vietnam veterans' compensation, II: 28-29;
    III: 26-27
Vietnamese civilians exposure, II: 108-109,
    148; III: 156-157; IV: 116-117, 148-149
wasting syndrome, I: 160-161, 162-166; II:
    76-77; III: 80-83; IV: 25, 31, 57
    See also Herbicides; Serum levels, TCDD;
        TCDD biologic plausibility
12-O-Tetradexanoylphorbol-13-acetate (TPA),
    II: 76
Texas, I: 60, 403-404, 696; III: 243
TGF. *See* Transforming growth factor
T-H Agricultural & Nutrition Company, I: 35
Thailand, I: 26, 90
Thompson Chemicals Corporation, I: 35
Thyroid
    TCDD effects, I: 168-169; IV: 135, 386-387
    thyroiditis, I: 697, 698
Times Beach, Missouri, I: 40-42, 268, 368-370,
    693-694; II: 113, 144, 184; III: 200-201,
    234, 283; IV: 115-116, 133, 148
Tissue distribution, TCDD, I: 129-131, 259

INDEX 595

TNF. *See* Tumor necrosis factor
Tobacco exposure and use, I: 11, 223, 442, 461, 463; II: 190-191, 197; III: 299, 377
 perinatal mortality and, I: 619-620
 respiratory cancer and latency, II: 268; III: 418
Tollerud, David, III: 25
Topography, I: 25
Tordon 101, IV: 117-118. *See also* 2,4-Dichlorophenoxyacetic acid (2,4-D); Picloram
Toxic equivalency factors (TEFs), II: 45, 52, 63; III: 37, 105, 106, 108; IV: 83-84
Toxic equivalent concentration (TEC), III: 105, 107
Toxicity
 2,4-D profile update, II: 46-49; III: 43-47; IV: 33-37
 2,4,5-T profile update, II: 49-50; III: 47-48; IV: 37-38
 cacodylic acid profile update, II: 50-51; III: 48-50; IV: 38-40
 contributing factors, III: 105-108
 definition, II: 35
 health risk estimation, III: 105-108
 picloram profile update, II: 51; III: 50; IV: 40-41
 TCDD profile update, II: 51-77; III: 50-108; IV: 41-81
Toxicokinetics, III: 32-36
 2,4-D, II: 46-47; III: 32-33, 43-44; IV: 24, 33
 2,4,5-T, II: 49; III: 47; IV: 24, 37
 cacodylic acid, II: 50; III: 32-33, 48; IV: 24, 38-39
 definition, II: 35
 literature update, II: 36; III: 36-37
 picloram, IV: 24
 previous reports summary, II: 38-39
 TCDD, II: 53-54; III: 33, 53, 161; IV: 23-24, 27-28, 41-46, 85-86
Toxicology
 cacodylic acid profile update, II: 50-51; III: 48-50
 2,4-D profile update, II: 46-49; III: 43-47
 disease outcomes, II: 37, 48-49, 50-51, 65-77; III: 33-35, 38-43, 44-47, 48, 50, 71-105
 earlier reports summary, II: 37-42; III: 36
 evaluation issues, III: 108-110
 human health relevance, III: 35-36; IV: 43
 literature update, II: 43-45; III: 36-43

 mechanisms of toxic action, II: 36, 47-48, 50, 54-65; III: 33, 38, 44, 47-48, 49-50, 53-71; IV: 24
 picloram profile update, II: 51; III: 50
 studies evaluation, III: 128-129
 summary, II: 35-37; III: 3-5, 32-36; IV: 24-25
 TCDD profile update, II: 51-77; III: 50-108
 toxicity profiles update, II: 45-77; III: 45-108
 2,4,5-T profile update, II: 49-50; III: 47-48
TPA. *See* 12-O-Tetradecanoylphorbol-13-acetate
Trail-Making Test, II: 308
Transforming growth factor, I: 145; II: 59, 74
2,4,5-Trichlorophenol (TCP), I: 28; II: 319; III: 152, 153, 219, 220, 223, 515; IV: 16, 134, 136, 138, 186, 251, 268, 292, 500
2,4,5-Trichlorophenoxyacetic acid (2,4,5-T); II: 4, 18; III: 5, 19, 218, 219, 220, 223, 224, 226, 234; IV: 2, 22, 110, 251, 268, 292, 474, 478, 479
 acute toxicity, I: 184
 Agent Orange and, I: 27; II: 26
 animal studies, I: 181-185; II: 49-50; III: 47-48, 396, 462; IV: 34, 426, 434-435, 458, 459, 512, 517
 birth defects and, II: 287; III: 462; IV: 404, 405n
 calcium homeostasis and, II: 4
 carcinogenicity, I: 37, 118, 119, 182-184; II: 40; III: 396; IV: 387
 chemical properties, I: 114, 182; II: 38; III: 32
 chemical structure, I: 111, 114
 chloracne and, I: 36; IV: 135, 500
 chronic exposure, I: 184
 circulatory disorders and, I: 700-701
 development of, I: 24, 26, 35, 181; III: 135, 136, 137, 138, 140
 developmental toxicity, I: 185; II: 42, 49-50
 disease outcomes, III: 48
 domestic use, I: 181
 environmental exposure events, I: 42-43
 genotoxicity, I: 119, 184
 half-life of, II: 4
 infertility and, II: 280-282
 liver toxicity, I: 125; II: 42; III: 524
 mechanisms of action, III: 33, 38, 47-48
 mechanisms of toxicity, II: 49-50
 metabolism, I: 115, 116
 military applications, I: 26, 88; II: 26

myelotoxicity, IV: 5, 31
neurobehavioral toxicity, III: 475
pharmacokinetics, I: 182
porphyria cutanea tarda and, II: 322
reproductive toxicity, I: 185; II: 42; III: 462; IV: 407, 413, 416, 426, 431, 434-435
respiratory disorders and, I: 709
suspension of use, I: 1, 39, 42-43, 92, 181-182
TCDD contamination of, I: 2, 3, 27, 91, 114, 126, 182; III: 140
teratogenicity, I: 30, 92, 373-374
toxicity profile update summary, II: 49; IV: 22-24, 28-29, 31, 37-41
toxicokinetics, II: 49; III: 47
volume used in Operation Ranch Hand, data, III: 136
See also Herbicides; 2,3,7,8-Tetrachloro-dibenzo-*p*-dioxin (TCDD)
Triglyceride levels, I: 688-689; III: 520-521
Trinoxol, I: 91; III: 137; IV: 119
Tuberculosis, I: 711
See also Respiratory disorders
Tumor necrosis factor (TNF), I: 148; II: 59, 60; III: 87, 88
Twin studies, I: 398-399, 406, 703, 711

U

UDP glucuronyl transferase (UGT1), II: 74; III: 37, 52
Uerdingen, Germany, III: 154; IV: 124
UGT1. *See* UDP glucuronyl transferase
Ulcers, gastrointestinal, I: 690-692
epidemiologic studies, II: 334; III: 510-513; IV: 500-504
epidemiology, II: 334; III: 508-509; IV: 498-499
herbicide exposure association with, II: 334; III: 510-514; IV: 505
herbicide occupational exposure and, III: 510-512; IV: 500-501
scientific literature update, II: 334; III: 510-513; IV: 500-504
Vietnam veterans and, III: 512-513; IV: 502-505
See also Metabolic and digestive disorders
Umea, Sweden, III: 228, 229
Uniroyal Inc., I: 35

United Kingdom, I: 315-316, 340, 382, 444, 462-463, 464, 477, 479, 537, 565, 595, 689; II: 194, 196, 269; III: 223, 224, 420
England National Cancer Register, III: 232; IV: 144
herbicide exposure assessment, III: 151; IV: 139
Parkinson's Disease Society Brain Bank, IV: 445
See also Yorkshire, England
United Nations, I: 45
United Paperworkers International Union, III: 232
Update 1996. See Veterans and Agent Orange: Update 1996 (Update 1996)
Uppsala, Sweden, III: 228
Urinary bladder cancer. *See* Bladder cancer
Uroporphyrinogen decarboxylase (UROD), II: 321; III: 480, 481
U.S. Air Force, I: 81, 113; III: 29, 138, 218, 237, 239, 339, 513, 517
Armstrong Laboratory, Population Research Branch, III: 29
Baseline Morbidity Report, II: 32
Baseline Mortality Report, 1982, II: 31
Follow-Up Examination Results, 1985, 1987, 1992, II: 32
Human Resources Laboratory records, II: 150, 152; III: 237
Military Personnel Center records, II: 151; III: 238; IV: 151
Mortality Updates, 1984, 1985, 1986, 1989, 1991, II: 32
Reproductive Outcomes, II: 32
Serum Dioxin Level Follow-Up Examination Results, II: 32
TCDD half-life investigations, II: 104-105
Vietnam casualties, I: 83
women veterans mortality studies, II: 152-153
See also Air Force Health Study (AFHS); Operation Ranch Hand
U.S. Army, I: 81, 280, 281, 702; II: 140, 185; IV: 121-22, 126
Army Chemical Corps Vietnam Veterans Health Study proposal, II: 24
Army I Corps, IV: 157
Environmental Support Group (ESG), II: 152
Vietnam casualties, I: 83

Vietnam veteran studies, II: 201, 226, 244; III: 240, 241, 283, 294, 298, 313, 315, 318, 338, 339, 344, 346, 348, 365, 373, 380, 485, 512, 517; IV: 21
women veterans mortality studies, II: 152-153, 201
See also U.S. Army Chemical Corps; U.S. Special Forces
U.S. Army Chemical Corps, I: 13, 15, 16-17, 94-95, 272, 273, 286, 394, 470, 571, 703-704, 705, 711, 722-725; II: 5, 23, 24, 101, 103, 104, 201-202, 245; III: 6, 23, 138-139, 146-147, 241, 272, 298, 309, 314, 344, 358-359, 385, 389, 485, 512, 517; IV: 120-124, 157, 287
U.S. Coast Guard, I: 81
U.S. Congress, I: 2, 31, 46-52; III: 25-28, 237, 240
See also Congressional hearings; Legislation
USDA. *See* Department of Agriculture, U.S.
U.S. Marine Corps, I: 81, 96, 280, 545, 702, 710; II: 185, 201, 226, 244; III: 140; IV: 121
non-Hodgkin's lymphoma in, I: 542, 545, 546-547
Vietnam casualties, I: 83
Vietnam veterans studies, III: 241, 242, 283, 294, 298, 309, 313, 315, 338, 339, 346, 348, 365, 373, 380, 485, 489, 512, 517; IV: 287, 298, 339
women veterans mortality studies, II: 152-153
U.S. Military Assistance Command, III: 138; IV: 119
U.S. Navy, I: 81, 280-281, 286; II: 185, 228; III: 339, 344
herbicide use in, I: 95; II: 104; III: 135, 139, 140
non-Hodgkin's lymphoma odds ratio in, I: 542
Vietnam casualties, I: 83
women veterans mortality studies, II: 152-153
U.S. Special Forces, I: 286; II: 103-104; III: 138
USSR, I: 317; III: 224
See also Russia
Utah, I: 560; II: 241
Uterine cancer, I: 506; III: 329, 333
herbicide association evidence, I: 13; II: 6, 211, 213; III: 333; IV: 323-324
See also Reproductive system cancers, women

V

VAO. *See* Veterans and Agent Orange: Health Effects of Herbicides Used in Vietnam
Verona, Missouri, II: 128-129; III: 219, 220; IV: 135, 148
Very low density lipoprotein (VLDL) receptors, II: 333; III: 503
VES. *See* Vietnam Experience Study
Veterans. *See* Foreign veterans; Vietnam veterans; Women veterans
Veterans Administration. *See* Department of Veterans Affairs (DVA)
Veterans and Agent Orange: Health Effects of Herbicides Used in Vietnam (VAO), II: 1, 2, 5, 8, 10, 11, 12, 35, 45, 63, 65, 71, 89, 90, 91, 96, 97, 99, 101, 102, 104, 107, 112, 132, 176, 179, 180, 181, 187, 190, 196, 207, 209, 210, 214, 218, 225, 228, 232, 236, 237, 246, 247, 249, 250, 266, 271, 278, 279, 286, 293, 296, 300, 305, 312, 323, 328, 357; III: 1, 2, 3, 5, 12, 32, 43, 85, 124, 125, 126, 132, 150, 157, 169, 220, 221, 223, 286, 303, 311, 320, 359, 389, 390, 416, 434, 435, 519, 522; IV: 5, 156-159
background, II: 17-19; III: 17-23; IV: 15, 103-104, 110, 132, 137, 249, 268, 351
basal/squamous cell skin cancer studies summary, III: 317-318, 321, 323; IV: 308, 312-313
birth defects studies summary, III: 436-439; IV: 400-401, 404, 435
bladder cancer studies summary, II: 225-226; III: 347-348, 350-351; IV: 340, 343-345
bone cancer studies summary, II: 204; III: 302, 305; IV: 288, 290-291
brain tumor studies summary, II: 229; III: 356-357, 360, 361; IV: 351, 353-355
breast cancer studies summary, III: 324-326, 328; IV: 314-315, 319-320
childhood cancer studies summary, II: 299; IV: 418, 429
chloracne studies summary, II: 318; III: 479-480; IV: 465
chronic persistent peripheral neuropathy studies summary, II: 310; IV: 454
circulatory disorders studies summary, II: 335-336; III: 514; IV: 506

cognitive and neuropsychiatric disorders studies summary, II: 307; III: 468-469; IV: 441-442
congressional hearings on Agent Orange, II: 27-28; III: 25
Department of Veterans Affairs Task Force, II: 4-26; III: 24-25
diabetes mellitus studies summary, II: 330; III: 496-497; IV: 482, 487, 488, 490, 492
federal government response to concerns over military use of herbicides in Vietnam, II: 27-32; III: 25-30
female reproductive cancers studies summary, II: 211-212; III: 330-331, 332, 333; IV: 321, 324-325
gastrointestinal tract tumors studies summary, II: 177-178; III: 268, 274-281; IV: 251, 256
gastrointestinal ulcers studies summary, II: 334; III: 510; IV: 500
health outcomes conclusions, II: 19-23; III: 19-20; IV: 11, 18-19, 20, 21, 384, 385, 414, 465, 467, 471, 513, 514
hepatobiliary cancers studies summary, III: 282-283, 287-288; IV: 268, 269
herbicide environmental exposure studies, II: 142-143, 144, 145-146; III: 197-202, 203-205, 275, 277, 279, 281, 283, 288, 291, 301, 316, 323, 328, 336, 342, 345, 350-351, 354, 369, 382, 392, 437, 454, 455, 456, 459, 479, 520; IV: 147-149, 261, 264, 266-267, 271-272, 276, 286, 291
herbicide occupational exposure studies, II: 114, 115-116, 117-118, 119-120, 121-126; III: 170-174, 176-178, 180-182, 183-185, 188-196, 274-275, 276-277, 278-279, 280, 282-283, 286, 291, 294, 300-301, 305, 310, 312, 316, 317, 321, 323, 324-326, 328, 332, 333, 335-336, 345, 350, 354, 360, 367-369, 374-376, 381-382, 391-392, 454, 455, 456, 459, 496, 520; IV: 137, 139, 140-142, 144-146, 257-261, 263, 265-266, 271, 276, 280, 285, 290
Hodgkin's disease studies summary, II: 235; III: 372, 374-375, 376; IV: 365, 368
immune system disorders, studies summary, II: 327; III: 488-489; IV: 477

impact of report, II: 24-26; III: 23-25
infertility studies summary, II: 280; III: 445-446, 450; IV: 406, 409
laryngeal cancer studies summary, III: 293, 294; IV: 277, 280
legislation on Agent Orange, II: 28-29; III: 26-27
leukemia studies summary, II: 245; III: 385-386, 391-392; IV: 378-379, 381, 383
lipid abnormalities studies summary, II: 333; III: 504, 520, 521; IV: 483
liver toxicity studies summary, II: 332; III: 510; IV: 500
low birthweight studies summary, III: 456-457, 459; IV: 399, 400, 412
lung cancer studies summary, III: 296, 300-301; IV: 281, 285-286
melanoma studies summary, III: 313-314, 316, 317; IV: 302, 306
metabolic and digestive disorders, studies summary, II: 330, 332, 333, 334; IV: 500
motor/coordination dysfunction studies summary, II: 309; III: 469-470; IV: 443-444
multiple myeloma studies summary, III: 377-378, 381-382; IV: 372, 375-376
nasal/nasopharyngeal cancer studies summary, III: 290, 291; 274; IV: 274
non-Hodgkin's lymphoma studies summary, II: 231-232; III: 362-363, 367-369, 370-371; IV: 356, 360-363
perinatal death studies summary, II: 285; III: 451, 454, 455, 456; IV: 412
peripheral neuropathy studies summary, III: 470-471, 473; IV: 454
porphyria cutanea tarda studies summary, II: 321-322; III: 481-482; IV: 467
prostate cancer studies summary, III: 335-336, 341, 342; IV: 327, 333-335
renal cancer studies summary, II: 224; III: 352-353, 354, 355; IV: 346, 349-350
research recommendations, II: 23-24; III: 23; IV: 21
respiratory disorders studies summary, II: 324-325; III: 483; IV: 471
sex ratios of offspring, IV: 429-430
skin cancer studies summary, III: 312; IV: 299-314
soft-tissue sarcomas studies summary, II: 205-206; III: 306-308; IV: 292, 297-299

spontaneous abortion studies summary, II: 283; IV: 410
summary of, II: 37-42
testicular cancer studies summary, III: 343-344, 345-346; IV: 336, 338-339
toxicology, overview, III: 36; IV: 22, 38, 41
Veterans and Agent Orange: Herbicides/ Dioxin Exposure and Type 2 Diabetes (Type 2 Diabetes), IV: 1, 10-11, 16, 104
Veterans and Agent Orange: Update 1996 (Update 1996); III: 1, 2, 3, 6, 8, 10, 32, 37, 43, 44, 50, 85, 106, 109, 125, 126, 132, 150, 157, 159, 169, 220, 221, 222, 223, 266, 286, 295, 298, 303, 309, 311, 319, 320, 339, 349, 359, 389, 390, 416, 417-418, 424, 426, 428, 434, 435, 444, 458, 519, 522, 533; IV: 1
background, III: 17-23; IV: 15-21, 110, 132, 137, 247, 251
basal/squamous cell skin cancer studies summary, III: 317-318, 321, 323; IV: 308-314
birth defects studies summary, III: 436-439; IV: 400-401, 435
bladder cancer studies summary, III: 347-348, 350; IV: 330-345
bone cancer studies summary, III: 302, 305; IV: 287-291
brain tumor studies summary, III: 356-357, 360, 361; IV: 350-355
breast cancer studies summary, III: 324-326, 327, 328; IV: 314-320
childhood cancers, IV: 418
chloracne studies summary, III: 479-480; IV: 465
circulatory disorders studies summary, III: 514; IV: 506
cognitive/neuropsychiatric disorders studies summary, III: 468-469; IV: 441-442
congressional hearings on Agent Orange, III: 25
Department of Veterans Affairs Task Force, III: 24-25
diabetes mellitus studies summary, III: 496; IV: 482-483, 490
federal government response to concerns over military use of herbicides in Vietnam, III: 25-30
female reproductive system cancers studies summary, III: 330-331, 332, 333; IV: 321-326
gastrointestinal tract tumors studies summary, III: 268, 274-281; IV: 257-264
gastrointestinal ulcers studies summary, III: 510; IV: 500
health outcomes conclusions, III: 19-20
hepatobiliary cancers studies summary, III: 282-283, 287-288; IV: 267-272
herbicide environmental exposure studies, III: 197, 201, 203, 275, 277, 279, 283, 288, 323, 328, 336, 342, 345, 354, 369, 375, 382, 392; IV: 147, 149
herbicide occupational exposure studies, III: 170, 172, 174, 175-176, 179, 183, 186-187, 274, 276, 278, 280, 282-283, 286, 291, 294, 300, 305, 316, 317, 321, 324-326, 328, 332, 333, 335-336, 345, 350, 354, 360, 367, 374, 381, 391, 496; IV: 135-137, 140-142, 144
Hodgkin's disease studies summary, III: 373, 374, 375, 376; IV: 364-371
impact of report, III: 23-25
infertility studies summary, III: 445-446; IV: 406-408
laryngeal cancer studies summary, III: 293, 294; IV: 277-281
legislation on Agent Orange, III: 26-27
leukemia studies summary, III: 385-386, 391, 392; IV: 377-383
lipid abnormalities studies summary, III: 504; IV: 493
liver disorders studies summary, III: 510; IV: 500
low birthweight studies summary, III: 456-457; IV: 412
lung cancer studies summary, III: 296, 298, 300; IV: 281-287
melanoma studies summary, III: 313-314, 316, 317; IV: 302-308
motor/coordination dysfunction studies summary, III: 469-470; IV: 444
multiple myeloma studies summary, III: 377-378, 381, 382; IV: 371-377
nasal/nasopharyngeal cancer studies summary, III: 290, 291; IV: 273-276
non-Hodgkin's lymphoma studies summary, III: 362-363, 367, 369, 370; IV: 355-364
pancreatic cancer, IV: 264-267
perinatal death studies summary, III: 451; IV: 412

peripheral neuropathy studies summary, III: 470-471, 473; IV: 18
porphyria cutanea tarda studies summary, III: 481-482; IV: 467
prostate cancer studies summary, III: 335-336, 341, 342; IV: 326-335
renal cancers studies summary, III: 352-353, 354, 355; IV: 345-350
research recommendations, III: 23
respiratory disorders studies summary, III: 483; IV: 471-472
sex ratios of offspring, IV: 429-430
skin cancer, IV: 299-301
soft-tissue sarcoma studies summary, III: 306-308; IV: 291-299
testicular cancer studies summary, III: 343-344, 345; IV: 335-339
toxicology, overview, III: 36; IV: 22

Veterans and Agent Orange: Update 1998 (Update 1998)
Australian Veterans, IV: 159
background of, IV: 1, 3, 8-10, 110, 132, 247, 251, 399-400
basal/squamous cell skin cancer studies summary, IV: 308-314
birth defects studies summary, IV: 400-401, 435
bladder cancer studies summary, IV: 330-345
bone cancer studies summary, IV: 287-291
brain tumor studies summary, IV: 350-355
breast cancer studies summary, IV: 314-320
childhood cancers, IV: 418, 426
hepatobiliary cancers studies summary, IV: 267-272
Hodgkin's disease studies summary, IV: 364-371
infertility studies summary, IV: 406-408
mortality in, IV: 254
Department of Veterans Affairs and, IV: 157-158
environmental exposure, IV: 148-149
epidemiology, IV: 257
female reproductive system cancers studies summary, IV: 321-326
gastrointestinal tract tumors studies summary, IV: 257-264
laryngeal cancer studies summary, IV: 277-281
leukemia studies summary, IV: 377-383
low birthweight studies summary, IV: 412
lung cancer studies summary, IV: 281-287
melanoma studies summary, IV: 302-308
multiple myeloma studies summary, IV: 371-377
nasal/nasopharyngeal cancer studies summary, IV: 273-276
non-Hodgkin's lymphoma studies summary, IV: 355-364
occupational exposure, IV: 135-137, 139-142, 144
Operation Ranch Hand, IV: 150, 152
pancreatic cancer, IV: 264-267
prostate cancer studies summary, IV: 326-335
renal cancers studies summary, IV: 345-350
sex ratios of offspring, IV: 429-430
skin cancer; IV: 299-301
soft-tissue sarcoma studies summary, IV: 291-299
spontaneous abortion, IV: 408-412
testicular cancer studies summary, IV: 335-339
toxicology overview, IV: 22
Veterans' benefits. *See* Compensation, veterans
Veterans' compensation. *See* Compensation, veterans
Veterans' Dioxin and Radiation Exposure Compensation Standards Act of 1984. *See* Public Law 98-542
Veterans' Health Care Eligibility Reform Act of 1996. *See* Public Law 104-262
Veterans' Health Care, Training, and Small Business Loan Act of 1981. *See* Public Law 97-72
Veterans' Health Programs Extension and Improvement Act of 1979, III: 240
Vietnam, III: 533
herbicide latency issues, methodology, II: 13; III: 12-14
herbicide targeting in, I: 99-106; IV: 116-117
herbicide use in, concerns about, I: 29-32, 45; II: 1, 2, 4, 11, 17, 18, 26; III: 1, 2, 5, 12, 13, 17, 18, 25
research in, I: 30-31
troop movements in, I: 52-53, 96, 287
U.S. casualties in, I: 82-83
U.S. involvement, I: 75-76, 84
U.S. military herbicide use in, I: 1, 3, 24, 27, 84-85, 89-93, 94-96, 98-107, 286; II: 17, 18, 26, 27-32; III: 135-142

See also Ca Mau peninsula; Con Thieu province, Vietnam; Hanoi, Vietnam; Ho Chi Minh City, Vietnam; Khe Sanh-Thonh Son Lam area; Mekong Delta; Rung Sat Special Zone; Vietnamese
Vietnam Experience Study (VES), III: 26, 240, 512
 birth defects in offspring, II: 288, 289, 290; III: 436, 438, 439, 445
 cancer mortality in, I: 444-445
 childhood cancer in, I: 629; II: 300
 chloracne in, I: 677
 circulatory disorders in, I: 702
 exposure assessment use, II: 101; III: 146
 hepatobiliary cancers, II: 185; III: 283
 Hodgkin's disease in, I: 556
 immune system disorders in, I: 696
 infertility in, II: 280
 liver cancer in, I: 455
 low birthweight outcomes in, I: 626
 lung cancer in, I: 469
 methodology, I: 57-58, 281, 284, 389-391
 multiple myeloma, II: 244
 neonatal death in, I: 622
 neurologic/neuropsychiatric outcomes in, I: 656
 non-Hodgkin's lymphoma in, I: 542-543
 origins, I: 50
 reproductive outcomes in, I: 601, 609, 610-611, 626, 632
 respiratory cancer in, II: 201
 respiratory disorders in, I: 710-711
 spina bifida in offspring, II: 9; IV: 8
Vietnam herbicides use by military, II: 26-27
Vietnam Veteran Agent Orange Health Study, I: 741
Vietnam veterans, I: 1; II: 2
 acute and subacute transient peripheral neuropathy, II: 313; III: 473; IV: 6, 459
 advocacy groups, I: 60-61
 Air Force research activities, II: 31-32; III: 28-29; IV: 13, 42-43, 150-156, 160-161
 altered sperm parameters in, I: 632, 634; III: 445, 446, 450; IV: 7
 amyloidosis, IV: 7
 Australian, I: 61, 91, 406, 418, 444, 470, 496-497, 546, 614-615, 633, 702, 710; II: 113, 149, 160, 202, 293; III: 9, 216-217, 218, 237, 244-245, 273, 285-286, 290, 294, 295, 298, 299, 303, 310, 311, 314, 315, 327, 329, 339, 340, 343, 346, 349, 353, 355, 359, 365, 380, 389, 413, 424, 425, 469, 486, 489, 500, 506, 512-513, 517; IV: 9, 10, 159-160, 322-333, 402, 421-422
 autoimmune disease in, I: 698, 699
 basal/squamous cell skin cancer in, III: 323; IV: 309-310
 birth defects in children of, I: 609-615, 618; II: 288-296, 298, 300; III: 435, 436, 437-438; IV: 7, 402
 bladder cancer in, I: 517; II: 223-224; III: 349, 351; IV: 7, 342
 bone cancer in, I: 473, 474-475; II: 204; III: 303, 305; IV: 7, 289
 brain tumors in, I: 522, 523, 525; III: 358-359, 361; IV: 7, 352
 breast cancer in, II: 213, 217, 218; III: 326, 328, 329; IV: 7, 316
 cancer expected incidence, I: 439-440, 442, 446, 452, 461, 501, 505, 513, 522, 526, 564; II: 176-177; III: 266-267, 430-431; IV: 249-250
 cancer in children of, I: 629, 630-631; II: 299; IV: 7, 420-422
 cancer mortality, I: 444-445
 cancer studies, I: 391-393, 401, 402-403, 405, 436-438; II: 176-177; III: 266-267, 430-431
 chloracne in, I: 677-679; II: 317, 318, 321; III: 479-480; IV: 6, 135, 485
 chronic persistent peripheral neuropathy in, II: 311; IV: 7, 456
 circulatory disorders in, I: 702-705; II: 336; III: 516-518; IV: 7, 508-509
 class action suit, I: 34-35
 cognitive/neuropsychiatric disorders in, II: 318; III: 469; IV: 7, 443
 compensation for, I: 34-35, 47, 50-51, 55-56; II: 28-29, 30-31; III: 26-27, 28
 congressional responses to concerns of, I: 46-52; II: 27-29; III: 25-28
 defining, I: 78
 demographics, I: 79, 80-84
 developmental toxicity, II: 72
 diabetes mellitus in, I: 684, 685, 698; II: 330; III: 495, 497, 498, 500, 502; IV: 6, 485-487
 disabilities discharges, I: 32
 disease increased risk for, I: 14-15, 221, 225-226, 247-248, 578; II: 14, 22-23, 88, 89, 91, 218, 223, 251, 276, 298, 300-301, 314, 321, 323; III: 14-15, 22-

23, 124, 127-128, 329, 334, 343, 397, 430-431, 444, 462, 475-476, 491, 503, 507-508, 525; IV: 12, 256, 270, 275, 279, 284, 290, 296, 305-306, 311, 318, 323-324, 332, 338, 343, 348, 353, 359, 367, 374, 381, 403, 407, 411-412, 413, 417, 426, 466, 468, 475, 489, 495, 505, 510, 513
distribution by branch of service, I: 81
Environmental Protection Agency research activities, II: 32; III: 29-30
epidemiologic studies, I: 50, 57-59, 62-63, 384-418; II: 3, 6-7, 28, 113, 149-161; III: 26, 206-217, 236-245, 272-273, 275, 277-278, 279, 281, 283, 285-286, 288, 290, 291, 294-295, 298, 301, 303, 305, 309-310, 312, 316, 317, 323, 326, 328, 333, 336, 338, 339, 340, 342, 343-344, 345-346, 349, 351, 353, 355, 358-359, 361, 363, 365, 370-371, 372, 373, 376, 380, 382, 385, 386, 389, 392, 435, 436, 437-438, 445, 446, 450, 454, 455, 456, 457, 459, 467, 468, 469, 470, 473, 479, 480, 481, 482, 485-486, 489, 491, 495, 497, 498, 500, 502, 505-506, 512-513, 516-518, 521; IV: 150-160, 255, 269, 275, 278, 283, 294-295, 303-304, 309-310, 316, 322-323, 329, 336-337, 342, 347, 357-358, 366-367, 373, 380, 402, 411, 420-422, 474, 485-487, 494, 502-504, 508-509
federal government activities/research on military use of herbicides, II: 27-32; III: 25-30
female reproductive system cancers in, I: 505, 511-512, 577; II: 211, 212; III: 333; IV: 7, 322-323
gastrointestinal tract cancers in, I: 446; II: 177, 180-181; IV: 7, 255
gastrointestinal ulcers in, I: 691, 692; III: 512-513; IV: 502-504
genitourinary tract cancers in, I: 513, 518, 522; II: 223-224; III: 272-273, 275, 277-278, 279, 281; IV: 7, 342
health care of, II: 28, 29; III: 26, 27
health concerns of, I: 1, 32-34, 46-47; II: 17-24, 26-27; III: 17-30
hepatic enzyme disorders in, I: 687
hepatobiliary cancers in, I: 455, 457; II: 181, 185, 187; III: 283, 285-286, 288; IV: 7, 269

herbicide exposure assessment issues, II: 4-5, 14, 17-24, 26-27; III: 2, 5-6, 142, 143, 146-150; IV: 122-127
herbicide exposure assessment strategies for, I: 270-284; II: 99-109; III: 144-145
Hodgkin's disease in, I: 526, 554-556, 557; II: 235, 236; III: 372, 373, 376; IV: 6, 366-367
immune modulation in, I: 695-696, 699; III: 489, 491
infertility, I: 632, 633, 634; II: 280; III: 445, 446, 450; IV: 7
International Agency for Research on Cancer research activities, III: 30
laryngeal cancer in, III: 294-295; IV: 6, 9, 278
latency relevance for assessing herbicides effect on cancer risk in, II: 276; III: 12-13, 430-431
legislation concerning herbicide exposure and health of, II: 28-29; III: 26-27
leukemia in, I: 13, 564, 570, 571-572; II: 245, 246; III: 385, 386, 389, 392; IV: 7, 380
lipid abnormalities in, I: 689, 692; II: 333; III: 505-506, 521; IV: 7, 494
liver toxicity in, II: 332; III: 512-513; IV: 502-504
low birthweight outcomes for, I: 626, 628; III: 457, 459; IV: 7
lung cancer in, III: 298, 301; IV: 6, 283
melanoma in, III: 316, 317; IV: 303-304
military experiences, I: 75, 82, 272, 286, 399
motor/coordination dysfunction in, I: 659-660, 662; II: 309, 310; III: 469, 470; IV: 7, 448
multiple myeloma in, I: 526, 562, 563; II: 244; III: 380, 382; IV: 6, 10, 373
nasal/nasopharyngeal cancer in, I: 459, 460; II: 189; III: 290, 291; IV: 7, 275
National Personnel Records Center listing, I: 17
neural tube defects in offspring, numbers, II: 297; IV: 7, 18, 404-405
neurobehavioral disorders in, II: 305, 308, 309, 310, 311, 313, 314; III: 467, 468; IV: 457-459
neuropsychiatric outcomes, I: 653-656, 658; II: 308; III: 469; IV: 443
non-Hodgkin's lymphoma in, I: 526, 541-

548, 549; II: 234; III: 363, 365, 370-371; IV: 6, 357-358
number of, I: 3, 4, 74, 75-80
outreach activities; II: 31; III: 28
Parkinson's disease in, II: 309-310
perinatal deaths in offspring, II: 285; III: 454, 455, 456; IV: 7
peripheral nervous system disorders in, I: 665, 666; II: 311, 313; III: 473, 475; IV: 6, 7, 456
porphyria cutanea tarda in, I: 681, 682-683; II: 321-322, 323; III: 481, 482; IV: 6, 8
prostate cancer in, I: 513, 518, 519, 522; II: 9, 217-218, 221, 223; III: 336, 338, 339, 340, 342; IV: 6, 8, 10, 329
records-based exposure assessment, I: 271-280; IV: 121-126
records identification, II: 24-25
renal cancers in, III: 352, 353, 355; IV: 7, 347
reproductive outcomes, I: 405-406, 418, 601-603, 609-615, 618, 620-622, 625; II: 71, 278, 300-301; III: 435, 436, 437-438, 445, 446, 450, 454, 455, 456, 457, 459; IV: 7, 402
research recommendations, II: 23-25; III: 23
respiratory cancers in, I: 469-470, 472; II: 190, 201-202, 203; IV: 6, 283
respiratory disorders in, I: 710-712, 713-714; III: 485-486; IV: 7, 474
risk assessment for, I: 14-15, 221, 225-226, 247-248, 578; II: 14, 22-23, 89, 91, 251, 276, 298, 300-301, 314, 321, 323, 349-357; III: 14-15, 22-23, 124, 127-128, 430-431; IV: 20, 105-108
serum testing, I: 20-21
skin cancer in, I: 501, 505; II: 209; III: 312; IV: 7, 301
soft-tissue sarcoma in, I: 475, 492-498, 500; II: 205, 208; III: 309-310; IV: 6, 294-295
South Korea, I: 61-62
spina bifida in offspring, II: 9-10, 296, 298, 301; III: 7, 8, 9-10, 21, 24-25, 437-438; IV: 7, 10, 18, 402
spontaneous abortions in, I: 601-603, 605; II: 283; IV: 7, 411
state-sponsored studies of, II: 152-153, 158-159, 161, 202, 292; III: 213-215, 243-244; IV: 158-159
suicide incidence, I: 655-656

testicular cancer in, II: 153; III: 343-344, 345-346; IV: 7, 336-337
twin studies, I: 398-399, 406, 703, 711
Vietnamese veterans, Vietnamese studies of, III: 245
women, I: 50, 83-84; II: 152-153, 180, 181, 190, 201, 204, 205, 209, 211, 212, 213, 216-217, 218, 223, 226, 228, 229, 231, 245, 278, 280; III: 326-329, 333, 434-435; IV: 316
See also Air Force Health Study (AFHS); Compensation, veterans; Demographic data, Vietnam veterans; Operation Ranch Hand; Risk assessment, Vietnam veterans
Vietnam veterans' exposure studies, II: 154, 156-157, 158-159; III: 206-209, 210-217, 275, 278, 279, 281, 283, 288, 291, 305, 310, 312, 316, 317, 323, 326, 328, 336, 342, 345-346, 351, 355, 370-371, 376, 382, 437-438, 450, 454, 455, 456, 459, 497, 521; IV: 150, 156-158, 262, 264, 272-273, 276-277
Vietnam veterans' increased disease risk, II: 22-23; III: 22-23
Vietnam Veterans of America, I: 60
Vietnamese
birth defects and herbicide exposure, II: 287-288
cancer in, II: 148; III: 283
epidemiologic studies, I: 599-601; II: 113, 144-145, 148, 184, 287-288; III: 202, 234, 283
herbicide environmental exposure, II: 144-145, 148, 287-288; III: 283
herbicide exposure assessment, I: 269, 370-372; II: 4-5, 108-109; III: 156-157; IV: 116-117
herbicide exposure indices development, II: 107-108
reproductive outcomes, I: 599-601, 608-609; IV: 148-149
research recommendations, I: 731
scientists in, studies of Vietnamese veterans, III: 245
Vietnamese Veterans, IV: 160
Viral infection
immune system response, I: 692-693
TCDD-enhanced susceptibility, I: 149
teratogenic potential, I: 607
See also Immune system disorders

Vitamin A, I: 174
VLDL. *See* Very low density lipoprotein (VLDL) receptors

W

Wales. *See* United Kingdom
War Research Service, I: 25
Washington, D.C., II: 343; III: 533
Washington state, I: 336-338, 341, 487-488, 535; II: 149, 241; III: 229, 230, 232, 234; IV: 149, 215
Wasting syndrome, TCDD-induced, I: 162-166; II: 76-77; III: 80-83; IV: 25, 31, 57, 76
Wechsler Adult Intelligence Scales, I: 641
Western Europe, II: 268; III: 510
West Germany, II: 328-329; III: 223, 337, 379, 387, 483, 506, 511, 515
West Virginia, I: 60, 404, 470, 496, 546, 621, 662-663, 686, 689, 700; II: 202; III: 243; IV: 364, 371
See also Nitro, West Virginia
Wilm's tumor, I: 594
See also Children, cancer in; Kidney cancer
Wisconsin, I: 37, 60, 336, 404-405, 445, 455, 470, 496, 517, 523, 534, 546, 556, 560, 702, 710; II: 185, 202, 226, 229, 239, 241; III: 229, 243, 283, 313, 348; IV: 259, 262, 264, 267, 272, 291, 299, 301, 335, 339, 345, 350, 355, 361, 363-364, 371, 375
Women. *See* Breast cancer; Cervical cancer; Demographic data, Vietnam veterans; Gender; Ovarian cancer; Reproductive system cancers, women; Reproductive system disorders; Uterine cancer; Women veterans
Women veterans, I: 79; II: 30
breast cancer estimated risk, II: 218; III: 329; IV: 318
breast cancer expected incidence, I: 440, 461, 501, 505, 513, 522, 526, 564; II: 213; IV: 314
breast cancer in, II: 213, 216-217; III: 322, 324-328, 329; IV: 314-320
circulatory disease in, I: 702
epidemiologic studies, I: 50, 81; II: 28, 152-153, 180, 181, 190, 201, 204, 205, 209, 211, 212, 213-217, 218, 219-223, 226, 228, 229, 231, 245, 278, 280; III: 324-328, 333; IV: 314-320
mortality studies, I: 394-395, 470, 545; II: 152-153, 180, 201
reproductive outcomes, III: 434-435; IV: 399-400
reproductive system cancers in, II: 211, 212; III: 333; IV: 320-326
research recommendations, I: 728
statistics, I: 83-84
See also Reproductive system cancers, women
Women Veterans Health Programs Act of 1992. *See* Public Law 102-585
World Health Organization, II: 282; III: 30, 454, 492; IV: 413, 415
Mortality Data Bank, I: 314; II: 132; III: 223, 378, 484-485, 512, 516
World War II; I: 25, 32, 82; II: 150, 268; III: 237, 420

X

Xenobiotic responsive elements (XREs), II: 56, 57, 58, 71; III: 66, 67, 104

Y

Yorkshire, England, III: 234; IV: 149